Current Trends in
Labor
Management

Current Trends in
Labor
Management

Series Editor
Narendra Malhotra
MD FIAJAGO FICMU FICOG FICMCH FRCOG FICS FMAS AFIAP
Managing Director
Department of IVF and Infertility
Global Rainbow Healthcare, Agra
Director
ART Rainbow IVF
Agra, Uttar Pradesh, India

Advisor Editor
Kawita Bapat
MS FICOG
Renowned Vaginal Surgeon
Department of Obstetrics and Gynecology
Director, Bapat Hospital
Indore, Madhya Pradesh, India

Editors

Poonam Goyal MD FICOG FICMCH
Director
Department of Obstetrics/Gynecology and IVF
Panchsheel Hospital, New Delhi
Head, IVF Unit
Max Super Speciality Hospital
Ghaziabad, Uttar Pradesh, India

Kavita Mandrelle Bhatti
MD FICOG FMAS ACME FRM
Professor and Head
Department of Obstetrics and Gynecology
Christian Medical College and Hospital
Ludhiana, Punjab, India

Bhavana Mittal
DNB FNB MNAMS FICOG
Director
Department of Obstetrics/Gynecology and IVF
Shivam IVF and Infertility Centre, New Delhi
Consultant, Max Super Speciality Hospital
New Delhi, India

Forewords
Padma Shri Alka Kriplani
S Shantha Kumari

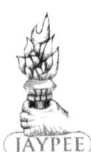

JAYPEE BROTHERS MEDICAL PUBLISHERS
The Health Sciences Publisher
New Delhi | London

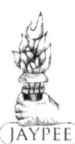 **Jaypee Brothers Medical Publishers (P) Ltd**

Headquarters

Jaypee Brothers Medical Publishers (P) Ltd
EMCA House, 23/23-B
Ansari Road, Daryaganj
New Delhi 110 002, India
Landline: +91-11-23272143, +91-11-23272703
+91-11-23282021, +91-11-23245672
Email: jaypee@jaypeebrothers.com

Corporate Office

Jaypee Brothers Medical Publishers (P) Ltd
4838/24, Ansari Road, Daryaganj
New Delhi 110 002, India
Phone: +91-11-43574357
Fax: +91-11-43574314
Email: jaypee@jaypeebrothers.com

Overseas Office

JP Medical Ltd
83 Victoria Street, London
SW1H 0HW (UK)
Phone: +44 20 3170 8910
Email: info@jpmedpub.com

EU GPSR Authorised Representative

Logos Europe, 9 rue Nicolas Poussin
17000, La Rochelle, France
Phone: +33 (0) 6 67 93 73 78
E-mail: Contact@logoseurope.eu

Website: www.jaypeebrothers.com
Website: www.jaypeedigital.com

Current Trends in Labor Management

First Edition: **2022**

ISBN: 978-93-5465-653-8

Dedication

We dedicate the book to
God's most wonderful creation
"MOTHER"
and all the Obstetricians taking care of her.

Contributors

Aarti Chitkara MD DNB
Senior Resident
Department of Obstetrics and Gynecology
All India Institute of Medical Sciences
New Delhi, India

Aashima Arora MD DNB
Associate Professor
Department of Obstetrics and Gynecology
Postgraduate Institute of Medical
Education and Research
Chandigarh, India

Aditee Goyal
LLB LLM Diploma in Healthcare Management
Admin Head and Manager Operations
Department of Administration
Panchsheel Hospital
New Delhi, India

Ajay Kumar Gupta MBBS MD DNB
Director and Pediatrician
Department of Pediatrics
Muskan Clinic
New Delhi, India

Akanksha Dwivedi MBBS MS
Senior Resident
Department of Obstetrics and Gynecology
VMMC and Safdarjung Hospital
New Delhi, India

Alok Basu Roy MBBS MD
Senior Consultant
Department of Anesthesia
Max Superspeciality Hospital
Ghaziabad, Uttar Pradesh, India

Alok Sharma MBBS MD MICOG FICOG DHA
Consultant
Department of Obstetrics and Gynecology
Civil Hospital
Mandi, Himachal Pradesh, India

Amogh Natchandra Chimote MBBS MD
Medical Director
Department of Reproductive Medicine
Vaunshdhara Fertility Centre
Nagpur, Maharashtra, India

Anita Rajorhia MBBS MD FICOG
Head and Senior Consultant
Department of Obstetrics and Gynecology
Dr Hedgewar Aarogya Sansthaan
New Delhi, India

Ankita Bansal Goyal MD DNB FMAS PGDS
Consultant
Department of Obstetrics and Gynecology
Sankalp Hospital
Raipur, Chhattisgarh, India

Ankita Srivastava MBBS MS DNB MRCOG
Clinical Assistant
Department of Obstetrics and Gynecology
Sir Ganga Ram Hospital
New Delhi, India

Anusha Devalla MBBS MS DNB
Consultant
Department of Obstetrics and Gynecology
Gayatri Hospital
Hyderabad, Telangana, India

Arati C Koregol MDS
Professor
Department of Dental
PM Nadagouda Memorial Dental College
and Hospital
Bagalkot, Karnataka, India

Aruna Singh MBBS MD MICOG FICOG DHA
Consultant
Department of Obstetrics and Gynecology
Postgraduate Institute of Medical
Education and Research
Chandigarh, India

Ashish R Kale MD DNB MNAMS FICOG FICS FICMCH
Director and Consultant
Department of Obstetrics and Gynecology
Ashakiran Hospital and Asha IVF Centre
Pune, Maharashtra, India

Ashwini Kale DGO DNB FICMCH
Director and Consultant
Department of Obstetrics and Gynecology
Ashakiran Hospital and Asha IVF Centre
Pune, Maharashtra, India

Asmita Kaundal MS DNB MNAMS
Assistant Professor
Department of Obstetrics and Gynecology
All India Institute of Medical Sciences
Bilaspur, Chhattisgarh, India

Bhagyashree Bijjaragi MS DNB FFM
Assistant Professor
Department of Obstetrics and Gynecology
Al-Ameen Medical College
Vijayapur, Karnataka, India

Bhavana Mittal DNB FNB MNAMS FICOG
Director
Department of Obstetrics and Gynecology and IVF
Shivam IVF and Infertility Centre, New Delhi
Consultant, Max Super Speciality Hospital
New Delhi, India

Chandana S Bhatt MBBS MS DNB MCH
Senior Resident
Department of Obstetrics and Gynecology
Sri Ramachandra Medical College
Chennai, Tamil Nadu, India

Charmila Ayyavoo MD DGO DFP FICOG PGDCR
Director Consultant
Department of Obstetrics and Gynecology
Aditi Hospital, Southern Railway Hospital
Trichy, Tamil Nadu, India

Chhavi Gupta MBBS MS
Senior Resident
Department of Obstetrics and Gynecology
VMMC and Safdarjung Hospital
New Delhi, India

Deeba Khanam MBBS MD
Assistant Professor
Department of Obstetrics and Gynecology
Jawaharlal Nehru Medical College, AMU
Aligarh, Uttar Pradesh, India

Deepa Gupta MBBS MS DNB MANAMS FICMCH
Medical Superintendent
Department of Obstetrics and Gynecology
Sree Krishna Medical and Research Centre
New Delhi, India

Deepa Gupta MBBS DGO FICOG
Director
Department of Obstetrics and Gynecology
Muskan Clinic
New Delhi, India

Dolly Mehra MBBS MS FICOG
Consultant
Department of Obstetrics and Gynecology
Mehra Nursing Home
Ratlam, Madhya Pradesh, India

Gunjan Kumari Bhagwat MBBS MD FMAGS RM
Consultant
Department of IVF
Max Superspeciality Hospital
Ghaziabad, Uttar Pradesh, India

Jaideep Malhotra
MD FRCOG FRCPI FICS FMAS FICMCH FIVMB
Managing Director
Department of IVF and Infertility
Global Rainbow Healthcare
Agra, Uttar Pradesh, India

Jayam Kannan MD DGO FICOG
Director
Department of IVF and Infertility
GFC Fertility Centre
Chennai, Tamil Nadu, India
Vice President, FOGSI–2018

Jaydeep Tank MD DGO FCPS
Consultant
Department of Obstetrics and Gynecology
Ashwini Maternity and
Nursing Home, Thane
Profert IVF Clinic
Mumbai, Maharashtra, India

Jyoti Bhaskar MD MRCOG FICOG
Clinical Director
Department of Obstetrics and Gynecology
Apollo Cradle Children's Hospital
Ghaziabad, Uttar Pradesh, India

K Aparna Sharma MD DNB FICOG
Additional Professor
Department of Obstetrics and Gynecology
All India Institute of Medical Sciences
New Delhi, India

Kartik Syal MD
Associate Professor
Department of Anesthesia
Indira Gandhi Medical College
Shimla, Himachal Pradesh, India

Kavita Mandrelle Bhatti
MD FICOG FMAS ACME FRM
Professor and Head
Department of Obstetrics and Gynecology
Christian Medical College and Hospital
Ludhiana, Punjab, India

Kawita Bapat MS FICOG
Renowned Vaginal Surgeon
Department of Obstetrics and Gynecology
Director, Bapat Hospital
Indore, Madhya Pradesh, India

Komal Chavan
MD DNB MNAMS FCPS DGO FICOG DRM
Senior Consultant and DNB Teacher
Department of Obstetrics and Gynecology
VN Desai Hospital
Mumbai, Maharashtra, India

Kunal Doshi MBBS DGO DFP FCPS
Consultant
Department of Obstetricsand Gynecology
and IVF
Ashish Maternity and Nursing Home, Mumbai
Profert IVF Clinic
Mumbai, Maharashtra, India

Mahesh Koregol MBBS MS FICOG Fellow
Consultant
Department of IVF and Infertility
Nova IVF
Bengaluru, Karnataka, India

Mala Srivastava DGO DNB
Professor and Senior Consultant
Department of Obstetrics and Gynecology
The Ganga Ram Institute for Postgraduate
Medical Education and Research
New Delhi, India

Meenakshi Sharma MBBS MD FICOG FICMCH
Consultant
Department of Obstetrics and Gynecology
Yashoda Superspeciality Hospital
Ghaziabad, Uttar Pradesh, India

Mitra Saxena MD DNB FICMCH Diploma in Endoscopy
Director and Head
Department of Obstetrics and Gynecology
Shri Ashwini Saxena Hospital
Rewari, Haryana, India
Chairperson, Practical Obstetrics Committee FOGSI

Mohita Agarwal MBBS MS FMAS
Associate Professor
Department of Obstetrics and Gynecology
SN Medical College
Agra, Uttar Pradesh, India

Monisha Singh MBBS MD
Consultant
Department of Obstetrics and Gynecology
Parul Hospital
Varanasi, Uttar Pradesh, India

Narendra Malhotra
MD FIAJAGO FICMU FICOG FICMCH FRCOG
FICS FMAS AFIAP
Managing Director
Department of IVF and Infertility
Global Rainbow Healthcare, Agra
Director
ART Rainbow IVF
Agra, Uttar Pradesh, India

Naveen Gupta MBBS MD
Consultant
Department of Anesthesia
Max Superspeciality Hospital
Ghaziabad, Uttar Pradesh, India

Nazia Ishrat MD
Assistant Professor
Department of Obstetrics and Gynecology
Jawaharlal Nehru Medical College, AMU
Aligarh, Uttar Pradesh, India

Neema Tufchi PhD (Biotechnology)
Scientist
Department of Obstetrics and Gynecology
Sir Ganga Ram Hospital
New Delhi, India

Neha Kapoor MBBS MD
Associate Consultant
Department of Obstetrics and Gynecology
Cloudnine Hospital
New Delhi, India

Neharika Malhotra
MBBS MD DRMDMIS FICMCH FMAS
Consultant
Department of IVF and Infertility
Malhotra Nursing Home and Rainbow IVF
Agra, Uttar Pradesh, India
Chairperson, FOGSI Young Talent Promotion
Committee FOGSI

Pallavi Goel MBBS
Resident
Department of General Medicine
Mahatma Gandhi Medical College
Jaipur, Rajasthan, India

Parul Gupta Khanna
MBBS DGO DNB MNAMS FRM
Consultant
Department of IVF
Nova and Southend IVF
Noida, Uttar Pradesh, India

Pavika Lal MD CIMP
Assistant Professor
Department of Obstetrics and Gynecology
GSVM Medical College
Kanpur, Uttar Pradesh, India

Poonam Goyal MD FICOG FICMCH
Director
Department of Obstetrics and Gynecology
and IVF
Panchsheel Hospital, New Delhi
Head, IVF Unit
Max Super Speciality Hospital
Ghaziabad, Uttar Pradesh, India

Prerna Keshan MBBS DGO FICOG
Consultant
Department of Obstetrics and Gynecology
Horizon Maternity and Fertility Clinic
Tinsukia, Assam, India

Preeti Gaur DNB
Director
Department of Obstetrics and Gynecology
Capital Nursing Home
New Delhi, India

Raji Cheriyan MSc
Senior Program Officer
Department of Obstetrics and Gynecology
JHPIEGO
Lucknow, Uttar Pradesh, India

Rajesh Kumar Verma MD
Associate Professor
Department of Anesthesia
Indira Gandhi Medical College
Shimla, Himachal Pradesh, India

Ramandeep Bansal MD
Assistant Professor
Department of Obstetrics and Gynecology
Postgraduate Institute of Medical Education
and Research
Chandigarh, India

Ramya VM DGO DNB
Senior Resident
Department of Obstetrics and Gynecology
KC General Hospital
Bengaluru, Karnataka, India

Ranjana Khanna MBBS MS DGO FICOG
Senior Consultant and Director
Department of Obstetrics and Gynecology
Ranjana Hospital
Allahabad, Uttar Pradesh, India

Renu Yadav MBBS MS FIAMS
Consultant
Department of Obstetrics and Gynecology
Sharbati Surgical and Maternity Home
Mahendragarh, Haryana, India

Richa Sharma MS MNAMS FICOG FICMCH FMAS
Professor
Department of Obstetrics and Gynecology
University College of Medical Sciences and
Guru Teg Bahadur Hospital
New Delhi, India
FOGSI MTP Committee

Rohini Rao MD
Associate Professor
Department of Obstetrics and Gynecology
Indira Gandhi Medical College
Shimla, Himachal Pradesh, India

Ruchika Garg
MD FICOG FICMCH FMAS MAMS FIAOG
Professor
Department of Obstetrics and Gynecology
SN Medical College
Agra, Uttar Pradesh, India

Sahir Bhatti MBBS
Demonstrator
Department of Physiology
Christian Medical College and Hospital
Ludhiana, Punjab, India

Sangeeta Rai MS FMAS PhD FICOG FICMCH
Professor
Department of Obstetrics and Gynecology
Banaras Hindu University
Varanasi, Uttar Pradesh, India

Seema Prakash MBBS MD FICOG
Consultant
Department of Obstetrics and Gynecology
University College of Medical Sciences and
Guru Teg Bahadur Hospital
New Delhi, India

Shaheen Anjum MBBS MS
Professor and In-Charge
Department of Obstetrics and Gynecology
ART Unit
Aligarh Muslim University
Aligarh, Uttar Pradesh, India

Shama Batra MBBS MD FICOG
Director
Department of Obstetrics and Gynecology
Patel Hospital
New Delhi, India

Shashibala Bhonsale Sao MS
Consultant Gynecologist
Department of Obstetrics and Gynecology
President Elect, Gwalior Obs and Gyne
Society 2022-2023
Obs and Gyne Specialist in Public Health and
Welfare Department
Co-ordinator, Rajyog IAEC Committee FOGSI
2021-22
Gwalior, Madhya Pradesh, India

Sheeba Marwah MBBS DNB Fellowship
Associate Professor
Department of Obstetrics and Gynecology
VMMC and Safdarjung Hospital
New Delhi, India

Sheela Mane MD FICOG FICMCH
Professor
Department of Obstetrics and Gynecology
KCG Hospital
Bengaluru, Karnataka, India

Shreya Prabhoo DNB DGO MNAMS
Consultant
Department of Obstetrics and Gynecology
Mukund Hospital, Surya Hospital
Mumbai, Maharashtra, India

Soumya Mahesh Koregol MBBS MS
Consultant
Department of Obstetrics and Gynecology
Hospitec Hospital
Bengaluru, Karnataka, India

Srishti Prakash MBBS MS
PG Resident
Department of Obstetrics and Gynecology
VMMC and Safdarjung Hospital
New Delhi, India

Surekha Tayade
MBBS MD DNB MNAMS FICOG PGDHHM FIME
FAIMER Fellow PhD
Consultant
Department of Obstetrics and Gynecology
Jawaharlal Nehru Medical College
Wardha, Maharashtra, India

Uma Jain
MS FMAS FART Fellowship (Colposcopy)
Professor
Department of Obstetrics and Gynecology
DH Shivpuri
New Delhi, India

Vaidehi Marathe
MBBS DGO FICOG FICMCH CIMP
Director
Department of Obstetrics and Gynecology
Maher Maternity and Nursing Home
Nagpur, Maharashtra, India

Vanita Jain MD DNB
Professor
Department of Obstetrics and Gynecology
Postgraduate Institute of Medical
Education and Research
Chandigarh, India

Vanita Suri MD
Professor and Head
Department of Obstetrics and Gynecology
Postgraduate Institute of Medical
Education and Research
Chandigarh, India

Vibhavaree Dandawate MD
Associate Professor
Department of Obstetrics and Gynecology
Al-Ameen Medical College
Vijayapur, Karnataka, India

Vidya A Thobbi MD FICOG
Professor
Department of Obstetrics and Gynecology
Al-Ameen Medical College
Vijayapur, Karnataka, India

VK Goyal MD
Director
Department of Pediatrics
Panchsheel Hospital
New Delhi, India

Yukti Bhardwaj MBBS DNB
Senior Resident
Department of Obstetrics and Gynecology
VMMC and Safdarjung Hospital
New Delhi, India

Foreword

It gives me immense pleasure to write a series forward for the PK series of books. This series of books aims at bringing light to important areas of obstetrics and gynecology.

This first book of this series has the blessings of Dr Narendra Malhotra and Dr Kawita Bapat as Senior Advisors. This book has been compiled and edited by senior gynecologists and academicians—Dr Poonam Goyal, Dr Kavita Mandrelle Bhatti, and Dr Bhavna Mittal.

It is totally dedicated to intranatal care and throws light on tackling labor patients in different conditions and situations. The book aims to provide uniform evidence-based protocols all over India. Sole aim is to bestow respectable maternal care to all the laboring patients. There are contributions from over 70 authors from all over the country who have immense experience and knowledge on the subject.

I give my best wishes to the editors, publishers and the readers who are devoted to promote academics and knowledge.

Padma Shri Alka Kriplani
MD FRCOG FAMS FICOG FIMSA FICMCH FCLS
Director and Head
Department of Gynecology, Obstetrics and ART
Paras Hospitals
Gurugram, Haryana, India
Former Professor and Head
Department of Obstetrics and Gynecology
All India Institute of Medical Sciences (AIIMS)
New Delhi, India
Former Director In-Charge, WHO-CCR, HRRC, and Family Planning
"Padma Shri", distinguished service in Medicine by President of India—2015

Foreword

I am extremely delighted to write a foreword for this first book *Current Trends in Labor Management* of the PK series. This book has been compiled and edited by senior gynecologists and academicians—Dr Poonam Goyal, Dr Kavita Mandrelle Bhatti, and Dr Bhavna Mittal. There are contributions from all over the country who have immense experience and knowledge. I congratulate the editors for bringing out a complete book on the very much-needed topic of intrapartum care. Actually, medical science is improving 24/7 and newer concepts are laid from evidence and experience. The traditional labor care approach has taken a new turn for the better. A recent simple and guidelines-based book on labor is the need of the hour.

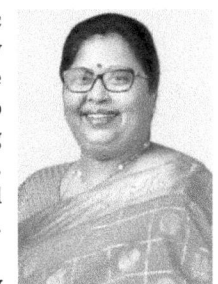

This book has come up very well. The title and the subtopics have been very carefully chosen to throw light on this important area of any obstetrician's practice. I also appreciate the vision of senior advisors Dr Narendra Malhotra and Dr Kawita Bapat without whose help this venture would not have taken shape. I hope that the readers of this book will enjoy and benefit from the concise but updated content.

I give my best wishes to all those associated with publishing this book.

S Shantha Kumari MD DNB FICOG FRCPI FRCOG
Senior Consultant
Obstetric and Gynecologist and
Laparoscopic Surgeon
Yashoda Hospitals, Hyderabad, Telangana
President, FOGSI 2021-22
Treasurer FIGO

Preface

The ability to reduce maternal and neonatal mortality is dependent on trained personnel who attend women in labor and during delivery.

The care that a woman receives during labor and delivery can affect the woman's physical and emotional health, and also have short- and long-term effects on the outcome. Intrapartum care aims to avert delivery-related complications and improve maternal and neonatal health.

This book is the first of a series of handbooks on important topics related to Obstetrics and Gynecology. It covers a large range of chapters related to basics of intrapartum care for normal and abnormal labor as well as complicated and uncomplicated cases during labor and delivery.

The book is a culmination of chapters which are authored by acknowledged masters in obstetrics. The authors have used best available evidence and standardized as much as possible the way we care for our antenatal mothers in labor. The practical manual is a comprehensive and easy reference book for undergraduates, postgraduates and colleagues practicing obstetrics. It is a user-friendly resource for how to care for patients in labor.

The topics have been organized sequentially into 14 sections and 60 chapters which include setting up of an ideal labor room, triaging patients, care during normal and abnormal labor, labor in medical disorders during pregnancy, vaginal and operative delivery, counseling and medicolegal aspects pertaining to labor and delivery.

In producing this series of handbooks and practical manuals, the editors and authors sincerely hope that the healthcare professionals and trainees will benefit and the practical information provided in the book will help in rendering high quality, respectful maternal care to our patients.

Narendra Malhotra
Kawita Bapat
Poonam Goyal
Kavita Mandrelle Bhatti
Bhavana Mittal

Acknowledgments

We have the pleasure of introducing this *Current Trends in Labor Management.*

We thank God Almighty for helping us throughout the journey of completing this task.

Our heartfelt gratitude and indebtedness to Dr S Shantha Kumari for her guidance and for being a constant pillar of support and strength to us in this academic initiative.

We are grateful to Dr Alka Kriplani for accepting to write the foreword of this book and also for sharing her expertise and pearls of wisdom.

It is with utmost pleasure that we thank Dr Narendra Malhotra and Dr Kawita Bapat, our mentors and guides for this practical manual which is the first of the 'PK Series' of books in Obstetrics and Gynecology. Their enthusiasm and encouragement kept us motivated to accomplish this task.

We wish to thank all the authors who responded to our requests with promptness and have contributed immensely by writing the chapters timely, and for sharing their knowledge and expertise.

We wish to appreciate the efforts of M/s Jaypee Brothers Medical Publishers (P) Ltd, New Delhi, India, for publishing this book so well. We also thank Shri Jitendar P Vij (Group Chairman), Mr Ankit Vij (Managing Director), Mr MS Mani (Group President), Ms Chetna Malhotra Vohra (Associate Director—Content Strategy), and Ms Pooja Bhandari (Production Head).

Our special appreciation and thanks to all our colleagues, friends and students who supported our idea of bringing out this practical manual and gave us the confidence to finish the book.

Most importantly, none of this could have happened without the support and co-operation of our family. We acknowledge the love and encouragement of all our near and dear ones which strengthened us and kept us going to finish this work of ours.

Contents

SECTION 5: Dysfunctional Labor

SECTION 6: Instrumental Delivery

SECTION 7: Operative Delivery

SECTION 8: Dreadful Complications

SECTION 9: Medical Disorders in Labor

1

Ideal Labor Room Set up and Prerequisites

Surekha Tayade

INTRODUCTION

Labor room is a place for the care and admission of women in the process of childbirth. In conventional labor rooms, a pregnant woman is admitted to labor room at or near full dilation of cervix and is shifted to the postpartum ward after 2 hours. In labor-delivery-recovery (LDR) unit, a pregnant woman spends the duration of labor, delivery, and 4 hours postpartum in the same bed.

WHAT IS LABOR-DELIVERY-RECOVERY?

A birthing unit that is:
- Standardized
- Provides privacy and comfort
- Eliminates the need to shift mother in different stages of labor
- Includes all the support areas
- Catering to a mother exclusively during labor and immediate postpartum.

FOCUS AREAS IN LABOR ROOM DESIGNING

- Space and layout
- Equipment and accessories
- Consumables
- Human resources
- Practices and protocols

Location and Layout

Labor room should be located:
- In a designated maternity services area with a central nursing area preferably at ground floor for safety and comfort.
- There should be adjoining operation theater, neonatal intensive care unit (NICU), and high-dependency unit (HDU).

- The galleries and doors should be smooth and broad at all entry and exit points with large double doors for easy transit of large trolleys and personnel.
- There should be close connectivity to prelabor ward and cesarean operation theater.

Dimensions of Labor Room

- Consider present and potential of next 20 years of workload while designing.
- Even in single practitioner set up, consider space needed for managing life-threatening emergencies.
- Each LDR unit should have four laboring areas with one labor table each, one nursing area, two toilets, one newborn care unit, and two wash areas **(Table 1)**.

Annexure for Labor Room

- Prelabor ward
- Emergency obstetric room
- Doctor/Staff room
- Scrub area
- Wash area

Prelabor Ward

- It should have 3–6 beds with bedside lockers, settees, and stools for attendants

Function	Net floor space (square feet)
1. Labor	100–160 per bed
2. Labor, delivery, and recovery	256
3. Vaginal delivery	350
4. Cesarean delivery	400 per bed

TABLE 1: Dimensions of labor room.

- Intravascular (I/v) drip stands, oxygen cylinder/central oxygen with tubing and mask, suction machine should be available
- There should be adequate running space and appropriate toilet area.

Emergency Obstetric Room

Emergency obstetric room specification and need has been described in **Table 2**.

Scrub Area

- Two elbow-operated taps with running water having mixer and good drainage
- There should be place for soaps, antiseptic solution, and towel handle
- Facility of 10 liter geyser
- Hand washing protocol should be displayed.

Wash Area

Labor room can become messy with blood and body fluid spillage. A wash area in close connection to labor room will make rapid cleaning possible. This should have:
- Place for taps

- Low set railings for drying
- Option for washing linen according to local needs
- Hooks for plastic aprons
    There should be dirty utility area to store soiled instruments, linen, etc., and a clean utility area to store clean and autoclaved supplies.
    Separate store-room is needed with adequate racks and cabinets to store supplies.

Doctors/Staff Room

- Allows area for rest and relaxation to the team
- Area should have sofa set, one small table, 2–3 chairs, and a bed for off-duty staff to have quick nap
- Personal lockers/cabinets should be provided
- There should be attached toilet with one western style WC and one wash basin
- Separate nurse's duty room should be designed
- A built-in shoe rack can allow shoe change into labor room shoes before entry.

Waiting/Registration and Triage

Waiting or registration and triage have been described in **Table 3**.

▥ LABOR ROOM INTERIOR

- While designing labor room interior, keep in mind possible number and size of labor tables with adequate running space.
- Adequate sunlight in day through glazed glass makes a positive environment and also saves electricity.
- Place for all necessary equipment should be marked beforehand in consultation with anesthetist and neonatologist.
- Efficient utilization of space and free movement space for nursing staff between labor tables should be planned

TABLE 2: Specification of emergency obstetric room.

Need	Specifications
• For patient who require close observation before or after labor • It helps in isolation from other patients • Adequate focus of staff for intensive monitoring • Assures relatives of due care and concern	• Good quality bed for quick change of position preferably hydraulic • All life-saving equipment should be available • Facility to do obstetric examination and minor procedure • There should be close connectivity to labor room, operation theater and ICU

TABLE 3: Difference between waiting area and triage.

Waiting area	Triage
• It should be at the entry of labor room complex and separate for regular in patient waiting • Ambulance approach should be feasible • Registration desk, seating area for 10 people and separate toilets for men and women	• Preferably at the entry for easy accessibility to patient and relatives • Examination room for risk stratification with examination bed and provision for privacy • A table for nurse, chairs and counter to store supplies • Emergency calling bell

- The walls should be tiled, white/light colored with seamless joints extending up to the ceiling, and floor should have vitrified tiles or natural stones with seamless joints.
- Air-handling unit (AHU) in labor room complex to provides proper quality and conditioned air and should ensure six air changes/hour.
- In case AHU not feasible, proper ventilation should be planned and temperature should be kept below 25°C. Split AC can also be used.
- A granite counter running the full length of shortest wall of labor room should be built in, to keep equipment and supplies. The space below it can be used to store crash trolley.
- Autoclaved delivery tray, baby tray, episiotomy tray, normal drug tray, and emergency drug tray can also be stored here.

Lighting

Apart from ambient light, provision should be made for focus lights to be used during obstetric procedure.

- Good shadowless ceiling lights—1 for two tables with 500 Lumens for labor area, to be calculated depending upon carpet area.
- Goose necked focus, LED, shadowless stand light for each labor table
- Assure power backup for continuous running of radiant warmer, lights, and fan. Solar panels are desirable.

Labor Table

- It may not necessarily be very costly or fashionable
- Good size and comfortable mattress is imperative
- Hydraulic/electronic/electric (best in maintenance) tables are available and should be chosen to allow quick change of position
- It should have side support railing, stirrups with knee and ankle support for lithotomy position
- An in-built I/V fluid stand and bucket place is preferred
- Labor table should be 3' from side wall, 2' from head end wall, and at least 6' from the second table.

Newborn Care Area (NBCA)

- Placed within labor room area and designated for resuscitation of newborn
- Within easy reach of labor table with no obstruction
- *Equipment needed:* Radiant warmer, oxygen cylinder/concentrator, functioning resuscitation kit, prewarmed towels, shoulder rolls, mucus extractor, clock with second hand, and pediatric stethoscope
- Pediatric laryngoscope with endotracheal tubes of different size
- Low pressure suction
- Baby weighing machine

Equipment and Accessories

Equipment and accessories required for labor room are described in **Table 4.**

Necessary Instruments

Necessary instruments required for delivery and baby has been shown in **Table 5.**

Consumables

Consumables should be available in adequate quantity, at all the time and adequate supplies lasting for at least a month should be kept in store, taking into consideration the use of items over past 6 months.

- *General consumables:* Cotton, gauze, IV drip sets, needles, syringes, IV fluids, leukoplast, oxytocics, soap, hand-wash, betadine solution, alcohol hand rub, suture material, gloves, antiseptics, etc.
- Disposables per delivery
  - Sterile disposable draw sheet to cover labor table
  - Two baby sheets, one to receive baby and another to dry baby
  - Leggings and other linen

Sterilization

- Independent sterilization facility for labor room is preferred
- Autoclave of two different size for quick and efficient working are recommended
- Tubs for bleaching powder, soap and water as universal work precaution are prescribed

TABLE 4: Equipment for labor room.

Life support equipment	Equipment for LR	Desirable equipment
• Boyles trolley with necessary accessories • Pulse oximeter • Cardiac monitor • Oxygen generator with back up of oxygen cylinder, with accessories • Suction machine • Crash cart with emergency drugs and fluids, and others like extra endotracheal tubes, mouth gag	• Two good quality adult stethoscope • Two BP apparatus • Fetal Doppler-2 • Cardiotocography machine • Small pulse oximeter • Digital thermometer • IV stands • Sterile delivery sets according to workload • PPH tray • Cervical and vaginal exploration set • Glucometer and urine examination sticks	• Syringe infusion pumps • Epidural infusion for continuous labor analgesia • Oxytocin infusion drip counters • Kelly's pad • Puncture proof container • Hub cutter/needle destroyer • MVA/EVA tray • PPIUCD tray

(BP: blood pressure; EVA: electric vacuum aspiration; IV: intravascular; MVA: manual vacuum aspiration; PPH: postpartum hemorrhage; PPIUCD: postpartum intrauterine contraceptive device)

TABLE 5: Instruments for delivery and baby.

Instrument list for delivery	Instrument for baby
• Cord clamps = 2/3 • Episiotomy scissor • Needle holder, scissors • Obstetric forceps of different sizes • Ventouse • Sponges-holding forceps, straight as well as angled • Varying size of Sims speculum • Anterior vaginal wall retractor • Artery forceps/mosquito forceps/Allis forceps • Adequate sponge holders (four at least) • Ribbon gauze for packing	• Baby trays of adequate size • Mucous extractor for suction • Ambu bag for IPPR with masks of different sizes • Baby laryngoscope with endotracheal tubes of different size *Others* • Surgeon's and patient's gown • Sterilized draping for conduct of delivery • Adequate quantity of disposable cap, mask, plastic aprons, slippers/shoes in adequate numbers

- Sterile and autoclaved supplies including linen and instruments should be provided by central sterilization and supply department in large hospitals
- However, primary cleaning and decontamination should be done at source.

HUMAN RESOURCES

- *Doctors*
  - Junior resident doctor round the clock
  - Senior obstetrician on call and for management of laboring women
  - Pediatrician on call/round the clock
  - Anesthetic on call/round the clock
- *Paramedical staff per laboring women*
  - One senior nursing staff trained in fetal and maternal monitoring
  - Two–three junior nurses
  - Attendants and trained paramedics as per need

Nurse to Patient Ratio for Labor and Delivery

Clinical setting and nurse to patient ratio has been described in **Table 6**.

DISPLAYS

Emergency phone number lists:
- Obstetricians/Registrars
- Anesthetist
- Pediatrician
- Blood bank
- Police

TABLE 6: Clinical setting and nurse to patient ratio.

Nurse to patient ratio	Clinical setting
1:2	Patient in labor
1:1	Patient in second stage of labor
1:1	Patient with medical or obstetrical complication
1:2	Oxytocin induction/augmentation
1:1	Initiation of epidural analgesia

All emergency protocols should be displayed:
- Partograph and maternofetal monitoring
- Hand washing
- Active management of the third stage of labor (AMTSL)
- Triage
- Biomedical waste management
- Essential newborn care

Labor room is a unique place. Knowledge, skill, and experience of obstetrician requires a well located, equipped, illuminated, and clean labor room and appropriate facilities to deliver appropriate care to laboring women.

BIBLIOGRAPHY

1. Maternal Health Division (2018). Resource Package for Quality Improvement in LaQshya Program [online]. Available from:http://gmch. gov.in/sites/default/files/documents/Revised_ material.pdf. [Last accessed on December 17, 2021].
2. National Health Mission (2016). Labor Room Guideline. cdr [Online]. Available from: https://nhm.gov.in/images/pdf/programmes/ maternal-health/guidelines/Labor_Room%20 Guideline.pdf. [Last accessed on December 17, 2021]
3. National Health Mission (2013). Maternal and Newborn Health Toolkit [online]. Available from:https://nhm.gov.in/index1.php? lang=1&level=3&sublinkid=839&lid=377. [Last accessed on December 17, 2021]

2

Tertiary Obstetric Care

Mala Srivastava, Neema Tufchi, Ankita Srivastava

INTRODUCTION

Maternal mortality and severe maternal morbidity, among women, have increased in India. The leading medical causes of maternal mortality include cardiovascular disease, infection, and common obstetric complications such as hemorrhage, and vary by timing relative to the end of pregnancy. Maternal mortality rate (MMR) in India has been recorded as 113 per 100,000 live births (2016-18) and 211 per 100,000 live births globally during 2000-2017. Although specific modifications in the clinical management of some of these conditions have been instituted, more can be done to improve the system of care for high-risk women at facility and population levels. The goal of levels of maternal care is to reduce maternal morbidity and mortality, including existing disparities. To standardize a complete and integrated system of perinatal regionalization and risk-appropriate maternal care, this classification system establishes levels of maternal care that pertain to basic care (level I), specialty care (level II), subspecialty care (level III), and regional perinatal health care centers (level IV).

ACCREDITED BIRTH CENTER

Care for low-risk women with uncomplicated singleton term vertex pregnancies, who are expected to have an uncomplicated birth.

Level I (Basic Care)

Care of low- to moderate-risk pregnancies with ability to detect, stabilize, and initiate management of unanticipated maternal-fetal or neonatal problems that occur during the antepartum, intrapartum, or postpartum period until the patient can be transferred to a facility at which the specialty maternal care is available. This includes:

- Ability to begin emergency cesarean delivery within a time interval that best incorporates maternal and fetal risks and benefits.
- Obstetric ultrasonography should be available all the time.
- Support services including laboratory testing and blood bank should be available all time.
- Capability to implement patient safety bundles for common causes of preventable maternal morbidity, such as management of maternal venous thromboembolism, obstetric hemorrhage, and maternal severe hypertension in pregnancy.
- Ability at all times to initiate massive transfusion protocol, with process to obtain more blood and component therapy as needed.
- Stabilization and the ability to facilitate transport to high-level hospital when necessary.
- Professional midwife, physician, or obstetrician-gynecologist should be available 24 × 7.
- Physician should be able to perform emergency cesarean delivery.
- Anesthesiologists should be readily available at all times.

Level II (Specialty Care)

Definition: Level I facility plus care of appropriate moderate to high-risk antepartum, intrapartum, or postpartum conditions.

- Computed tomography scan, magnetic resonance imaging, nonobstetric ultrasound imaging, and maternal echocardiography with interpretation readily available daily.
- Obstetric ultrasound imaging with interpretation readily available 24 × 7.
- Physician obstetric leadership is a board-certified, obstetrician-gynecologist with experience in obstetric care.

- An MFM should be available all the times for consultation onsite, by phone, or by tele-medicine as needed.
- Anesthesiologist should be available 24 × 7
- Internal or family medicine physicians and general surgeons readily available all the time for obstetric patients.

Level III (Subspecialty Care)

Definition: Level II facility plus care of more complex maternal medical conditions, obstetric complications, and fetal conditions
- In-house availability of all blood components.
- Computed tomography scan, magnetic resonance imaging, maternal echocardio-graphy and nonobstetric ultrasound imaging services and interpretation readily available at all the times.
- Specialized obstetric ultrasound and fetal assessment including Doppler studies, with interpretation readily available at all times.
- Basic interventional radiology (capable of performing uterine artery embolization) available 24 × 7.
- Ventilators and other equipment to monitor women in labor and delivery should be present.
- Medical and surgical ICUs for pregnant women and women in postpartum period should be present. The ICUs should have adult critical care providers physically present at all the times.
- Documented mechanism to facilitate and accept maternal transfers or transports.
- Full complement of subspecialists, such as subspecialists in critical care, general surgery, infectious disease, hematology, cardiology, nephrology, neurology, gastroenterology, internal medicine, behavioral health, and neonatology, readily available for inpatient consultation at all times.

Level IV (Regional Perinatal Health Care Centers)

Definition: Level III facility plus on-site medical and surgical care of the most complex maternal conditions and critically ill pregnant women and fetuses throughout antepartum, intrapartum, and postpartum cares.

It provides level III facilities plus on-site medical and surgical care of complex maternal conditions with the availability of critical care unit or ICU beds. On-site ICU care for obstetric patients with primary or comanagement by maternal-fetal medicine team. Comanagement includes at least daily rounds by an MFM with interaction with the ICU team and other subspecialists with daily documentation. Perinatal system leadership, including facilitation of collaboration with facilities in the region, analysis, and review of system perinatal outcome and quality data, provision of outreach education, and assistance with quality improvement as needed.

In level-IV healthcare providers provides:
- Maternal-fetal medicine care team with expertise to manage highly complex, critically ill, or unstable maternal patients. A board certified MFM attending with full inpatient privileges is readily available at all times for consultation and management. This includes comanagement of ICU admitted obstetric patients.
- Nursing Service Line leadership with advanced degree and national certification.
- Continuous availability of adequate numbers of registered nurses who have experience in the care of women with complex medical illnesses and obstetric complications with close collaboration between critical nurses and obstetric nurses with expertise in caring for critically ill women.
- Board certified anesthesiologist with obstetric anesthesia fellowship training or experience in obstetric anesthesia physically present at all times.
- At least one of the following adult subspecialties readily available at all times for consultation and treatment as needed onsite: neurosurgery, cardiac surgery, or transplant. If the facility does not have all three subspecialties available, there should be a process in place to transfer women to a facility that can provide the needed service.

The specified person should be physically present and readily available at all times where perinatal care is provided, i.e., 24 hours a day, 7 days a week. All facilities need to have the capability to stabilize and provide initial care for any patient while being able to accomplish transfer

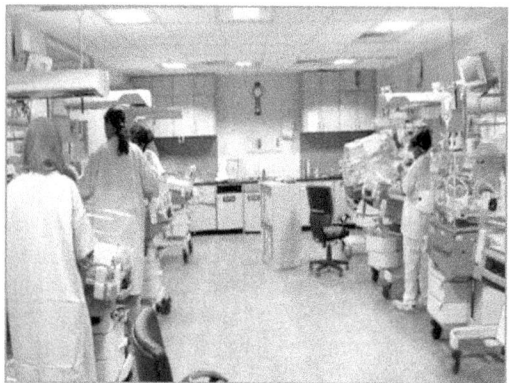

Fig. 1: Neonatology care.

if needed and, thus, must have resources to manage the most common obstetric emergencies such as hemorrhage and hypertension. To ensure optimal care of all pregnant women, all birth centers, basic (level I), and specialty care (level II) hospitals should collaborate with subspecialty care and regional perinatal health facilities to develop and maintain maternal transport plans and cooperative agreements to meet the health care needs of women who develop complications.

Regional centers, which include all level IV facilities and any level III facility that functions in this capacity, should develop relationships with level I and level II hospitals in their referral network. Likewise, level I and II hospitals should be open to collaboration and establishing relationships with a level III or IV facility in their region. Birth centers, according to the AABC 2017 Standards, should have relationships with a higher-level facility **(Fig. 1)**. The regional center should coordinate access to risk-appropriate health services, provide support for quality and safety monitoring, and provide outreach education. These functions are ideally accomplished in collaboration with, and supported by, public health agencies.

▒ BIBLIOGRAPHY

1. American Academy of Pediatrics, American College of Obstetricians and Gynecologists. Guidelines for Perinatal Care, 8th edition. Elk Grove Village (IL): AAP; Washington, DC: American College of Obstetricians and Gynecologists; 2017.
2. American Hospital Association. AHA guide to the health care field. 2014 edition. Chicago (IL): AHA; 2013.
3. Association of Maternal and Child Health Programs (2018). Building U.S. Capacity to Review and Prevent Maternal Deaths. Report from nine maternal mortality review committees. [online] Available from: http://reviewtoaction.org/sites/default/files/national-portal-material/Report%20from%20Nine%20MMRCs%20final_0.pdf [Last accessed on December 18, 2021]
4. Burgansky A, Montalto D, Siddiqui NA. The safe motherhood initiative: the development and implementation of standardized obstetric care bundles in New York. Semin Perinatol 2016;40:124-31.
5. Callaghan WM, Creanga AA, Kuklina EV. Severe maternal morbidity among delivery and postpartum hospitalizations in the United States. Obstet Gynecol. 2012;120:1029-36.
6. Centers for Disease Control and Prevention (2017). Severe maternal morbidity in the United States. [online]. Available from: https://www.cdc.gov/reproductive health/maternalinfanthealth/severe maternalmorbidity.html. [Last accessed on December 18, 2021].
7. Gortmaker S, Sobol A, Clark C, Walker DK, Geronimus A. The survival of very low-birth weight infants by level of hospital of birth: a population study of perinatal systems in four states. Am J Obstet Gynecol. 1985;152:517-24.
8. https://www.pib.gov.in/PressReleasePage.aspx?PRID=1697441
9. Hung P, Henning-Smith CE, Casey MM, Kozhimannil KB. Access to obstetric services in rural counties still declining, with 9 percent losing services, 2004-14 [published erratum appears in Health Aff 2018;37:679]. Health Aff (Millwood). 2017;36:1663-71.
10. Kozhimannil KB, Hung P, Henning-Smith C, Casey MM, Prasad S. Association between loss of hospital-based obstetric services and birth outcomes in rural counties in the United States. JAMA. 2018;319:1239-47.
11. Lasswell SM, Barfield WD, Rochat RW, Blackmon L. Perinatal regionalization for very low-birth-weight and very preterm infants: a meta-analysis. JAMA. 2010;304:992-1000.
12. Levels of neonatal care. American Academy of Pediatrics Committee on Fetus And Newborn. Pediatrics. 2012;130:587-97.

13. Main EK, Cape V, Abreo A, Vasher J, Woods A, Carpenter A, et al. Reduction of severe maternal morbidity from hemorrhage using a state perinatal quality collaborative. Am J Obstet Gynecol. 2017;216:298.e1-11.

14. Main EK. Maternal mortality: new strategies for measurement and prevention. Curr Opin Obstet Gynecol. 2010;22:511-6.

15. March of Dimes (2010). Toward improving the outcome of pregnancy III: enhancing perinatal health through quality, safety and performance initiatives. [online] Available from: https://www.marchofdimes.org/toward-improving-the-outcome-of-pregnancy-iii.pdf. [Last accessed on December 18, 2021].

16. Menard MK, Liu Q, Holgren EA, Sappenfield WM. Neonatal mortality for very low birth weight deliveries in South Carolina by level of hospital perinatal service. Am J Obstet Gynecol. 1998;179:374-81.

17. Obesity in pregnancy. Practice Bulletin No. 156. American College of Obstetricians and Gynecologists [published erratum appears in Obstet Gynecol 2016;128:1450]. Obstet Gynecol. 2015;126:e112-26.

18. Paneth N, Kiely JL, Wallenstein S, Marcus M, Pakter J, Susser M. Newborn intensive care and neonatal mortality in low-birth-weight infants: a population study. N Engl J Med. 1982;307:149-55.

19. Petersen EE, Davis NL, Goodman D, Cox S, Mayes N, Johnston E, et al. Vital signs: pregnancy-related deaths, United States, 2011-2015, and strategies for prevention, 13 states, 2013-2017. MMWR Morb Mortal Wkly Rep. 2019;68:423-9.

3

Initial Assessment, Management, and Triage of Patients in Labor

Seema Prakash, Srishti Prakash

▉ INTRODUCTION

The initial assessment, screening, and management of patients in labor is crucial in improving overall maternal and fetal outcome. Whenever a patient in labor comes to healthcare facility it becomes very important to provide evidence-based quality care in an environment of minimal risk.

▉ RECEIVING AND INITIAL ASSESSMENT

In emergency receiving area, doctors, and paramedical staff should quickly assess the general condition of patient in a designated room in complete privacy including general physical examination, assessment of vitals—Pulse, BP, RR, SpO_2, temperature, and obstetric examination. A provisional diagnosis should be made as soon as possible so that treatment may be prioritized and complications are identified quickly and managed promptly. Most hospitals and health facilities have formulated guidelines for management of patients in labor.

Fetal status must be assessed on every patient who is evaluated or admitted in a labor triage unit in consultation with pediatrician or neonatologist. Classify the case as high-risk or low-risk category according to condition of patient, associated complications, and expected outcome.

The clinician's initial evaluation and documentation in labor and delivery shall include:
- Documentation of personal details of patient
- Reviewing the patient's prior pregnancy(s)
- Reviewing and summarizing the antenatal course

▉ HISTORY

Detailed history is important to identify patients in low-risk or high-risk group and also to ascertain that patient is in labor or not. History in an obstetric patient should be quick and conclusive. It should include sociodemographic profile of patient, chief presenting complaints, and confirmation of period of gestation. Important events of present pregnancy and previous obstetric history, medical and surgical history should be elicited. Certain factors, which are known to increase risk of maternal and fetal morbidity and mortality, should be taken into consideration.

▉ PHYSICAL EXAMINATION

- Taking appropriate precautions for COVID assess general condition, evaluate status of labor (description of uterine activity, cervical dilation and effacement, and fetal station and presentation) and confirm stage of labor-latent or active phase.
- Abdominal or obstetric examination to assess fundal height, lie, and presentation should be done. The level of presenting part in pelvis and frequency and duration of uterine contractions must be noted.
- *Per speculum examination:* If there is history of bleeding or leaking per vaginally to look for color of liquor or meconium.
- Vaginal examination should be performed under aseptic conditions to note consistency, effacement, dilatation of cervix, position, and station of presenting part, check for caput or molding, assess bony pelvis.
- Assessment of progress of labor is done by observing contractions and decent of presenting part and cervical changes.

Fetal Surveillance

Evaluation of fetal status, including interpretation of auscultation or electronic fetal monitoring (Intermittent or continuous fetal heart monitoring). On admission nonstress test or contraction stress test should be performed. Auscultation of fetal heart sounds should be done for minimum 1 minute postcontraction.

The Plan for Delivery

Take consent, counsel the attendants, explain present situation and further plan of action. For patients in labor or those with complications mode of delivery should be planned.

▨ INVESTIGATIONS

Basic antenatal investigation to be checked and if not available all requisite investigations should be sent.

Any special investigations should be done identifying high-risk maternal or fetal situation.

Evaluation During First Stage Labor

The patient should be evaluated by the obstetrician during labor at appropriate intervals. Each evaluation should include:

- Assessment of maternal status
- Description of uterine activity
- Assessment of fetal status
- Description of findings on vaginal examination, including cervical dilation and effacement, fetal station, change in status of membranes, and progress since last examination
- Summary of maternal and fetal status
- Plan, including plans for or performance of clinical interventions and pain management

Each evaluation should be recorded in the medical record.

Evaluation During Second Stage Labor

The monitoring clinician should document in the medical record at the time of identification of second stage, after 2 hours of second stage, and hourly thereafter. This documentation, which should be dated and timed, should include:

- Assessment of maternal status
- Assessment of fetal status

- Description of uterine activity
- Fetal station and, if known, position
- Assessment of progression and a plan for delivery. For a patient without complications, fetal heart rate (FHR) monitoring is done intermittently by fetal handheld Doppler every 5–15 minutes FHR should be evaluated and recorded at least every 5–15 minutes and 30 seconds postcontraction depending on the risk status of the patient. Continuous FHR monitoring should be done for patients with any of these indicators:
  - History of an abnormal antepartum FHR or rhythm
  - Abnormal presentation,
  - History of prior cesarean delivery
  - Multiple gestation
  - Nonreassuring fetal assessment
  - Significant maternal illness
  - Abnormality of active or second stage labor
  - Thick meconium
  - Heavy vaginal bleeding

Electronic fetal monitoring is also preferred when auscultation is not feasible as in case of COVID infection.

Triage for Stage of Labor

Triaging of patients in labor is described in **Table 1**.

▨ ACTION ON ALERT SIGNS

Prompt action is required in case there are any of the alert signs in patient.

During First Stage of Labor

Action on alert sign during first stage of labor is shown in **Table 2**.

During Second Stage of Labor

Action on alert sign during second stage of labor is shown in **Table 3**.

▨ OUTLINE OF MANAGEMENT DURING LABOR

Management during labor is described in **Flowchart 1**.

TABLE 1: Triaging of patients in labor.

Latent phase <5 cm	Active phase >5 cm
• Admit in ward • Supportive care • Ambulation • Pain relief • Hydration • Nutrition • Reassurance • Reassessment	• Admit in labor room • Supportive care • Vital monitoring • Fetal heart rate monitoring • Progress of labor chart • Contractions • Descent of presenting part

Contractions subside	Contractions increase	Protracted active phase	Arrest of active phase
↓	↓	↓	↓
False labor	Reassess for active phase	Augmentation of labor	Cesarean section

TABLE 2: Action on alert sign during first stage of labor.

Maternal	Cervical dilatation	Progress of labor
Pulse <60/min or >120/min SBP < 80/>140 mm Hg Urine ketones 2+ *Fetal* Baseline FHR < 110/min or >160/min Late deceleration	5 cm > 6 hours 6 cm > 5 hours 7 cm > 3 hours 8 cm > 2.5 hours 9 cm > 2 hours	• Contractions ≤2 or >5 contractions duration/second <20 or >60 • Fetal position—posterior or transverse • Caput +++ • Molding +++ • Liquor-meconium stained

TABLE 3: Action on alert sign during second stage of labor.

Maternal	Fetal	Progress of labor
Pulse <60 or >120 min SBP <80 or >140 mm Hg Urine ketones 2+	Baseline FHR <110 or >160/min Late decelerations	• Contractions <2 >5 <20 >60 seconds duration • Fetal position • Posterior or transverse • Caput+ • Molding+ • Liquor-meconium stained

▨ TRIAGE IN LABOR

In centers where there is a heavy load of patients in emergency department, it becomes mandatory to screen patients in receiving area. The healthcare professionals should have clear understanding of triage of patients on the basis of severity, complications and urgency of treatment.

Patients Requiring Immediate Care

• Patients presenting with abnormal vital signs
• Maternal HR <40 or >130, apneic, SpO$_2$ <93%, SBP ≥160 or DBP ≥110 or <60/palpable,
• No FHR detected by Doppler or FHR <110 bpm for >60 seconds
• In most of such cases immediate lifesaving intervention required.

Flowchart 1: Management of during labor.

First stage
- Quick assessment of fetus and maternal status
- Supportive care
- Make provisional diagnosis—classify case as low/high risk
- Document early labor—Plan for delivery

↓

Second stage
- Labor progress monitoring
- Maternal vitals 1 hourly
- Fetal monitoring 5–15 minutes
- Contractions and descent half hourly
- Follow alert threshold

↓

Third stage
AMTSL
- Delayed cord clamping
- Maternal and newborn care
- Delay in third stage—retained placenta

↓

Fourth stage management
- 1 Hourly maternal and newborn monitoring
- Early initiation of breastfeeding

Maternal

- Cardiac compromise
- Severe respiratory distress
- Seizures
- Hemorrhage
- Acute mental status change
- Signs of placental abruption
- Signs of uterine rupture
- Prolapsed cord

Imminent Birth

- Fetal parts visible on the perineum
- Active maternal bearing-down efforts

Women in Labor who Require Prompt Attention

- Signs of active labor ≥34 weeks

- Early labor signs and/or SROM/leaking 34–36.6 weeks
- ≥34 weeks with regular contractions and HSV lesion
- ≥34 weeks planned, elective, repeat cesarean with regular contractions
- ≥ 34 weeks multiple gestation pregnancy with irregular contractions

Patients who do not Require Urgent Attention

- ≥37 weeks early labor signs and/or c/o SROM/leaking
- Non-urgent symptoms may include common discomforts of pregnancy, vaginal discharge, constipation, ligament pain, nausea, anxiety
- Prescription refill
- Outpatient service that was missed
- Scheduled procedure when the patient has no complaint

Triage of Patients in Labor According to Fetomaternal Condition

According to fetomaternal condition, triage of patients in labor has been described in **Table 4**.

PRIORITY OF PATIENTS IN EMERGENCY

Priority of patients in emergency has been shown in **Flowchart 2**.

Emergency obstetrics departments of tertiary care hospitals have structured guidelines that aid in determining which patients must be evaluated promptly and which may wait safely and aid in determining anticipated course of care. Color coding of triage units is a good concept in which critically sick patients are kept in red zone requiring immediate care, less sick patients requiring emergency care are kept in yellow zone and managed, and those who are stable are kept in green zone are mostly managed as outpatient.

TABLE 4: Triage of patients in labor according to fetomaternal condition.

Zone	Action	Conditions	Management area
Red	Immediate/ Life saving	**Maternal** HR <40 or >130, Apneic, SpO$_2$ <93%, SBP ≥160 or DBP ≥110 or <60/palpable, No FHR detected by Doppler Urine ketones 2+ **Fetal** • Baseline FHR <110/min or >160/min • Late deceleration • Immediate lifesaving intervention required, such as: *Maternal:* – Cardiac compromise – Severe respiratory distress – Seizures – Hemorrhage – Acute mental status change – Signs of placental abruption – Signs of uterine rupture – Prolapsed cord *Imminent birth:* – Fetal parts visible on the perineum – Active maternal bearing-down efforts	ICU/HDU/OT
Yellow	Prompt	• Signs of active labor ≥34 weeks • Early labor signs and/or SROM/leaking 34–36.6 weeks • ≥34 weeks with regular contractions and HSV lesion • ≥34 weeks planned, elective, repeat cesarean with regular contractions • ≥34 weeks multiple gestation pregnancy with irregular contractions • ≥37 weeks early labor signs and/or c/o SROM/leaking	LR/OT
Green	Non-urgent	Common discomforts of pregnancy, vaginal discharge, constipation, ligament pain, nausea, anxiety. • Prescription refill • Outpatient service Scheduled procedure	Ward/OPD

Flowchart 2: Priority of patient in emergency.

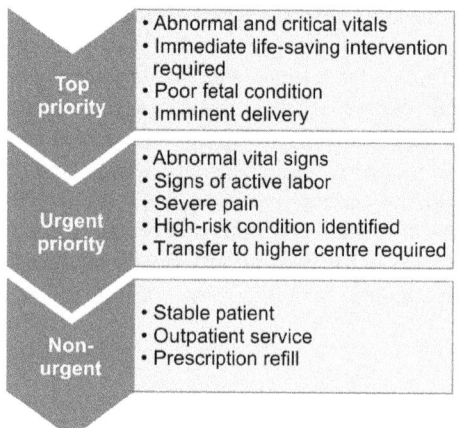

Top priority
• Abnormal and critical vitals
• Immediate life-saving intervention required
• Poor fetal condition
• Imminent delivery

Urgent priority
• Abnormal vital signs
• Signs of active labor
• Severe pain
• High-risk condition identified
• Transfer to higher centre required

Non-urgent
• Stable patient
• Outpatient service
• Prescription refill

■ BIBLIOGRAPHY

1. NICE Guidelines. Surveillance of Intrapartum Care for Healthy Women and Babies. London CG-190.UK: National Institute for Health and Care Excellence; 2019.
2. World Health Organization. WHO Labor care guide: Users Manual. Geneva: World health Organization;2020.
3. World Health Organization. WHO Recommendations: Intrapartum care for a Positive Childbirth Experience. Geneva: World Health Organization; 2018.

Communication, Consent, and Counseling of a Woman in Labor

Richa Sharma

COMMUNICATION

Labor and childbirth is a very dynamic experience involving not only the woman and her family members, but also the entire healthcare team. An effective communication between healthcare team members, laboring mother and her family members is pivotal for ensuring safety. The skills which are required to provide good and effective communication should be present in each team member. They should have proper knowledge as well as skills related to leadership, mutual support, and anticipation of situations. Focusing on appropriate communication, language barriers, and care practices can build an environment full of confidence as well as strengthen the women's childbirth experience. Ideally communication should be direct, patient-centered, specific and timely occurring between the mother, her close family members, and staff of the healthcare team. The effectiveness of communication can be influenced by courtesy, prior experiences with team members, and body language. Various other factors that influence an effective communication are:

- Skills of listening which are equally important as skills to speak.
- An ability of a woman to deal with her pain, anxiety, fears, or discomfort. It is also contributed by the support of her family members through managing strategies.
- Long hours fasting, fatigue, lack of sleep, and sleep inertia.
- Development of better systemic strategies can help in providing an effective communication and improve in responding to quick changes in woman's status. Such systematic strategies that can be applied to maternal care are:
  - Situation-Background-Assessment-Recommendation (SBAR) communication tool

- Training in tool management principles
- Training health workers and other staff members through workshops and drills
- Systematic ward rounds and bedside rounds
- Formulating checklists and developing standard order sets

For effective communication with a distressed woman in labor:

- Healthcare provider should remain calm and focused while maintaining his/her professional relationships.
- Voice should not be raised under any circumstances. Healthcare worker should deal with empathy and politeness keeping her respect and dignity in mind.
- Constant praising, encouragement, and reassurance can lead to better results and help in decreasing her anxiety and distress.
- Respect and appropriate care should be given throughout labor.

SHARED DECISION MAKING

Before making choices and final decisions, it is essential for an obstetrician to acknowledge the patient's own values, priorities, and cultures. These choices and decisions are reflection of healthcare's own beliefs, and cultures. Shared decision making is based on the best available evidences and being mutually formulated through a process involving woman, her family, and healthcare team. The information about the effect of the decisions on women's future should be thoroughly discussed. Many benefits are obtained through shared decision making like increasing woman's engagement, better compliance to the treatment, and outcomes as well as sense of satisfaction.[1] A "SHARE" approach can be used for making shared decisions as illustrated in **Figure 1**.[2]

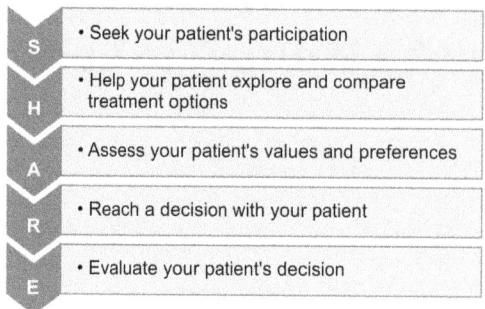

S • Seek your patient's participation

H • Help your patient explore and compare treatment options

A • Assess your patient's values and preferences

R • Reach a decision with your patient

E • Evaluate your patient's decision

Fig. 1: "SHARE" approach for decision making.

TEAM WORK

A good quality of team members results in less clinical faults with better outcomes and satisfaction. Perinatal care improvement can be achieved through training of interdisciplinary team as they better address woman centered care needs. Mother and child healthcare team should involve training in some important areas such as healthcare team member leadership, support and performance monitoring mutually, respect for all the individuals, effective communication, adaptability, and avoiding hierarchy. Ideally, the team should incorporate following aspects.[1]

• Immediate and suitable response to an emergency situation
• Effective communication
• Friendly environment amongst the team members and ability to share all the problems faced during provision of healthcare services
• Anticipation of difficult situations
• Scrutinizing all the procedures
• Debriefing all the team members after any event irrespective of the outcomes for identifying different ways that may improve maternal safety and health
• Proper mutual understanding amongst the team members and ability to recognize each other's weaknesses and strengths.

CONSENT

The health worker should ensure proper understanding and shared decision making before obtaining informed consent. Before taking consent from a woman, it is important to ensure that the woman is fully aware about the procedure or test, its consequences, benefits, complications or risks, alternative interventions, and understands the nature of the situation for which it is being done. Any doubts regarding the management protocols should be discussed and cleared before the consent.[3]

Consent in Labor

Consent during labor should be taken with care especially if a woman is under the influence of narcotic analgesics or in pain. The women should be informed in the antenatal period itself regarding anticipatory situations during labor. However, she may not be able to recall some information provided before labor. Therefore, it is important to provide again the proper and full information along with necessary explanation during labor. During labor, information should be given in-between the contractions. Provision of a brief summary regarding possible interventions and operations can be considered at admission in labor or during induction of labor. Before making any final decision, it is always a good practice to encourage women for giving their opinions. Consent for sterilization should not be taken from the women during labor except if the women was being provided full information during antenatal visit and had agreed upon provisionally.[3]

Consent for Assisted Vaginal Deliveries, Emergency Cesarean Section, and Perineal Repair

There is a scope to allow verbal consent to be obtained before any emergency procedure if it benefits the mother or baby. However, written consent should always be taken for all the procedures done under regional or general anesthesia if time permits. Verbal consent should be obtained in the presence of a professional care witness in emergency cases. The reasons for emergency delivery without having written consent as well as all the consents obtained verbally must be recorded. If a woman refuses assisted vaginal delivery or emergency cesarean section even after being explained about all the consequences for her and the baby, her decision should be respected. For episiotomy/perineal repair under local anesthesia following a normal or assisted vaginal delivery, verbal consent is acceptable. However, written consent should be obtained for more extensive repair under local anesthetic or for those under regional or general anesthesia.[3]

COUNSELING

For women especially primigravida, labor can be a very petrifying experience. Moreover, they can encounter various physical and mental emotions ranging from discomfort to severe pain. Counseling during labor thus plays an important role in helping the women in overcoming such situations. It is very crucial to counsel the women in labor about all the anticipatory situations and solutions to prevent or treat them. The counseling should be done in a friendly and empathic way keeping all her values, beliefs, and cultures in mind. Ideally, counseling process should be started right from the preconception period till her discharge. Counseling should involve not only the mother but also her family members. All the staff members of healthcare team should equally participate in counseling process. An effective counseling can motivate the woman as well as her family members and help in building trust between them. This can lead to better outcomes and satisfaction. The counseling includes:[4]

- Making the woman relax as much as possible.
- Being well aware of her situation can help in diminishing her pain and emotional distress during the process of labor and childbirth.
- An effective counseling go hand to hand with a good quality care, adequate comfort and support, timely information, and reassurance childbirth.
- The counseling process should take place while maintaining the respect of the women.
- Proper explanation should be given before any intervention. What step you are going to perform, why it is being done, and what will be the consequences of doing or not doing should be detailed to the women and her family members.
- Confidentiality and privacy should be carried out throughout the labor and childbirth including use of curtains, and keeping women covered as much as possible.
- Preferences of the women should be acknowledged and accordingly birth and emergency plan should be formulated.
- Self-care should be encouraged which includes:
  - Keeping her genitals clean by taking bath/shower/washing at the onset of labor and later on whenever she feels like.

Do not administer any local herbs or medicine	Do not ecourage the woman to push
Do not keep the woman in bed if she wants to move around	Do not give advice other than that given by the health worker

Fig. 2: Instructions for the birth companions.

- Ambulate frequently during initial stage and choose position in labor of her choice.
- Drinking fluids or having meals as per her comfort and wishes.
- Other effective strategies of encountering pain like breathing techniques. Teaching her to breathe out more slowly, or to pant at the end of the first stage or at the height of a painful contraction to prevent pushing.

ROLE OF A BIRTH COMPANION

It is advantageous to have a birth companion of women's choice during labor. The birth companion can be any member of her family with which she is most comfortable with. The main role of the companion is to provide support, compassion, motivation, and reassurance during the labor. The companion can help the woman in performing some basic steps like breathing and relaxing or rub her back, providing sips of water as allowed, wiping her brow with a wet cloth, or doing other supportive actions. It is crucial to guide birth companions as shown in **Figure 2**.[4]

REFERENCES

1. Lichtmacher A. Quality Assessment Tools: ACOG Voluntary Review of Quality of Care Program, Peer Review Reporting System. Obstet Gynecol Clin North Am. 2018;35(1):147-62.
2. American College of Obstetrician and Gynaecologists: Informed Consent and Shared Decision Making in Obstetrics and Gynaecology. Committee Opinion No. 819, February 2021.
3. College of Obstetricians and Gynaecologists: Obtaining Valid Consent. Clinical Governance Advice Royal No. 6, January 2015.
4. World Health Organization. Counselling for maternal and newborn health care: a handbook for building skills. World Health Organization; 2013.

Referral and Transport of High-risk Patients

Seema Prakash, Srishti Prakash

■ INTRODUCTION

It is a proven fact that appropriate antenatal care (ANC) improves pregnancy outcomes. In India, routine ANC is provided at primary care facilities and women with high-risk pregnancy or with complications which may lead to poor maternal or fetal outcomes are referred to advanced centers with facility to manage high-risk cases.

The primary care facilities include sub-health centers, primary health centers, and community health centers, in ascending order of level of obstetric care provided. The latter two should provide basic and comprehensive obstetric care, respectively. Besides this, a large number of health-care supports is provided by private sector and private health facilities play an important role in health scenario of India. The management and referrals during pregnancy with high-risk condition and/or complications need to be streamlined in India.

■ PATIENT TRANSFER PROTOCOL

- Every healthcare facility and hospitals should have guidelines for transfer of patients.
- There must be reasonable ground for transfer of patients, which should be clearly recorded in the transfer summary.
- Patient should be transferred with a transfer summary/referral slip.
- Patients' relatives/attendants should be informed and explained about the condition of patient and reason for transfer to other health facility.
- Patients who are hemodynamically unstable should first be stabilized before transfer.
- In cases where it is difficult to stabilize the patient she should be transferred in a fully equipped ambulance accompanied by a trained staff.
- Inform and take permission of senior obstetrician before transfer
- Maintain records of all transferred patients
- The health care provider should ensure that proper history is elicited and complete general physical, systemic, and abdominal examinations are performed on the pregnant women during each ANC visit. Though any case could develop complication during or after pregnancy or childbirth, a pregnancy with a high-risk factor poses higher than normal risk for the pregnant women.

Some common high risk conditions of pregnancy are enumerated in **Table 1**.

Personal or Past History

- Young primigravida (less than 18 years) or elderly gravida (more than 35 years)
- Short stature < 140 cm.
- Parity > 5
- History of consanguinity
- Smoking/alcoholism/drug/substance abuse
- Bad obstetric history (History of still birth, abortion, and congenital malformation)
- Previous LSCS/uterine surgery
- Patient with history of any current/past history of systemic illness(es).

Ongoing Maternal/Fetal Complications

- Postdated pregnancy
- Preterm labor/PPROM
- Malpresentation
- Maternal weight > 90 kg or < 45 kg.
- FGR/Uteroplacental insufficiency
- Cephalopelvic disproportion/Obstructed labor

TABLE 1: High-risk pregnancy to be referred to tertiary care hospitals.

Obstetric complications	Pregnancy with medical conditions
Accidental hemorrhage, placenta previa, abruption	Severe anemia (Hb < 7 g/dL)
Postpartum hemorrhage	Gestational diabetes mellitus
Adherent placenta or other placental abnormalities	Diabetic ketoacidosis
Sepsis	Cardiac disease
HELLP syndrome	Jaundice/Liver disease
Pre-eclampsia/Eclampsia/Hypertensive crisis	Thyrotoxicosis/thyroid storm
Multiple gestation with complications	Disseminated intravascular coagulopathy (DIC)
Uterine anomalies complicating pregnancy	Pheochromocytoma
Ruptured ectopic	Bleeding disorders
Obstetric hysterectomy	Dengue/Malaria
Hydatidiform mole	Chronic Kidney disease (CKD)
Patients requiring intensive care/ monitoring	

- Placenta previa/Abruption
- Severe anemia
- Twin/Multiple pregnancy
- Syphilis/HIV/Hepatitis
- Medical disorders (Heart, liver, kidney disease)
- Gestational diabetes mellitus
- Hypothyroidism
- Pregnancy-induced hypertension, pre-eclampsia, eclampsia
- Rh-negative/Hydrops

An appropriate medical screening examination must be done to determine whether the patient has an emergency medical condition taking into account the health of the woman as well as the fetus.

All obstetrics emergencies should be managed in HDU/ICU of labor room where available. A decision to transfer patient must be taken, if facilities are not available and per transfer policy of health care facility.

- If an emergency medical condition is determined to exist, stabilize the patient or transfer her if the obstetric care provider certifies that the benefits of transfer outweigh the risks. In such cases counseling and written informed consent is required. Details about maternal and fetal condition, pregnancy complications, benefit/risks of transfer, and any alternatives available to them should be explained in their own language. Also explain about risks involved in transfer of these patients

- When necessary, arrange for transfer to another appropriate facility, if the patient is stabilized or if the benefits of transfer outweigh the risks. Transfer should be carried out by qualified personnel and fully equipped ambulance [Basic life support (BLS) or advanced life support (ALS)] depending on condition of patient.
- In private health care facilities appropriate medical screening and management should not be delayed to inquire about payment method or insurance status.

SUMMARY

Transfer summary must contain:
- History
- Clinical examination
- Investigation reports
- Treatment provided
- Reason for transfer
- Enumerate what facilities are required for patient, which are not available in transferring hospital
- Whether a referral call was made to transferring hospital
- Transfer summary must contain legible name and designation of transferring doctor
- In case of patients insisting on transfer without indication or low-risk patients going against advice of treating doctors it should be mentioned in the summary that it is being done on patient/attendants request.

- For patients belonging to Economically Weaker Sections (EWS) the guidelines issued by government should be followed.

COMPLICATIONS

Complications can occur during pregnancy and affect the health and survival of the mother and the fetus. As suggested by Government of India every pregnant woman must receive at least four check-ups during pregnancy (Registration and 1st check-up within 12 weeks, 14–26 weeks, 28–32 weeks, and 36–40 weeks). A woman in labor is considered unstable from the latent phase through delivery of the placenta, if there is inadequate time to safely transfer her to another hospital before delivery or if that transfer may pose a threat to health or safety of mother and fetus.

WARNING SIGNS

Warning signs should be explained to each pregnant woman using the safe motherhood booklet. Delivery of a woman with high-risk/complicated pregnancy must be planned in institute with facilities to manage such cases. The Indian health system should improve the provision of obstetric care by standardizing services at each level of health care and increasing the focus on emergency treatment for complications, appropriate decision-making for referral, and improving referral communication and staff support.

BIBLIOGRAPHY

1. Hospital disaster preparedness for obstetricians and facilities providing maternity care. Committee Opinion American College of Obstetricians and Gynecologists. Obstet Gynecol. 2013;121:696-9.
2. Maternal–fetal triage index. (Reprinted from Ruhl C, Scheich B, Onokpise B, Bingham D. Content validity testing of the maternal fetal triage index. J Obstet Gynecol Neonatal Nurs. 2015;44:701-9.
3. Paisley KS, Wallace R, DuRant PG. The development of an obstetric triage acuity tool [published in MCN Am J Matern Child Nurs 2012;37:72]. MCN Am J Matern Child Nurs. 2011;36:290-6.
4. Ruhl C, Scheich B, Onokpise B, Bingham D. Content validity testing of the maternal fetal triage index. J Obstet Gynecol Neonatal Nurs. 2015;44:701-93.

Sheeba Marwah, Chhavi Gupta

CHAPTER 6

Management of Normal Labor

INTRODUCTION

Labor or parturition is the process of expulsion of a viable fetus from the uterus per vaginum. While over enthusiastic management of labor can lead to unnecessary interventions that may add to the cost, discomfort, and anxiety of the patient, missing the warning signs can lead to complications. Thus, management of normal labor requires a balance of good practices, careful monitoring, and readiness to intervene as and when necessary.

PREREQUISITES OF NORMAL LABOR[1]

- Spontaneous in onset.
- Between 37 and 41 completed weeks of gestation.
- Low-risk to start with and remaining so throughout parturition.
- In vertex position
- Good condition of mother and baby after birth.

AIMS OF LABOR CARE

- Safe delivery for the mother.
- Alive and healthy baby.
- Pleasurable and fulfilling experience of childbirth for both the parents.

GOALS OF LABOR CARE

Respectful maternity care, effective communication, companion of choice, and continuity of care are the four pillars that form the basis of labor care **(Fig. 1)**.

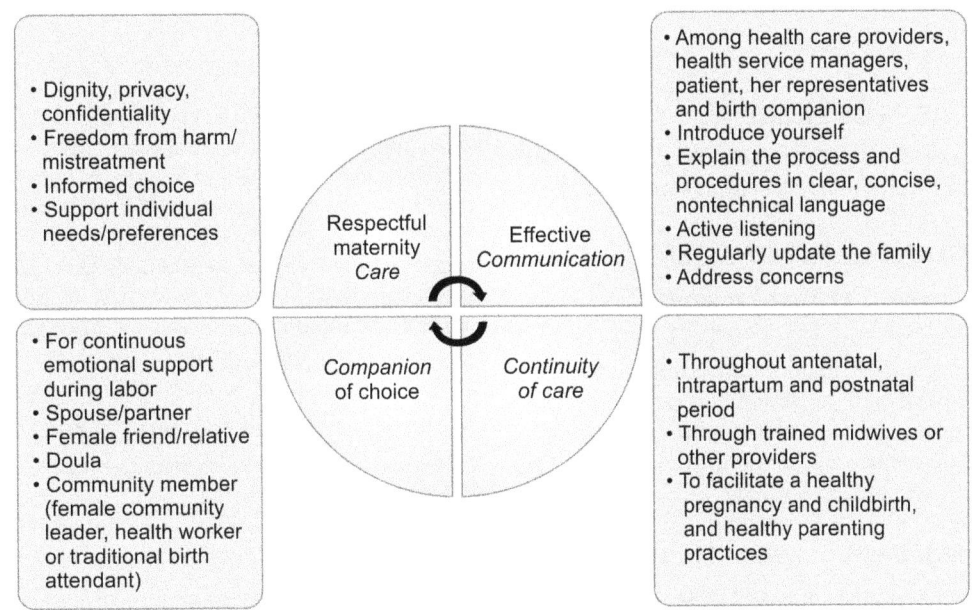

- Dignity, privacy, confidentiality
- Freedom from harm/mistreatment
- Informed choice
- Support individual needs/preferences

Respectful maternity Care

Effective Communication

- Among health care providers, health service managers, patient, her representatives and birth companion
- Introduce yourself
- Explain the process and procedures in clear, concise, nontechnical language
- Active listening
- Regularly update the family
- Address concerns

- For continuous emotional support during labor
- Spouse/partner
- Female friend/relative
- Doula
- Community member (female community leader, health worker or traditional birth attendant)

Companion of choice

Continuity of care

- Throughout antenatal, intrapartum and postnatal period
- Through trained midwives or other providers
- To facilitate a healthy pregnancy and childbirth, and healthy parenting practices

Fig. 1: Pillars of labor care that can be memorized as 4 C.

Flowchart 1: Stages of labor.

```
                          ┌─────────────────┐
                          │ Stages of labor │
                          └─────────────────┘
```

1st stage of labor	2nd stage of labor	3rd stage of labor	4th stage of labor

Latent phase Cervical dilatation up to 5 cm	*Active phase* Cervical dilatation from 5 cm until full dilatation	Full cervical dilatation till birth of baby	Delivery of baby to delivery of placenta-membranes	Delivery of placenta up to 2 hours after delivery
Variable as it is difficult to ascertain the actual onset of labor	Up to 12 hours in primiparous, 10 hours in multiparous (95th percentile)	3 hours in primiparous; 2 hours in multiparous. However, actual onset of 2nd stage is difficult to establish, and overall duration can differ	Usually 15 minutes; but can vary; 5–6 minutes with active management of 3rd stage of labor[2]	2 hours

TABLE 1: Initial assessment in labor room.		
Maternal vital parameters • Pulse rate • Blood pressure • Temperature • Respiratory rate	*Per abdominal examination* • Fetal lie • Fetal size • Fetal heart rate (FHR) • Uterine contractions—frequency, quality, duration	*Digital cervical examination* after excluding placenta previa and prelabor rupture of membranes (PROM) • Cervical dilation—effacement • Fetal presentation, station, position • Pelvic capacity Routine clinical pelvimetry has been replaced by clinical trial of labor[2]

STAGES OF LABOR

The process of labor is one of the continuum, but can be divided into four stages **(Flowchart 1)**.

MANAGEMENT OF NORMAL LABOR

Assessment at First Presentation

All women presenting in labor should have comprehensive maternal and fetal assessment by a health care professional to exclude previous undiagnosed or new developing complications, establish baseline cervical status and triage laboring women accordingly.[2]

Management of Latent First Stage

Healthy women in this stage can wait in waiting rooms with their companions, on-site midwife-led birthing units (OMBUs) or can be admitted to the labor ward. Labor ward admission policy in this stage remains variable and should be tailored to the individual needs and institutional protocols. However, unnecessary medical interventions to accelerate labor should be avoided. Alternatively, they can wait at home, if the woman desires and is motivated enough to follow-up. Though, this approach is not yet completely established.[2]

Management of Active First Stage

All women in active first stage and beyond have to be admitted to labor room.[2,3]

Initial Assessment in Labor Room

This establishes a baseline for future examinations **(Table 1)**.

TABLE 2: Laboratory investigations.

Hemoglobin/ hematocrit	Blood type and screen	Screen for *HIV, hepatitis B* surface antigen, *Syphilis* if not already screened
	• Low risk—Rh typing[4-7]	
	• Moderate risk[*]—type and screen	
	• High risk[†]—type and crossmatch[8]	

[*]Multiple gestation, trial of labor after cesarean, pre-eclampsia/HELLP without coagulopathy, grand multiparity, intra-amniotic infection, large fibroids.

[†]Placenta previa or accreta, pre-eclampsia/HELLP with coagulopathy, severe anemia, congenital or acquired bleeding diathesis, previous postpartum hemorrhage.

Flowchart 2: Good clinical practices.

Not Recommended	Recommended
Enforcing Bed Rest	**Upright Position** Position of woman's choice or comfort Mobility[11,12]
Restricted Oral Intake causes hypovolemia, ketosis, longer duration of labor	**Oral Fluid-Food Intake** (Myometrial requirement of glucose in labor is analogous to that in sustained and vigorous exercise)[13,14]
Intravenous Fluid For shortening the duration of labor as it restricts woman's motility, increases risk of fluid overload, particularly with intravenous oxytocin infusion[14,15]	**Intravenous Fluids** For supportive care or when oral intake is restricted for risk for cesarean delivery
Bladder Catheterization for preventing labor delay	**Pain Relief** Pharmacological/ nonpharmacological methods
Enema as it is invasive, discomfortable[19]	**Encourage regular voiding**[17,18]
Antispasmodic Agents for preventing labor delay	**Usual Daily Medications** can take medication orally; however, if unpredictable gastric absorption is a concern, prefer nonoral route
Antacids—not required	
Perineal/Pubic Shaving woman's personal choice[2,20]	
Vaginal Irrigation with Chlorhexidine for preventing infectious morbidities[21]	

Laboratory Investigations

Laboratory investigations have been described in **(Table 2)**.

Good Clinical Practices

These ensure mother is comfortable and safe and has a pleasurable birthing experience **(Flowchart 2)**.

Monitoring

Frequent maternal-fetal assessment is important as 20–25% intrapartum complications can arise rapidly even in low-risk women **(Table 3)**.[9]

Maternal vital parameters can be recorded in CEMACH MEOWS or Carle's Obstetric Early Warning Score Charts to ensure timely detection of deteriorating mother and need for stepping up care.[10,11]

TABLE 3: Monitoring in active first stage of labor.	
Maternal wellbeing	Record maternal pulse rate, blood pressure, temperature, respiratory rate, percentage oxygen required to maintain saturation of 95% and above
Fetal wellbeing	*Intermittent auscultation* of FHR with Doppler ultrasound device or Pinard fetal stethoscope every 15–30 minutes. Auscultate during a uterine contraction and continue for at least 30 seconds after the contraction with each auscultation lasting for at least 1 minute[2]
	Continuous cardiotocography is not recommended in healthy pregnancies for the risk of increased rate of cesarean section and other medical interventions[2]
Labor progress	*Uterine contractions:* Frequency, duration, strength[2] • Manual palpation • External tocodynamometry Internal pressure transducer (if tracing is inadequate)
	Digital Vaginal Examination every 4 hours or more frequently if maternal-fetal condition demands.[12]
	However, keep examinations to a minimum to avoid patient discomfort and iatrogenic infections, particularly in prolonged rupture of membranes and long duration of labor[2]
	Unlike previous recommendations, a minimum cervical dilatation rate of 1 cm/hour throughout active first stage (as depicted by the partograph alert line) is not always possible and a slower rate should not raise false alarm prompting obstetric intervention (oxytocin augmentation or cesarean section) provided fetal-maternal conditions are reassuring, cephalopelvic disproportion have been excluded, maternal emotional, psychological and physical needs are being met[2]

Fetal wellbeing and labor progress can be recorded on partogram. The utility of WHO partogram to alert obstetrician, especially in low resource settings, cannot be overlooked, but now plotting should commence from a cervical dilatation of 5 cm.[2] Hence, these partogram need to be revised.

WHO has instituted a new Labor Care Guide for all women in active first stage of labor and beyond for use at all levels of health care. Though, high-risk women may still necessitate additional monitoring (**Fig. 2**).[13]

Active Management of Labor (Early Amniotomy, Oxytocin)

This reduces the duration of labor and possible cesarean section rate, but is not advised as it is interventional, undermines women's autonomy and needs resources. *Continuous one-to-one support* during labor, is the only component that is beneficial.[2]

Management of Second Stage of Labor

Transportation

Transportation of woman from labor room to a specific delivery room at beginning of the second stage when labor is progressing normally is not preferred as it is unpleasant and unnecessary.[2]

Birth Position

Encourage position of woman's choice and comfort.[2]

- *Upright positions (walking, standing, sitting, supported kneeling):* Pelvis is in a vertical plane that increases pelvic dimensions and aligns fetus with the birth canal that might reduce episiotomy and instrumental vaginal births but is associated with PPH and second-degree tears.
- Upright position is possible with current "low dose" and "mobile" epidural analgesia but not with traditional epidural analgesia that provides dense neuroaxial block.
- *Semirecumbent or all-fours position just before expulsion of fetus:* Facilitates perineal techniques to reduce perineal tears and blood loss.
- *Lithotomy:* Useful if fetal manipulation or optimal surgical exposure is anticipated.
- *Supine position:* Causes aortocaval compression and should be avoided.
- *Left/Right lateral (Sims) position:* Avoids aortocaval compression and is preferred.[2]

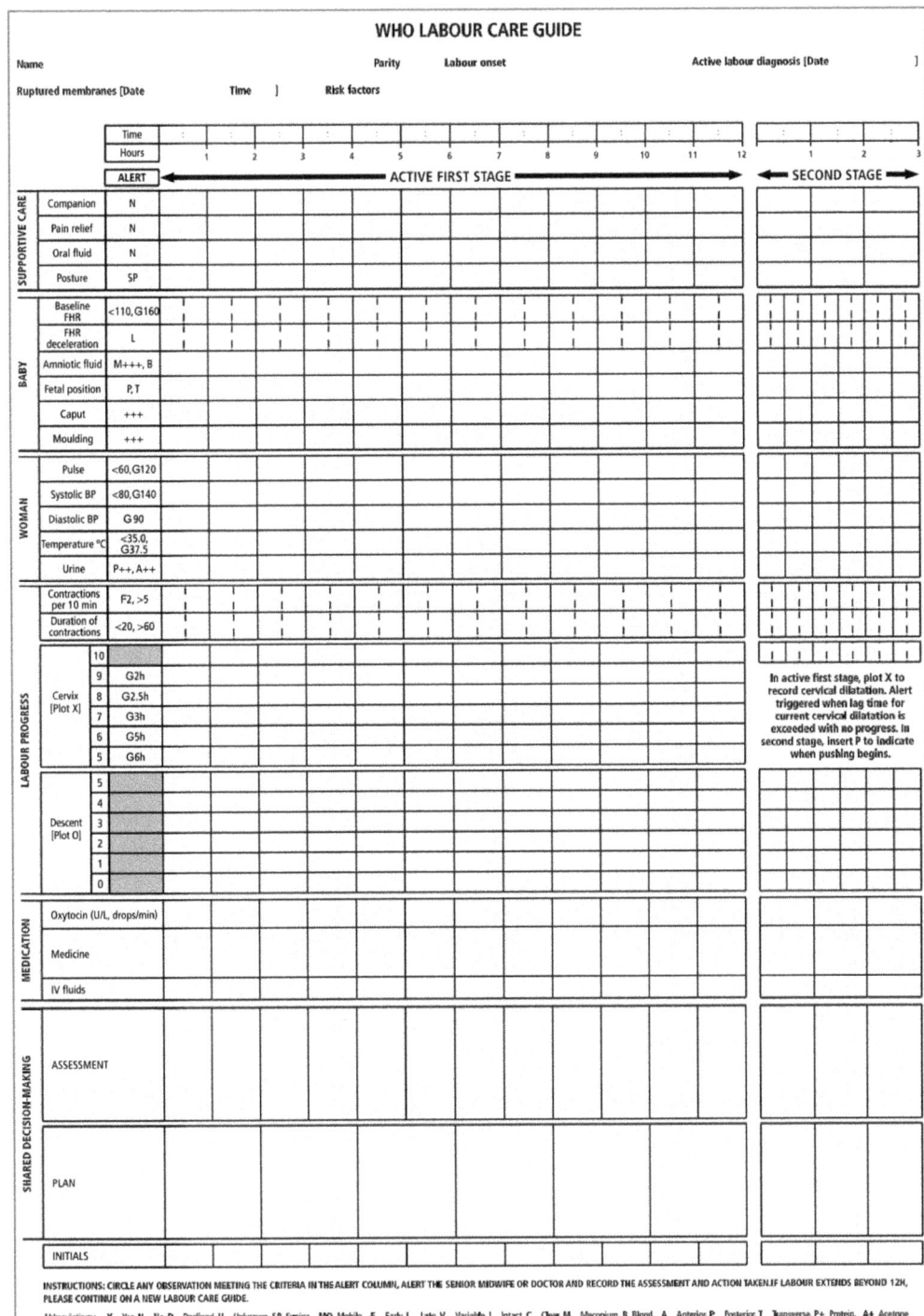

Fig. 2: WHO labor care guide.

Monitoring

- Intermittent auscultation of FHR every 5 minutes.
- Digital vaginal examination at 2 hour interval.[2]

Pushing

Avoid immediate pushing or directed pushing with valsalva maneuver and encourage woman to follow their own urge to push.[14,15]

With epidural analgesia, delay pushing for 1–2 hours after full dilatation or until the woman regains the sensory urge to bear down.[2]

Reduce Perineal Trauma

- Avoid manual fundal pressure.[2] However, the results of gentle-assisted pushing (gap) trial are awaited.[16]
- Routine or liberal use of mediolateral episiotomy is not recommended and is reserved for deliveries with a high risk of severe perineal laceration, significant soft tissue dystocia. It can be used in obstetric emergencies, such as fetal distress requiring instrumental vaginal birth.[2]
- Perineal massage with two fingers of the lubricated gloved hand moving from side to side just inside the patient's vagina and exerting mild, downward pressure.[17,18]
- Warm perineal compresses (up to 110°F/ 43°C).[19,20]
- "Hands on" guarding of the perineum reduces 1st degree perineal tears. One hand flexes the head and controls the speed of crowning, other hand eases the perineum away from the path of emerging head.[2]
- Ask woman to pant or make only small expulsive efforts when the head is fully crowning.[2]
- Avoid ritgen's maneuver/hands-off technique (one hand placed on fetal occiput to control speed of birth, fingers of other hand placed between the maternal anus and coccyx to actively lift the fetal chin anteriorly).[2]

Routine Antibiotic Prophylaxis

Itis not required. Antibiotics are given only if there are risk factors or clinical signs of peripartum infection, infection of an episiotomy wound, prophylactically for 3rd or 4th degree perineal tear.[2]

No Intervention

No intervention is required if the mother-fetus are in good condition, there is descent of fetal head and the duration is well within the standard duration.[2]

Management of Third Stage of Labor

Active Management of Third Stage of Labor

This helps to prevent PPH:[21]

- *Prophylactic uterotonic agent* before delivery of placenta, preferably Oxytocin (10 IU, IM/ IV), else Ergometrine/Methylergometrine (contraindicated in hypertension) or oral misoprostol (600 microgram).
- Controlled cord traction
- It is done only if skilled birth attendants are available and the care provider/parturient woman regard a small reduction in blood loss (average 11 mL) and a small reduction in the duration (average 6 minutes) of the third stage of labor as important.
  - *With oxytocin use:* CCT may add small benefit.[21]
  - *With ergot alkaloids:* CCT is essential.
  - *With misoprost:* Role of CCT is under evaluation.

  CCT is the first intervention to treat retained placenta.
- *Sustained uterine massage* is not required if prophylactic oxytocin is given.[22,23] Its role is uncertain if no uterotonic or uterotonic other than oxytocin is used.

Delayed Umbilical Cord Clamping (Table 4)[2]

Delay cord clamping for at least 60 seconds (even in HIV positive woman), except when mother or newborn is unstable or when the newborn-placental circulation is not intact (e.g., abruption, previa, cord avulsion). 75% of blood available for placenta-to-fetus transfusion is transfused in the 1st minute after birth.[24]

Current data suggest equipoise between DCC and cord milking in preterm births.[26]

Examine the Placenta, Umbilical Cord, and Fetal Membranes

Succenturiate placental lobe and number of vessels in the cord.

Flowchart 3: Management of normal labor.

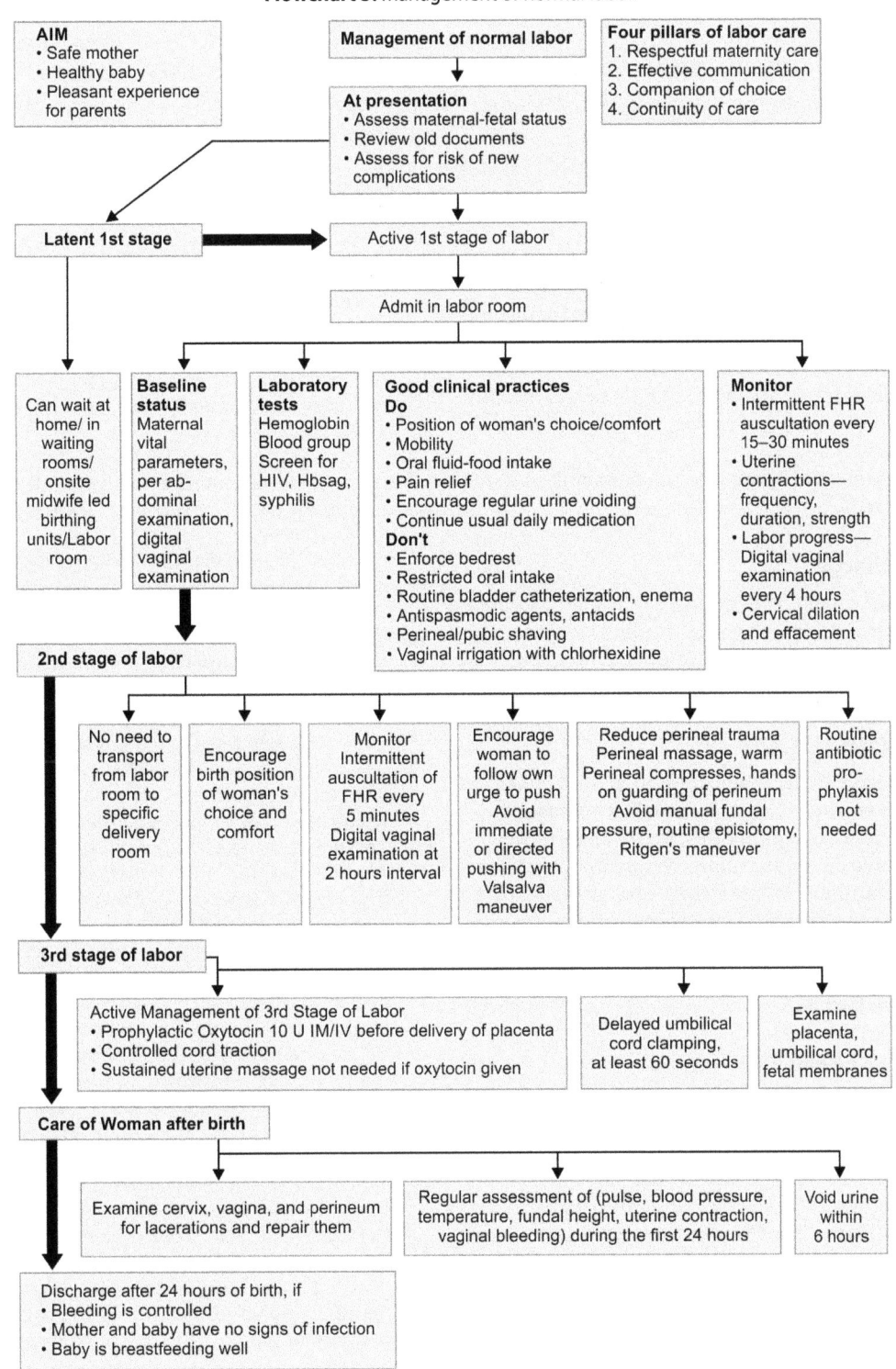

TABLE 4: Benefits and drawbacks of delayed cord clamping.

Benefits	Drawbacks
Facilitates transition from fetal to newborn life	Causes hyperbilirubinemia
Reduces intraventricular hemorrhage (IVH) and necrotizing enterocolitis in preterm infants	Reduces volume of blood available for stem cell harvesting
Ensures higher infant iron stores at 6 months of age that prevents impaired neurodevelopment[25]	

Care of Woman after Birth

- Examine cervix, vagina, and perineum for lacerations and repair them.
- Regular assessment of (pulse, blood pressure, temperature, fundal height, uterine contraction, and vaginal bleeding) during the first 24 hours.
- Urine void should be documented within 6 hours. [2]

Discharge

Patient should be discharged only after 24 hours of birth, if bleeding is controlled, mother and baby have no signs of infection, and baby is breastfeeding well.[2]

CONCLUSION

Management of labor aims to achieve healthy mother and baby, imparting pleasurable experience to parents. Respectful maternity care, effective communication, companion of choice, and continuity of care form the basis of labor care. A systematic approach, watchful expectancy, good clinical practices and management based on established guidelines ensure a good outcome **(Flowchart 3)**.

REFERENCES

1. Technical Working Group, World Health Organization. Care in normal birth: A practical guide. Birth. 1997;24(2):121-3.
2. WHO. WHO Recommendations: Intrapartum Care for a Positive Childbirth Experience. Geneva: World Health Organization; 2018.
3. Lagrew DC, Low LK, Brennan R, Corry MP, Edmonds JK, Gilpin BG, et al. National partnership for maternal safety: consensus bundle on safe reduction of primary cesarean births-supporting intended vaginal births. Obstet Gynecol. 2018;131(3):503-13.
4. Palmer RH, Kane JG, Churchill WH, Goldman L, Komaroff AL. Cost and quality in the use of blood bank services for normal deliveries, cesarean sections, and hysterectomies. JAMA. 1986;256(2):219-23.
5. Ransom SB, Fundaro G, Dombrowski MP. Cost-effectiveness of routine blood type and screen testing for cesarean section. J Reprod Med. 1999;44(7):592-4.
6. Cousins LM, Teplick FB, Poeltler DM. Pre-cesarean blood bank orders: a safe and less expensive approach. Obstet Gynecol. 1996; 87(6):912-6.
7. Ransom SB, Fundaro G, Dombrowski MP. The cost-effectiveness of routine type and screen admission testing for expected vaginal delivery. Obstet Gynecol. 1998;92(4 Pt 1):493-5.
8. Goodnough LT, Daniels K, Wong AE, Viele M, Fontaine MF, Butwick AJ. How we treat: trans-fusion medicine support of obstetric services. Transfusion (Paris). 2011;51(12): 2540-8.
9. Zapata-Vázquez RE, Rodríguez-Carvajal LA, Sierra-Basto G, Alonzo-Vázquez FM, Echeverría-Egíluz M. Discriminant function of perinatal risk that predicts early neonatal morbidity: its validity and reliability. Arch Med Res. 2003;34(3):214-21.
10. Singh S, McGlennan A, England A, Simons R. A validation study of the CEMACH recommended modified early obstetric warning system (MEOWS). Anaesthesia. 2012;67(1):12-8.
11. Carle C, Alexander P, Columb M, Johal J. Design and internal validation of an obstetric early warning score: secondary analysis of the Intensive Care National Audit and Research Centre Case Mix Programme database. Anaesthesia. 2013;68(4):354-67.
12. Downe S, Gyte GML, Dahlen HG, Singata M. Routine vaginal examinations for assessing progress of labour to improve outcomes for

women and babies at term. Cochrane Database Syst Rev. 2013;(7):CD010088.

13. WHO. WHO labour care guide: user's manual. Geneva: World Health Organization; 2021.

14. Di Mascio D, Saccone G, Bellussi F, Al-Kouatly HB, Brunelli R, Benedetti Panici P, et al. Delayed versus immediate pushing in the second stage of labor in women with neuraxial analgesia: a systematic review and meta-analysis of randomized controlled trials. Am J Obstet Gynecol. 2020;223(2):189-203.

15. Lemos A, Amorim MM, Dornelas de Andrade A, de Souza AI, Cabral Filho JE, Correia JB. Pushing/bearing down methods for the second stage of labour. Cochrane Database Syst Rev. 2017;3:CD009124.

16. Hofmeyr GJ, Singata M, Lawrie T, Vogel JP, Landoulsi S, Seuc AH, et al. A multicentre randomized controlled trial of gentle assisted pushing in the upright posture (GAP) or upright posture alone compared with routine practice to reduce prolonged second stage of labour (the Gentle Assisted Pushing study): study protocol. Reprod Health. 2015;12:114.

17. Aasheim V, Nilsen ABV, Reinar LM, Lukasse M. Perineal techniques during the second stage of labour for reducing perineal trauma. Cochrane Database Syst Rev. 2017;6: CD006672.

18. Beckmann MM, Stock OM. Antenatal perineal massage for reducing perineal trauma. Cochrane Database Syst Rev. 2013; (4): CD005123.

19. Albers LL, Sedler KD, Bedrick EJ, Teaf D, Peralta P. Midwifery care measures in the second stage of labor and reduction of genital tract trauma at birth: a randomized trial. J Midwifery Womens Health. 2005; 50(5):365-72.

20. Dahlen HG, Homer CSE, Cooke M, Upton AM, Nunn R, Brodrick B. Perineal outcomes and maternal comfort related to the application of perineal warm packs in the second stage of labor: a randomized controlled trial. Birth Berkeley Calif. 2007;34(4):282-90.

21. Gülmezoglu AM, Lumbiganon P, Landoulsi S, Widmer M, Abdel-Aleem H, Festin M, et al. Active management of the third stage of labour with and without controlled cord traction: a randomised, controlled, non-inferiority trial. Lancet. 2012;379(9827):1721-7.

22. Hofmeyr GJ, Abdel-Aleem H, Abdel-Aleem MA. Uterine massage for preventing postpartum haemorrhage. Cochrane Database Syst Rev. 2013;(7):CD006431.

23. Chen M, Chang Q, Duan T, He J, Zhang L, Liu X. Uterine massage to reduce blood loss after vaginal delivery: a randomized controlled trial. Obstet Gynecol. 2013;122(2 Pt 1):290-5.

24. Lainez Villabona B, Bergel Ayllon E, Cafferata Thompson ML, Belizán Chiesa JM. [Early or late umbilical cord clamping? A systematic review of the literature]. An Pediatr Barc Spain 2003. 2005;63(1):14-21.

25. Andersson O, Lindquist B, Lindgren M, Stjernqvist K, Domellöf M, Hellström-Westas L. Effect of delayed cord clamping on neurodevelopment at 4 years of age: A randomized clinical trial. JAMA Pediatr. 2015; 169(7):631-8.

26. Rabe H, Jewison A, Fernandez Alvarez R, Crook D, Stilton D, Bradley R, et al. Milking compared with delayed cord clamping to increase placental transfusion in preterm neonates: a randomized controlled trial. Obstet Gynecol. 2011;117(2 Pt 1):205-11.

CHAPTER 7

Analgesia in Labor

Alok Basu Roy, Naveen Gupta

■ INTRODUCTION

The pain of childbirth is the most severe pain; most women will endure in their lifetimes. The delivery of the infant into the arms of a conscious and pain-free mother is one of the most exciting and rewarding moments in medicine. Pain relief in labor has always been surrounded with myths and controversies.

Providing effective and safe analgesia during labor has been a challenge for the anesthesiologist.

■ HISTORY

The modern era of childbirth analgesia began in 1847 when JY Simpson administered ether to a woman in childbirth.

Queen Victoria was given chloroform by John Snow (1853) for the birth of her eighth child Prince Leopold and this did much to popularize the use of pain relief in labor.

■ PHYSIOLOGY OF PAIN

- *1st stage of labor:* Visceral pain
  - Pain is caused by stretching of lower uterine segment and cervix
  - A delta and C fibers carry noxious stimulus
  - Accompanied with sympathetic nerve endings, they enter spinal cord at T10 to L1
  - Poorly localized, primarily in lower abdomen, referred to lumbosacral area, gluteal and thigh region
- *2nd stage of labor:* Somatic pain
  - Distention of the pelvic structures and perineum
  - Sharp, severe and well localized
  - Rapidly conducting A-delta fibers enter spinal cord via pudendal nerve at S2–S4.

Systemic Effects of Labor Pain on Mother and Fetus

- Labor pain and stress cause sympathetic stimulation and increased circulating catecholamines, which increases cardiac output, peripheral resistance, and blood pressure.
- This is of importance in parturients with cardiac disease.
- Delay in gastric emptying
- Hyperventilation associated with labor pain leads to hypocarbia and respiratory alkalosis with shift in the oxyhemogobin curve to left causing increased maternal affinity for oxygen and thereby reducing fetal oxygen supply
- Hyperglycemia and lipolysis with production of fatty acids, ketones and lactate leads to metabolic acidosis
- Decrease uterine contractions and placental perfusion
- This leads to fetal hypoxemia and fetal acidemia.
- Mental disturbance-postpartum depression and post-traumatic stress disorder.

Anatomic Changes of Pregnancy

The anatomic changes of pregnancy are as follows:
- Engorgement of epidural veins due to uterine enlargement and vena cava compression
- Hormonal changes make ligamentum flavum softer and less dense so more chances of dural punctures
- Less dose requirement for spinal anesthesia
- Intercristal line (Tuffiers line) assumes more cephalad relationship to vertebral column
- Apex of lumbar lordosis shifts caudad and reduces thoracic kyphosis during pregnancy

and reduces space between adjacent lumbar spinous process
- Labor pain makes it difficult for women to maintain ideal position during neuraxial anesthesia.

Ideal Obstetric Analgesic

- Attenuates maternal anxiety and fear
- Provides good analgesia
- Is safe for the mother and baby
- Is predictable and constant in its effects
- Is easy to administer
- Should not cause loss of maternal consciousness
- Should not interfere with uterine contractions or progress of labor
- Should not interfere with mobility

▨ TECHNIQUES OF LABOR ANALGESIA

Techniques of labor analgesia are:
- Nonpharmacological
- Pharmacological

Nonpharmacological Methods

Mind-body Interventions

- Psychoprophylactic methods
  - Breathing exercises
  - Deep abdominal breathing
  - Prepared childbirth method
- Biofeedback
- *Aromatherapy:* Improves mood and anxiety levels
- *Energy yoga:* Relaxation, concentration, meditation
- *Physical methods:* Helps to relax tense muscles and soothe and calm the individual
  - Massage, heating pads, warm bath
- *Alternative methods:* Acupuncture, hypnosis
- *Haptonomy:* Science of affectivity
- Music therapy

Transcutaneous Electrical Nerve Stimulation (TENS)

- *Mechanism of action:* Gate theory of pain
- Electrical impulses are applied to skin via electrode.
- Electrodes are applied in both stages of labor
- 1st stage electrodes are placed at T10–T11 on either side of spinous process

- 2nd stage electrodes are placed at S2–S4
- Allows mother to mobilize
- Variable success rate

Water Blocks

- Mechanism similar to TENS
- 0.1 mL saline water injections at four spots over the sacrum
- Intense burning seems to relieve pain

Pharmacological Methods

- Inhalational analgesia
- Systemic analgesia
- Regional analgesia

Inhalational Agents

- *Entonox:* 50% nitrous oxide in oxygen
  - *Nitrous oxide:* Administered via face-mask/mouth piece connected to a breathing circuit with a demand valve
  - Provide analgesia within 20–30 seconds of inhalation
  - Maximum or peak effect within 45 seconds
- *First stage*: Inhale 30 seconds before the onset of contractions
- *Second stage:* 2-3 breaths before each expulsive force
- Disadvantages
  - Increased rate of maternal O_2 desaturation
  - Respiratory depression
  - Drowsiness
  - Environmental pollution

Volatile halogenated agents: The usual range of concentrations of volatile inhalational agents administered with oxygen:
- Desflurane 0.2%
- Enflurane 0.25–1.25%
- Isoflurane 0.2–0.25%
- Sevoflurane 0.8% (Sevox)
- Sevoflurane/Sevox:
  - 0.8% Sevoflurane with oxygen in Oxford Miniature Vaporizer
  - Good analgesia with minimal sedation
  - Pleasant odor, nonirritant to the respiratory tract
  - Useful pain relief during the first stage of labor
  - Greater analgesia than Entonox

- Preferred over Entonox
- More sedation with sevoflurane

Systemic Analgesia

Indications: Regional contraindicated or technically difficult or not available

Systemic opioids:
- Most commonly used class of drugs
- *Primary mechanism of action:* Analgesia and/or heavy sedation.
- Drugs can be given in intermittent doses or via patient-controlled analgesia (PCA)
- Inexpensive
- Significantly higher VAS scores compared with regional anesthesia.
- *Disadvantages*:
  - Dose dependent respiratory depression of mother and neonate
  - Delayed gastric emptying, increased gastric volume, nausea, and vomiting
  - Sedation, dysphoria, euphoria, and amnesia
  - Hypotension

Fentanyl:
- Short T1/2 and no active metabolites
- Can be used as IV bolus or as PCA
- *Usual dose 25–50 μg IV; peak effect:* 3–5 minutes
- *Analgesic effect:* 30–60 minutes
- Suitable for prolonged use in labor
- Minimal neonatal respiratory depression
- Adverse effects
  - Short duration
  - Sedation
  - Transient decrease in fetal heart rate (FHR) variability

Remifentanyl:
- Ideal labor analgesic when used via PCA pump to manage the pain of labor without neonatal depression being major problem.
- Ultra short-acting opioid derivative of fentanyl
- Metabolism is independent of hepatic or renal function
- *T1/2:* 1.3 minutes
- Prolonged administration doesn't cause any accumulation
- Fetal exposure minimal
- *PCA:* 0.25–0.5 μg/ kg; lockout—2 minutes

- *Infusion:* 25 μg bolus; 0.05μg/kg/min infusion; lockout—5 minutes
- Dose-dependent maternal sedation

Regional Analgesia

Regional techniques provide excellent analgesia with minimal depressant effects on mother and fetus.

Techniques:
- Most commonly performed regional techniques for labor are:
  - Epidural analgesia
  - Subarachnoid block
  - Combined spinal-epidural blocks.
- Less frequently performed regional techniques:
  - Lumbar sympathetic block
  - Paracervical block
  - Pudendal block

INDICATIONS FOR NEURAXIAL ANALGESIA

Indications for neuraxial analgesia are as follows:
- Maternal request
- Hypertensive disorders of pregnancy
- Pre-existing medical disease
- Multiple pregnancy
- Previous cesarean section
- Prolonged labor
- Deterioration in fetal wellbeing.

CONTRAINDICATIONS FOR NEURAXIAL ANALGESIA

Contraindications for neuraxial analgesia are as follows:
- Maternal refusal
- Coagulopathy and thrombocytopenia
- Local or systemic infection
- Inadequate staffing or facilities
- Actual or anticipated serious maternal hemorrhage
- Fixed cardiac output disease
- History of allergy to local anesthetics
- Refractory maternal hypotension

DRUGS IN THE EPIDURAL SPACE

Drugs used in the epidural space are described as:
- Local anesthetic drugs

- Racemic bupivacaine
- Levobupivacaine
- Ropivacaine
- Lidocaine
- Opioids
  - Morphine
  - Fentanyl
- Adjuvants
  - Clonidine
  - Adrenaline
  - Neostigmine
  - Ketamine

LUMBAR EPIDURAL ANALGESIA

- Gold standard technique for pain control in obstetrics.
- Provide excellent analgesia with minimal depressant effects in mother and fetus.
- Aims to provide selective sensory block from T10–L1
- Sparing motor blockade.

MAINTENANCE OF EPIDURAL ANALGESIA

- Labor lasts several hours in most parturient
- Single intrathecal or epidural injection of local anesthetic and/or opioid typically does not provide adequate analgesia for the duration of labor.
- Supplemental doses are needed to maintain analgesia in most women **(Table 1)**.
- Single epidural shot
- Intermittent bolus/regular top up:
  - Simple method of delivery

TABLE 1: Maintenance of epidural analgesia.	
Anesthetic solutions for maintenance of epidural analgesia: continuous infusion or patient-controlled epidural analgesia	
Drug	*Concentration*
Local anesthetics	
Bupivacaine	0.05–0.125%
Ropivacaine	0.08–0.2%
Levobupivacaine	0.05–0.125%
Lidocaine	0.5%–1.0%
Opioids	
Fentanyl	1.5-3 µg/mL
Sufentanil	0.2-0.4 µg/mL

- No need for complex infusion device
- Better spread of the local anesthetic in the epidural space with better analgesia
- *Disadvantage*
  - Breakthrough pain
  - Hypotension
  - Risk of high block
  - Local anesthesia toxicity
- *Drug regimen*:
  - Bupivacaine 0.125% with fentanyl 2 mcg/mL, 10 mL injected once in 60-90 minutes
  - Ropivacaine 10 mL of 0.125%–0.2% with fentanyl 2 mcg/mL once in 60-90 minutes
- *Continuous infusion epidural*
  - Advantages:
    - Maintenance of a stable level of analgesia
    - More stable maternal heart rate and blood pressure with decreased risk of hypotension.
    - Less frequent need to give bolus doses of local anesthetic, which may reduce the risk of systemic local anesthetic toxicity
    - Satisfactory perineal analgesia
  - Drug regimen:
    - 0.0625% Bupivacaine 8–15 mL/hours with fentanyl 2 mcg/mL

PATIENT-CONTROLLED EPIDURAL ANALGESIA

- Advantages
  - Effective labor analgesia
  - Excellent patient satisfaction
  - Decreases the total amount of LA used
  - Lessens unwanted effects like hypotension and motor block
  - Reduces the demands on staff
  - Gives many parturients with a feeling of empowerment
- Drug regimen:
  - Initial block:
    - *Bupivaciane:* 0.125% (10–15 mL) with fentanyl 2 mcg/mL of Bupivacaine.
    - *Ropivacaine:* 0.125-0.2% with fentanyl (10–15 mL)
  - *Basal infusion:* 6 mL/hour of Bupivacaine 0.0625% with fentanyl 2 mcg/mL
  - *Demand bolus dose:* 3-5 m:—Bupivacaine 0.062-0.125% with fentanyl 2 mcg/mL

- *Lock out interval:* 10 minutes
- Ropivacaine 0.125% with fentanyl 2 mcg/mL can also be used instead of Bupivacaine in the same dose

TIMING FOR ANALGESIA

- No fetal distress
- Good regular contractions 3–4 minutes apart and lasting about 1 minute.
- Adequate cervical dilatation, i.e., 3–4 cm
- Engagement of the fetal head.

TEST DOSE FOR EPIDURAL LABOR ANALGESIA

- Purpose is to exclude or confirm intravascular or intrathecal placement after initial catheter placement.
- An ideal test dose should be able to detect both accidental intravascular and subarachnoid injections of local anesthetics.
- The choice of drugs for the test dose is controversial.
- A typical test dose is 3 mL of either 1.5% lignocaine with epinephrine 1:200,000 (i.e., lignocaine 45 mg and epinephrine 15 μg) or bupivacaine 7.5–12.5 mg with epinephrine.
- Many anesthesiologists have argued for a "no test dose" technique (considering the concentration of local anesthetic used to maintain labor epidural analgesia has been decreased to 0.0625–0.125%), in which "every dose is a test dose".
- Signs and symptoms of intravascular injection are sought every time a bolus of local anesthetic is administered.

SPINAL ANALGESIA

- Used mainly for very late in labor because it has limited duration of action.
- Faster onset than epidural
- Amount of local anesthetic used is much smaller.
- Opioid alone or low dose local anesthesia + opioid.
- Low-dose combination (fentanyl 25 μg, bupivacaine 2.5 mg, and morphine 250 μg) in one injection provides up to 4 hours of ambulatory pain control

- Continuous spinal analgesia with a "micro-catheter" may be considered in cases of accidental dural puncture.
- Labor is unpredictable and the process of labor is unique to parturients, a second spinal block may be required, when the effect of the first dose wears off.

Continuous Spinal Analgesia (CSA)

- *Indications:*
  - Parturients in whom epidural catheter placement is difficult due to morbid obesity
  - Anatomical deformities
  - *Previous spinal surgery:* Identification and spread of the drug in the epidural space are challenging in such patients. CSA can be helpful
  - *Significant cardiac disease:* Intrathecal opioids alone which usually have negligible hemodynamic effects.
  - Salvage technique after an unintentional dural puncture, while attempting epidural
  - For CSA, pediatric epidural catheters size 24G or 20G epidural catheters may be used
  - Technically more difficult
  - High chances of catheter failures.

Combined Spinal Epidural Analgesia (CSE)

- The CSE technique is widely used in obstetric practice.
- CSE has added advantages of both spinal (rapid onset and dense block) and epidural (prolonged duration of block and postoperative analgesia) blocks
  - Rapid onset analgesia with intense analgesia
  - Early sacral analgesia
  - Additional flexibility epidural
  - Very low failure rate
  - Less need for supplemental boluses
  - Minimal motor block (walking epidural)
  - Reduced total local anesthetic dose with intrathecal administration of opioid.
  - Supplemental analgesia supplied by epidural catheter.

- *IT opioids:* Fentanyl 5–25 µg, sufentanil 5–10 µg
- *Early labor:* Opioid ± 0.125 mg bupivacaine
- *Advanced labor:* opioid ± 2–2.5 mg bupivacaine
- High-maternal satisfaction.
- *Can be placed in lateral or sitting position*

▨ MOST COMMON TECHNIQUE

Needle-through-needle (NTN) in mid lumbar interspinous space, which involves identification of epidural space and insertion of a long fine-bore pencil point spinal needle through the epidural needle until the tip of spinal needle pierces the dura.

- *Indications:*
  - Late labor
  - Parous female with rapid progress of labor
  - Severe pain
  - Second stage fetal distress
  - Unsatisfactory previous epidural

Walking Epidural

Use of opioid only to allow parturients to ambulate during labor because there is little or no interference with motor function.

Criteria for Ambulation during Labor with Neuraxial Analgesia

- Reassuring fetal status
- Engagement of fetal presenting part and no obstetric contraindication
- Ability to perform bilateral straight-leg raises in bed against resistance
- Ability to step up on a step stool with either leg taking the first step, without assistance
- Satisfactory trial of walking accompanied by a nurse
- Patient must be accompanied by a companion at all times
- Intermittent FHR monitoring every 15 minutes.

▨ DURAL PUNCTURE EPIDURAL (DPE) TECHNIQUE

- Technical modification of the CSE in which the dura is perforated with a Whitacre spinal needle (CSE technique), but direct administration of medications into the subarachnoid space is not done
- Intrathecal transfer of injectate from the epidural space via the dural hole, allowing for more rapid onset and symmetrical analgesia

Paracervical Block

- Block transmission through paracervical ganglion, which lies immediately lateral and posterior to the cervicouterine junction.
- Good for first stage of labor not for second stage
- 5–10 mL of local anesthetic injected through a needle introduced into left or right lateral vaginal fornix, near the cervix, at 4 o'clock and 8 o' clock position
- Now rarely used because of its association with a high incidence of fetal asphyxia and poor neonatal outcome.

Pudendal Nerve Block

- Block the pudendal nerve distal to its formation by anterior divisions of S2–S4 but proximal to its division into terminal branches immediately before delivery
- Repeated on both sides
- Provide adequate anesthesia for outlet forceps delivery and episiotomy repair

Lumbar Sympathetic Block

- Analgesia during first stage of labor only
- Analgesia comparable to paracervical block
- Less risk of fetal bradycardia

▨ RECENT ADVANCES

Computer Integrated Patient Controlled Epidural Analgesia (CI-PCEA)

- Patient-controlled epidural analgesia (PCEA) is safe and effective method for maintaining epidural analgesia for the patients in labor
- A novel epidural drug delivery system has been developed
- A laptop computer with a programmed algorithm is connected to a standard epidural pump
- The computer program automatically adjusts the background infusion rate based

on the analysis of patient's local anesthesia requirement in the last 1 hour
- CI-PCEA is associated with lesser incidence of breakthrough pain
- Increased maternal satisfaction.

Programmed Intermittent Epidural Boluses (PIEB)

- PIEB is an automated method of administration that delivers identical volume doses of epidural medication intermittently at scheduled periods of time.
- Provide more extensive spreading of local anesthetic in the epidural space compared to continuous administration.
- Lower anesthetic consumption
- Higher patient satisfaction scores.

Ultrasound-guided Neuraxial Technique

- Ultrasound imaging is becoming an increasingly popular aid for performing neuraxial blockade.
- Helps to identify the midline, localize the epidural space, measure the skin-to-epidural space distance and estimate the angle of needle insertion.
- Useful in obese pregnant women and patients with scoliosis.
- Ultrasonography used as a teaching tool, increases epidural success rate
- Reduces the number of epidural attempts and catheter replacement for failed labor analgesia.

Epidurals that do not Work

- There is a well-recognized failure rate with epidural blockade, even in experienced hands.
- Failure is much higher among obstetric patients than other surgical patients.

Reasons why the Epidural Fails

- The catheter has never been in the epidural space. Possible locations include the subcutaneous tissues, interspinous ligament, and paravertebral space.
- The catheter was once in the epidural space, but has migrated out. This includes transforaminal escape.

- The catheter has gone beyond the epidural space into the subdural space.
- There is inadequate spread of the drug.
- Not enough volume of drug.
- Presence of anatomical barriers within the epidural space.
- Blocked epidural catheter.
- Abnormal spinal anatomy, e.g., scoliosis.

■ COMPLICATIONS (TABLE 2)

- The mainstay of labor analgesia is regional analgesia.
- Major complications related to it are:
    - Inadequate and failed block
    - Hemodynamic instability (hypotension and bradycardia)
    - Respiratory depressions
    - Total spinal anesthesia
    - Intravascular injection of LA
    - Fetal bradycardia

Inadequate Analgesia

Inadequate analgesia has been described in **Table 3**.

Intravascular Injection of LA

- Serious toxicity from labor analgesia follows accidental intravenous injection or by overdose of local anesthetic drug.
- Usually manifests in the CVS and CNS

CVS

- Toxicity includes hypotension, tachycardia, arrhythmias, and cardiac arrest
- Hypotension is the most common effect that needs immediate treatment
- Treatment includes:
    - O$_2$ administration
    - Maternal repositioning
    - Left uterine displacement by wedge application
    - IV boluses of ephedrine (5–10 mg)
    - Rapid fluid boluses

CNS

Toxicity includes dizziness, tinnitus, metallic taste, numbness of tongue and mouth, slurred speech, bizarre behavior, muscle fasciculation and excitation, convulsion, or loss of consciousness.

TABLE 2: Complications of analgesia.

Problems	Treatments	Comments
Pruritus	• Naloxone 40–100 µg IV • Nalbuphine 5–10 mg IV • Diphenhydramine 25 mg IV • Propofol 10 mg IV • Droperidol 0.0625 mg IV • Ondanestron 8 mg IV	10–25% may need some therapy, but few (<5%) have severe pruritus; more problematic with intrathecal morphine; treat early if patient is concerned
Hypotension	IV fluids, maternal positioning (LUD), and vasopressors (ephedrine, phenylephrine). As usual	Occurs in 5–10% of laboring women with intrathecal opioids; probably catecholamine mediated but cause unproven
Respiratory depression	• O$_2$ as needed (ventilation rarely necessary) • Naloxone 40–100 µg or more as indicated when previously opioids administered	Rarely clinically significant but has occurred with sufentanil 10 µg (lower dose [5 µg] may decrease incidence); depression immediately or at 0.5–5]; more common
Nausea and vomiting	• Naloxone 40–100 µg, IV • Metoclopramide 5–10 mg, IV • Droperidol 0.625 mg, IV • Other agents—ondansetron, Dolasetron, propofol (also see Pruritus above)	Often hard to differentiate from obstetric causes; use lowest effective dose of opioid
PDPH	Postpartum management as needed; epidural blood patch highly effective	Headache uncommon (<1%); incidence similar to that with the use of routine epidural technique
Urinary retention	• Catheterization • Naloxone 400–800 µg may be required for treatment	Catheterization (single time) often provides resolution
FHR	• Maintain maternal BP, saturation, LUD • Fluids and ephedrine • Nitroglycerin (50–200 µg IV or 400–800 µg [1–2 puffs] sublingual)	Incidence unclear; mechanism not defined—sudden catecholamine changes and/or increased uterine tone implicated

TABLE 3: Inadequate analgesia.

Total failure	Catheter in wrong place
	Given too late in labor
Partial failure	Unilateral block
	Missed segment
	Inadequate dose/concentration
	Low backache
	Full bladder
	Rectal pain
	Pathological pain—uterine rupture
	Failure to give top-ups

MYTHS AND CONTROVERSIES

- *Increased incidence of cesarean delivery:* Neuraxial analgesia does not increase the risk of cesarean delivery. Initiation of neuraxial analgesia in the latent phase of labor (cervical dilation, 4 cm) does not increase the risk of cesarean delivery.
- *Increased incidence of instrumental vaginal delivery:*
  - Conflicting evidence, not yet assessed as primary outcome in any trial.
  - Outcome is affected by multiple confounding factors (e.g., degree of analgesia during second stage of labor, LA

concentration, method of epidural analgesia maintenance, neuraxial analgesic technique, and obstetric factors).

- *Increased duration of first stage of labor:* Conflicting evidence. Overall evidence from literatures suggests no difference in the duration of the first stage of labor.
- *Increases the duration of second stage of labor:* Effective neuraxial analgesia increases duration of second stage of labor
- *Associated with future back pain:* Epidural analgesia is not associated with increased incidence of back pain after child birth.
- *Associated with maternal pyrexia:*
  - Minimal increase in body temperature after induction
  - Little clinical significance
  - Not associated with neonatal infection
- *Impaired breastfeeding:* Low-dose local anesthetic/low-dose fentanyl epidural labor analgesia regimens do not clinically affect breastfeeding.

BIBLIOGRAPHY

1. Cambic CR, Wong CA. Labor analgesia and obstetric outcome. BJA. 2010;105(S1): i50-6.
2. Chestnut DH, Wong CA, Tsen LC, Ngan Kee WD, Beilin Y, Mhyre J. Chestnut's Obstetric Anesthesia: Principles and Practice, 5th edition. Philadelphia, United States: Elsevier-Saunders; 2014.
3. Collis R, Harries S, Theron A. Oxford Specialist Handbooks in Anaesthesia, Obstetric anaesthesia, 2nd edition. Oxford: Oxford University Press; 2020.
4. Gropper M, Eriksson L, Fleisher L, Wiener-Kronish J, Cohen N, Leslie K. Anesthesia for obstetrics. In: Miller's Anaesthesia, 9th edition. Netherlands: Elsevier; 2019.
5. Pandya ST. Labour analgesia: Recent advances. Indian J Anaesth. 2010;54:400-8.

Cervical Ripening and Induction of Labor

Vanita Suri, Ramandeep Bansal

█ DEFINITION

Induction of labor (IOL) means methods or techniques or active induction of uterine contractions for delivery of fetus before spontaneous onset of labor.[1]

When is IOL Indicated?

World health organization (WHO) recommends IOL for women at gestational age (GA) of 41 weeks. At present, WHO does not recommend IOL at GA of <41 weeks in women having uncomplicated pregnancy.[2]

Induction of labor at GA of <41 weeks is done for medical or obstetric indication provided the likely benefit of shortening the duration of pregnancy exceeds potential harms which may occur if pregnancy is allowed to continue.[2] Some common indications for IOL are given here:[1]

- Post-term pregnancy
- Premature rupture of membranes
- Hypertensive disorders during pregnancy—gestational hypertension, pre-eclampsia, eclampsia, HELLP syndrome
- Fetal death, fetal growth restriction
- Diabetes during pregnancy
- Oligohydramnios, chorioamnionitis
- Abruption placenta
- Intrahepatic cholestasis in pregnancy
- Alloimmunization with fetal anemia
- Twin pregnancy

What are Contraindications for IOL?[1]

- Placenta or vasa previa
- Abnormal fetal lie or presentation (e.g., transverse lie, footling breech or cord presentation)
- Prior classical or inverted T-shaped uterine incision
- Significant prior uterine surgery (Full thickness myomectomy)
- Previous uterine rupture
- Active genital herpes
- Pelvic deformities—cephalopelvic disproportion
- Invasive carcinoma cervix

What is Cervical Ripening (CR) and why is it Necessary?

An important prerequisite for IOL is CR, i.e., softening, effacement, and dilatation of cervix prior to beginning of uterine contractions during labor.

Cervical ripening is done before IOL to reduce time between induction and delivery of baby and enhance chances of vaginal delivery.[3,4]

When is CR done?

Cervical ripening is done if status of cervix is unfavorable before IOL. There is no consensus on definition of unfavorable cervix. We use Bishop's score to assess status of cervix in our institute. If score is <6, then cervix is taken as unfavorable and we proceed to use ripening agent. If score is ≥6, we proceed to IOL without CR.[3,4]

What is Bishop's Scoring System?

Bishop's scoring system is given in **Table 1**.

TABLE 1: Bishop's scoring system.

	Score			
Factor	0	1	2	3
Cervical dilatation (centimeter)	Closed	1–2	3–4	≥5–6
Cervical effacement (percentage)	0–30	40–50	60–70	≥80
Cervical consistency	Firm	Medium	Soft	
Position of cervix	Posterior	Midposition	Anterior	
Station*	–3	–2	–1,0	+1, +2

*Station is defined by position of fetal head in relation to distance from ischial spines. It is graded on a scale and ranges from –3 to +3.
Total score: 13; *Favorable score*: 6–13; *Unfavorable score*: <6

What is the Checklist for CR and IOL?

- Recheck history and redo examination—general physical, systemic, and abdominal
- Estimate gestational age accurately
- Check for any contraindication and review indication of IOL
- Recheck pregnancy specific parameters such as fundal height, presentation, uterine contractions and baseline fetal heart rate, etc.
- Review ultrasonography for location of placenta, fetal weight and presentation, etc.
- Assessment of cervical status using Bishop's score
- Discuss need for and details of procedure, expected outcomes and potential harms with patient and caregivers and obtain a written informed consent
- *All patients needs to be admitted to hospital before IOL (WHO recommendation 2014[5])*

What is Appropriate Agent for CR?

There is no consensus regarding ideal method for CR. The chosen method depends upon patient preference and personal experience. The various methods available for CR include:
- *Mechanical methods:* Use of double balloon/Foley's catheter, hygroscopic dilators[6]
- *Pharmacological methods:* Use of drugs such as prostaglandins and low-dose oxytocin[6]

What are Mechanical Methods for CR?

Currently used double and single balloon (Foley's catheter) **(Boxes 1 and 2)** catheters have similar efficacy and safety profile.[7] We use Foley's catheter as 1st choice for CR as it is cheap, freely available,

BOX 1: Procedure of Foley's catheter (18F) insertion.

- Make sure urinary bladder is empty
- Insert Foley's catheter into cervix under direct supervision with a speculum using all aseptic precautions
- Pass deflated catheter through internal cervical os (ICO)
- Place Foley's bulb in extra-amniotic space just above ICO
- Inflate balloon with normal saline. Use of both small (30 mL) as well as large volume (60 mL) is reasonable. We prefer 30 mL in our institute
- Tap catheter to inner side of thigh with gentle traction and leave it
- Perform fetal nonstress test immediately following balloon placement and frequently thereafter
- If it expels spontaneously, no further action is needed. If membranes rupture spontaneously or catheter does not expel at 12 hours, deflate and remove it

and accessible. These act though local release of prostaglandins and mechanical dilation.

Mechanical methods should not be used in women with rupture of membranes and undiagnosed vaginal bleeding.[6]

What are Pharmacological Methods for CR?

These include prostaglandins and low-dose oxytocin.

Prostaglandins (Table 2)

Prostaglandins (PGs) result in several biochemical and biophysical changes in uterine milieu, which lead to softening of cervical tissue along with increased contractility of uterine myometrium. Two PG preparations, which are used commonly include: Prostaglandin E_2 (PGE$_2$) (Dinoprostone) and Prostaglandin E_1 (PGE$_1$) (Misoprostol).[6]

- *PGE$_2$ (Dinoprostone):* Currently two preparations of PGE$_2$ are available in India for CR. These include:
  1. *Dinoprostone gel (0.5 mg dinoprostone in 3 g gel):* It is placed inside the cervix but not above internal os. If required, it can be reinserted at 6–8 hours intervals, but total dose should not exceed 1.5 mg (three doses) in 24 hours.[6]
  2. Dinoprostone vaginal pessary has 10 mg dinoprostone embedded in a mesh. Entire pessary is placed transversely in posterior fornix of vagina for 24 hours.[6]

Both vaginal pessary and cervical gel are equally effective and result in significantly lower rates of cesarean delivery (CD) rates and increased proportion of vaginal deliveries.[10]

Some more considerations while using dinoprostone are given here:

- Women can be ambulated within 30 minutes of insertion of either preparation
- Careful and strict monitoring of maternal and fetal status with special attention to vitals (pulse rate, blood pressure, vaginal bleeding, etc.) should be done immediately after insertion and then at 4–6 hourly
- If additional dose of gel is necessary, check for uterine contractions and fetal heart before administering next dose
- In women with uterine hyperstimulation and changes in fetal heart rate remove pessary or give vaginal wash for gel preparations. Note that vaginal wash is not of much use and this may be considered a disadvantage of gel use
- Both gel and pessary are not very effective in women with rupture of membranes[11,12]
- *PGE$_1$ (Misoprostol):* It is synthetic prostaglandin used for CR. It is still not approved by Drug Controller General of India, for use in India[9]

BOX 2: Procedure of double balloon catheter insertion (distal and proximal balloons)[8].

- Insert the catheter under full aseptic precautions till proximal (vaginal) balloon is in external cervical os. At this point, distal (uterine) balloon is just above ICO in extra-amniotic space
- Now inflate distal catheter with 40 mL normal saline. Pull it gently and allow it to rest against ICO
- Now inflate proximal balloon with 20 mL saline
- Ensure that both balloons are placed correctly at either end of cervix
- Now inflate each balloon with saline up to 80 mL
- Now remove the speculum
- Perform fetal nonstress test immediately following balloon placement and frequently thereafter
- Tap catheter to inner side of thigh with gentle traction and leave it
- If it expels spontaneously, no further action is needed. If membranes rupture spontaneously or catheter does not expel at 12 hours, deflate and remove it

---

TABLE 2: Comparison of two preparations of dinoprostone.[9]

Parameter	Dinoprostone gel	Dinoprostone vaginal pessary
Storage	In refrigerator at 2–8°C	In freezer at –10 to –25°C
Frequency of administration	Repeated after 6–8 hours if needed (maximum three doses)	Placed only once: releases PGE$_2$ at constant rate of ~0.3 mg/hr for 24 hours
Need for removal	No need	Should be removed after 24 hours or at onset of active labor
Timing of oxytocin infusion	If required oxytocin is given 6–12 hours after last dose	If required oxytocin is given 30 minutes after removal of pessary
Ease of administration	Difficult	Easy
Vaginal delivery within 24 hours of use	Lower than vaginal pessary	Higher that cervical gel

TABLE 3: Rate of infusion of oxytocin.

Units of oxytocin added to 500 mL of Ringer lactate	Oxytocin infusion in drops per minute and equivalent dose in mU (milli-units) per minute (one mL = 16 drops)							
	Number of drops (mU)/ minute							
1 unit	8 (1 mU)	16 (2 mU)	24 (3 mU)	32 (4 mU)	40 (5 mU)	48 (6 mU)	56 (7 mU)	64 (8 mU)
2 units	8 (2 mU)	16 (4 mU)	24 (6 mU)	32 (8 mU)	40 (10 mU)	48 (12 mU)	56 (14 mU)	64 (16 mU)

It is however recommended as CR agent by WHO both as an oral preparation in dose of 25 µg every 2 hourly and as low dose vaginal preparation in dose of 25 µg every 6 hourly) for IOL. This low-dose regimen recommended by WHO is associated with reasonable efficacy and safety profile and results in lower rates of uterine hyperstimulation and CD.[13,14]

Recent trials have used buccal preparation also for CR. However, vaginal route is better in terms of reduction in time to vaginal delivery.[15] Common adverse effects of PG use include fever, chills, vomiting, and diarrhea. Another important side effect includes uterine hyperstimulation which may cause fetal distress. Tocolytic drugs such as terbutaline can be used in dose of 250 ug as subcutaneous injection, if in utero resuscitation is needed.

Low Dose Oxytocin

Oxytocin is used for CR only if PGs are not available or contraindicated. It is used in a starting dose of 1–2 mU/min infusion, which is increased by 1–4 mU/min at every 30 minutes interval.[9]

Other Methods

Several authors have used alternative methods for CR such as mifepristone, nitric oxide donors, relaxin, hyaluronidase, or breast stimulation, etc. However, these are not recommended for use at present due to insufficient data.

How to Perform IOL?

Induction of labor: Most common method for IOL is administration of oxytocin in form of Intravenous (IV) infusion.

How to make Oxytocin Infusion?

- Oxytocin is administered as dilute solution.
- Isotonic solutions [Ringer lactate (RL) or normal saline (NS)] are preferred over dextrose solutions for preparation of infusion. This prevents electrolyte imbalance like hyponatremia and volume overload
- Oxytocin is available as 1 mL ampoule, which has 5 units
- 1st dilute 2 ampoules (2 mL—10 units) of oxytocin with 8 mL of normal saline in 10 mL syringe
- Now syringe has 10 mL of normal saline having 10 units of oxytocin or in other words, 1 mL of this saline solution has 1 unit of oxytocin
- Add 1 mL of above solution to 500 mL of normal saline to get 1 unit solution or add 2 mL of above solution to 500 m of NS to get 2 unit solution (1 unit and 2 unit solution has 1 and 2 units or 1000 milli-units and 2000 milli-units of oxytocin in 500 mL of NS, respectively)
- Rate of infusion is given in **Table 3**.

How to Administer Oxytocin?[9]

Our protocol: We add 30 units (6 ampoules) to 500 mL of RL. So we have 30 units of oxytocin in 500 mL RL = 30,000 mU in 500 mL RL = 60 mU in 1 mL RL.

Rate of infusion used: 1 mL/hr = 1 mU in 60 minutes = 1 mU/ minute.

We use infusion pump to provide continuous and precise flow rate of 1 mL per hour.

WHO does not recommend enema prior to IOL.[2]

- Several randomized controlled trails/meta-analyses have compared combination techniques (e.g., Misoprostol + Foley's catheter insertion; Foley's catheter insertion + oxytocin, etc.) with Foley's catheter or prostaglandins alone[16]
- WHO recommends balloon catheter + oxytocin as an alternative method for IOL when PGs are not available or contraindicated. Its use is associated with lower risk of uterine hyperstimulation. It reduces rate of CD when compared to oxytocin alone[13]

TABLE 4: Oxytocin infusion regimens.

Regimen	Starting dose (mU/ min)	Increase (mU/min) (increment)	Time interval (minutes)
Low dose	0.5–1	1	30–40
Alternate low dose	1–2	1–2	15–30
High dose	6	6 Reduced to 3 if uterine hyper-stimulation present and reduced to 1 if hyperstimulation is recurrent	15–40
Alternate high dose	4	4	15

In high-dose regimen, some obstetricians do not administer cumulative dose of >10 units and limit duration of infusion to ≤6 hours.
Most obstetricians do not recommend >40 mU/min infusion.[1]
Rates of maternal and fetal complications are similar with both low- and high-dose regimens. High-dose regimens reduce induction to delivery interval but at expense of high rate of tachysystole than low-dose protocols.[1]

What are Different Oxytocin Infusion Regimens?

Different oxytocin infusion regimens are described in **Table 4**.

Rate of oxytocin infusion is increased until labor progress is normal or uterine activity reaches at least 200–250 Montevideo units (i.e., good regular uterine contractions: at least three contractions in 10 minutes, each lasting for 40–45 seconds duration).

During oxytocin infusion, continuously monitor uterine contractions and well as maternal and fetal well being including fetal heart rate by cardiotocography.

There is no general consensus about whether to continue or discontinue oxytocin in active labor. In our institute, we continue to give oxytocin till delivery.[17]

What are Side Effects of Oxytocin and their Management?

Major side effects of oxytocin include:
- Oxytocin shares structural homology with vaso-pressin (antidiuretic hormone). Thus its use may result in water retention (intoxication) and electrolyte imbalance, i.e., hyponatremia. Hypo-natremia is rare and is seen when high dose are given (50 mU/min) for prolonged period (≥7 hour) or when oxytocin is administered in large quantities (>3 L) of hypotonic solutions such as 5% dextrose. Management includes stopping oxytocin, and restricting water intake. If symptomatic consider administration of hypertonic saline[18]
- Tachysystole (>5 contractions in 10 minutes averaged over 30 minutes) is seen in <5% of women. It occurs either with high dose oxytocin or when oxytocin is used in conjunction with PGs.

Management includes reducing dose or stopping oxytocin altogether. Severe tachysystole may result in fetal hypoxia and rarely uterine rupture. If uterine resuscitation is attempted, consider administration of tocolytics such as terbutaline
- Hypotension
- Amniotic fluid embolism (rare—1/10,000 live births)

What is the Role of Amniotomy in IOL?

In women with favorable cervix, amniotomy may be used for IOL, especially if head is opposed to cervix. However, when compared to amniotomy alone, combination of oxytocin infusion and amniotomy is more efficacious.[19]

What is Membrane Stripping/ Sweeping?

- It is used in outpatient setting to fasten onset of spontaneous labor in women with partially dilated cervical canal
- Here clinician inserts his/her finger beyond ICO to reach lower uterine segment. Then he rotates it circumferentially so that fetal membranes are detached from decidua
- It enhances rate of spontaneous labor without any effect of maternal and fetal outcomes[20]

Points to Ponder
- There has to be a strong indication for IOL
- IOL for maternal request alone has to be discouraged
- Preinduction counseling of couple is important
- Patient should be informed about need for and method of IOL and written informed consent should be obtained
- Continuous fetal monitoring is mandatory during IOL
- Proper analgesia should be provided to patient during IOL. Keep in mind that induced labor is prolonged and more painful than natural labor
- The discharge slip shall have details of IOL for guidance in next pregnancy

REFERENCES

1. ACOG Committee on Practice Bulletins—Obstetrics. ACOG Practice Bulletin No 107: Induction of Labour. Obstet Gynecol. 2009;114: 386.
2. WHO. WHO recommendations: Induction of labour at or beyond term. Geneva: World Health Organization; 2018.
3. Bernardes TP, Broekhuijsen K, Koopmans CM, Boers KE, van Wyk L, Tajik P, et al. Caesarean section rates and adverse neonatal outcomes after induction of labour versus expectant management in women with an unripe cervix: a secondary analysis of the HYPITAT and DIGITAT trials. BJOG. 2016;123:1501.
4. Tajik P, van der Tuuk K, Koopmans CM, Groen H, van Pampus MG, van der Berg PP, et al. Should cervical favourability play a role in the decision for labour induction in gestational hypertension or mild pre-eclampsia at term? An exploratory analysis of the HYPITAT trial. BJOG. 2012;119:1123.
5. WHO. WHO Recommendations for Augmentation of Labour. Geneva: World Health Organization; 2014.
6. Grobman W (2021). Induction of labour: techniques for preinduction cervical ripening. [online]. Available from: https://www.uptodate.com/contents/induction-of-labor-techniques-for-preinduction-cervical-ripening. [Last accessed on December 23, 2021].
7. Yang F, Huang S, Long Y, Huang L. Double-balloon versus single-balloon catheter for cervical ripening and labor induction: a systematic review and meta-analysis. J Obstet Gynaecol Res. 2018;44:2.
8. NICE (2015). National Institute for health care and excellence guidelines: Insertion of a double balloon catheter for induction of labour in pregnant women without previous caesarean section Interventional procedures guidance. [online] Available from: nice.org.uk/guidance/ipg528. [Last accessed on December 23, 2021]
9. Good clinical practice recommendations FOGSI-ICOG (2018). Induction of labour (Good clinical practice recommendations) [online]. Available from: https://www.fogsi.org/wp-content/uploads/2018/09/XGCPR-IOL-26July.pdf. [Last accessed on December 23, 2021].
10. Kelly AJ, Malik S, Smith L, Kavanagh J, Thomas J. Vaginal prostaglandin (PGE2 and PGF2a) for induction of labour at term. Cochrane Database Syst Rev. 2009;(4):CD003101.
11. Smith CV, Rayburn WF, Miller AM. Intravaginal prostaglandin E2 for cervical ripening and initiation of labor. Comparison of a multidose gel and single, controlled-release pessary. J Reprod Med. 1994;39:381.
12. Witter FR, Rocco LE, Johnson TR. A randomized trial of prostaglandin E2 in a controlled-release vaginal pessary for cervical ripening at term. Am J Obstet Gynecol. 1992;166:830.
13. WHO. WHO Recommendations for Induction of Labour. Geneva, World Health Organization; 2011.
14. Kerr RS, Kumar N, Williams MJ, Cuthbert A, Aflaifel N, Haas DM, et al. Low-dose oral misoprostol for induction of labour. Cochrane Database Syst Rev. 2021;6:CD014484.
15. Haas DM, Daggy J, Flannery KM, Dorr ML, Bonsack C, Bhamidipalli SS, et al. A comparison of vaginal versus buccal misoprostol for cervical ripening in women for labor induction at term (the IMPROVE trial): a triple-masked randomized controlled trial. Am J Obstet Gynecol. 2019;221:259.e1.
16. Levine LD, Downes KL, Elovitz MA, Parry S, Sammel MD, Srinivas SK. Mechanical and pharmacologic methods of labor induction: a randomized controlled trial. Obstet Gynecol. 2016;128:1357.
17. Boie S, Glavind J, Velu AV, Mol BWJ, Uldbjerg N, de Graaf I, et al. Discontinuation of intravenous oxytocin in the active phase of induced labour. Cochrane Database Syst Rev. 2018;8:CD012274.
18. Bergum D, Lonnée H, Hakli TF. Oxytocin infusion: acute hyponatremia, seizures and coma. Acta Anaesthesiol Scand. 2009;53:826.
19. Howarth GR, Botha DJ. Amniotomy plus intravenous oxytocin for induction of labour. Cochrane Database Syst Rev. 2001:CD003250
20. Finucane EM, Murphy DJ, Biesty LM, Gyte GM, Cotter AM, Ryan EM, et al. Membrane sweeping for induction of labour. Cochrane Database Syst Rev. 2020;2:CD000451.

Intrapartum Fetal Monitoring

Ruchika Garg, Pavika Lal

INTRODUCTION

One of the greatest challenging tasks faced by an obstetrician regularly is the responsibility of delivering a vigorous and neurological intact fetus. The importance of intrapartum fetal monitoring has been emphasized since ages as uterine contractions adversely affect the fetus, especially if it is already compromised due to utero placental insufficiency, cord compression associated with oligohydramnios and iatrogenic hyperstimulation. Even an apparently normal fetus in antenatal period may develop distress during labor.

OBJECTIVES OF INTRAPARTUM FHR MONITORING[1]

- Identification of fetal heart rate (FHR) changes potentially associated with inadequate fetal oxygenation may enable timely intervention to reduce the likelihood of hypoxic injury or death.
- Accurate identification of appropriately oxygenated fetuses may prevent unnecessary intervention.

The procedure for intrapartum FHR monitoring, physiology behind FHR accelerations and decelerations, classification of FHR tracings, and use of ancillary tests to evaluate the fetus will be described here.

WHY INTRAPARTUM FETAL MONITORING IS NECESSARY?

Intrapartum fetal monitoring was developed in 1960s to identify the events that might result in hypoxic-ischemic encephalopathy (HIE), cerebral palsy or fetal death, and it became an integral part of routine maternity care in 1970s.[2] *The FHR pattern is an indirect marker of fetal cardiac and* central nervous system responses to changes in blood pressure, blood gases, and acid-base status.

Poor fetal oxygenation can be demonstrated by documentation of metabolic acidosis in the umbilical cord immediately after birth or in the newborn circulation during the first minutes of life, although very few develop short- or long-term complications. *HIE is the short-term neurological dysfunction caused by inadequate intrapartum fetal oxygenation, and cerebral palsy of the spastic quadriplegic or dyskinetic types is the long-term neurological complication most commonly associated with it.[3]*

Although there is insufficient evidence from randomized controlled trials to demonstrate that any form of intrapartum fetal monitoring reduces the incidence of adverse outcomes, reports from the clinical setting have documented a decrease in metabolic acidosis, HIE and intrapartum death over the last decades, *thereby all obstetric societies recommend monitoring of FHR during labor.[3]*

CONTINUOUS VERSUS INTERMITTENT INTRAPARTUM FHR MONITORING (TABLE 1)

For both low- and high-risk pregnancies, *continuous electronic FHR monitoring is not superior to intermittent auscultation* with respect to preventing death or poor long-term neurologic outcome and has a high false-positive rate.[4-6]

A 2017 meta-analysis that compared continuous electronic FHR monitoring with intermittent auscultation (13 randomized trials, >37,000 low- and high-risk pregnancies) reported the following major findings.[5] No statistically significant differences between techniques were noted for the following newborn/childhood outcomes:

TABLE 1: Surveillance during low- and high-risk pregnancies.		
Surveillance	*Low-risk pregnancies*	*High-risk pregnancies*
Evaluation intervals	Evaluation intervals	Evaluation intervals
First stage labor (active)	30 minutes	15 minutes
Second stage labor	15 minutes	5 minutes

- Acidemia (measured in cord blood) [relative risk (RR) 0.92, 95% CI 0.27–3.11]
- Apgar score <4 at five minutes (RR 1.80, 95% CI 0.71–4.59)
- Neonatal intensive care unit admission (RR 1.01, 95% CI 0.86–1.18)
- Hypoxic-ischemic encephalopathy (RR 0.46, 95% CI 0.04–5.03)
- Perinatal mortality (RR 0.86, 95% CI 0.59–1.24)
- Neurodevelopmental impairment at ≥12 months of age (RR 3.88, 95% CI 0.83–18.2)

GUIDELINES FOR METHODS OF INTRAPARTUM FHR MONITORING

- ACOG:[7]
  - Either continuous electronic FHR monitoring or intermittent auscultation—acceptable in uncomplicated patients.
  - High-risk pregnancies (preeclampsia, suspected growth restriction, type 1 diabetes mellitus) should be monitored continuously during labor.
- National Institute for Health and Care Excellence:[8]
  - In all birth settings, offer intermittent auscultation to low-risk women in the first stage of labor.
  - Advise continuous cardiotocography, if any of the following risk factors occur during labor:
    - Suspected chorioamnionitis, sepsis, or temperature ≥38°C
    - Severe hypertension (≥160/110 mm Hg)
    - Oxytocin use
    - Significant meconium
    - Fresh vaginal bleeding

If continuous cardiotocography was used because of concerns arising from intermittent auscultation but the tracing is normal after 20 minutes of observation, remove the cardiotocograph and return to intermittent auscultation.

METHODS OF FHR MONITORING AND THEIR INDICATIONS

Structured Intermittent Auscultation (SIA)

It employs the systematic use of a Doppler assessment of FHR during labor at defined timed intervals and is equivalent to continuous EFM in screening for fetal compromise in low-risk patients.[4]

Safety in using structured intermittent auscultation is based on a nurse-to-patient ratio of 1:1 and an established technique for intermittent auscultation for each institution.

Frequency: Every 15–30 minutes of active phase of first stage of labor, every 5 minutes in second stage of labor with pushing (**Table 2**).

Continuous Electronic Fetal Monitoring

Continuous EFM should be used when there are abnormalities in structured intermittent auscultation or for high-risk patients.

ANTENATAL

Maternal and fetal high-risk factors that indicate use of continuous electronic fetal monitoring (**Table 3**).

Tracing Acquisition

Maternal Position

Lateral recumbent, half-sitting is the preferred position for prolonged monitoring rather than supine recumbent position as it results in aorto-caval compression by the pregnant uterus, affecting placental perfusion and fetal oxygenation.[9]

Paper Scales for CTG

- The horizontal and vertical scals available for CTG registration are usually 1, 2, or 3 cm/min and 20 or 30 bpm/cm, respectively, and is commonly called "paper speed".

TABLE 2: Frequency, indications, and procedure of SIA.

Indications of SIA	Procedure of SIA
Assess FHR before: Initiation of labor enhancing procedure, ambulation of patient, administration of medication, or initiation of analgesia or anesthesia *Assess FHR after:* Admission of patient, artificial or spontaneous rupture of membranes, vaginal examination, abnormal uterine activity, or evaluation of analgesia or anesthesia	• Palpate the abdomen to determine the position of the fetus (Leopoid maneuvers) • Place the Doppler over the area of maximum intensity of fetal heart tones • Differentiate maternal pulse from fetal pulse • Palpate for uterine contraction during period of FHR auscultation to determine relationship • Count FHR between contractions for ≥60 seconds to determine average baseline rate • Count FHR after uterine contraction for ≥60 seconds (at 5 second intervals) to identify fetal response to active labor (this may be subject to local protocols)

TABLE 3: Maternal and fetal high risk factors that indicate use of continuous electronic fetal monitoring.

Fetal risk factors	Maternal risk factors
• Abnormal fetal heart rate on auscultation or admission • Tracing (20-minute strip) • Meconium-stained amniotic fluid	• Hypertonic uterus • Induced or augmented labor • Intrauterine infection or chorioamnionitis • Post-term pregnancy (>42 weeks gestation) • Preterm labor (<32 weeks gestation) • Previous cesarean delivery • Prolonged membrane rupture >24 hours at-term • Regional analgesia, particularly after initial bolus and after top-ups (continuous electronic fetal monitoring is not required with mobile or continuous-infusion epidurals) • Vaginal bleeding in labor
• Abnormal umbilical artery Doppler velocimetry • Breech presentation • Intrauterine growth restriction • Multiple pregnancies • Oligohydramnios • Rh-immunization	• Anemia • Antepartum hemorrhage • Cardiac diseases • Diabetes • Hypertension (pre-eclampsia or eclampsia)

- Some experts feel that 1 cm/min provide records of sufficient detail for clinical analysis, and has the advantage of reducing tracing length but the small details are better evaluated using higher paper speeds.
- It is very important that the healthcare professionals should be familiar with paper speed because tracing interpretation depends on pattern recognition, which appears very different with the use of different paper scales.

EXTERNAL VERSUS INTERNAL FHR MONITORING

External FHR monitoring uses a Doppler ultrasound transducer to detect the movement of cardiac structures. The resulting signal requires modulation and autocorrelation which results in an approximation of the true heart rate intervals, which is considered to be sufficiently accurate for analysis.[10]

External FHR monitoring is more prone to signal loss, to inadvertent monitoring of the maternal heart rate (MHR) and to signal artefacts especially during the second stage of labor.[11] It may also not record fetal cardiac arrhythmias accurately.

Internal FHR monitoring uses a fetal scalp electrode (can also be applied to the breech) evaluates the time intervals between successive heart beats by identifying R waves on the fetal electrocardiogram QRS complex, and therefore measures ventricular depolarization cycles.

Essential prerequisites are:
- It requires a disposable electrode.
- Fetal electrode should be only applied after a clear identification of the presenting part and that delicate fetal structures such as sutures and fontanels should be avoided.
- Requires ruptured membranes.

Disadvantages of internal FHR monitoring:
- More expensive
- Has limitations due to contraindications:
  - Mainly related to the increased risk of vertical transmission of infections (patients with active genital herpes infection, those who are seropositive to hepatitis B, C, D, E, or to human immunodeficiency virus)[12,13]
- In suspected fetal blood disorders
  - When there is uncertainty about the presenting part, or when artificial rupture of membranes is inappropriate (i.e., an unengaged presentation).
  - Fetal electrode placement should also preferably be avoided in very preterm fetuses (under 32 weeks gestation).

External FHR monitoring is the recommended initial method for routine intrapartum monitoring, provided that a recording of acceptable quality is obtained, i.e., that the basic CTG features are identifiable. If an acceptable record cannot be obtained with external monitoring, then internal monitoring should be used in absence its contraindications.

Minimum requirements for using external FHR monitoring are:
- Careful repositioning of the probe is carried out during the second stage of labor.
- During atypical FHR tracings, MHR monitoring should be carried out.

EXTERNAL VERSUS INTERNAL MONITORING UTERINE CONTRACTIONS

External Monitoring of Uterine Contractions

- It uses a tocodynamometer evaluates increased myometrial tension measured through the abdominal wall.
- Incorrect placement, reduced tension applied to the supporting elastic band, or abdominal adiposity may result in inadequate registration of contractions.
- It only provides accurate information on the frequency of contractions and not possible to extract reliable information regarding the intensity and duration of contractions, nor on basal uterine tone.

Internal Monitoring of Uterine Contractions

- It uses an intrauterine catheter provides quantitative information on the intensity and duration of contractions, as well as on basal uterine tone.
- It is more expensive as the catheter is disposable, and requires ruptured membranes.
- Contraindications include uterine hemorrhage of unknown cause and placenta previa.
- It may also be associated with a small risk of fetal injury, placental hemorrhage, uterine perforation, and infection.[14]
- The use of intrauterine pressure catheters has not been shown to be associated with improved outcomes in induced and augmented labor, and so it is not recommended for routine clinical use.[15]

Terminologies used for Uterine Contractions

- Normal uterine activity—≤5 contractions in 10 minutes over a 30 minute window.
- Tachysystole more than 5 contractions in 10 minutes, averaged over 30 minutes.
- The term uterine hyperstimulation has been abandoned.

SIMULTANEOUS MONITORING OF THE MATERNAL HEART RATE

Useful in specific maternal health conditions and where it is difficult to distinguish between maternal and FHR (e.g., fetal heart block).[11] Some CTG monitors provide the possibility of continuous MHR monitoring, either by electrocardiography or pulse oximetry. In some models, it has been incorporated in the tocodynamometer, and therefore does not cause discomfort to the mother.

Simultaneous MHR monitoring should be considered when performing continuous CTG, especially during the second stage of labor, when tracings show accelerations coinciding with contractions and expulsive efforts,[11] or when the MHR is elevated.

STORAGE OF TRACINGS

In all CTG tracings patient name, place of recording, "paper speed", date and time when acquisition started and ended should be entered properly as a part of the patient record and preserved for future references, review, and audit by clinical staff and medicolegal purpose.

ANALYSIS OF TRACINGS

CTG analysis includes basic CTG features *baseline variability, accelerations, decelerations, and uterine contractions followed by CTG classification* and needs to be integrated with other clinical information for a comprehensive interpretation and adequate management.

As a general rule, if the fetus continues to maintain a stable baseline and a reassuring variability, the risk of hypoxia to the central organs is very unlikely.

The Advanced Life Support in Obstetrics (ALSO) curriculum developed the mnemonic *DR C BRAVADO* to teach a systematic, structured approach to continuous EFM interpretation that incorporates the NICHD definitions **(Table 4)**.

BASELINE

- All the three bodies (FIGO, NICE, ACOG) have similar consensus on baseline FHR **(Table 5)**.
- Defined as mean FHR rounded to increments of 5 bpm during a 10-minute segment, excluding: periodic or episodic changes, periods of marked FHR variability, segments of baseline that differ >25 bpm.
- In tracings with unstable FHR signals, review of previous segments and/or evaluation of longer time periods may be necessary to estimate the baseline,[18] in particular during the 2nd stage of labor and to identify the fetal behavioral state of active wakefulness that can lead to an erroneously high baseline estimation.
- Preterm fetuses tend to have values towards the upper end of this range and post-term fetuses toward the lower end.

CAUSES OF FETAL TACHYCARDIA

- Maternal pyrexia (most common cause)[19]
- Epidural analgesia[19]

TABLE 4: DR C BRAVADO mnemonic for interpretation of continuous electronic fetal monitoring.[16,17]

DR: Determine risk	High, medium, or low risk (i.e., risk in terms of the clinical situation)
C: Contractions	Rate, rhythm, frequency, duration, intensity, and resting tone
BRA: Baseline rate	Bradycardia (<110 bpm), normal (110–160 bpm), or tachycardia (>160 bpm); rising baseline
V: Variability	Reflects central nervous system activity: Absent, minimal, moderate, or marked
A: Accelerations	Spontaneous; stimulated; none Rises from the baseline of ≥15 bpm, lasting ≥15 seconds *Preterm:* ≥10 bpm, lasting ≥10 seconds
D: Decelerations	Absent, early, variable, late, or prolonged
O: Overall assessment and written plan	Stoplight algorithm

TABLE 5: Comparison of normal baseline, fetal bradycardia, and tachycardia by FIGO, NICE, and ACOG.

	FIGO	NICE	ACOG
Normal baseline	110–150 bpm	110–160 bpm	110–160 bpm
Tachycardia	No definition	>180 bpm (161–180 is moderate tachycardia)*	>160 bpm*
Bradycardia	<80 bpm	<100 bpm (100–109 bpm is moderate bradycardia)*	<110 bpm*

*Lasting for >10 minutes

TABLE 6: Comparison of normal, reduced, and increased variability by FIGO, NICE, and ACOG.

	FIGO	NICE	ACOG
Normal variability	Between 5 and 25 bpm	≥5 bpm between contractions	Amplitude range 6–25 bpm (moderate variability)
Reduced variability	<5 bpm for >50 min[23] (suspicious if variability 5–10 bpm for >40 min) Or decreased variability >3 min during deceleration[24]	<5 bpm for 40–90 min (nonreassuring) or >90 min (abnormal variability)	Amplitude range ≤5 bpm (minimal variability)
Increased variability	>25 bpm* (saltatory pattern)	—	Amplitude range >25 bpm (marked variability)*

*Lasting for >30 minutes.

- *Drugs:*[20]
  - Beta-agonist drugs (salbutamol, terbutaline, ritodrine, fenoterol)
  - Parasympathetic blockers (atropine, escopolamine)
- Fetal arrhythmias supraventricular tachycardia and atrial flutter.

CAUSES OF FETAL BRADYCARDIA

- Maternal hypothermia[21]
- Administration of beta-blockers[22]
- Fetal arrhythmias, e.g., atrial-ventricular block

VARIABILITY

- All the three bodies have similar consensus on variability of FHR **(Table 6)**
- Defined as minor fluctuation in baseline FHR occurring at three to five cycles per minute.
- Measured by estimating the difference in bpm between the highest peak and lowest trough of fluctuation in a 1-min segment of the trace.

Points to be Considered in Interpretation of Reduced Variability

- Careful re-evaluation is recommended in borderline situations due to high degree of subjectivity in the visual evaluation of this parameter.
- Reduced variability due to hypoxia is a rare occurrence without preceding or concomitant decelerations and a rise in the baseline following an initially normal CTG **(Fig. 1)**.
- During deep sleep, variability is usually in the lower range of normality, but the bandwidth amplitude is seldom under 5 bpm.

Causes of Reduced Variability[25]

- Central nervous system hypoxia/acidosis and resulting in decreased sympathetic and parasympathetic activity
- Previous cerebral injury
- Infection
- Administration of central nervous system depressants, parasympathetic blockers

Increased Variability (Saltatory Pattern)
Usually linked with recurrent decelerations, when hypoxia/acidosis evolves very rapidly due to fetal autonomic instability/hyperactive autonomic system **(Fig. 2)**.[26]

ACCELERATIONS

Comparison of accelerations by FIGO, NICE, and ACOG has been described in **(Table 7)**.

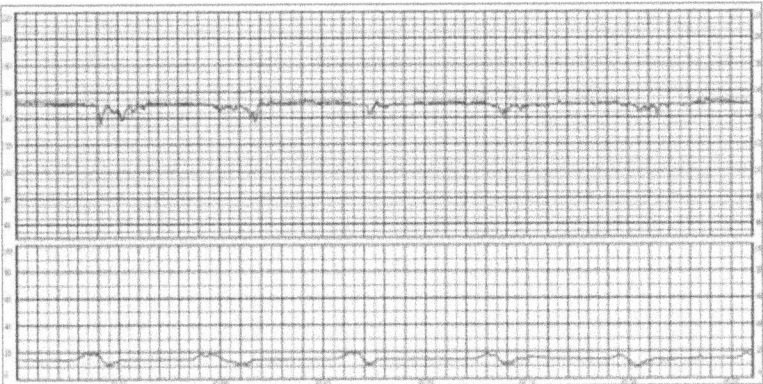

Fig. 1: Reduced beat-to-beat variability.

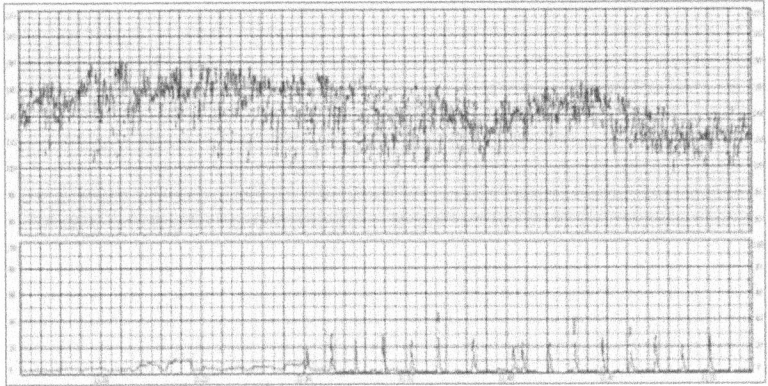

Fig. 2: Increased variability or saltatory pattern.

TABLE 7: Comparison of accelerations by FIGO, NICE, and ACOG.		
FIGO	**NICE**	**ACOG**
FIGO transient increase in heart rate of ≥15 bpm and lasting ≥15 seconds	Transient increases in FHR of ≥15 bpm and lasting ≥15 seconds	• ACOG A visually apparent abrupt increase (onset to peak in <30 seconds) in the FHR. Beyond 32 weeks of gestation, an acceleration has a peak of ≥15 bpm above the baseline, with a duration of ≥15 sec but <2 minutes from onset to return. • Prolonged accelerations last ≥2 min but <10 minutes

- Most accelerations coincide with fetal movements and are a sign of a neurologically responsive fetus that does not have hypoxia/acidosis.
- Before 32 weeks' gestation, their amplitude and frequency may be lower (10 seconds and 10 bpm of amplitude).
- After 32–34 weeks, with the establishment of fetal behavioral states, accelerations rarely occur during periods of deep sleep, which can last up to 50 minutes.[23]
- The absence of accelerations in an otherwise normal intrapartum CTG is of less significance, as it is unlikely to indicate hypoxia/acidosis.
- Accelerations coinciding with uterine contractions, especially in the second stage of labor, suggest possible erroneous recording of the

TABLE 8: Comparison of subtypes of decelerations by NICE and ACOG.

	NICE	ACOG
Early deceleration	Uniform, repetitive, periodic slowing of FHR with onset early in the contraction and return to baseline at the end of the contraction	• Visually apparent usually symmetrical gradual decrease and return of the FHR associated with a uterine contraction • A gradual decrease is defined as from the onset to the FHR nadir of ≥30 seconds. The decrease in FHR is calculated from the onset to the nadir of the deceleration. The nadir of the deceleration occurs at the same time as the peak of the contraction. In most cases, the onset, nadir, and recovery of the deceleration are coincident with the beginning, peak, and ending of the contraction, respectively
Late deceleration	Uniform, repetitive, periodic slowing of FHR with onset mid to end of the contraction and nadir >20 seconds after the peak of the contraction and ends after the contraction has subsided In the presence of a nonaccelerative trace with baseline variability <5 bpm, the definition would include decelerations 10–15 bpm	• Visually apparent usually symmetrical gradual decrease and return of the FHR associated with a uterine contraction • A gradual decrease is defined as from the onset to the FHR nadir of ≥30 seconds. The decrease in FHR is calculated from the onset to the nadir of the deceleration. The deceleration is delayed in timing, with the nadir of the deceleration occurring after the peak of the contraction • In most cases, the onset, nadir, and recovery of the deceleration occur after the beginning, peak, and ending of the contraction, respectively
Variable deceleration	Variable, intermittent periodic slowing of FHR with rapid recovery to baseline (onset to recovery in < 30 sec), good variability within the deceleration, varying size, shape and relationship to uterine contractions	Visually apparent abrupt decrease in FHR. An abrupt decrease is defined as from the onset of the deceleration to the beginning of the FHR nadir of < 30 seconds. The decrease in FHR is calculated from the onset to the nadir of the deceleration. The decrease in FHR is ≥15 bpm, lasting ≥15 seconds, and <2 min in duration. When variable decelerations are associated with uterine contractions, their onset, depth, and duration commonly vary with successive uterine contractions
Prolonged deceleration	An abrupt decrease in FHR to levels below the baseline that lasts at least 60–90 seconds. These decelerations become pathological, if they cross two contractions (i.e., >3 min)	Visually apparent decrease in the FHR below the baseline. Decrease in FHR from the baseline that is ≥15 bpm, lasting ≥2 min but <10 min in duration. If a deceleration lasts ≥10 min, it is a baseline change

maternal heart rate, as FHR more frequently decelerates with a contraction, while the maternal heart rate typically increases.[11]

≥10 seconds or more. FIGO does not subcategorize deceleration into various subtypes whereas NICE and ACOG does **(Table 8)**.

DECELERATIONS

FIGO: Transient episodes of slowing of FHR below the baseline level of >15 bpm and lasting

Early Decelerations

They are caused by fetal head compression[27] and do not indicate fetal hypoxia/acidosis **(Fig. 3)**.

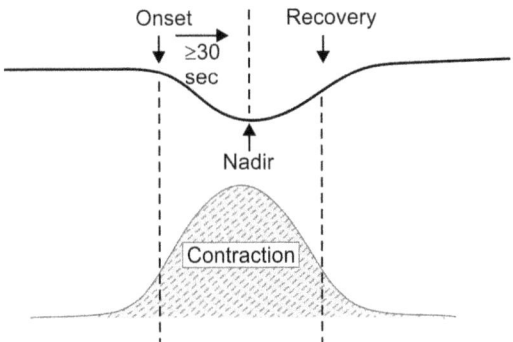

Fig. 3: Features of early deceleration.

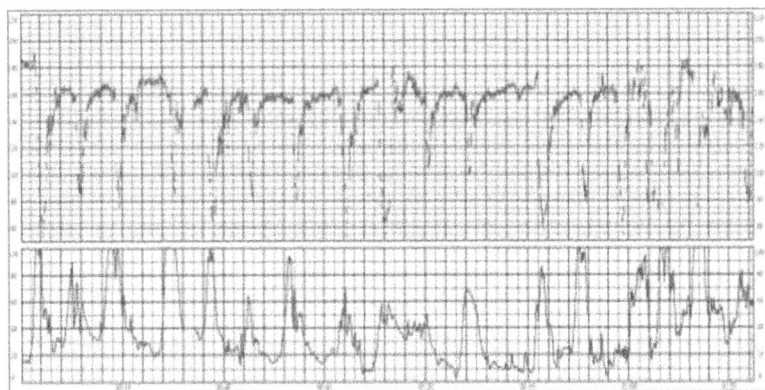

Fig. 4: Variable decelerations.

Variable Decelerations (V-shaped)

- Constitute majority of decelerations during labor, and they translate a baroreceptor-mediated response to increased arterial pressure, as occurs with umbilical cord compression **(Fig. 4)**.[28]
- Seldom associated with severe degree of fetal hypoxia/acidosis unless
  - Evolve to exhibit a U-shaped component
  - Reduced variability within the deceleration
  - Individual duration exceeds 3 minutes[24,29]

Late Decelerations (U-shaped and/or with Reduced Variability)

These decelerations are indicative of a chemoreceptor-mediated response to fetal hypoxemia **(Fig. 5)**.[27,29]

Prolonged Decelerations

These are likely to include a chemoreceptor-mediated component and thus to indicate hypoxemia. Decelerations exceeding 5 minutes, with FHR maintained <80 bpm and reduced variability within the deceleration are frequently associated with acute fetal hypoxia/acidosis[24,30,31] and require emergent intervention **(Fig. 6)**.

◼ SINUSOIDAL PATTERN

Comparison of sinusoidal pattern is described in **Table 9**.

Additional features of sinusoidal pattern (Fig. 7):
- Stable baseline heart rate of 120–160 bpm with regular oscillations
- Fixed or flat short-term variability
- Oscillation of sinusoidal waveform above or below a baseline
- Absent accelerations.

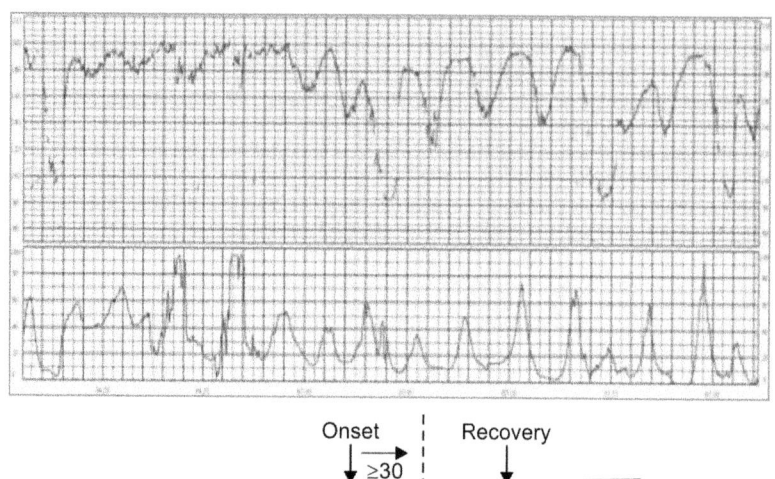

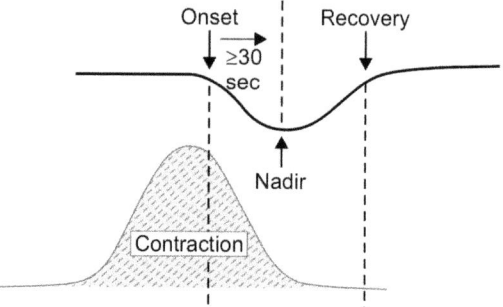

Fig. 5: Late decelerations.

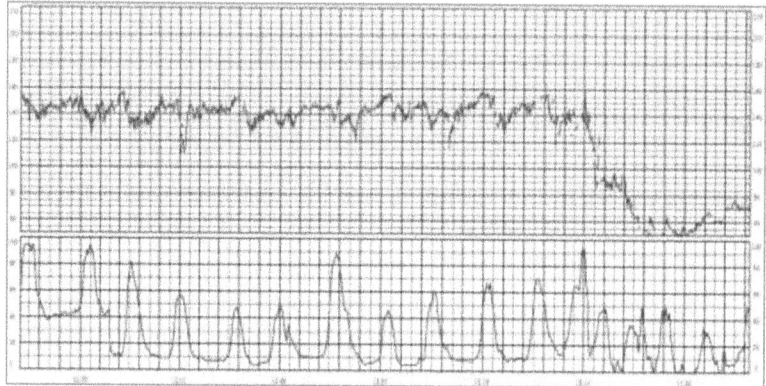

Fig. 6: Prolonged decelerations.

TABLE 9: Comparison of sinusoidal pattern by FIGO, NICE, and ACOG.			
	FIGO	*NICE*	*ACOG*
Frequency	< 6 cycles/min	3–5 cycles/min	3–5 cycles/min
Amplitude	At least 10 bpm	5–15 bpm	
Duration	≥20 min	At least 10 min	≥20 min

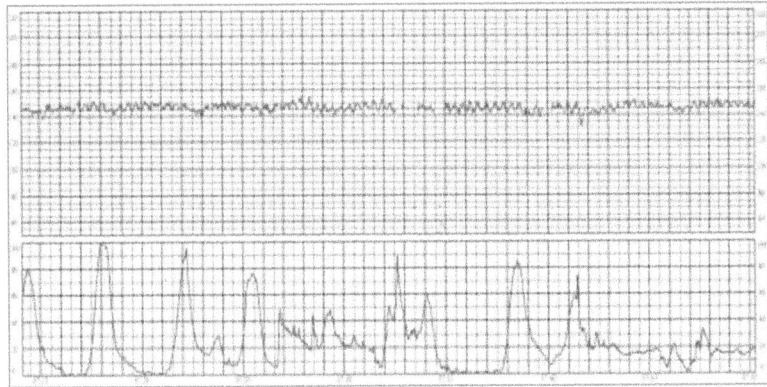

Fig. 7: Sinusoidal pattern.

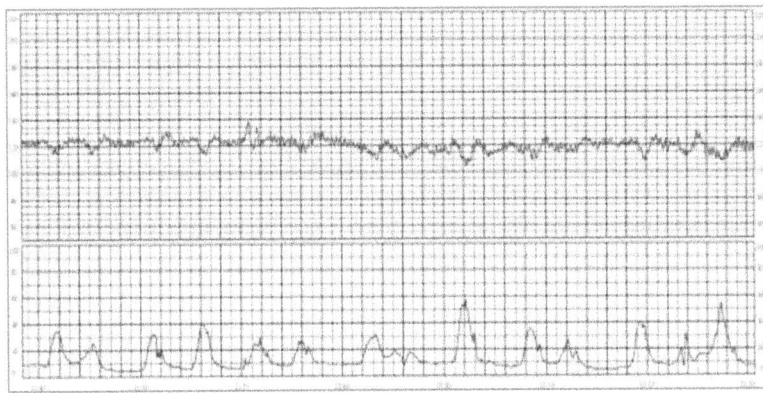

Fig. 8: Pseudosinusoidal pattern.

Causes of Sinusoidal Pattern[32]

- Severe fetal anemia:
    - Anti-D alloimmunization
    - Fetal-maternal hemorrhage
    - Twin-to-twin transfusion syndrome
    - Ruptured vasa previa
- Acute fetal hypoxia
- Infection
- Cardiac malformations
- Hydrocephalus and gastroschisis

Pseudosinusoidal Pattern

- A pattern resembling the sinusoidal pattern, but with a more jagged "saw-tooth" appearance, rather than the smooth sine-wave form.
- Duration seldom exceeds 30 minutes and it is characterized by normal patterns before and after.

- Occurs after analgesic administration to the mother, and during periods of fetal sucking and other mouth movements[33]
- Pseudosinusoidal pattern is differentiated from the true sinusoidal pattern, by the duration as it is the most important variable to discriminate between the two **(Fig. 8)**.

FETAL BEHAVIORAL STATES

- Refers to periods of fetal quiescence reflecting deep sleep (no eye movements), alternating with periods of active sleep (rapid eye movements) and wakefulness[34,35]
- Deep sleep can last up to 50 minutes[23] and is associated with a stable baseline, very rarely accelerations, and borderline variability.
- Active sleep is the most frequent behavioral state, and is represented by a moderate number of accelerations and normal variability.

- Active wakefulness is rarer and represented by a large number of accelerations and normal variability. In the latter pattern, accelerations may be so frequent as to cause difficulties in baseline estimation.

CONTRACTION

Contractions are essential for the progression of labor, but they compress the vessels running inside the myometrium and may transiently decrease placental perfusion and/or cause umbilical cord compression. With the tocodynamometer, only the frequency of contractions can be reliably evaluated, but increased intensity and duration can also contribute to FHR changes.

CLASSIFICATION OF FHR PATTERNS (TABLES 10 TO 12 AND FIG. 9)

- Interpretation of an FHR tracing includes four components:
  1. Qualitative and quantitative descriptions of baseline rate and variability
  2. Presence/absence of accelerations, decelerations, or sinusoidal pattern
  3. Changes or trends of the FHR over time
  4. Assessment of uterine activity
- Standard definitions of FHR baseline, variability, accelerations, decelerations, and sinusoidal pattern were proposed by the National Institute of Child Health and Human Development (NICHD) in 1997 and reaffirmed in 2008. They are used clinically throughout the United States, and have been endorsed by ACOG. The International Federation of Gynecology and Obstetrics (FIGO) published a similar consensus guideline in 2015 (FIGO 2015), which is used in many other countries.

Agreement and accuracy using the FIGO, ACOG, and NICE cardiotocography interpretation guidelines:[36]

- This study compares the agreement, reliability, and accuracy of FIGO, ACOG, and NICE guidelines for CTG interpretation and showed that attribution of category II is very frequent with the ACOG guidelines, leading to a high overall interobserver agreement, a low reliability, a low sensitivity and a high

specificity of category III tracings in the prediction of fetal acidemia.

- With the FIGO and NICE guidelines, a more balanced distribution of classifications is seen, and there appears to be a higher sensitivity and a lower specificity of pathological tracings in prediction of fetal acidemia (**Tables 10 to 12**).
- It also confirms that there is strong agreement in identification of normal baseline, tachycardia, normal variability, and presence of accelerations and decelerations. It was not possible to evaluate the classification of decelerations, as these events are defined differently in the three guidelines.

Continuous Electronic Fetal Monitoring Stoplight

Stoplight algorithm for continuous electronic fetal monitoring has been shown in **Figure 10**.

LIMITATIONS

- CTG analysis is subjected to *considerable intra- and interobserver differences*, even with experienced clinicians using widely accepted guidelines[37-39] especially with:
  - Identification and classification of decelerations
  - Evaluation of variability[38]
  - Classification of tracings as suspicious and pathological[38,39]
- Suspicious and pathological tracings have a limited capacity to predict metabolic acidosis and low Apgar scores[40]
- Only significant improvement was a 50% reduction in neonatal seizures (HIE was not evaluated in most trials), and no differences were found in the incidences of overall perinatal mortality and cerebral palsy. However, it is widely recognized that the trials were underpowered to detect differences in these outcomes.[41] Only a small proportion of perinatal deaths and cerebral palsies are caused by intrapartum hypoxia/acidosis, so a large number of cases is needed to show any significant benefit.

TABLE 10: Classification of CTG features by FIGO and NICE.

	Normal	Suspicious	Pathological
FIGO	• Baseline heart rate between 110 and 150 bpm • Amplitude of heart rate variability between 5 and 25 bpm	• Baseline heart rate between 150 and 170 bpm or between 100 and 110 bpm • Amplitude of variability between 5 and 10 bpm for more than 40 min • Increased variability above 25 bpm • Variable decelerations	• Baseline heart rate 170 bpm • Persistence of heart rate variability of 40 min • Severe variable decelerations or severe repetitive early decelerations • Prolonged decelerations • *Late decelerations:* The most ominous trace is a steady baseline without baseline variability and with small decelerations after each contraction • A sinusoidal pattern

NICE	*Baseline rate:* 110–160 bpm
	• *Variability:* ≥5 bpm
	• No decelerations
	• *Accelerations:* Present
		Suspicious (a CTG, where one of the following features is present and all others fall into the reassuring category):
		• *Baseline rate:*
		  – 100–109 bpm
		  – 161–180 bpm
		• *Baseline variability:*
		  – 50% of contractions occurring for >90 min
		  – Single prolonged deceleration for up to 3 min
		• *Accelerations:*
		  – The absence of accelerations with an otherwise normal trace is of uncertain significance
			A CTG with one or more of the following features or two or more features in the previous category:
			• *Baseline rate:*
			  – <100bpm
			  – >180 bpm
			  – Sinusoidal pattern ≥10 min
			• *Baseline variability:* <5 bpm for ≥90 bpm
			• *Decelerations:*
			  – Atypical variable decelerations with >50% contractions for >30 min
			  – Late decelerations for >30 min
			  – Prolonged deceleration >3 min

• Continuous CTG was associated with a 63% increase in cesarean delivery and a 15% increase in instrumental vaginal deliveries.[42]

LESS USEFUL ANCILLARY TESTS FOR INTRAPARTUM FETAL EVALUATION

• Fetal scalp blood sampling
• Scalp stimulation
• Vibroacoustic stimulation
• Fetal pulse oximetry
• Intrapartum Doppler velocimetry

Maternal operative interventions did not decrease and neonatal outcomes were not significantly improved with addition of these techniques to standard continuous EFM by cardiotocograph and therefore not routinely recommended.

FETAL STAN[43]

• Fetal STAN needs little consideration and therefore discussed in detail. It combines standard CTG monitoring with concurrent assessment of fetal ECG and the rationale behind this technique is based on the observation that the mature fetus exposed to hypoxemia develops an elevated ST segment with progressive increase in T-wave height that can be expressed as T:QRS ratio which reflect fetal cardiac ability to adapt to hypoxia and appears before neurological damage.
• Worsening hypoxia results in increasingly negative ST segment deflection such that it appears biphasic form (**Figs. 11A and B**).
• NICE and ACOG does not recommend its routine use.
• None of the studies have found a significant benefit with addition of ST segment.

TABLE 11: NICHD classification of CTG features (endorsed by ACOG).

	Category I	Category II	Category III

ACOG	Category I FHR tracings include all of the following:
	• *Baseline rate:* 110–160 bpm
	• *Baseline variability:* 6–25 bpm
	• *Late or variable decelerations:* Absent
	• *Early decelerations:* Present or absent
	• *Accelerations:* Present or absent
		Category II FHR tracings include all FHR tracings not categorized as Category I or Category III. Examples of Category II FHR tracings include any of the following:
		• *Baseline rate:*
		  – Bradycardia not accompanied by absent baseline variability
		  – Tachycardia
		• *Baseline variability:*
		  – Minimal variability
		  – Absent variability with no recurrent decelerations
		  – Marked variability
		• *Accelerations:* Absence of induced accelerations after fetal stimulation
		• *Periodic or episodic decelerations:*
		  – Recurrent variable decelerations accompanied by minimal or moderate baseline variability
		  – Prolonged deceleration 2–10 min
		  – Recurrent late decelerations with moderate baseline variability
		  – Variable decelerations with other characteristics such as slow return to baseline, overshoots or shoulders
			Category III FHR tracings include either:
			• Absent baseline FHR variability and any of the following:
			  – Recurrent late decelerations
			  – Recurrent variable decelerations
			  – Bradycardia
			• Sinusoidal pattern

TABLE 12: Management of various categories by intrapartum tracings (NICHD).

Continuous EFM findings	Significance	Management
Category 1	Normal pH and fetal well being	Continue current monitoring method (SIA and EFM)
Category 2 1. Baseline FHR changes (<110 bpm) not accompanied by absent baseline variability or tachycardia (>160bpm) 2. Changes in FHR variability (absent and not accompanied by decelerations minimal and marked) 3. No FHR stimulations after fetal stimulation 4. FHR decelerations without absent variability	1. Tachycardia medications, maternal anxiety, infections, fever. *Bradycardia:* Rupture of membranes, occipitoposterior position, post-term pregnancy, congenital anomalies 2. Medications, sleep cycle change in monitoring, fetal hypoxia, academia 3. Possible fetal hypoxia or academia 4. Variable cord entrapment or prolapse Late possible uteroplacental insufficiency, epidural hypotension, tachysystole	1. General measure, consider expedited delivery if abnormalities persist 2. General measures + change fetal monitoring method internal monitoring if doing continuous EFM or EFM if doing SIA + consider expedited delivery if abnormalities persist 3. General measures + discontinue oxytocin + consider expedited delivery, if abnormalities persist 4. General measures + amnioinfusion (for recurrent decelerations) + discontinue oxytocin + consider expedited delivery, if abnormalities persist
Category 3 1. Absent baseline FHR variability with recurrent decelerations (variable or late) and/or bradycardia 2. Sinusoidal FHR pattern	1. Uteroplacental insufficiency, fetal hypoxia or academia	1. General measures 2. Discontinue oxytocin + expedite delivery

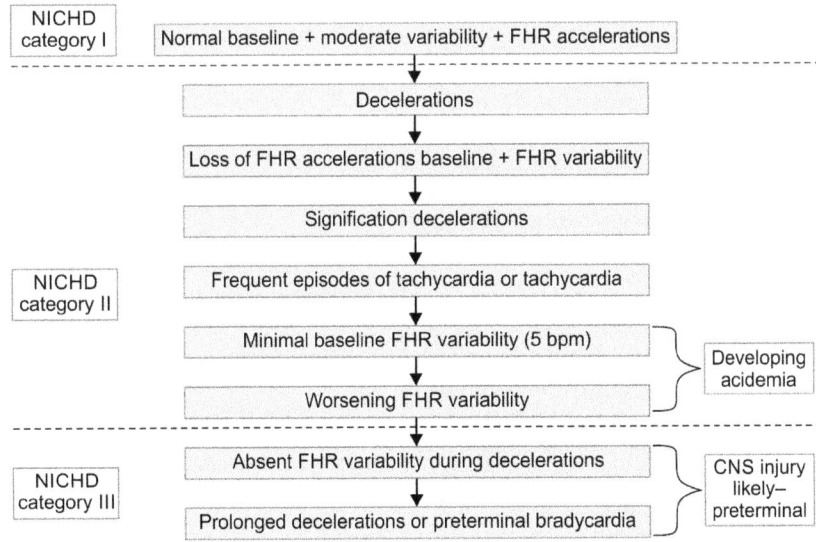

Fig. 9: Evolving FHR pattern during intrapartum fetal distress.

NICHD category III (abnormal)	NICHD category II (indeterminate)	NICHD category I (normal)
• Absent baseline FHR variability with recurrent late or variable decelerations and/or bradycardia, or with a sinusoidal pattern • General measures; discontinue oxytocin (Pitocin); expedite delivery by operative vaginal or cesarean delivery • NICHD	• FHR patterns that are concerning enough to warrant increased frequency in monitoring, but that respond to interventions provided • General measures; consider discontinuing oxytocin; consider potential need to expedite delivery if abnormalities persist or worsen	• Normal baseline FHR, moderate variability, and lack of concerning decelerations • Continue monitoring

Fig. 10: Stoplight diagram for intrapartum surveillance of fetal heat rate (FHR) (NICHD).

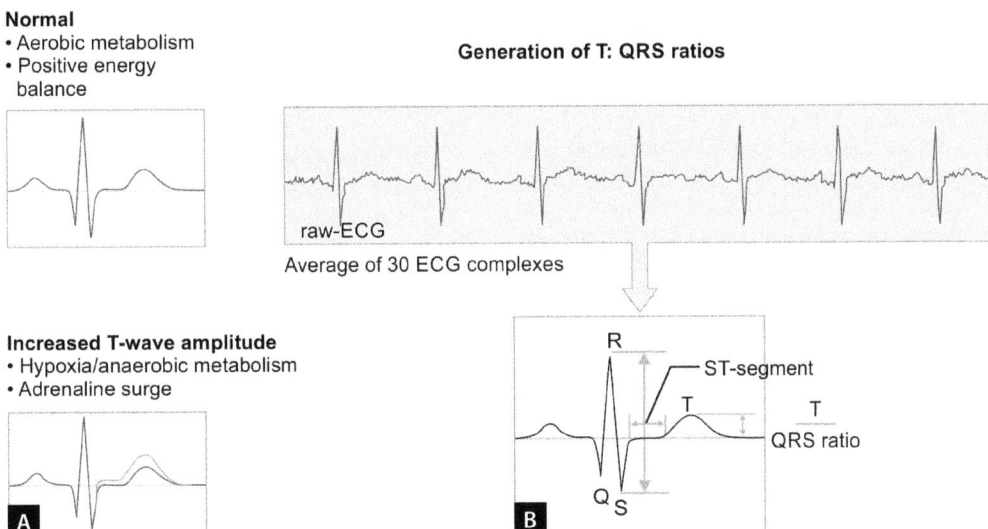

Figs. 11A and B: (A) ST segment changes in normal and hypoxic conditions; (B) Generation of T:QRS ratios.
Source: Redrawn from Devoe, 2006, with permission.

• It is not indicated for monitoring initiated in the second stage of labor, since there may not be enough time to establish the baseline fetal ECG data required for automatic ST event signals. Transcutaneous Electrical Nerve Stimulation (TENS) for analgesia during labor is another contraindication because TENS may interfere with acquisition of the fetal ECG signal.

CONCLUSION

Intrapartum fetal monitoring should be used judiciously along with its proper interpretation so that unjustified and unnecessary interventions can be avoided. Simultaneously, it is equally important that CTG picks up the cases of fetal distress timely to improve the neonatal outcome.

REFERENCES

1. Miller DA (2021). Intrapartum fetal heart rate monitoring: overview. [online] Available from: https://www.uptodate.com/contents/intra-partum-fetal-heart-rate-monitoring-overview. [Last accessed on December 24, 2021].
2. Martin JA, Hamilton BE, Sutton PD, Ventura SJ, Menacker F, Munson ML. Births: final data for 2002. Natl Vital Stat Rep. 2003; 52(10):1-113.
3. Diogo ayres-de-campos. Introduction: Why is intrapartum foetal monitoring necessary: Impact on outcomes and interventions? Best Pract Res Clin Obstet Gynaecol. 2016:30:3-8.
4. Grimes DA, Peipert JF. Electronic fetal moni-toring as a public health screening program: the arithmetic of failure. Obstet Gynecol. 2010; 116:1397.
5. Alfirevic Z, Devane D, Gyte GM, Cuthbert A. Continuous cardiotocography (CTG) as a form of electronic fetal monitoring (EFM) for fetal assessment during labour. Cochrane Database Syst Rev. 2017;2:CD006066.
6. Al Wattar BH, Honess E, Bunnewell S, Welton NJ, Quenby S, Khan KS, et al. Effectiveness of intrapartum fetal surveillance to improve maternal and neonatal outcomes: a systematic review and network meta-analysis. 2021;193: E468.
7. American College of Obstetricians and Gynecologists. ACOG Practice Bulletin No. 106: Intrapartum fetal heart rate monitoring: nomenclature, interpretation, and general management principles. Obstet Gynecol. 2009; 114:192. Reaffirmed 2019.
8. NICE (2014). Intrapartum care for healthy women and babies. [online] Available from: https://www.nice.org.uk/guidance/cg19 0/chapter/1-Recommendations#monitoring-during-labour.[Last accessed on December 24, 2021].
9. Carbonne B, Benachi A, Leveque ML, Cabrol D, Papiernik E. Maternal position during labor: effect on fetal oxygen saturation measured by fetal pulse oximetry. Obstet Gynecol. 1996; 88:797-800.
10. Carter MC. Signal processing and display—cardiotocographs. Br J Obstet Gynaecol. 1993;100(Suppl 9):21-3.
11. Nurani R, Chandraharan E, Lowe V, Ugwumadu A, Arulkumaran S. Misidentification of maternal heart rate as fetal on cardiotocography during the second stage of labour: the role of the fetal electrocardiograph. Acta ObstetGynecol Scand. 2012; 91(12):1428-32.
12. Maiques V, Garcia-Tejedor A, Perales A, Navarro C. Intrapartum fetal invasive procedures and perinatal transmission of HIV. Eur J Obstet Gynecol Reprod Biol. 1999;87:63-7.
13. Kaye EM, Dooling EC. Neonatal herpes simplex meningoencephalitis associated with fetal monitor scalp electrodes. Neurology. 1981; 31:1045-7.
14. Handwerker SM, Selcik AM. Placental abruption after insertion of catheter tip intrauterine pressure transducers: a report of four cases. J Reprod Med. 1995;40:845-9.
15. Bakker JJ, Janssen PF, van Halem K, van der Goes BY, Papatsonis DN, van des Post JA, Mol BW. Internal versus external tocodynamometry during induced or augmented labour. Cochrane Database Sys Rev. 2013;8:CD006947.
16. Bailey RE. Intrapartum fetal surveillance. In: Leeman L (Ed). Advanced Life Support in Obstetrics Program: Provider Course Syllabus. Leawood, Kan.: American Academy of Family Physicians; 2009.
17. Macones GA, Hankins GD, Spong CY, Hauth J, Moore T. The 2008 National Institute of Child Health and Human Development Workshop Report On Electronic Fetal Monitoring: update on definitions, interpretation, and research guidelines. Obstet Gynecol. 2008;112(3):661-6.
18. Ayres-de-Campos D, Bernardes J, Marsal K, Nickelsen C, Makarainen L, Banfield P, et al. Can the reproducibility of fetal heart rate

baseline estimation be improved? Eur J Obstet Gynecol Reprod Biol. 2004;112:49-54.

19. Segal S. Labor epidural analgesia and maternal fever. Anesth Analg. 2010;111: 1467-75.

20. Neilson JP, West HM, Dowswell T. Betamimetics for inhibiting preterm labour. Cochrane Database Syst Rev. 2014;2: CD004352.

21. Jadhon ME, Main EK. Fetal bradycardia associated with maternal hypothermia. Obstet Gynecol. 1988;72(3 Pt 2):496-7.

22. Boutrov MJ. Fetal and neonatal effects of the beta-adrenoreceptor blocking agents. Dev Phamacol Ther. 1987;10:224-31.

23. Suwanrath C, Suntharasaj T. Sleep–wake cycles in normal foetuses. Arch Gynecol Obstet. 2010;281:449-54

24. Hamilton E, Warrick P, O'Keeffe D. Variable decelerations: do size and shape matter? J Matern Fetal Neonatal Med. 2012;25:648-53.

25. Nelson KB, Dambrosia JM, Ting TY, Grether JK. Uncertain value of electronic fetal monitoring in predicting cerebral palsy. N Engl J Med. 1996;334(10):613-8.

26. Nunes I, Ayres-de-Campos D, Kwee A, Rosen KG. Prolonged saltatory fetal heart rate pattern leading to newborn metabolic acidosis. Clin Exp Obstet Gynecol. 2014; 41(5):507-11.

27. Court DJ, Parer JT. Experimental studies of fetal asphyxia and fetal heart rate interpretation. In: Nathanielsz PW, Parer JT (Eds.). Research in Perinatal Medicine (I). New York: Perinatalogy Press; 1984. pp.113-69.

28. Ball RH, Parer JT. The physiologic mechanisms of variable decelerations. Am J Obstet Gynecol. 1992;166:1683-9.

29. Holzmann M, Wretler S, Cnattingius S, Nordstrom L. Cardiotocography patterns and risk of intrapartum fetalacidemia. J Perinat Med. 2015;43(4):473-9.

30. Cahill AG, Roehl KA, Odibo AO, Macones GA. Association and prediction of neonatal acidemia. Am J ObstetGynecol. 2012;207:206. e1-8.

31. Takano Y, Furukawa S, Ohashi M, Michikata K, Sameshima H, Ikenoue T. Fetal heart rate patterns related to neonatal brain damage and neonatal death in placental abruption. J ObstetGynecol Res. 2013;39:61-6.

32. Modanlou HD, Murata Y. Sinusoidal fetal heart rate pattern: reappraisal of its definition and clinical significance. J Obstet Gynaecol Res. 2004;30:169-80.

33. Graça LM, Cardoso CG, Clode N, Calhaz-Jorge C. An approach to interpretation and classification of sinusoidal fetal heart rate patterns. Eur J Obstet Gynecol Reprod Biol. 1988;27:203-12.

34. Nijhuis JG, Prechtl HF, Martin CB, Bots RS. Are there behavioural states in the human fetus? Early Hum Dev. 1982;6:177-95.

35. de Vries JIP, Visser GHA, Prechtl HFR. The emergence of fetal behaviour. II. Quantative aspects. Early Hum Dev. 1985;12:99-120.

36. Santo S, Ayres-de-campos D, Costa-santos C, Schnettler W, Ugwumadu A, Da Graça LM, et al. Agreement and accuracy using the FIGO, ACOG and NICE cardiotocography interpretation guidelines. 2016 Nordic Federation of Societies of Obstetrics and Gynecology. Acta Obstet Gynecol Scand. 2017;96:166-75.

37. Blackwell SC, Grobman WA, Antoniewicz L, Hutchinson M, Gyamfi-Bannerman C. Interobserver and intraobserver reliability of the NICH 3-tier fetal heart rate interpretation system. Am J Obstet Gynecol. 2011;205:378. e1-5.

38. Ayres-de-Campos D, Arteiro D, Costa-Santos C, Bernardes J. Knowledge of adverse neonatal outcome alters clinicians' interpretation of the intrapartum cardiotocograph. BJOG. 2011; 118:978-84.

39. Spencer JA. Clinical overview of cardiotocography. Br J Obstet Gynaecol. 1993;100(Suppl 9):4-7.

40. O'Mahony F, Hofmeyr GJ, Menon V. Choice of instruments for assisted vaginal delivery. Cochrane Database Syst Rev. 2010;11:CD005455

41. Royal College of Obstetricians and Gynaecologists. The use of electronic fetal monitoring. Evidence-based clinical guideline, number 8. London: RCOG Press; 2001

42. Alfirevic Z, Devane D, Gyte GM. Continuous cardiotocography (CTG) as a form of electronic fetal monitoring (EFM) for fetal assessment during labour. Cochrane Database Syst Rev. 2013;5:CD006066.

43. Sacco A, Muglu J, Navaratnarajah R, Hogg M. ST analysis for intrapartum fetal monitoring. Obstet Gynaecol. 2015;17:5-12.

CHAPTER 10

Managing Third Stage of Labor

Ankita Bansal Goyal, Jaideep Malhotra

INTRODUCTION

The third stage is one of the most crucial stages of labor and is referred to as period following the completed delivery of the fetus until the completed delivery of the placenta, known as placental stage of labor.[1]

The third stage of labor is very important to record as there is significant risk of postpartum hemorrhage. All women need vigilant monitoring during third stage to avoid significant morbidity and mortality. It usually lasts for 5-10 minutes.[2] However, it may be prolonged in cases of preterm delivery, and if there is no bleeding then expectant management can be done till 30 minutes.

The third stage of labor may be managed expectantly or actively. During physiological management, the process is allowed to take its natural course to not requiring uterotonics prophylactically, the cord may or may not be clamped early, and the placenta is delivered by maternal efforts with minimal assistance, if required. It is considered "prolonged" if the placenta and membranes are not delivered within 30 minutes of the birth.[3] In active management, uterotonic drugs are given prophylactically, cord clamping is done within 2-3 minutes after delivery of the fetus,[1] and placenta is delivered by controlled cord traction. This becomes "prolonged" if the placenta and membranes are not delivered within 60 minutes of the birth.[3]

METHODS

The two methods currently in practice are:[1]
1. *Expectant management*: It follows natural physiological process of spontaneous delivery of placenta and membranes. However, minimal assistance may be given for the placental expulsion, if needed.

Prerequisites:
- Uncomplicated pregnancy
- Uncomplicated labor
- Cervix must remain open.
- Good uterine contraction.
- Constant watch.

In the majority, this occurs in following sequential order:
A. *Separation of the placenta:* The placenta separates from the myometrium as a result of abrupt decrease in size of the uterine cavity as the retraction process accelerates leading to formation of retroplacental clot.

There are two methods of placental separation:
1. *Schultze method*: Separation starts in the middle portion of the placental bed (**Fig. 1**). The entrapped retroplacental blood will facilitate the placental separation, so that separation is more complete and rapid and will deliver like a parachute. The amount of blood loss is less.
2. *Duncan's method*: Placental separation start at the edge with no retroplacental clot to facilitate the separation as a result the separation is slow and less complete (**Fig. 2**). The amount of blood loss in more as compared to Schultze method.

Signs of placental separation:
- *Per abdomen*:
  - Uterus becomes firm, globular, and ballotable.
  - Fundal height is slightly raised
  - Suprapubic bulging.
- *Per vaginum examination*:
  - Slight gush of vaginal bleeding
  - Permanent lengthening of cord.
B. *Descent of the placenta:* After separation, the placenta moves down the birth canal and through the dilated cervix.

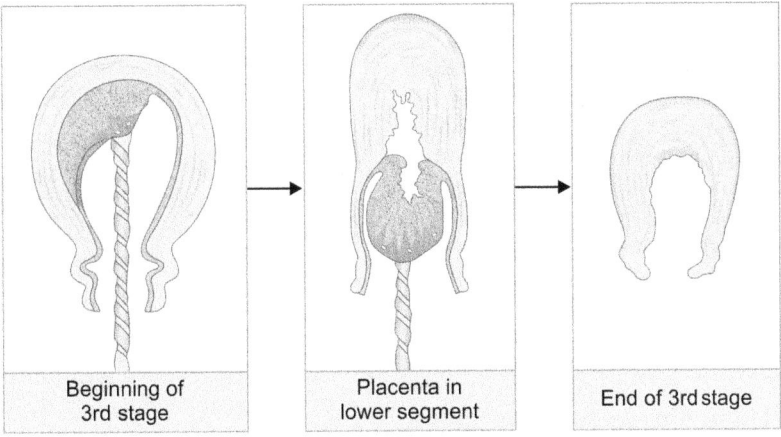

Fig. 1: Schultze method.

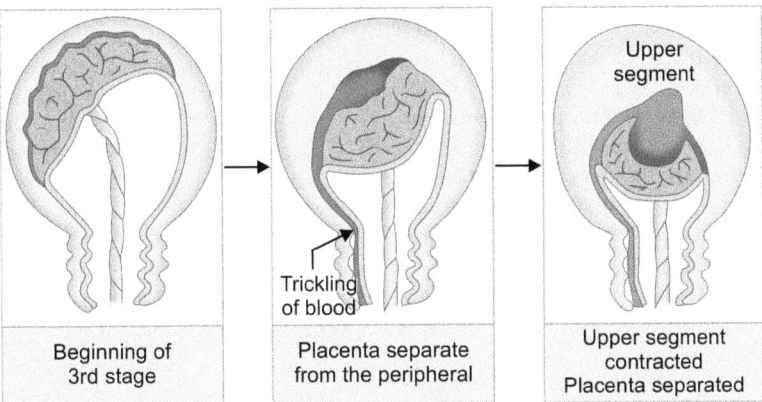

Fig. 2: Duncan method.

Descent of placenta occurs due to:

- Spontaneous uterine contractions
- Downward pressure due to retroplacental clot
- Increase in intra-abdominal pressure.

C. *Expulsion of the placenta:* The placenta is completely expelled from the birth canal with or without minimal assistance.

Steps: This provides constant support to the patients.

Patient should be encouraged to lie in dorsal position to note the features of placental separation and to assess the amount of bleeding.

A hand is placed over the fundus to recognize the signs of separation of placenta and to assess the state of uterine activity. Uterine massage should be strongly avoided.

When the features of placental separation and its descent into lower segment has been confirmed patient is asked to bear down during uterine contraction, placenta is expelled usually within 20 minutes, and once the placenta passes through the introitus, it should be grasped with hands and twisted round with gentle traction in downward and backward direction to avoid tearing of membranes. If membranes are torn or threaten to tear, they should be grasped with sponge holding forceps and in similar twisting movement the rest of the membranes are delivered.

If this physiological process is failed to completion or is not possible due to certain reasons, i.e., during anesthesia, then any of the following steps can be taken to expedite placental delivery.

- *Assisted expulsion[1] (controlled cord traction):* When the uterus is hard and contracted left hand is placed over the symphysis pubis (at the junction of upper and lower third of the uterine body) with its palmer surface facing the uterus and pushing it toward the umbilicus with simultaneous firm traction with right hand holding the clamp at umbilical cord in downward and backward direction. It should basically work on uterine elevation rather than downward pulling of the placenta **(Fig. 3)**.
- *Fundal pressure:[1]* Uterine fundus is grasped at front with the thumb and four fingers at the back and is pushed in downward and backward direction as a piston only when uterus is hard. Pressure should be released as soon as the placenta passes the introitus to avoid inversion. This method is usually preferred in cases of compromised cord strength, such as in cases of macerated fetus or extreme preterm delivery. Sometimes the cord is accidently torn in that case right hand is inserted inside the vagina, placenta is grasped and is extracted **(Fig. 4)**.

After placental expulsion uterus is massaged to make uterus hard and thus facilitating removal of clots, if any.

Placenta and its membranes are examined for its completeness and anomalies.

2. *Active management (preferred):*
   Benefits: There are certain additional benefits of active management of third stage of labor in terms of:
   - Reducing additional blood loss and need of further blood transfusion

- Decrease in duration of second stage of labor.
- Reduces the need of additional uterotonics for postpartum hemorrhage.

Components:[4]
- Administration of a uterotonic drug within 0 minutes after the baby's birth and after ruling out multiple pregnancy
- Clamping and cutting the cord after cord pulsations have ceased or approximately 2–3 minutes after birth of the baby, whichever comes first.
- CCT during a contraction with counter traction to stabilize the uterus towards the umbilicus, including gentle twisting movement to deliver the placenta so to avoid tearing of the membranes.
- Massaging the uterus immediately after delivery of the placenta. Clinical guidelines for management of the third stage of labor will generally also include careful inspection of the placenta and genitalia to rule out retained placenta/placental fragments and genital lacerations, and careful monitoring of the woman and her new-born for at least the first 6 hours postpartum.

Use Uterotonic Agents[5]

- Immediately after delivery, palpate the abdomen to rule out the presence of multiple pregnancies and give oxytocin 10 units IM.
- Oxytocin is preferred over other uterotonic drugs because it is effective 2–3 minutes after

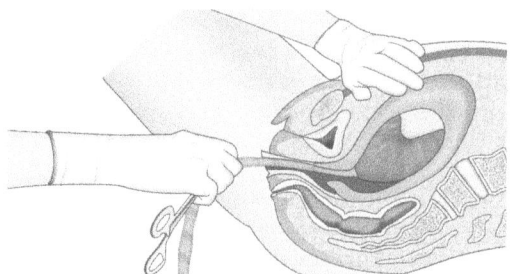

Fig. 3: Assisted expulsion.

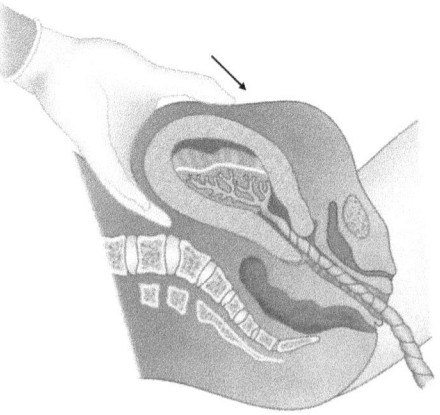

Fig. 4: Fundal pressure.

injection (mean half-life of 3–7 minutes, has minimal side effects and can be used in all women.

- Oxytocin when given intravascular as a bolus can cause profound hypotension. So, preferred mode of administration is lighter intramuscular or slow intravenous infusion.
- Alternative to oxytocin other uterotonics can be used such as: ergometrine 0.2 mg IM, syntometrine (1 ampoule) IM or misoprostol 400–600 mcg orally. Whether given intramuscularly or orally, both are powerful stimulants of myometrial contractions, exerting an effect that persists for hours. Ergometrine derivative scan be harmful for the fetus and mother when given before delivery.
- Ergot alkaloids are not superior as compared with oxytocin; moreover safety and tolerability are greater with oxytocin. Therefore ergot alkaloids are still preferred as second line for third stage management.
- Ergot alkaloids are to be avoided in patient with severe hypertension to avoid the risk of severe vasoconstriction.
- Oral administration of misoprostol drugs are to be given only in conditions when oxytocin and ergot derivatives, cannot be given or are contraindicated and in case of unfavorable storage environment.

Controlled Cord Traction

Place the left hand over the symphysis pubis, pushing and stabilizing the uterus toward the umbilicus hold the cord clamp with right hand as close to perineum as possible. Exert firm but gentle tension on the cord but avoid pulling while waiting for strong uterine contraction. Encourage the mother to push along with strong uterine contraction while exerting traction at the cord and counter traction at the uterine fundus. If placenta does not descent for 30–40 seconds of controlled cord traction continue with gentle holding of the cord and repeat the same procedure with another contraction. As the placenta delivers, hold it and remove it with gentle twisting movement to avoid tearing of membranes. If the membranes tear then hold it with sponge holding forceps and remove with gentle twisting.

Uterine Massage

Massage the fundus of the uterus until the uterus is contracted. Continue palpating the uterine fundus every 1 minute and continue with uterine massage, if needed, during first 2 hours.

Examination of the Placenta

Examine the placenta carefully to ensure its complete removal, as placental bits can cause secondary hemorrhage and infection.

Flowchart 1: Expectant management.

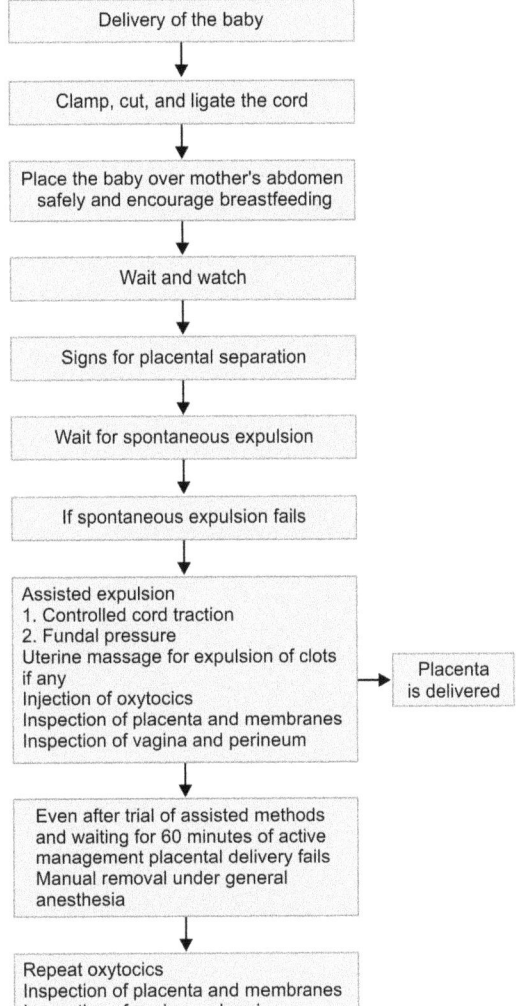

Flowchart 2: Active management.

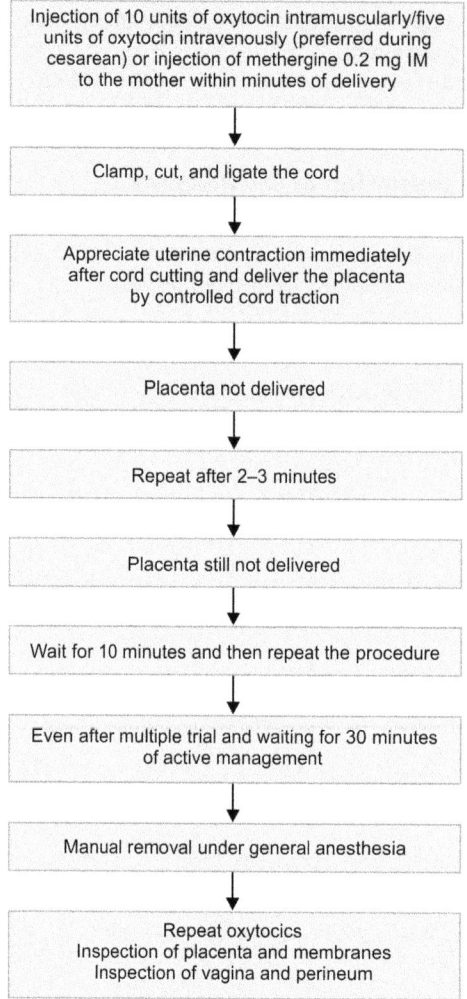

Injection of 10 units of oxytocin intramuscularly/five units of oxytocin intravenously (preferred during cesarean) or injection of methergine 0.2 mg IM to the mother within minutes of delivery

↓

Clamp, cut, and ligate the cord

↓

Appreciate uterine contraction immediately after cord cutting and deliver the placenta by controlled cord traction

↓

Placenta not delivered

↓

Repeat after 2–3 minutes

↓

Placenta still not delivered

↓

Wait for 10 minutes and then repeat the procedure

↓

Even after multiple trial and waiting for 30 minutes of active management

↓

Manual removal under general anesthesia

↓

Repeat oxytocics
Inspection of placenta and membranes
Inspection of vagina and perineum

■ CONCLUSION

Third stage of labor can be very devastating, if not managed properly as there can be several complications like postpartum hemorrhage, uterine inversion, hematoma formation, retained placenta, shock, etc., so vigilant monitoring is crucial in its management.

Management of third stage of labor (**Flowcharts 1 and 2**).

■ REFERENCES

1. Konar H. DC Dutta's Textbook of Obstetrics Including Perinatology and Contraception. Kolkata, India: New Central Book Agency; 2011.
2. GLOWM (2021). The Active Management of the Third Stage of Labor. [online]Available from: https://www.glowm.com/resource_type/resource/wall_chart/title/active-management-ofthe-third-stage-of-labor/resource_doc/535. [Last accessed on December 22, 2021]
3. Prendiville WJP, Elbourne D, McDonald SJ. Active versus expectant management in the third stage of labour. Cochrane Database Syst Rev. 2000;(3):CD000007.
4. World Health Organization. WHO Recommendations for the Prevention and Treatment of Postpartum Haemorrhage. Geneva, Switzerland: WHO; 2012.
5. Güngördük K, Olgaç Y, Gülseren V, Kocaer M. Active management of the third stage of labor: A brief overview of key issues. Turk J Obstet Gynecol. 2018;15(3):188-92.

CHAPTER

11

Prolonged Labor

Anita Rajorhia, Yukti Bhardwaj

▓ DEFINITION

Labor is defined as "prolonged", when its duration is more than 20 hours in nulliparas and more than 14 hours in multiparas. The term prolonged labor is considered at or after 5 cm dilatation and patient having three contractions per minute. It is also known as "Protracted Labor" and is a clinical diagnosis in active labor.[1]

▓ INCIDENCE

It occurs in 8% of primigravida and 2% of multigravidas.

Prolonged Latent Phase of First Stage

It is also called "false labor" and is hallmarked by latent phase, which exceeds more than 20 hours in primigravida or 14 hours in multigravida.

Prolonged Active Phase First Stage

Active first stage of labor is considered to be prolonged when its duration is more than 12 hours and rate of cervical dilation < 1 cm/hour in primigravida and < 1.5 cm/hour in multigravida.

Disorder of Active Phase

The diagnosis of active phase arrest is made when the woman has 6 cm or more of cervical dilation with membrane rupture and one of the following:
- 4 hours or more of adequate contractions (i.e., more than 200 Montevideo units) or 6 hours or more of inadequate contractions.

Prolonged Second Stage

It is divided into two phases (NICE-2014):
1. *Pelvic phase*: It is the extension of first stage that begins with full dilatation of cervix and lasts till

bearing down efforts start. This usually is not defined unless frequent vaginal examinations are performed.
2. *Perineal phase*: It is hallmarked by bearing down efforts and lasts till baby is delivered. For diagnosing prolongation of this phase, timing of urge of push has to be exactly noted.[2]

Second stage of labor is said to be prolonged when it exceeds >2 hours in primigravida, >1 hour in multigravida.

As per the latest American College of Obstetrician and Gynecologist (ACOG) and National Institute of child health and development (NICHD) 2012 recommendations, the duration of second stage is 3+1 hours (additional 1 hour for epidural analgesia) for primigravida and 2+1 hours (additional 1 hour for epidural analgesia) for multigravidas. Allowing this duration is used as a strategy to reduce LSCS rates provided fetal and maternal condition remains alright.

As per Federation of International Gynecologist and Obstetricians (FIGO) 2012 recommendation, primiparous women should not push for more than 2 hours and multiparous women not more than 1 hour, to prevent birth asphyxia and maternal infection.

The prolonged second stage is of two types and both maybe an indicator of prolonged/obstructed labor requiring prompt intervention.
1. Protracted descent
2. Arrest of descent
1. *Protracted descent*: It is defined as failure of descent of presenting part by less than 2 cm/hour for multiparous women and less than 1 cm/hour for primiparous women.
2. *Arrest of descent*: The head of the fetus is found at the same place or station during the first and second vaginal examination done at least 1 hour apart.

CAUSES OF PROLONGED LABOR

They can be mainly of two types:
1. *Dynamic dystocia*: It is due to poor, inadequate, or incoordinate uterine action.
2. *Mechanical dystocia*: It is caused by fetopelvic disproportion.[3]

Causes of Prolonged First Stage of Labor

The cause may lie in 4 P's—the power (contractions), the passage (pelvic shape and size) and the passenger (fetus) during 1st stage
1. *P—Fault in "Power"*: Abnormal uterine contractions
   - Uterine inertia or poor uterine contractions
   - Incoordinate uterine contractions
2. *P—Fault in "Passage"*:
   - Contracted pelvis
   - Cervical dystocia
   - Pelvic tumor
   - Full bladder
3. *P—Fault in "Passenger"*:
   - *Fetal malposition*: Occipitoposterior, occipitotransverse
   - Fetal malpresentation—face presentation, brow presentation, breech
   - Congenital anomalies of fetus—fetal ascites, hydrocephalus, sacrococcygeal tumor
   - Multiple pregnancies
   - Large for date baby.[4]
4. *P—Use of "Pain" killers* or administration of *sedatives* before active labor.

Causes of Prolonged Second Stage of Labor

1. 1P—Fault in power
   - Uterine inertia
   - Inability to bear down or poor expulsive efforts due to maternal exhaustion
   - Epidural analgesia
   - Constriction ring
2. 2P—Fault in passage
   - Cephalopelvic disproportion
   - Android pelvis
   - Contracted pelvis
   - Pelvic tumor
   - Pelvic floor resistance
   - Full bladder

3. 3P—Fault in passenger
   - Large baby
   - Deflexed head
   - Malposition—occipitoposterior, occipitotransverse
   - Malpresentation—mentoposterior
   - Congenital malformation of baby

COMPLICATIONS OF PROLONGED LABOR

- Fetal complications:
  - Low APGAR score
  - Hypoxia
  - Intrauterine infection
  - Intracranial hemorrhage
  - Fetal acidosis
  - NICU admissions
  - Birth trauma
  - Birth depression
- Maternal complications:
  - Maternal dehydration, distress and exhaustion
  - Chorioamnionitis
  - Increased operative delivery
  - Postpartum hemorrhage
  - Genital trauma—cervical and vaginal injuries
  - Third- and fourth-degree perineal tear
  - Puerperal sepsis
  - Subinvolution
  - Paralytic ileus

DIAGNOSTIC FEATURES

- Arrest of cervical dilatation for 4 hours during active phase of labor
- Nondescent of presenting part, even after full dilation of cervix, for more than 2 hours in multipara and more than 3 hours in primipara.
- Variable degree of molding and caput

PREVENTION OF PROLONGED LABOR

- Antenatal or early intranatal detection of factors likely to cause prolonged labor and timely intervention
- Careful clinical assessment for ruling out cephalonpelvic or fetopelvic disproportion continuous moral support during labor

- Allowing patient to remain mobile, upright, or in lateral position as per her convenience
- Judicious use of partograph
- Timely "augmentation of labor" by low rupture of membranes followed by oxytocin drip
- Allowing birth companion in labor suite
- Avoiding labor dehydration
- Use of just adequate analgesia
- Thorough clinical assessment to rule out:
  - Full bladder
  - Cephalopelvic disproportion
  - Malpresentation of the fetal head, e.g., occipitoposterior, occipitotransverse or deflexed fetal head
  - Inadequate uterine activity
  - Poor pushing efforts
- Being vigilant for signs of obstructed labor.

MANAGEMENT OF PROLONGED LABOR

All necessary general care and support in labor is given which is beyond the scope of this chapter.

Managing First Stage Delays

- Re-verify the fetal presentation, position, and station. Clinical pelvimetry to be done.
- If pelvis is adequate and uterine activity is good, do "Amniotomy and/or Oxytocin augmentation" in gradually increasing concentrations by Lowden's method.
- Remember that oxytocin is contraindicated in any kind of fetopelvic disproportion, due to fear of rupture of uterus.
- It is prudent to rule out any sign of fetal distress before oxytocin use.
- Reassess after 2–4 hours of good uterine contractions for progress of labor. Use partograph judiciously and intervene timely.
- Good pain relief may help.
- Cesarean to be done, if malpresentation or malposition is diagnosed, labor is not progressing despite good uterine contractions or vaginal delivery is considered unsafe.
- Avoid LSCS as far as possible, if fetus is dead and allow more time for dilatation and descent.
- Fetal destructive procedures may be tried in intrapartum fetal demise if expertise for same is available and prerequisites are conforming.

Managing Second Stage Delays

- Assisted vaginal delivery with forceps or ventouse is tried.
- Thorough clinical assessment is re-done to rule out:
  - Full bladder-patient is encouraged to pass urine or catheterization may be required, which may itself be difficult due to pressure and kinking of urethra
  - Cephalopelvic disproportion
  - Malpresentation of the fetal head, e.g., occipitoposterior, occipitotransverse-manual or Kielland forceps rotation followed by forceps/vacuum extraction may be tried. Deflexed fetal head-oxytocin drip may help in increasing flexion and descent of head. LSCS to be performed as a safer option or if above fail.
  - Inadequate uterine activity may warrant use of oxytocin drip.
  - Poor pushing effort—mother is given lot of moral support and a gentle "lift out forceps" or vacuum may be tried if conditions are ideal for instrumental delivery.
- An informed-written consent is must before operative vaginal delivery which should ideally be tried in operation theater. The use of sequential instruments is not recommended.
  - Signs of obstructed labor— LSCS to be planned at earliest.
  - Consider embryotomy, if fetus is dead and skill for same is there.

TECHNIQUE OF LSCS IN PROLONGED LABOR

- First stage LSCS are performed in usual way.
- *Second stage LSCS*: As the head may be impacted deep down in the pelvis in second stage LSCS, there have been two techniques described for the purpose of delivery of fetal head.
- *"Push technique"*: In push technique, an assistant is required to push the head of the fetus from below after uterine incision has been given.
- *"Pull technique"*: In pull technique however, the limbs and trunk of the baby are delivered before delivery of the head.

- Based on position of the back, pull technique may be of three types:
  1. For "back lying anteriorly", "Patwardhan maneuver" is used, wherein both shoulders are delivered first, followed by delivery of the trunk by flexion, then the legs are delivered, and finally head is lifted out.
  2. "For back lying posteriorly", "reversed breech extraction" is performed, wherein both legs are delivered first, followed by delivery of trunk by flexion, then both shoulders are delivered and finally head is lifted out.
  3. In occipitotransverse position, anterior shoulder is delivered first, followed by delivery of the posterior shoulder, then trunk is delivered by flexion, followed by legs and finally the head is lifted out.

RECENT ADVANCES

"The Fetal Pillow" is an innovative device invented by Rajiv Varma in 2007. It is used for disimpaction of the deeply engaged fetal head. It is a soft silicone balloon device that is inserted below the baby's head and inflated using saline with a syringe. It inflates only in one direction upward and elevates the fetal head.

CONCLUSION

Prolonged labor is an important cause of fetal and maternal morbidity.

Diagnosing and managing prolonged labor is often challenging. We must individualize care of patients with labor prolongation. In the absence of any complications, we may wait in latent phase or augment active phase.

If fetal compromise is suspected or other features point towards cephalopelvic disproportion or malposition, as cause of undue prolongation, intervention earlier is justified.

Prolonged second stage may be managed by oxytocin augmentation, instrumental delivery or caesarean section.

Delivery of a deeply impacted head may pose a problem even during caesarean section.

Skilled birth attendants and experienced obstetricians should conduct these deliveries.

REFERENCES

1. Merck Manual Professional version; Moldenhauer JS (2021). Protracted Labor [online]. Available from: msdmanuals.com/en-in/professional/gynecology-and-obstetrics/abnormalities-and-complications-of-labor-and-delivery/protracted-labor. [Last accessed on December 23, 2021].
2. Singh S, Kohli UA, Vardhan S. Management of prolonged second stage of labor. Int J Reprod Contracept Obstet Gynecol. 2018;7:2527-31
3. Médecins Sans Frontières. Labor dystocia and malpresentations/Prolonged labor. In: Essential Obstetric and Newborn Care. Geneva: Médecins Sans Frontières; 2019.
4. Merck Manual Professional version; Moldenhauer JS (2020). Fetal Dystocia [online]. Available from: https://www.msdmanuals.com/en-nz/professional/gynecology-and-obstetrics/abnormalities-and-complications-of-labor-and-delivery/fetal-dystocia. [Last accessed on December 23, 2021].

Obstructed Labor

Anita Rajorhia, Yukti Bhardwaj

INTRODUCTION

Obstructed labor is obsolete in the developing world with improved maternal health care services. It is a life-threatening obstetrical complication associated with high maternal and fetal morbidity and mortality. The strategy of early diagnosis and prompt action are the mainstay to prevent associated complications to both mother and baby.

DEFINITION

Obstructed labor is considered when the presenting part of the fetus cannot progress into the birth canal due to mechanical reasons, despite strong uterine action.

INCIDENCE

It is the fifth major cause of maternal death after hemorrhage, infection, unsafe abortions, and hypertensive disorders of pregnancy. The incidence is 5% in worldwide pregnancies and causes 8% maternal deaths besides other associated maternal morbidities.[1] It is more common in resource limited and underdeveloped countries when maternal undernutrition is common.

Precipitating factors leading to higher risk for obstructed labor:
- Rural setup with poor health facilities
- Early marriage and social taboos and beliefs
- Teenage pregnancy—smaller developing pelvis make them more prone to obstructed labor
- Short stature
- Lower socioeconomic status and marginalization
- Poor nourishment causes poor development of pelvis leading to decreased size or altered shape.
- Ignorance and poor educational status make them unaware to seek health care in time.
- *Poor antenatal care due to poor access or high cost of medical care*: It can lead to missed diagnosis of multiple pregnancies, big baby, fetal anomalies, other risk factors and fetopelvic disproportion.
- Poor birth preparedness and riot being aware of danger signs of pregnancy can lead to poor coping in case of any exigency or eventuality.
- Home delivery by unskilled birth attendants often leads to delay in diagnosis and management. Trying to achieve vaginal delivery at any cost may cause delay in referral.
- The three level delays:
  1. *Level 1 delay*: Delay in deciding about seeking health care by patient and attendants
  2. *Level 2 delay*: Nonavailability transport or accompanying persons to reach health care facility.
  3. *Level 3 delay*: Poorly equipped primary or secondary level with lack of infrastructure health care facilities may add on to the delay before patient can be referred to tertiary care hospital. Poor and delayed decision by health care provider, lack of transport ambulances and refusal by families at times adds to further problems.
- Fear of operative/instrumental deliveries or LSCS by patient or relative may cause problem.
- Lost art of destructive operations.

MEDICAL CAUSES OF OBSTRUCTED LABOR

- Cephalopelvic disproportion, e.g., macrosomia increased baby size in pre-existing diabetes in pregnancies or gestational diabetes mellitus or decreased pelvis size or altered

shape, which may be constitutional (short stature) or acquired due to medical problems, e.g., rickets, poliomyelitis, deformity, sickle cell disease, teenage pregnancies
- *Malpresentations*: Breech presentations, transverse lie, face (mentoposterior) or brow presentation.
- *Malposition*: Persistent occipitoposterior, deep transverse arrest
- Locked twins
- Pelvic tumors
- *Congenital malformations*: Hydrocephalus, fetal ascites, conjoint twins, sacrococcygeal teratoma, etc.

COMMON COMPLICATIONS OF OBSTRUCTED LABOR

Maternal

- Sepsis and septic shock (38.8%)
- Anemia and need for multiple blood transfusions
- Maternal dehydrations and exhaustion
- Postpartum hemorrhage (33.54%)
- Rupture of uterus (29.84%)
- Maternal death (7.5–17.27%)—confounding as death may be reported due to sepsis, PPH, anemia, rupture uterus, and shock
- Urological injuries—development of stress incontinence or urinary continence caused by vesicovaginal obstetrical fistulae or fetal incontinence due to development of rectovaginal fistulae.
- Pelvic floor dysfunction and predisposition to uterovaginal prolapse
- Complications of instrumental deliveries and operative delivery by LSCS (7.5%)—wound infections, sepsis/septic shock, bust abdomen, prolonged hospital stays, paralytic ileus, puerperal sepsis, and subinvolution
- Operative destructive operations, currently a lost art, may cause complications (2.7%) in form of uterine rupture (2.6–9.1%), PPH (4.5%), cervical or vaginal lacerations (1–3%), and maternal mortality (0–2.7%).
- Psychosocial and economic fallouts—vesicovaginal fistula (VVF) and rectovaginal fistula (RVF) may lead to abandonment, divorce, not able to attend religious and social functions, broken families, poverty, malnutrition, depression, and suicide.

Complication to Baby

- Poor Appearance, Pulse, Grimace, Activity, and Respiration (APGAR) score
- Cerebral palsy due to birth asphyxia
- Birth fractures—clavicle, humerus, or femur
- Brachial plexus injury
- Klumpke's paralysis
- Still birth (38.59%)

RECOMMENDATIONS TO PREVENT OBSTRUCTED LABOR

- Promotion of antenatal care services institutional deliveries
- Proper implementation of maternal healthcare schemes
- Robust referral system linkages
- Comprehensive obstetrical care units
- Good intrapartum care with use of partogram properly
- Early diagnosis and timely interventions for prolonged/protracted labor
- Good communication and transport services between linkage health care units
- Prevention of three delays
- Delivery by trained and skilled birth attendants or obstetricians
- Effective emergency obstetric care services
- Regular drills for development of skilled labor room staff and capacity building.

DIAGNOSIS OF OBSTRUCTED LABOR

- The cases are usually referred from lower health care facilities.
- It is diagnosed by usually by a labor, which is prolonged for more than 24 hours with insurmountable barrier to fetal descent.
- Mother is often dazed, anxious, agitated, prostrated, not able to move and take care of herself due to pain, exhaustion, and dehydration.
- The mother is having tachycardia, tachypnea and hypotension.[2] There may be hyperthermia or hypothermia.
- Bladder is over-distended.
- The uterus feels tonically contracted with a pathological retraction ring known as Bandl's ring, which causes an "hour-glass uterus".
- Fetal heart auscultation or electronic fetal monitoring may reveal fetal bradycardia, variable deceleration or fetal heart sounds may not be heard.

- Features of rupture uterus in form of loss of fetal station, irregular shape of uterus with fetal parts palpable separately and maybe superficially in abdomen.
- There maybe signs of hemoperitoneum.
- The urine output is often decreased.
- Local examination reveals gross vulval edema, significant caput, irreducible molding, edematous cervix and vagina, which may feel hot and dry.
- Cervix is edematous and felt hanging loose over the presenting part like an empty sleeve and vagina is dry, edematous, fragile, and hot. Meconium is often present in liquor, which is usually drained out and foul-smelling discharge maybe present. There maybe retention of after coming head of breech or prolapsed arm maybe felt in neglected transverse lie. Neglected-obstructed labor may present with maternal and fetal death.[3]

MANAGEMENT OF OBSTRUCTED LABOR

- Start IV fluids—normal saline or Ringer lactate using a wide bore cannula.
- Foley's catheterization is done under aseptic conditions. It maybe difficult because urethra is obstructed by engaged baby's head.
- Preparations are made for referral to operation theater.
- IV antibiotics are started as there is prolonged rupture of membranes.
- Fetal destructive operation is safer than abdominal delivery in neglected obstructed labor with fetal demise provided there is no impending uterine rupture.
- Vaginal delivery is often abandoned for more progressive safe methods like lower segment cesarean section, as vaginal operative delivery may cause further maternal or fetal trauma.
- Rarely symphysiotomy maybe performed to alleviate obstruction but there is not much role in modern obstetrics.
- Emergency lower segment cesarean section is planned, which is often challenging and difficult to perform second stage arrest of labor with deeply impacted head.
- The delivery of baby maybe done by shoulder first method during LSCS. This method was introduced by Patwardhan in which delivery of

shoulder is done first, followed by trunk, feet, and lastly head by lifting the baby by legs. It has the advantage of causing less lateral or vertical extension of uterine incisions, bladder injury and neonatal asphyxia.
- If obstetrician is not properly skilled, Erb's palsy maybe caused due to Brachial plexus injury.
- Conventional methods of Push technique in which a second assistant disimpacts the head from vagina and pushes it upward, while the operating obstetrician brings out the head through uterine incision. This is associated with danger of lateral extension of uterine incision into broad ligament or vagina leading to profuse hemorrhage and increased operative time.
- Another technique used is operating obstetrician maneuvering the fingers head and pelvis until finger reach below presenting part, which is lifted upward gently.
- "Pull" or "reverse breech" or "lift out" technique has also been described.
- The obstetrician introduces hand in upper segment of uterus, searches for one fetal leg, brings it down and then other leg is brought done with gentle traction. The two legs are held together and the fetus is gently pulled up and out of uterine incision as in assisted breech delivery.
- Diagnosis of uterine rupture warrants immediate laparotomy with cesarean delivery followed by repair of uterus or hysterectomy as per need.
- Consider putting drains, if there are significant chances of infection but their role remains controversial. It may cause drain site hemorrhage, infection, intestinal perforation, and even visceral herniation from drain site.
- Some patients may need prolonged catheterization for 14 days.
- Good antibiotic cover is given postlaparotomy or LSCS.
- Consider early ambulation and thromboprophylaxis.
- Close maternal and neonatal monitoring is done for development of any complication and their timely treatment.
- Arrange for scheduled follow-up and contraception advice.

- Be vigilant and counsel the patient for development of delayed complications and timely intervention.

CONCLUSION

- Obstructed labor is a preventable obstetric complication, which is an important cause of maternal and fetal morbidity and mortality in developing world.
- Promoting good antenatal and intranatal services with robust referral linkage system and infrastructure development for institutional deliveries can decrease the incidence of obstructed labor.
- Early diagnosis and timely management of obstructed labor can improve maternal and fetal outcomes.

REFERENCES

1. Ayenew AA. Incidence, causes, and materno-fetal outcomes of obstructed labor in Ethiopia: systematic review and meta-analysis. Reprod Health. 2021;18: 61
2. Médecins Sans Frontières. Labor dystocia and malpresentations/Prolonged labor. In: Essential Obstetric and Newborn Care. Geneva: Médecins Sans Frontières; 2019.
3. Merck Manual Professional version; Moldenhauer JS (2020). Uterine rupture [online]. Available from: https://www.msdmanuals.com/en-nz/professional/gynecology-and-obstetrics/abnormalities-and-complications-of-labor-and-delivery/fetal-dystocia. [Last accessed on December 23, 2021]

CHAPTER 13

Abnormal Presentations

Shreya Prabhoo

BREECH

Incidence

The incidence of breech presentation varies with gestational age. Breech presentation at term occurs in 3–4% of pregnancies. As term approaches, the uterine cavity accommodates the fetus best in a longitudinal lie with cephalic presentation. Hence a lower incidence of breech presentation is observed at term **(Fig. 1)**.

Etiology

Various maternal, placental and fetal factors have been suggested which predispose to breech presentation.

- *Maternal:* High parity, polyhydramnios, oligohydramnios, uterine anomalies, e.g., bicornuate uterus, unicornuate uterus, septate uterus and tumors, e.g., uterine or pelvic neoplasm.
- *Placental:* Cornual-fundal insertion of placenta, placenta previa, short umbilical cord.
- *Fetal:* Prematurity, multiple pregnancy, congenital anomalies, and intrauterine fetal death.

Congenital anomalies associated with breech presentation:

- *Central nervous system:* Anencephaly, hydrocephalus, meningomyelocele, meningoencephalocele.
- *Genitourinary system:* Potter's syndrome, polycystic kidney, hydronephrosis.
- *Skeletal system:* Arthrogryposis, achondroplasia, osteogenesis imperfecta.
- *Cardiovascular system:* Patent ductus arteriosus, ventricular septal defect, and hypoplastic left heart.
- *Gastrointestinal system:* Diaphragmatic hernia, esophageal atresia, duodenal atresia, imperforate anus.
- *Chromosomal anomalies:* Down's syndrome, Turner's syndrome, Trisomy 18.

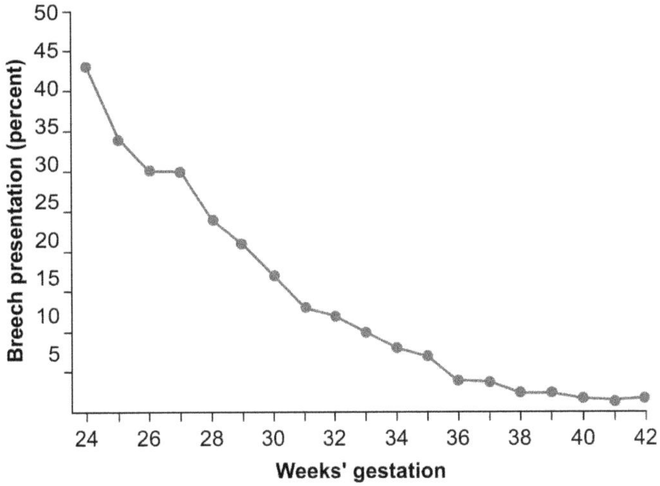

Fig. 1: Incidence of breech at weeks of gestation.

Types (Figs. 2A to C)

There are four types of breech presentations:
1. *Complete breech*: Flexion at hips and knees.
2. *Frank breech:* Flexion at hips and extension at knees.
3. *Footling breech:* Flexion at hips and knees. It can be single or double.
4. *Kneeling breech:* Flexion at hips and flexion at knees. It can be single or double.

Modes of Delivery

- Vaginal delivery
- Cesarean section

Vaginal Breech Delivery (Figs. 3A to C)

There are three methods:
1. *Spontaneous breech delivery:* The baby is expelled entirely by the natural forces of the mother, with no assistance other than support to the baby as it is being born.
2. *Assisted breech delivery:* The baby is delivered by natural forces of the mother up to the umbilicus. Rest of the baby is extracted by the assistant.
3. *Total breech extraction:* The entire baby is extracted by the accoucheur.

Criteria to be considered for vaginal trial in breech presentation:
- Breech with flexed head.
- Gestational age more than 36 weeks.
- Fetal weight > 1.5 kg < 3.0 kg. (All the patients considered in the study who were <1.5 kg and delivered vaginally had come with an intrauterine fetal death or were referred in a state where vaginal delivery was inevitable.)
- Adequate maternal pelvis on clinical pelvimetry.
- Fetal biparietal diameter less than 9.5 cm.
- Zatuchni and Andros breech score of 4 or more.
- No other maternal or fetal indication for cesarean section.
- Facilities for anesthesia, emergency cesarean section, and neonatal resuscitation should be available.

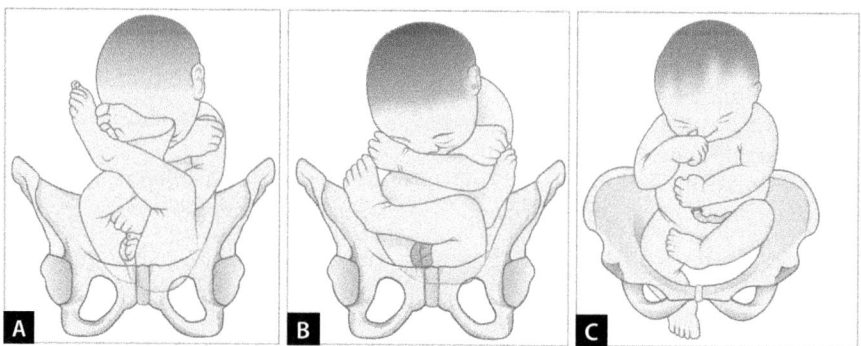

Figs. 2A to C: (A) Frank breech; (B) Complete breech; (C) Footling breech.

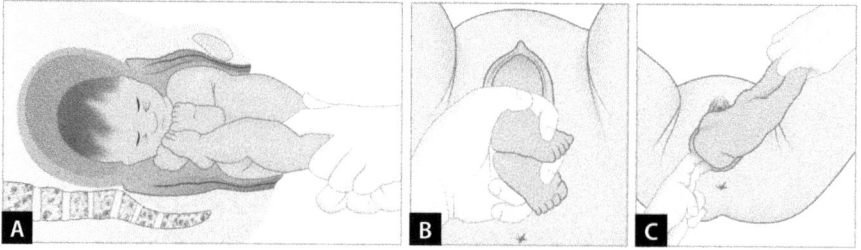

Figs. 3A to C: (A) Total breech extraction by groin traction; (B) Footling extraction; (C) Extraction of upper limbs.

TABLE 1: Zatuchni and Andros breech score*.			
	0 Point	*1 Point*	*2 Points*
Parity	Primigravida	Multipara	
Gestational age	39 weeks or more	38 weeks	37 weeks or less
Estimated fetal weight	> 8 lb	7–8 lb	< 7 lb
Previous breech > 2.5 kg	None	1	2 or more
Cervical dilatation on admission	2 cm or less	3 cm	4 cm or more
Station on admission	-3 or higher	-2	-1 or lower

*It is suggested that a score of 3 or less is an indication for cesarean section.

Breech score of Zatuchni and Andros: The breech score is a numerical summary of several important parameters **(Table 1).**

Role of pelvimetry: A patient might have a difficult vaginal delivery despite pelvimetry proved adequate pelvis. X-ray pelvimetry does not give information about soft tissue compliance.[1] Pelvic diameters are not rigid and both transverse and anterior-posterior measurements increase in 28% of the women between the supine and squatting positions.[2] Hence X-ray pelvimetry is unable to detect the actual pelvic diameters in labor.

Role of ultrasonography: Ultrasonography has a very important role to play in management of breech presentation. Besides confirming the presentation, it also detects the number of fetuses, site of placenta, congenital anomalies, biparietal diameter and estimated fetal weight. It can also detect extension of fetal head.

Mechanism of labor in breech presentation:
- *Descent:* With good uterine activity engagement occurs with bitrochanteric diameter in the right oblique diameter of the maternal pelvis. Since breech is poor dilator as compared to the head, the descent is slow.
- *Flexion:* Lateral flexion takes place at the waist and the anterior hip becomes the leading part.
- *Internal rotation of breech:* Anterior hip meets the resistance of the pelvic floor and rotates downward forward and toward the midline. The bitrochanteric diameter rotates 45° from the right oblique diameter of the pelvis to the anteroposterior diameter.
- *Birth of buttocks by lateral flexion:* The anterior hip impinges under the pubic symphysis,

lateral flexion occurs and posterior hip is born over the perineum. Buttocks then fall toward the maternal anus and anterior hip slips out under the symphysis pubis.
- *Engagement of shoulder:* Engagement of shoulders takes place in the right oblique diameter of the maternal pelvis.
- *Internal rotation of shoulder:* Anterior shoulder rotates under the symphysis and the bisacromial diameter turns 45° from the right oblique diameter to the anteroposterior diameter of the outlet. The sacrum turns from right sacral anterior (RSA) to right sacral transverse (RST) toward the right maternal thigh.
- *Birth of shoulders by lateral flexion:* Anterior shoulders impinge under the symphysis and the posterior shoulders and arm are born over the perineum as the baby's body is lifted upward.
- *Descent and engagement of head:* Head enters the pelvis with the sagittal suture in the left oblique diameter.
- Flexion occurs.
- *Internal rotation:* Head strikes the pelvic floor and rotates internally so that sagittal suture comes in the anteroposterior diameter of the pelvis. Occiput comes under the symphysis. Back is anterior.
- *Birth of head by flexion:* Nape of the neck pivots under the symphysis and the chin, mouth, nose, forehead, bregma and occiput are born over the perineum by a movement of flexion.

Assisted Breech Delivery (Figs. 4A to F)
Delivery of breech:
- The patients are encouraged to bear down with contractions but must rest between them.

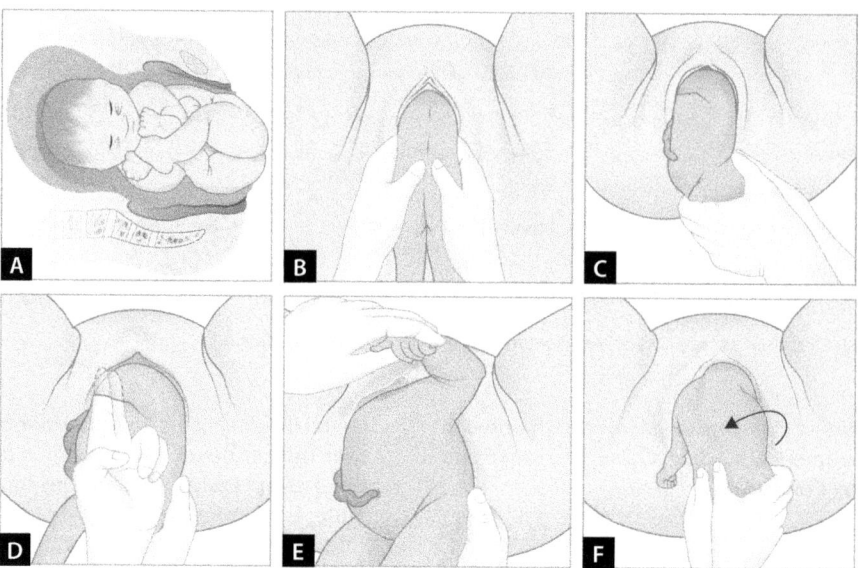

Figs. 4A to F: Assisted breech delivery.

- When the buttocks are ready to crown, a wide mediolateral episiotomy is made and hemostasis secured.
- As long as there is no fetal or maternal distress spontaneous delivery up to umbilicus is awaited, the operator should not interfere.
- Once the umbilicus has delivered, time becomes an important factor and remainder of the birth is expedited gently and skillfully.
- The obstetrician has 10 minutes to complete the delivery after birth of umbilicus to avoid anoxic brain damage.
- The legs usually deliver spontaneously.
- The baby is covered with warm towel and the body is supported, a loop of the umbilical cord is pulled down to minimize the traction on it in case it is caught between the head and the pelvic wall at the same time it is palpated for pulsation.
- The back should be kept anterior.
- If there is arrest at any state, the remainder of the breech is extracted.

Delivery of extended arm:
- Classical method:
  - Body of the baby is grasped by pelvic girdle
  - Gentle downward traction given and trunk is rotated, so as to make the inferior end of anterior scapula visible under the pubic arch and to place the posterior shoulder in sacral hollow.
  - Hand is introduced along the curve of sacrum along the back of posterior shoulder until the antecubital fossa of the posterior arm is reached.
  - With firm pressure on humerus the arm is pushed down over the child's face and delivered from the anterior aspect.
  - While trunk is depressed downward toward the perineum.
  - If this fails the body of the baby is rotated to make the anterior arm posterior and the arm is then disengaged in a similar manner.
- Lovset's maneuver **(Fig. 5)**:
  - The baby is lifted slightly to cause lateral flexion.
  - The trunk is then rotated through 180° keeping the back anterior and maintaining a downward traction.
  - This will bring the posterior arm under the symphysis pubis, which is then delivered.
  - The trunk is then rotated in the reverse direction keeping the back anterior to deliver the anterior shoulder under the symphysis pubis.

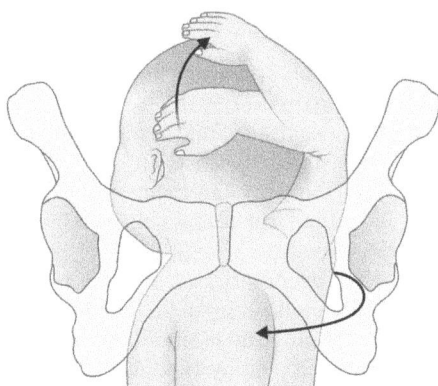

Fig. 5: Lovset's maneuver.

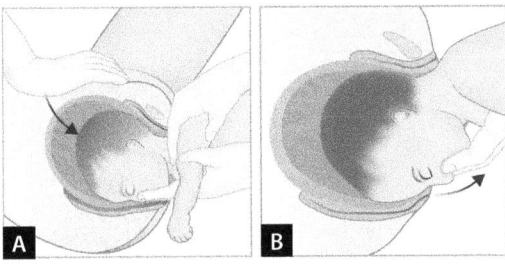

Figs. 6A and B: Mauriceau–Smellie–Veit maneuver.

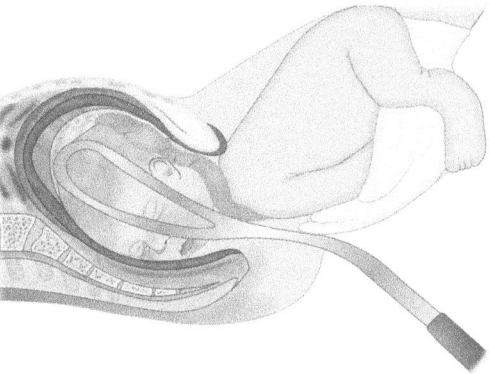

Fig. 7: Piper's forceps delivery.

Delivery of the after coming head:
- Burns Marshall maneuver:
  - The baby is allowed to hang by its own weight.
  - The assistant is asked to give suprapubic pressure in downward and backward direction toward the sinciput.
  - When the nape of the neck is visible under the pubic arch, the baby is grasped by the ankles with a finger in between the two.
  - Maintaining a steady traction and forming a wide arc of a circle, the trunk is swung in upward and forward direction.
  - When the mouth is cleared off the vulva, the trunk is depressed to deliver rest of the head.
- Mauriceau–Smellie-Veit maneuver **(Figs. 6A and B):**
  - The body of the baby rests upon the palm of the operator's hand and forearm.
  - The middle finger and index finger of the same hand is placed over the maxilla so as to maintain flexion.
  - Two fingers of the operator's other hand are hooked over the fetal neck and grasping the shoulders, downward traction is applied until nape of the neck is seen under the symphysis.
  - The body of the baby is then elevated toward the mother's abdomen and the chin, mouth nose, brow and occiput emerge successively over the perineum.
  - Gentle suprapubic pressure is given simultaneously by and assistant to keep the head flexed.

- Piper's forceps on the after coming head **(Fig. 7):**
  - Baby's feet are grasped by an assistant and body is raised.
  - A folded towel can be used to raise the body.
  - Right hand is placed in the vagina and the left forceps blade is guided into the place over the parietal bone.
  - The right blade is then applied using the left hand as a guide.
  - The forceps blades are applied along the occipitomental diameter.
  - Traction is given and head is extracted slowly.
  - Munro-Kerr advocated application of piper's forceps as the most reliable method for delivery of after coming head of the breech.
  - Forceps exert traction directly on the head, so damage to the structure in the neck is avoided.
  - Decompression of the head is controlled in forceps delivery.

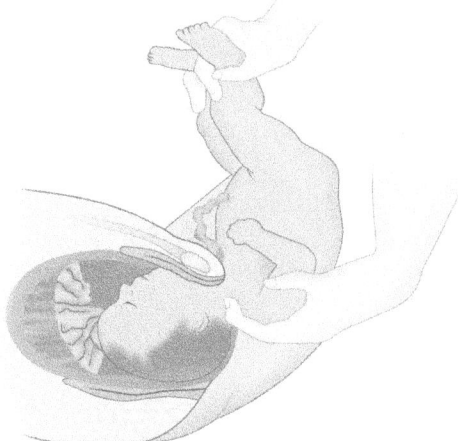

Fig. 8: Prague maneuver.

- Wigand–Martin maneuver:
  - The body of the baby is placed on the arm of the operator, with the middle finger of the hand of that arm place in the baby's mouth and index and ring fingers on the malar bones, so as to maintain flexion.
  - With the other hand suprapubic pressure is exerted on the head.
- Prague maneuver (**Fig. 8**):
  - This maneuver was recommended by Kiwisch (1846) who practised in Prague.
  - This is used when back of the fetus fails to rotate anteriorly.
  - In this, maneuver fingers are placed over shoulders and outward and upward traction is made.
  - The legs are grasped with the other hand and the baby is swung over the mother's abdomen.
  - By this procedure occiput is born over the perineum.
  - Since this procedure carries with it the risk of overstretching or breaking the neck of the infant, it is rarely used.
- Modified Prague maneuver/Van Hoorn's method:
  - This is used if occiput has not engaged in the pelvis, it is combined with pressure on the forehead from outside.
  - This pressure should accomplish most of the work.
  - The child is lifted up over the pubis to which its chest applies, and thus the

occiput comes to hollow of sacrum the physician flexes the head and Mauriceau method is performed in reverse.
- Kristeller maneuver:
  - Body is raised gently so that there is slight extension at the neck.
  - With the other hand, suprapubic pressure is exerted and head is delivered by flexion.
- Bracht maneuver:
  - The breech is allowed to deliver spontaneously up to the umbilicus.
  - The fetal body is then held against the maternal symphysis pubis.
  - The suspension of the fetus in this position along with the uterine.
  - Activity and moderate suprapubic pressure results in a spontaneous delivery
- Pinard maneuver (**Figs. 9A and B**):
  - Pinard maneuver is used to convert the frank breech into a footling breech.
  - This aids in bringing the fetal feet within reach of the operator.
  - The procedure is performed under anesthesia.
  - Two fingers of one hand are carried up along the thigh of one extremity until the popliteal fossa is reached.
  - Popliteal fossa is pressed and abducted.
  - Spontaneous flexion usually follows and the foot of the fetus is felt to impinge upon the back of the hand.
  - The fetal foot then may be grasped and brought down.
  - The other leg is similarly brought down.
  - Delivery is usually completed by breech extraction.

This procedure is rarely used in modern obstetrics. It may be justified in the following situations:
- Delivery of a breech/transverse lies of the second baby in twins
- Fetus in a transverse lie and facility for cesarean is not available
- Transverse lie with intrauterine fetal death

Indications for cesarean section for breech presentation:
- Large baby
- Contracted or borderline pelvis
- Hyperextended fetal head
- Footling or kneeling breech
- Preterm breech

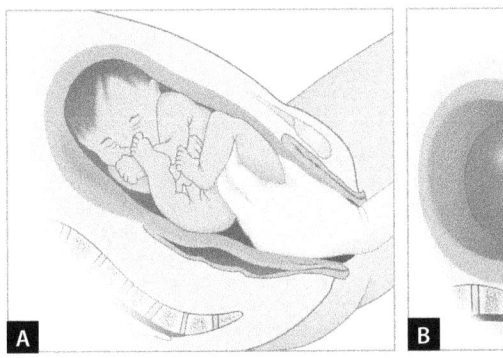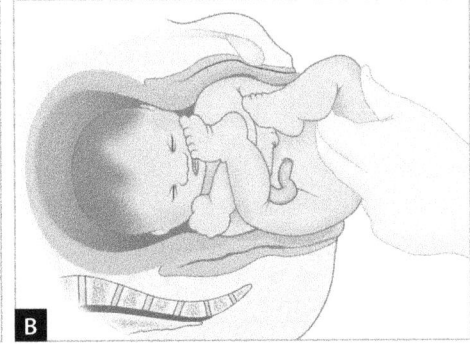

Figs. 9A and B: Role of internal podalic version and breech extraction.

- Low birth weight breech
- Bad obstetric history
- Placenta previa
- Previous cesarean section
- Infertility
- Associated medical problems
- Uterine dysfunction
- Primigravida with breech presentation, baby weight > 3 kg

EXTERNAL CEPHALIC VERSION

Definition

External cephalic version is the transabdominal manipulation of a noncephalic presenting fetus into a cephalic presentation.
- This has been practiced since the time of Hippocrates.
- With the decreasing morbidity of cesarean sections, this technique is practice to a lesser extent.
- Currently with the advent of ultrasonography, electronic fetal monitoring, and tocolysis, there is a renewed interest in this procedure.

Prerequisites

- Single fetus without any gross malformations
- Adequate liquor
- Gestational age more than 26 weeks
- Unengaged breech
- No cephalopelvic disproportion
- Nontender and relaxed uterus
- Facilities for electronic fetal monitoring and ultrasonography

- Facilities for immediate cesarean section
- Absence of any other obstetric contraindication
- Experienced obstetrician

Complication

- Abruptio placentae
- Preterm labor
- Premature rupture of membranes
- Fetomaternal hemorrhage and isoimmunization
- Fetal distress
- Uterine rupture
- Intrauterine fetal death

Contraindication

- *Absolute*
  - Placenta previa
  - Multiple gestations.
  - Vaginal bleeding in the 3rd trimester
  - Oligohydramnios
  - Cephalopelvic disproportion
  - Presence of uterine anomalies
  - Preterm labor
  - Deep engagement of the breech
  - Pre-eclampsia
- *Relative*
  - Previous cesarean section
  - Uteroplacental insufficiency

Transverse Lie (Figs. 10A to D)

Fetus is said to be in transverse lie when the fetal axis is at 90° to the maternal spine. When the axis is at an acute angle it is called as an oblique lie.

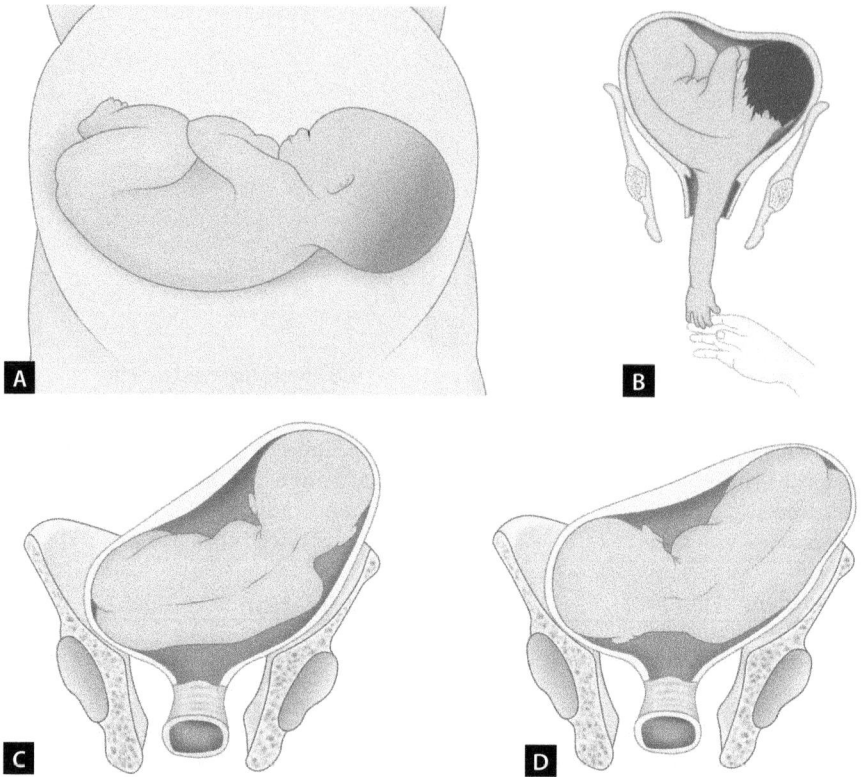

Figs. 10A to D: (A) Transverse lie; (B) Hand prolapse; (C) Breech in iliac fossa; (D) Head on in iliac fossa.

- Oblique lie is an unstable lie and either converts to a transverse lie or vertical when labor starts.
- The position of the shoulder is usually over the pelvic inlet.
- The head is felt one iliac fossa, and breech in the other.
- The maternal side on which the shoulder (acromion) rests determines the lie as right or left.
- Further the back may lie in anterior (dorsoanterior), posterior (dorsoposterior), superior (dorsosuperior) and inferior (dorsoinferior).
- The incidence is around 1:500, it is higher before term (around 1 in 50 at 32 weeks of gestation).[3]

Etiology

The common causes of transverse lie are:
- Laxed abdominal wall from high parity
- Preterm fetus
- Placenta previa
- Uterine anomaly
- Polyhydramnios
- Contracted pelvis

Diagnosis

A transverse lie usually can be recognized easily by inspection alone:
- The abdomen is wider than usual
- The uterine fundus is felt slightly above the umbilicus.

Palpation:
- The fetal pole is not detected in the lower part of the uterus.
- The head is ballotable on one side and the breech in the opposite iliac fossa.
- The back is felt anterior as a hard board like plane extending across the front of the abdomen.
- When the back is posterior, we can feel the limbs as nodular parts.

On vaginal examination the ribs, scapula, clavicle can be felt distinctly. The side on which the axilla is felt indicates the side toward which the fetal shoulder is directed.

Mechanism of labor:
- It is impossible to deliver a fetus vaginally in case of a persistent transverse lie.
- If labor continues and membranes rupture, the fetal shoulder may be forced into the pelvis, and the arm very frequently prolapses.
- If the labor is allowed to continue the shoulder gets arrested at the margins of the pelvic inlet, with the head lying in one iliac fossa and breech in another, the shoulder then gets impacted at the inlet.
- This frequently leads to hyperactivity in the uterus and results in a retraction ring which becomes more marked with time.
- This situation if neglected results in uterine rupture.
- Morbidity also increases because of the higher incidence of placenta previa and chances of cord prolapse which warrant immediate operative intervention.

Vaginal delivery is possible only:
- In cases of a wide pelvis with a very small fetus < 800 g in a transverse lie
- The fetus doubles up on itself (conduplicato corpore)
- The thorax is felt below the shoulder and appears at the vulva
- The head and thorax together pass through the pelvic cavity

Management
- Fetus in transverse lie in active labor is an indication for a cesarean section
- But prior to the commencement of labor, attempt can be made at external cephalic version if there is no other obstetric or maternal contraindication
- If the external cephalic version is successful it is advocated to induce labor so that the head fixes
- In case of a cesarean section, at times a delivery becomes difficult if the limbs are not felt, in such cases especially in dorsoanterior, it is recommended to take a vertical incision on the uterus

Brow Presentation (Figs. 11A to D)
The fetus is said to be in the brow presentation when the leading part of the fetal head is the area between the orbital ridges and the anterior fontanelle.
- The neck of the fetus in brow presentation is not extended as much as in face presentation.
- It is considered as the rarest malpresentation with a prevalence of 1 in 500 to 1 in 4,000 deliveries.[4]
- The fetal head is midway between full flexion (occiput) and extension (face).

Etiology
- The causes of a persistent brow presentation are same as the causes for face presentation.
- But brow presentation is usually unstable and often converts to an occiput or face presentation.[5]

Diagnosis
- The brow presentation can be diagnosed by abdominal palpation when we can palpate both the occiput and chin
- Vaginal examination is necessary to confirm the findings
- The parts felt on vaginal examination are the large anterior fontanelle, frontal sutures, orbital ridges, the root of the nose and eyes but the mouth or the chin are not palpable.

Mechanism of Labor
- Labor in a brow presentation is possible only if the fetus is very small fetus and the pelvis is roomy, but if the fetus is bigger, a vaginal delivery is very difficult.
- This is because the engaging diameter of the fetal head is the occipitomental (mentovertical) which is the longest diameter of the fetal skull (14 cm) and is the distance between the tip of the chin and midpoint between the fontanelles.
- The engagement is impossible until there is extreme molding which shortens this diameter or if the head undergoes flexion to attain an occiput presentation or extends completely to a face presentation.
- This extreme molding deforms the head.

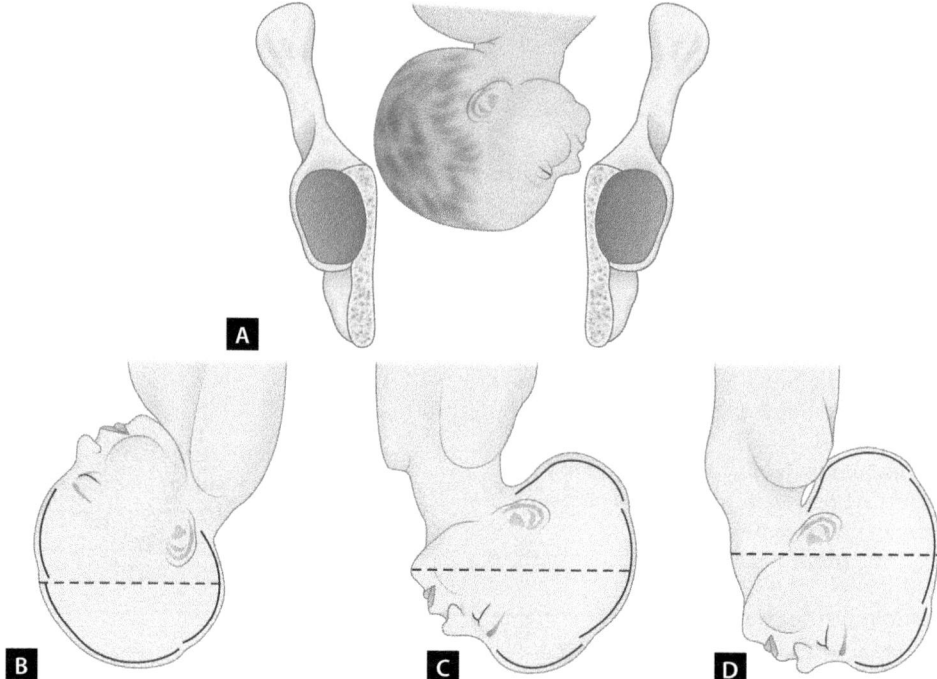

Figs. 11A to D: Brow presentation.

- The caput succedaneum is seen over the forehead, which makes the identification of brow difficult.
- In primary brow presentations, the outcome depends on the final presentation.
- Persistent brow presentation is a contra-indication for a vaginal delivery.

Face Presentation

Face presentation is a rare obstetric event where the fetus is in a longitudinal lie, fetal head is fully extended on the neck, and the occiput is abutting against the upper back.

- The fetal face may present with the chin (mentum) anteriorly or posteriorly, relative to the maternal symphysis pubis.
- Face presentation occurs in 0.1–0.2% of deliveries.[6]

Predisposing Factors

Any factor that favors extension and prevents flexion of the head results in a brow or face presentation.

The following risk factors predispose around 60% of face presentations:

- Fetopelvic disproportion either due to contracted pelvis or large fetus
- Small fetus
- High parity (due to pendulous abdomen)
- Polyhydramnios
- Multiple pregnancies
- Coils of cord around the neck
- Uterine or nuchal cord anomaly
- Enlargement of the neck
- Anenchephaly.

But 40% of face presentations occur with none of these above factors.[7]

Diagnosis

- Face presentation is diagnosed by vaginal examination and palpation of facial features.
- It is possible to mistake a breech for a face presentation as the anus can be mistaken for the mouth and ischial tuberosities for the malar prominences.
- Newborn infants with face presentation usually have severe facial edema, facial

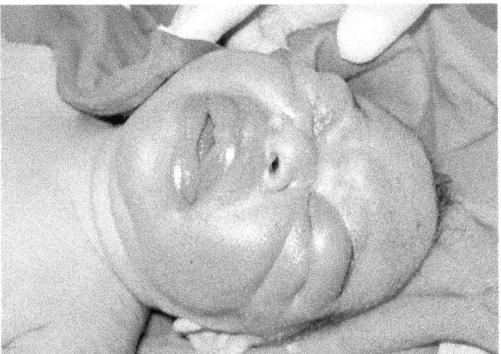

Fig. 12: Facial edema.

bruising or ecchymosis and damage to the eyes due to repeated vaginal examination to assess the presenting part and the progress of labor **(Figs. 12 and 13)**.[8]

Mechanism of Labor (Fig. 14)

- The engaging diameter of the fetal skull is submentobregmatic which is measured from the center of the bregma to the angle of the mandible, measuring 9.5 cm.
- Face presentations very rarely deliver vaginally. More than half of the cases are delivered by cesarean section.[9]
- A vaginal birth in a fetus with face presentation at term is possible only if the fetus is in the mentum anterior position.
- The mechanism of labor consists of the cardinal movements of descent, extension, internal rotation, flexion, extension and external rotation.
  - *Descent* is brought about by the mechanism same as in cephalic presentations.
  - *Extension* is due to the relation of the fetal body to the deflected head. When resistance is encountered, the occiput is pushed toward the back of the fetus while the chin descends.
  - *Internal rotation* of the face brings the chin under the symphysis pubis. In this way the neck can traverse the posterior surface of the symphysis pubis (mentum anterior). If the chin rotates posteriorly (mentum posterior), the relatively short neck cannot span the anterior surface of the sacrum, which measures about 12 cm in length.

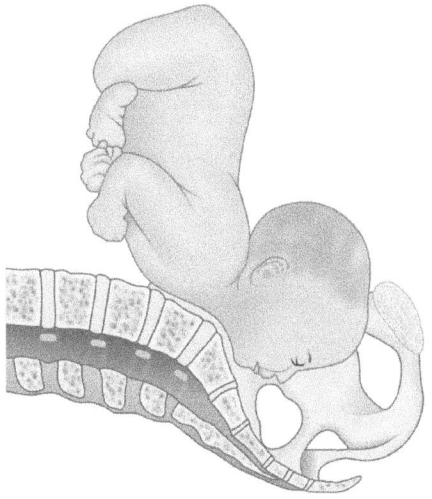

Fig. 13: Mento posterior position.

- *Flexion:*
  - The fetal brow (bregma) abuts against the maternal symphysis pubis followed by *flexion* which is necessary to negotiate the birth canal.
  - Hence, birth of a fetus in a mentum posterior position is not possible unless the shoulders enter the pelvis at the same time, which is possible only when the fetus is extremely small or macerated.
  - Following the anterior rotation and descent the chin and mouth appear at the vulva, the inferior surface of the chin hooks on the symphysis, and the head is delivered by flexion.
  - The nose, eyes, brow (bregma), and occiput then appear in succession over the anterior margin of the perineum.
  - After birth of the head, the occiput sags backward toward the anus.
  - The chin then rotates externally to the side toward which it was directed at the start, and the shoulders are born by the same mechanism as in cephalic presentations.

Edema may sometimes distort the face significantly and the skull undergoes considerable molding, which is manifested by an increase in the occipitomental diameter of the head.

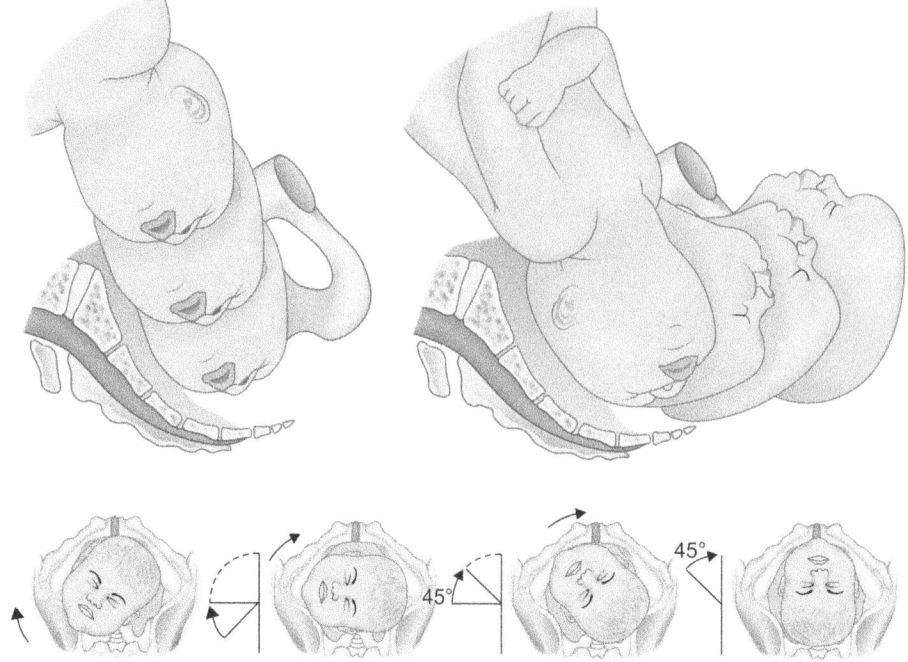

Fig. 14: Mechanism of labor.

Since face presentations are commonly seen in patients with pelvic contraction, attempt for a vaginal delivery should be made with caution. Attempts to manually convert face presentation to vertex, manual or forceps rotation of the persistent posterior chin to anterior are contraindicated as they can be dangerous.

OCCIPITOPOSTERIOR POSITION

Definition

The fetus is said to be in an occipitoposterior position when the fetal back is directed posteriorly and the occiput is directed toward the sacrum or the iliac fossa.

It is seen in about 10% of patients at the onset of labor. Right occipitoposterior (ROP) is more common than the left occipitoposterior (LOP) position because (**Figs. 15A to C**):
- The left oblique diameter is reduced by the presence of sigmoid colon
- The right oblique diameter is slightly longer than the left one
- Dextrorotation of the uterus favors occipitoposterior in ROP position

Etiology
- Anthropoid and android pelvises predispose an OP position due to a narrow fore-pelvis
- Maternal kyphosis
- Anterior placenta[10]
- Placenta previa
- Pelvic tumors
- Multiple pregnancy
- Pendulous abdomen
- Polyhydramnios[11]

Diagnosis

On inspection the abdomen looks flattened below the umbilicus, fetal movements are more in the midline.

On abdominal examination:
- In antenatal period mostly the head is not engaged due to deflexion
- The fetal limbs are easily felt on the anterior abdomen on either side of the midline
- The fetal heart is heard in the flank away from the midline

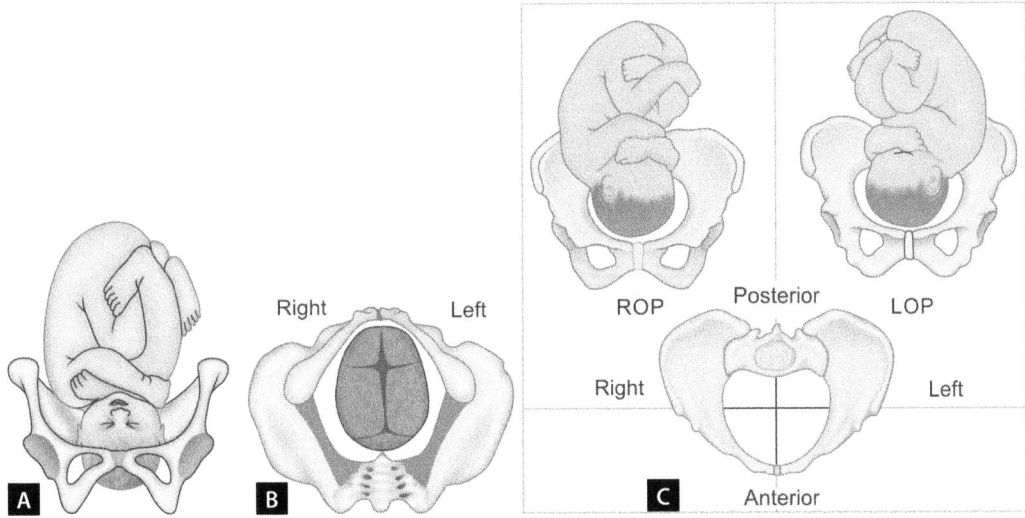

Figs. 15A to C: (A) Fetal occipitoposterior (OP) position; (B and C) Right and left occipitoposterior positions.

- During labor on vaginal examination, the degree of deflexion and the direction of the occiput can be determined

Mechanism of Labor (Fig. 16)

- In most of the occiput posterior presentations, the mechanism of labor is identical to that of the anterior occipital positions, except that in posterior positions the occiput has to internally rotate to the symphysis pubis through 135 degrees.
- A certain degree of deflexion is due to the opposition of the fetal convexity and convexity of maternal lumbar spine.
- The longer biparietal diameter (9.5 cm) enters the narrow sacrocotyloid diameter (9 cm) while the shorter bitemporal diameter (8 cm) enters the longer oblique diameter (12 cm).
- As a result of this the occipitofrontal diameter 11.5 cm enters the pelvis leading to delayed engagement.

Normal Mechanism (90%)

- Deflexion is corrected and complete flexion occurs.
- The occiput meets the pelvic floor first, long anterior rotation 3/8 circle occurs bringing the occiput anteriorly and the fetus is delivered normally.

Abnormal Mechanism (10%)

Incomplete forward rotation (1%): The occiput rotates 1/8 circle anteriorly and then the head gets arrested in the transverse diameter causing deep transverse arrest.

Nonrotation (3%): The occiput and sinciput meet the pelvic floor simultaneously, no internal rotation and the head persists in the oblique diameter causing persistent occipitoposterior position.

   In both these conditions spontaneous vaginal delivery is not possible and needs instrumental delivery.

Posterior rotation (6%): The sinciput meets the pelvic floor first, rotates 1/8 circle posteriorly and the occiput becomes direct posterior and the fetus is born face to pubis provided the pelvis is wide. Perineal injury is very common due to overstretching by the large occipitofrontal diameter (11.5 cm).

   Factors like well flexed head, good uterine activity, wide roomy pelvis, and intact membranes favor anterior rotation along the long axis.

   Methods of delivery in deep transverse arrest (1%) and persistent occipitoposterior (3%):

- *Vacuum rotation and vacuum extraction (ventouse):* Proper application of the ventouse as close to the occiput as possible will promote flexion of the head, then a gentle traction with

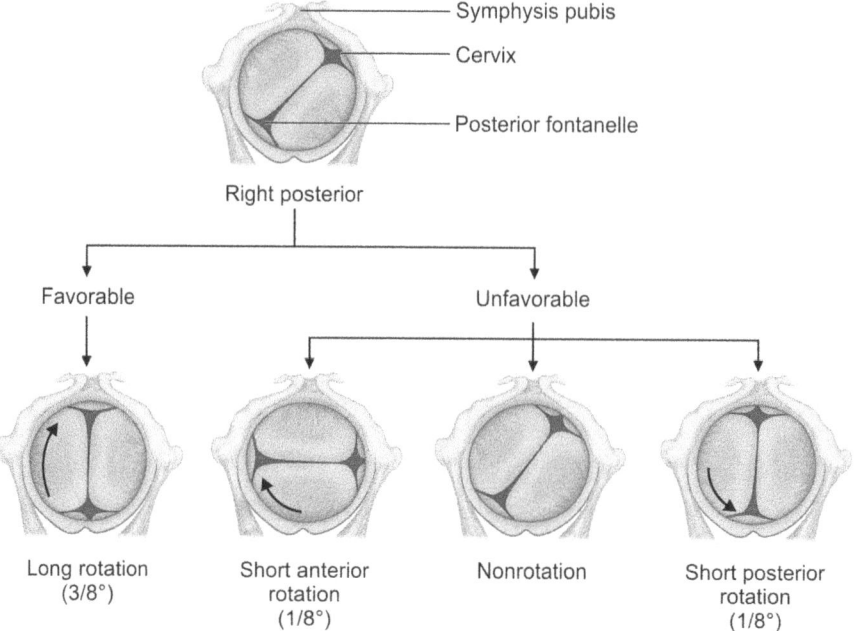

Fig. 16: Diagrammatic representation showing favorable and unfavorable rotation of occipitoposterior position.

contraction simultaneously rotating the head can bring about delivery.

- *Manual rotation and forceps extraction:* Under suitable anesthesia (general or Pudendal block)
  - Full hand method **(Fig. 17):**
    - *Disimpaction and flexion:* The head is held by the bitemporal diameter and disimpacted by pushing it slightly upward and then flexed.
    - *Rotation of the occiput anteriorly:* The rotation by the right hand vaginally is aided by, rotation of the anterior shoulder abdominally toward the middle line by the left hand or an assistant.
    - *Extraction:* Once the head is rotated the head is fixed by an assistant and then extracted with the help of forceps.
  - *Half hand method (Fig. 18):* The hand is placed in the posterior fornix and pressure is applied on the head in the direction to get the occiput anterior.
- Forceps rotation and forceps extraction:
  - *Kielland's forceps:* It has a minimal pelvic curve so single application is needed for rotation and extraction of the head.

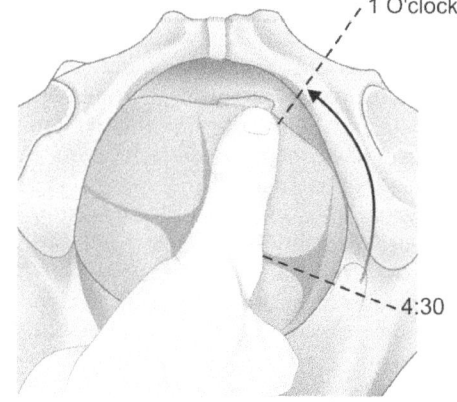

Fig. 17: Full hand method.

  - *Barton's forceps:* This forceps was originally designed for deep transverse arrest. It has a hinge in one of the blades between the blade proper and the shank to facilitate its application. The angle between the handle and the blades is 55° which is the angle between the pelvic inlet and the outlet. This forceps is used for rotation and then extraction as it has an axis traction device.

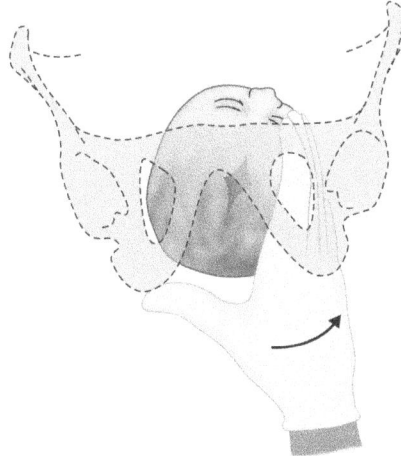

Fig. 18: Half hand method.

– *Scanzoni double application*: Here the conventional forceps is applied along the pelvic curve and rotated till the occiput is anterior, then the forceps is removed and reapplied so that it maintains the correct pelvic curve and head is extracted. This method is no longer used as it is traumatic to the mother and fetus.

• *Cesarean section:* It is indicated when the above methods fail, or there are contraindications to instrumental delivery such as contracted pelvis, placenta previa, cord prolapse, previous cesarean scar.

• *Craniotomy:* It can be done if the fetus is dead.

Though all these methods are available, the methods used in modern obstetrics are vacuum extraction and cesarean section.

REFERENCES

1. Varner MW, Cruikshank DP, Laube DW. X-ray pelvimetry in clinical obstetrics. Obstet Gynecol. 1980;56:296-300.
2. Russell JGB. Moulding of the pelvic outlet. J Obstet Gynecol Br Common W. 1969;76:817.
3. Posner G, Black A, Jones G, Dy J. Oxorn-Foote Human Labor and Birth, 6th edition. New York: McGraw-Hill Education/Medical; 2013.
4. Zayed F, Amarin Z, Obeidat B, Obeidat N, Alchalabi H, Lataifeh I. Face and brow presentation in northern Jordan, over a decade of experience. Arch Gynecol Obstet. 2008; 278(5):427-30.
5. Cruikshank DP, White CA. Obstetric mal-presentations: twenty years' experience. Am J Obstet Gynecol. 1973;116:1097.
6. Julien S, Lockwood CJ, Barss VA. Face and brow presentations in labor. Up to date. 2014.
7. Bashiri A, Burstein E, Bar-David J, Levy A, Mazor M. Face and brow presentation: independent risk factors. J Maternal-Fetal Neo Med. 2008;21(6):357-60.
8. Cunningham FG, Leveno JK, Bloom SL. Williams Obstetrics, 24th edition. New York: McGraw-Hill; 2014. pp. 466-7.
9. Gardberg M, Leonova Y, Laakkonen E. Malpresentations—impact on mode of delivery. Acta Obstet Gynecol Scand. 2011; 90(5):540-2.
10. Gardberg M, Tuppurainen M. Anterior placental location predisposes for occiput posterior presentation near term. Acta Obstet Gynecol Scand. 1944;73:151.
11. Cunningham FG, Leveno JK, Bloom SL. Williams Obstetrics, 24th edition (For images only). New York: McGraw-Hill; 2014.

Charmila Ayyavoo, Jayam Kannan

HAND PROLAPSE

Definition

If the hand is the first part of the fetus's body to emerge during childbirth, it is termed as hand prolapse.

Classification

Hand prolapse can happen as a part of fetal malpresentation which may be as shown in **Table 1**.[1]

Diagnosis

- On per abdominal examination, the fetus can be in transverse lie or in longitudinal lie.
- Per vaginal (PV) examination is to be done only after an ultrasound is done to rule out a placenta previa.
- In PV, the hand can be felt inside the vagina and sometimes seen outside the introitus. In an arm prolapse, hands can be shaken to identify whether it is the right or left arm.
- It is mandatory to rule out an associated cord prolapse in hand prolapse.

Management (Flowchart 1)

Ultrasound is done to identify whether the presenting part with the hand is the head, breech, or transverse lie and to rule out placenta previa, fibroid uterus, and fetal malformations.

Conclusion

Premature prolapse of fetal limbs before labor or during labor is very rare now-a-days because of optimum antenatal care in many centers with timely ultrasounds to diagnose fetal malpresentations when there is a clinical suspicion. Care is needed when dealing with prematurity, prematurely rupture membranes, polyhydramnios, masses, multiparous women, and twin pregnancy.

CORD PROLAPSE

Definition

The umbilical cord of the fetus is felt below the presenting part after the membranes have ruptured. The cord can be felt in the vagina or seen lying outside the vulva.

Classification[2]

Classification of cord prolapse has been described in **Table 2**.

Diagnosis

- It is done by vaginal examination. The membranes are absent and the cord can be felt

TABLE 1: Classification of hand prolapse.	
Type 1	*Type 2*
Transverse lie of the fetus	Compound presentation: It is associated with different combinations
	Cephalic presentation with prolapse of: • Upper limb (arm–hand), one or both • Lower limb (leg–foot), one or both • Arm and leg together
	Breech presentation with prolapse of the hand or arm

Flowchart 1: Management of hand prolapse.

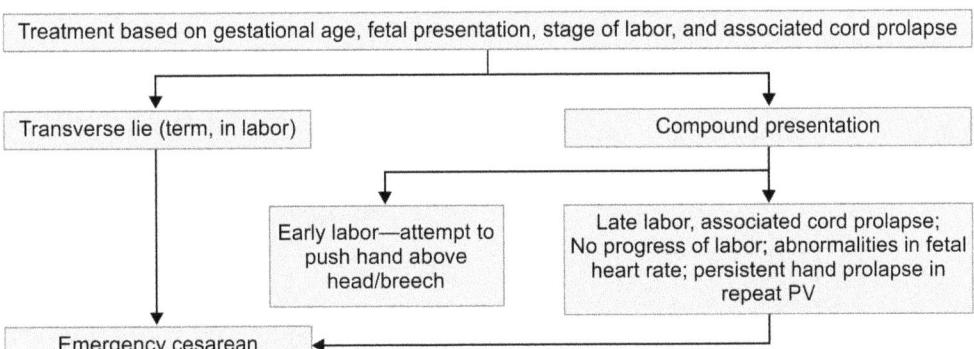

TABLE 2: Classification of cord prolapse.	
Type	**Presentation**
Cord presentation	The cord is palpated along the presenting part or below and the membranes are intact
Occult cord prolapse	After the rupture of the membranes, the cord can be felt alongside the presenting part of the fetus
Overt cord prolapse	The cord is seen below the presenting part and can be seen lying inside the vagina or outside the introitus

by the side of the presenting part. It should be palpated for cord pulsations.

- Cord prolapse is suspected, if there is sudden fetal bradycardia or there are variable decelerations after the membranes have ruptured.
- Occult cord prolapse is difficult to diagnose but must be looked for when there is a suspicion.

Management (Flowchart 2)

Cord prolapse is an emergency. Check for cord pulsations. If it is present, the baby is delivered at the earliest time possible as diagnosis to delivery time is very important.

Conclusion

Preventive measures to reduce the incidence of cord prolapse should be followed. After membranes rupture in preterm labor pains, polyhydramnios and malpresentations, cord prolapse is checked for. Artificial rupture of membranes (ARM) should be performed with care in floating head and polyhydramnios. Controlled ARM is practiced. Disengagement of the head with

subsequent cord prolapse can happen in vaginal procedures. This should be avoided.

▓ DEEP TRANSVERSE ARREST

Definition

It is the arrest of labor when the vertex of the fetus does not rotate after the occipitotransverse position and does not descend below the level of the ischial spines when there are optimum uterine contractions for at least one hour.

Causes

- *Abnormal position of the fetus:* Occipitoposterior position
- *Variations in the pelvis:* Android pelvis, anthropoid pelvis
- Cephalopelvic disproportion

Diagnosis[2]

- Fully dilated cervix
- Vertex at the level of ischial spines
- Sagittal suture in the transverse diameter of the pelvis

Flowchart 2: Management of cord prolapse.

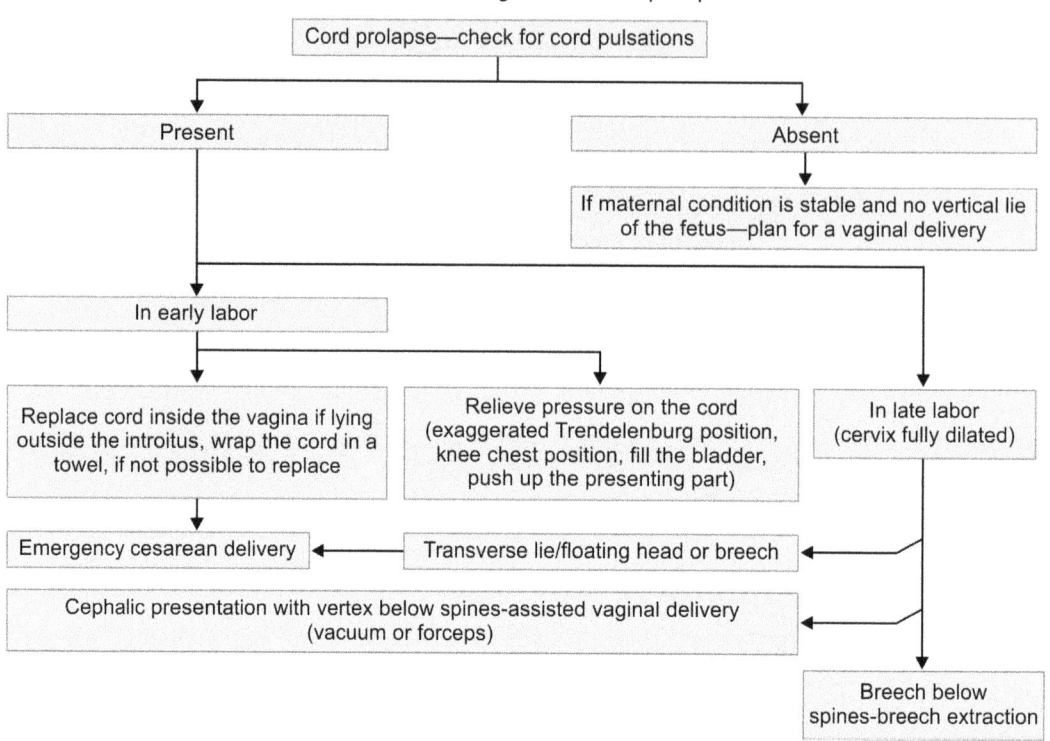

- Optimum uterine contractions
- No descent of vertex for 1 hour

Management

Care is needed, if the baby is in the occipito-posterior position.

If deep transverse arrest is diagnosed, cesarean section is the management.[3]

Conclusion

Poor uterine contractions, epidural analgesia, big-sized baby, and fault in the flexion of the head will contribute to deep transverse arrest. Effective contractions of the uterus are maintained to avoid the problem.

▣ IMPENDING UTERINE RUPTURE

Definition

The appearance of symptoms and signs of disruption of the layers of the uterine wall in a nonsurgical setting in a pregnant uterus is impending uterine rupture.

TABLE 3: Classification of uterine rupture.

Type	Presentation
Primary rupture	Rupture occurs in an unscarred uterus
Secondary rupture	Rupture occurs in a uterus with a scar

Classification

Classified as primary uterine rupture and secondary uterine rupture (**Table 3**).[3]

Diagnosis

- Fetal changes:
    - The most common and initial clinical presentation is a change in the fetal heart rate pattern.
    - There may be a loss of fetal station and the head retracts back.
- Maternal changes:
    - May be the onset of acute vaginal bleeding, constant abdominal pain, uterine tenderness, change in uterine shape,

Flowchart 3: Management of uterine rupture.

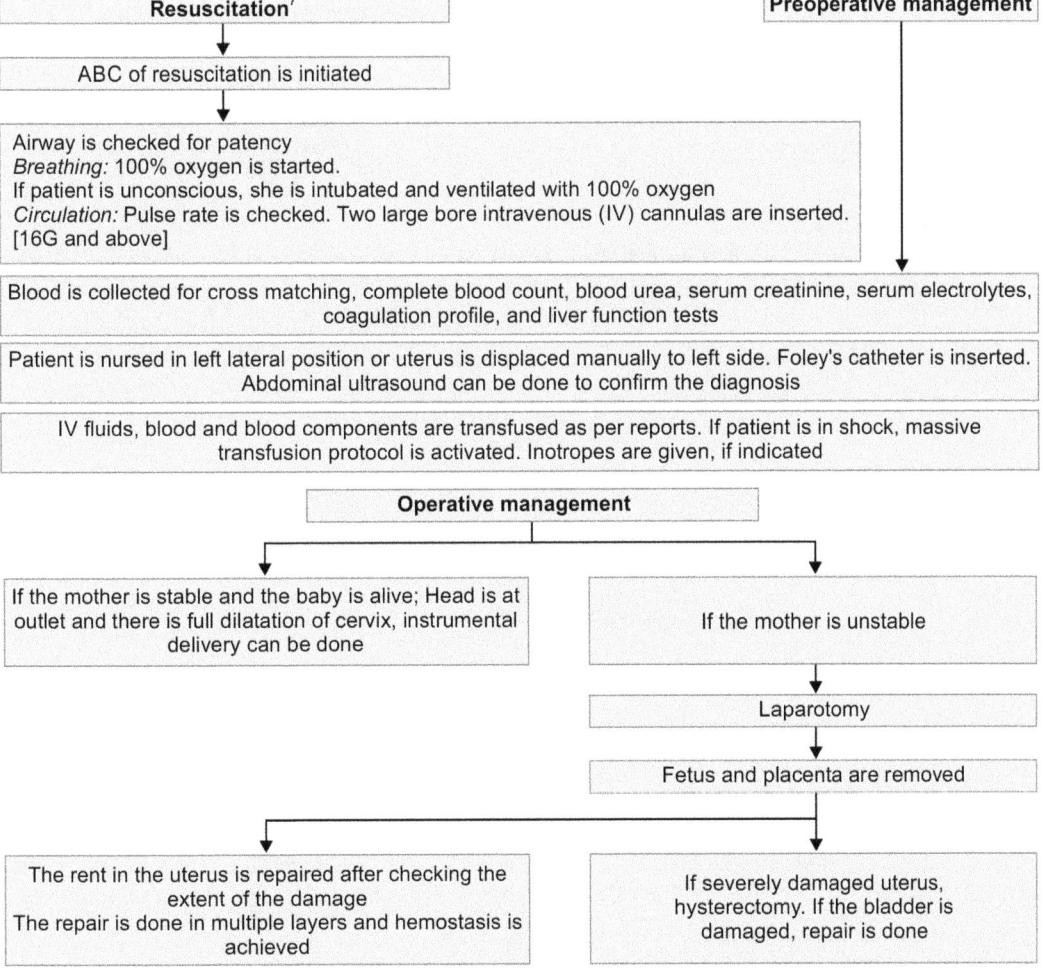

stoppage of uterine contractions, hematuria, if there is bladder extension and signs of hemodynamic compromise.
– There may be referred pain to the shoulder
• Scar dehiscence:
– May be asymptomatic in 49% of cases.[4]
– Scar dehiscence is manifested by gradual reduction in uterine contractions, maternal tachycardia, fetal decelerations and a gradual maternal deterioration.

Management (Flowchart 3)[5]
• Senior most multidisciplinary team is summoned.

• Emergency protocol for collapsed patient is activated.
• Preoperative and postoperative antibiotic prophylaxis with broad spectrum coverage are given.

Postoperative Management
• Depending on patient's condition, she is shifted to high-dependency unit or intensive care unit.
• Vital signs are monitored continuously with a multiparameter monitor.
• PV blood loss is assessed.
• Airway assessment is done. High flow oxygen is given through a reservoir face mask.

- Hourly urine output is measured.
- Coagulation status and renal function are assessed periodically.

Documentation

The events of labor and management of rupture uterus are documented.

TABLE 4: Classification of shoulder dystocia.

Type	Presentation
Unilateral	If posterior shoulder is felt in the sacral hollow
Bilateral	If both shoulders are arrested above pelvic brim

Flowchart 4: Management of shoulder dystocia.

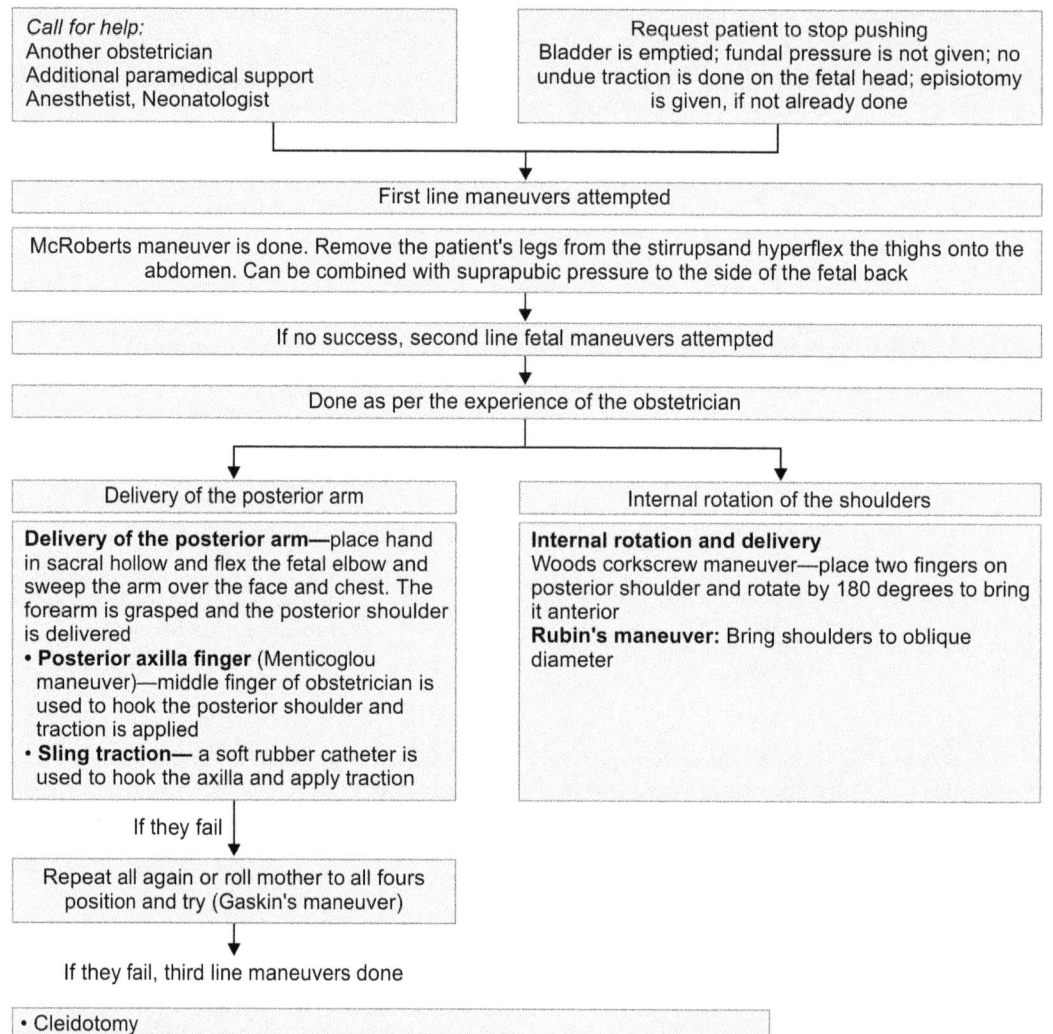

Conclusion

Uterine rupture is a catastrophe to the mother and her baby. Women at high risk need to be identified, diagnosed correctly, transferred urgently, and managed optimally for a favorable fetal and maternal outcome

SHOULDER DYSTOCIA

Definition[2]

The shoulders of the baby fail to deliver after the delivery of the head. There is impaction of the anterior shoulder behind the pubic symphysis

Classification

Classification of shoulder dystocia is shown in **Table 4.**

Diagnosis

- After delivery of head, external rotation does not occur, and head recoils back against the perineum. It is called as the "Turtle sign". It is the first warning sign of shoulder dystocia (SD).
- If the time interval between the delivery of the head to the body is more than 60 seconds, it is SD.[6,7]
- The baby's cheeks bulge out. There is failure of restitution

Risk Factors

- Significant:
  - Fetal macrosomia.
  - Maternal diabetes.
  - SD in previous pregnancy.
- Associated:
  - Baseline maternal obesity.
  - Excessive gestational weight gain.
  - Postdated pregnancy.

Management (Flowchart 4)[2,8]

- If Turtle sign is observed, one should wait for a contraction. There may be a spontaneous restitution with a contraction.
- The drill for delivery is activated after diagnosis
- Immediate management

Conclusion

It is difficult to predict or prevent the occurrence of shoulder dystocia. Vigilance of the obstetrician and the paramedical staff is of utmost importance to manage this complication.

REFERENCES

1. Tawagi G. Compound presentations; 6th edition. In: Oxorn-Foote Human Labor& Birth. NewYork: McGraw Hill Medical; 2013.
2. Seshadri L, Arjun G. Abnormal labour; malpositions and malpresentations, 2nd edition. In: Essentials of Obstetrics; Philadelphia: Wolters Kluwer Health; 2021. p. 539.
3. Cunningham FG. Normal labour, 24th edition. In: Williams Obstetrics; New York: McGraw-Hill Education; 2014. pp. 443-4; 790-91
4. Royal College of Obstetricians and Gynaecologists. Green-top Guideline No. 45. Birth after previous caesarean birth; 2015
5. management of ruptured uterus clinical guidelines register no: 04243 Intrapartum NICE Guidelines RCOG guideline; 2017
6. Aggarwal R, Soni KD, Trikha A. Initial management of a pregnant woman with trauma. J Obstet Anaesth Crit Care. 2018; 8(2):66.
7. Spong CY, Beall M, Rodrigues D, Ross MG. An objective definition of shoulder dystocia: prolonged head-to-body delivery intervals and/or the use of ancillary obstetric maneuvers. Obstet Gynecol. 1995; 86(3):433-6
8. Shoulder Dystocia. Green-top Guideline No. 42); 2012

CHAPTER

15

Abnormal Uterine Action

Vaidehi Marathe, Amogh Natchandra Chimote

DEFINITION

Any deviation of the normal pattern of uterine contraction affecting the course of labor is designated as disordered or abnormal uterine action.

CLASSIFICATION OF ABNORMAL UTERINE ACTION (FLOWCHART 1)

Why is it Important to know about Abnormal Uterine Action?

Any deviation from the normal contraction pattern of the uterus can cause and untoward outcome for the baby as well as the mother, so it is very important that a prompt diagnosis and early management is started to avert the complications and unwanted outcome of an abnormal uterine action.

DIAGNOSIS OF ABNORMAL UTERINE ACTION

Incoordinate Uterine Action

Spastic Lower Segment

Spastic lower segment condition is common in primigravida and is characterized by:

- Dominance of upper segment is lost and reversal of polarity from fundus to the lower segment (**Fig. 1**).

Flowchart 1: Classification of abnormal uterine action.

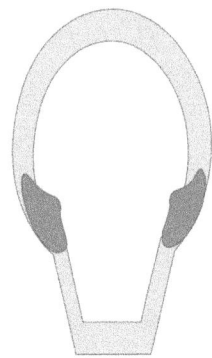

Fig. 1: Spastic lower segment.

Clinical picture
- Labor is prolonged
- Uterine contractions are irregular and painful
- Marked, prolonged, and consistent pain before and throughout the contraction with increased and significant pain, if the fetus is in occipitoposterior position.
- On tocography, a high-resting intrauterine pressure is noted in between two contractions (> 10 mm Hg)
- Rate of cervical dilation is slow
- Chances of premature rupture of membranes
- Fetal distress and maternal pain and change in the vitals

Diagnosis
- Nulliparous patient
- Sever pain in abdomen, which is referred to the back during and even after contraction
- Evidence of dehydration and ketoacidosis
- Distention of bladder with retention of urine
- Gaseous distention of bowel and stomach
- Premature attempts to bear down
- Early signs of fetal distress

P/A
- Tense
- Tender
- Hard
- Difficulty in palpating fetal parts
- Loss of fundal polarity
- Increased contractility at the lower segment

P/V
- Thick edematous and loose hanging cervix, which is not well applied to the presenting part
- Ruptured membranes

- Varying degree of caput succedaneum
- Meconium-stained liquor may be present

Management
- Cesarean section done after correction of dehydration and ketoacidosis by rapid infusion of RL
- Antibiotic cover

Generalized Tonic Uterine Contraction (Uterine Tetany)

The whole uterus upper as well as the lower segment is in a constant state of contraction with no physiological differentiation between upper and lower segment.

Etiology
- Cephalopelvic disproportion
- Obstruction not cleared even after powerful uterine contractions
- Nonjudicious use of oxytocin

Diagnosis
- General features
  - Prolonged labor
  - Severe and continuous pain
  - High-resting pressure of uterus on tocography

P/A
- Uterus appears to slightly smaller in size
- Tense and tender
- Fetal parts not well defined
- Fetal heart sound may not be easily audible
- Contractions lasting for >2 minutes or >5 contractions in 10 minutes
- Increase in intensity of pain with each contraction

P/V
- Vagina appears to be edematous and dry
- No change in decent of head for more than 2 hours
- Caput formation
- Molding

Management
- Cesarean section done after correction of dehydration and ketoacidosis by rapid infusion of RL
- Broad spectrum antibiotic cover
- Adequate pain relief (Pethidine, Fentanyl, Phenargan)

TABLE 1: Types of cervical dystocia and their characteristics.

Functional (Primary)	Organic (Secondary)
• No organic lesion present • Good effacement • Failure of dilatation of external os • Due to cervical spasm resulting from overactive sympathetic tone	• Previous history of cervical surgery, i.e., conization, cauterization, amputation or obstetrics trauma (Tear) • Cervical myoma or carcinoma

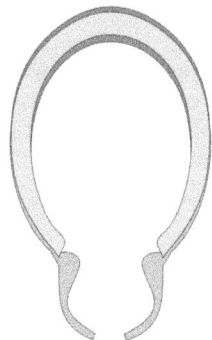

Fig. 2: Cervical dystocia.

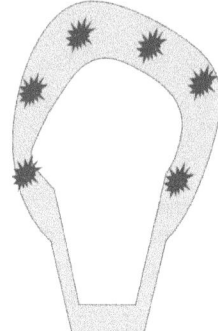

Fig. 3: Asymmetrical uterine contraction.

- Tachysystole induced by oxytocic can be managed by tocolytics (terbutaline 0.25 mg SC) and stopping oxytocin infusion.

Cervical Dystocia

Failure of the cervix to dilate at an expected rate in spite of good and regular uterine contractions.

Cervical dystocia can be further classified into two subgroups as show in **Table 1**.

Clinical picture and diagnosis: Abnormal relationship between the cervix and presenting part (malpresentation, malposition)
- No dilatation even after hours of labor
- Rigid edematous cervix
- Cervix is well effaced and well applied to the presenting part
- Presence of a firm ring over the external os
- Features of annular detachment or avulsion of anterior lip of cervix **(Fig. 2)**.

Management of primary cervical dystocia: In case of malposition and malpresentation cesarean section is the treatment of choice.

Head low down with rim of cervix:
- Push up the ring manually or Duhrssen's incision at 2 and 10 o'clock position can be

additionally one more incision at 6 o'clock position can also be given and deliver by Ventouse
- Resuturing of the incision is to be done like stitching a cervical tear.

Management of secondary cervical dystocia: Cesarean delivery

Asymmetrical Uterine Contraction

Asymmetrical contraction of the uterine segment due to multiple pacemakers in the uterus resulting in incoordinated action causing no downward movement of the fetus or cervical dilatation **(Fig. 3)**.

Clinical picture and diagnosis: Common in primigravida and nulliparous

P/A
- Poor and weak contraction
- The successive contractions are of increasing intensity
- Increased tone of the uterus at some parts only.

P/V
- Poor cervical dilation and effacement
- Station may be high up

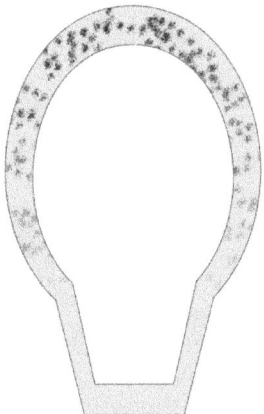

Fig. 4: Colicky uterus.

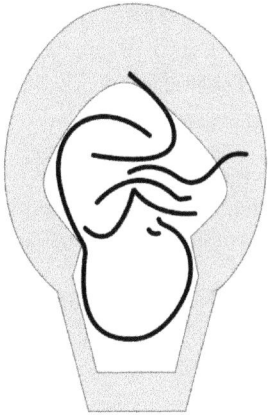

Fig. 5: Constriction ring.

- Very slow progress of labor for more than 2 hours

Management
- Cesarean section
- Normal delivery is possible with proper hydration and pain relief, if fetopelvic disproportion is ruled out.

Colicky Uterus

Lack of polarity leading to strong contraction of the uterus **(Fig. 4)**.

Clinical features and diagnosis: Strong and powerful contraction, pain generally in the hypogastrium

P/A
- High resting tone of uterus
- Irritable uterus, i.e., contractions start even with the slightest of stimuli.
- Tenderness

P/V
- Cervix uneffaced
- Thick and edematous cervix
- Presenting part poorly applied to the cervix

Management: Cesarean section

Constriction Ring (Schroeder's Ring, Physiological Ring, Hour Glass Contraction)

Form of incoordinate uterine action with localized area of tetanic contraction of a ring of circular muscle fibers of the uterus.

Forms at the junction of upper and lower segment and in the natural groove of the fetus like the neck **(Fig. 5)**.

Clinical presentation and diagnosis
- Sudden arrest of progress of labor in a previously normal progress
- Sudden fetal distress in the form of alternating tachy and bradycardia

P/A
- Normal uterine contour, no deformity felt per abdomen
- Can only be diagnosed on
  - Cesarean section in the first stage
  - Application of forceps in the second stage
  - In the third stage during manual removal of placenta

Management
- Cesarean section with deep anesthesia.
- If the ring persists during cesarean section then the ring is to be cut vertically and the baby delivered.
- If forceps are applied deepening the level of anesthesia will help in the ring passes off.

Hypotonic Uterine Inertia

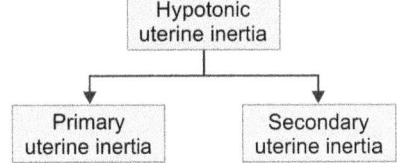

Primary Uterine Inertia

Cervical dilatation of <1 cm/hour following a normal latent phase of labor.

Diagnosis and clinical features:
P/A
- Less pain during contraction
- Less hardening of uterus on manual palpation
- Easily indentable uterine wall at the height of contraction
- Well relaxed uterus in between contractions

P/V
- Poor cervical dilatation < 1 cm/hour beyond 3 cm
- Contracted pelvis, if malposition can be diagnosed
- Membranes intact

Management: General measures
- Reassurance
- Low amniotomy (Artificial rupture of membranes)
- Catheterization
- Maintain hydration

Active measures
- Use of oxytocin and judicious titration
- Even after oxytocin if the cervical dilatation is unsatisfactory and fetal distress appears cesarean delivery is to considered.

Absolute indications for LSCS (lower segment cesarean section) in primary uterine inertia
- Contracted pelvis or fetopelvis disproportion
- Malpresentation
- Fetal/maternal distress
- Unsatisfactory progress on oxytocin

Secondary Uterine Inertia

A type of hypotonic uterine action with feeble uterine contraction and cervical dilatation of <1 cm/hr but is defined when cervical dilatation slows or stops after the normal start of active phase.

Diagnosis and clinical features

P/A
- Less pain during contraction
- Less hardening of uterus on manual palpation
- Easily indentable uterine wall at the height of contraction
- Well-relaxed uterus in between contractions

P/V
- Poor cervical dilatation < 1 cm/hour beyond 3 cm
- Contracted pelvis, if malposition can be diagnosed
- Membranes intact

Management
- Rule out cephalopelvis disproportion, malpresentation, and malposition
- Judicious use of oxytocin drip and titration
- Low amniotomy
- Incase of cephalopelvis disproportion, malpresentation and malposition LSCS is the preferred mode of delivery.

▚ HYPERTONIC DYSFUNCTION

Bandl's Ring (Retraction Ring, Pathological Ring) (Fig. 6)

Tonic uterine contraction due to obstructed labor.

Symptoms
- Nausea
- Dehydration and ketoacidosis
- Fever
- Severe and constant abdominal pain

Signs
- Febrile to touch
- Cold and calmy extremities
- Signs of dehydration

P/A
- Uterus is hard and tender
- Prominent and tender round ligaments

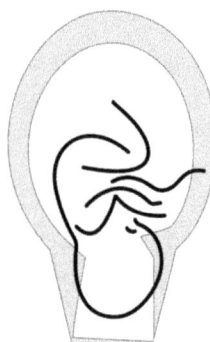

Fig. 6: Bandl's ring.

TABLE 2: Clinical picture and per abdomen findings in abnormal uterine action.

P/V findings	Spastic lower segment	Generalized tonic contraction	Cervical dystocia	Asymmetrical uterine action	Colicky uterus	Construction ring	Bandl's ring	Uterine inertia
Fetal parts	Palpable	Not well defined	Palpable	Difficult to palpate	Difficult to palpate	Palpable	Difficult to palpate	Felt easily
U. tenderness	Present	Present	Not present	Absent	Present	No	Hard and tender	Absent
Fetal heart	Heard	Difficult to appreciate	Heard	Heard with difficulty	Difficult to heard	Heard	Difficult to heard	Heard
Maternal dehydration	Present	No	Late	Late	No	No	Present with fever	No
Maternal exhaustion	Present	Present	Late	Late	No	Appears after sudden arrest of labor	Present	No
Contractions	Irregular, prolonged, before and throughout	Contractions lasting for >2 minutes or >5 contractions in 10 minutes	Inefficient and weak, less than 1 minute	Poor, weak initially, subsequent contraction increase in intensity	Contraction starts at the slightest of stimuli	Sudden increase in intensity after the arrest of progress of labor	Severe and constant	Diminished intensity with good and increased interval of relaxation
Tocodynamometry	High resting pressure >10 mm Hg	High resting pressure >15 mm Hg	Normal resting pressure	Poor and inconsistent resting pressure eventually rises >15 mm Hg	High resting tone of the uterus >20 mm Hg	High resting pressure and increase in intensity	High intensity and high resting pressure	Intrauterine pressure does not rise above 25 mm Hg at the height of contraction
Ketoacidosis	Present	No	Late onset	No	No	No	Present	
Fetal distress	Present	Late onset	Present	Present	Present	Sudden fetal distress	Present	No

Contd...

Contd...

P/V findings	Spastic lower segment	Generalized tonic contraction	Cervical dystocia	Asymmetrical uterine action	Colicky uterus	Construction ring	Bandl's ring	Uterine inertia
Specific finding	Bladder and bowel distention Increase lower segment contractity	Uterus slightly smaller due to tonic contraction	Malpresentation, malposition	Irregular areas of contraction on the surface of the uterus	Painful contraction felt more in the hypogastrium	Sudden arrest of progress of labor. Hour glass deformity seen only during cesarean section	Prominent tender round ligaments. Ring running transversely across the uterus	During contraction less hardening of the uterus Uterine wall easiy Indentable at the height of pain
Vagina	Normal	Edematous and dry	Cervix is	Normal	Congested and edematous	Ring can be felt vaginally	Dry and warm vagina with foul smelling discharge Ring can not be felt vaginally	Normal
Cervix	Thick edematous and loose hanging cervix	Edematous	Rigid and edematous Presence of a firm ring over the external os Features or annular detachment or avulsion of anterior lip of cervix	Thick and edematous	Thick and edematous cervix	As in normal labor	Eedematous cervix Caput succedaneum	Normal
Presenting part	Nol well applied	Well applied	Loosely applied	Loosely applied	Presenting part poorly applied to the cervix	Difficult to determine	Difficult to determine	High up
Dilatation	Poor, generally not more than 3–4 cm	Poor	No dilation even after hours of labor	Poor	Poor	Initially good then can be arrested	Poor	Poor

Contd...

Contd...

P/V findings	Spastic lower segment	Generalized tonic contraction	Cervical dystocia	Asymmetrical uterine action	Colicky uterus	Construction ring	Bandl's ring	Uterine inertia
Effacement	Poor, <25%	Varying degree	Well effaced and well applied to the presenting part	Poor	Uneffaced	Poor	Uneffaced	Uneffaced to just effaced
Membranes	Ruptured	Present	Present	May be present	May or may not be present	Present	Present, may be buldging	Present
Liquor	Meconium stained	Can be meconium stained	–	–	–	–	–	–
Caput/molding	Varying degrees	A fairly big caput with molding	Cannot evaluate	May or may not be present	–	Station high up, late onset caput	Present	Caput present
Progress of labor	Slow	No progress	Slow and may be arrested	Very slow progress or labor for more than 2 hours	Arrest of labor after initial slow progress	Obstructed	Obstructed	Slow
Rate of decent	<1 cm per hour	No change in rate for >2 hours	Slow or arrested without intervention	Station may be high up	No decent	Arrested	Arrested	<1 cm/hr

TABLE 3: Diagnostic questions in cases of suspected dysfunctional uterine contraction.

Question	Possible pathology	Treatment options
1. Is the patient in true labor?	Prelabor or false labor	Serial observation, simple enema, sedation
2. Is the progress tardy?	Inefficient pains, disproportionate occipitoposterior position and fetal macrosomia	Partogram shows tardy progress in active phase: Consider oxytocin drip, amniotomy, analgesics, LSCS for disproportion
3. Are the membranes ruptured?	Chorioamnionitis, cord prolapse	Antibiotics , labor induction, LSCS
4. Undiagnosed type of pelvis?	Android/anthropoid pelvis	TOL, Oxytocin stimulation, face to pubis delivery, forceps/ventouse or LSCS
5. Is the fetus macrosomic generalized or locally?	*Fetal weight:* > 3800 g Diabetic mother, post dated Hydrocephalus, sacral tumor Distended foetal bladder	TOL if no progress in 2 hours LSCS
6. Is there a obstructed labor?	Contracted pelvis, CPD, malpresentation, malposition, Müllerian anomaly, pelvic neoplasia, placenta previa	Avoid NVD LSCS first choice
7. Are the pains effective?	Hypotonic uterine contraction	Conisider augmentation with oxytocin or prostaglandins

TABLE 4: Abnormal labor patterns, diagnostic criteria, and methods of treatment.

Labor	Diagnostic criteria		Preferred treatment	Expectant management
	Nulliparas	Multiparas		
Prolongation disorder Prolonged latent phase	>20 hrs		Bed rest	Oxytocin augmentation if maternal and fetal parameters normal Fetal distress, maternal exhaustion: LSCS
Protraction disorder Protracted active phase dilatation Protracted descent	<1.2 cm/hr <1 cm/hr		Expectant and support	CPD, maternal exhaustion, dehydration, fetal distress : LSCS
Arrest disorder Prolonged deceleration phase Secondary arrest of dilatation Arrest of descent Failure of descent	>3 hrs >2 hrs >1 hr NO descent in deceleration phase or second stage		Evaluate and rule out CPD CPD+: LSCS CPD -: Oxytocin	LSCS

- A ring running obliquely or transversely across the uterus demarcating the upper and lower segment
- Difficult to palpate the fetal parts
- Difficult to auscultate fetal heart sounds

P/V

- Dry and warm vagina with foul smelling discharge
- Edematous cervix
- Difficult to determine the presenting part
- Caput succedaneum

Management

- Correction of dehydration and ketoacidosis with RL, crystalloids with or without sodium bicarbonate infusion
- Analgesics
- *Broad spectrum antibiotics:* Cefotaxime 1 g IV 12 hourly or Ampicillin 500 mg IV 6 hourly along with Metronidazole 500 mg 8 hourly
- Cross-matched blood two units PRC along with FFP two units
  - Mode of delivery
  - Cesarean section
  - Rule out and manage uterine rupture, if present

Precipitate Labor

When the combined duration of 1st and 2nd stage of labor is less than 2 hours.

Management

- In case of previous history of precipitate labor, admit the patient before the labor starts
- Suppression of the contraction by administering magnesium sulfate during the contractions
- Controlled delivery of the head
- Elective induction of labor by low rupture of membranes and careful conduction by low dose oxytocin
- Avoid augmentation by oxytocin
- Episiotomy to avoid cervical laceration and vaginal tears
- Examine the vagina and cervix for tears or injury
- Careful monitoring of 3rd and 4th stage of labor

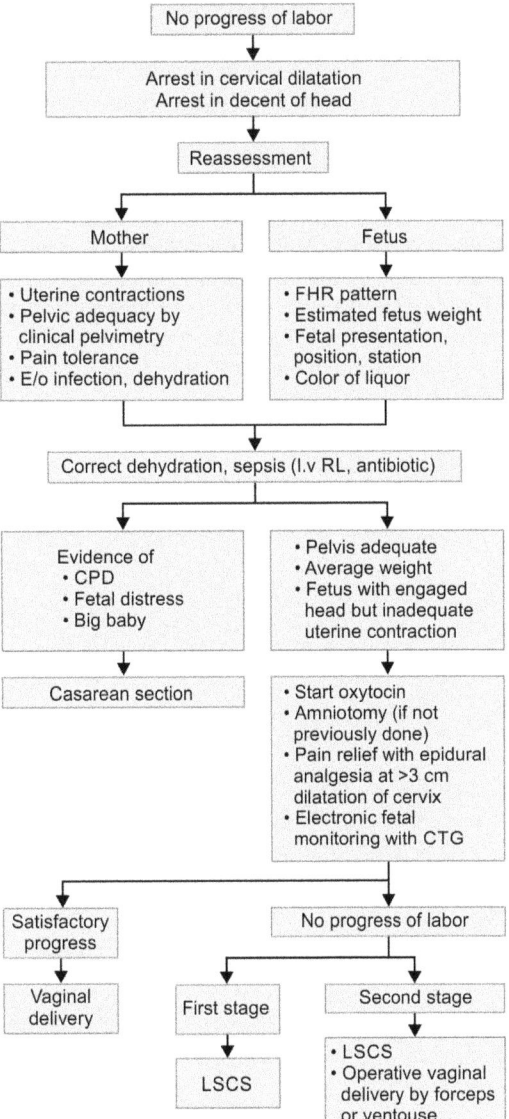

Flowchart 2: Management algorithm for abnormal uterine action.

Management of Dysfunctional Labor due to Abnormal Uterine Action

See **Flowchart 2**.

▦ CONCLUSION

Abnormal uterine actions are very tricky and difficult situations to manage and require a lot of attention to detail when looking for subtle signs of nonprogress of labor to determine the best course of action for the situation.

A judicious and controlled use of oxytocin and amniotomy can bring about normal vaginal delivery with good outcome in cases of hypotonic abnormalities once the CPD, malposition, and malpresentation have been rues out. On the other hand, it is very important to quickly identify the nonprogress of labor due to hypertonic action of the uterus and administer emergency care in the form of stabilization of the mother and the fetus. Most often then not cesarean section is the choice of route of delivery in such cases and should be done sooner rather than later, which may lead to a poor out come of the pregnancy both of for the mother as well as the fetus

▧ BIBLIOGRAPHY

1. American College of Obstetrics and Gynecology Committee on Practice Bulletins-Obstetrics. ACOG Practice Bulletin Number 49, December 2003: Dystocia and augmentation of labor. Obstet Gynecol. 2003;102(6):1445-54.
2. Konar H, Dutta DC. Abnormal uterine action. In: D.C DUTTA'S Text book of Obstetrics, 7th edition. New Delhi: Jaypee Brothers Medical Publishers (P) Ltd; 2013. pp. 357-63.
3. Ressel GW; American College of Obstetricians and Gynecologists. ACOG releases report on dystocia and augmentation of labor. Am Fam Physician. 2004;69(5):1290-2.
4. Sharma JB. Text book of Obstetrics. New Delhi: Avichal Publishing Company; 2017. pp.264-72.
5. Sharma A. Abnormal uterine action in labor. In: A Practical Guide to Third Trimester of Pregnancy and Puerperium, 1st edition. New Delhi: Jaypee Brothers Medical Publishers (P) Ltd; 2016.
6. Townsend L. Abnormal uterine action. In: Obstetrics for Students. London: Palgrave; 1978.

16 Precipitate Labor

Shama Batra, Preeti Gaur

INTRODUCTION

A precipitate labor can be among the most stressful events an emergency obstetrician encounters. Most of precipitous deliveries result in good outcomes for mother and baby but during emergency obstetrician must be prepared to manage framed complications, such as tight nuchal cord, shoulder dystocia, and breech presentation.

An understanding of labor process, as well as advanced planning, including delivery checklist, kits consultant lists can help decrease the stress and chaos inherent to any precipitous labor.

DEFINITION

- Not only can labor be too slow, but it also can be abnormally rapid.
- Precipitate labor has been defined as a labor that lasts not more than 3 hours from onset of regular contractions to delivery.
- Precipitate labor also called FAST or RAPID labor. It is the term given to the case when a woman goes into labor and has her baby within 3 hours.

INCIDENCE

- Only 2/100 women will end up experiencing precipitate labor.
- The incidence of precipitous labor in India is about 14% of all singleton deliveries, which seemed to be higher than those reported in the United States and other countries: 0.1–3%.

CAUSES OF PRECIPITATE LABOR

- Certain factors can precipitate labor.
- Strong uteri that contract with all its might when in labor.
- A smooth birth canal, abnormal low resistance of birth canal.

- Placental abruption
- Baby's size smaller than average size
- Chronic hypertension (gestational hypertension)
- Prostaglandins to induce precipitate labor

CONTRIBUTING FACTORS/RISK FACTORS

- Multiparous women
- Small fetus
- Relaxed pelvic and vaginal musculature
- History of rapid labor with previous deliveries
- A particular efficient uterus which contracts with great strength.
- Increased risk of precipitate labor, in patients conceived after infertility treatment.

Prevalence of intake of few herbs such as cinnamon is the one found associated with precipitate labor.

SIGNS

- Contractions that are very close together and that do not leave you with much recovery time between them.
- Intense pain throughout that feels like it is a one long contraction.
- An urge to push that emerges very suddenly and without warning.
- Often times this symptom is not accompanied by contractions as the cervix dilates very quickly.

DIAGNOSIS

- Retrospective diagnosis as the patient is usually seen in the 2nd or 3rd stages of labor.
- If seen delivery first stage of labor the pictograph will show rapid progress of cervical dilatation and effacement.

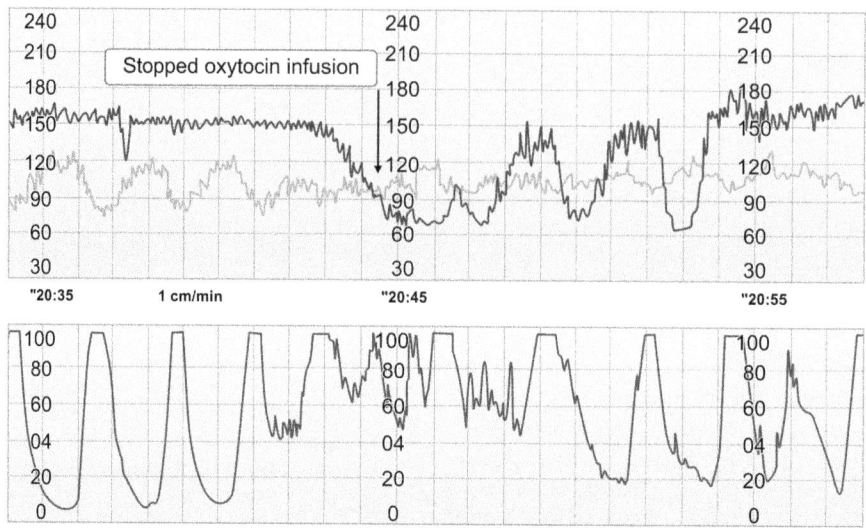

Fig. 1: Graph of precipitate labor.

TABLE 1: Management of precipitate labor.		
Before delivery	***During delivery***	***After delivery***
1. Patient who had previous precipitate labor should be hospitalized before expected date of delivery as she is more prone to repeated precipitate labor.	1. *Inhalation anesthesia:* As nitrous oxide and oxygen is given to slow the course of labor. 2. *Tocolytic:* As ritodrine (yutopar) may be effective. 3. *Episiotomy:* To avoid perineal lacerations and intracranial hemorrhage.	1. Examine the mother and fetus for injuries.

GRAPH

The graph of precipitate labor is shown in **Figure 1**.

COMPLICATIONS

Maternal Complications

- Laceration of the cervix, vagina, and perineum
- Shock
- Inversion of the uterus
- *Postpartum hemorrhage:* No time for retraction
- *Sepsis due to:* Lacerations inappropriate surroundings

Fetal Complications

- Intracranial hemorrhage due to sudden compression and decompression of the head.
- Fetal asphyxia due to strong frequent uterine contractions reducing placental perfusion, lack of immediate resuscitation
- Avulsion of the umbilical cord
- Fetal injury due to falling down

MANAGEMENT OF PRECIPITATE LABOR (TABLE 1)

Prophylaxis

- Patient with previous history of precipitate labor should be admitted to the hospital at the first perception of labor pains.
- Uterine contraction may be suppressed by administering nitrous, oxygen or sedation, or ether during contraction.
- Delivery of head should be controlled. Elective induction of labor by low rupture of membrane

and careful conduction of controlled delivery may be done.

- If patient seen after delivery exploration of birth canal for any injury and manage accordingly.
- Prophylactic antibiotics, if delivery occurred in unsuitable conditions.
- Proper examination of fetus for detection of any complication. Stop any oxytocin, if being administered.
- No significance of use of analgesia terbutaline or ritrodrine intravenously; physical attempts to retard delivery are absolutely contra-indicated.

Lax pelvic musculature and vagina is a cause for precipitate labor; so pelvic floor muscle exercises can be a preventive measurement.

Pelvic floor muscles are like any other muscle more you exercise them stronger they become.

BIBLIOGRAPHY

1. Cunningham FG, Leveno KJ, Bloom SL, Hauth JC, Rouse DJ, Spong CY. Abnormal labour. In: Cunningham FG, Leveno KJ, Bloom SL, Hauth JC, Rouse DJ, Spong CY (Eds). Williams Obstetrics, 23rd edition. New York: McGraw-Hill; 2009. pp. 464-89.
2. http/www.ncbinim.n.hgov>actively
3. http://mayoclinic.org>drs20376848nice.org. uk/guidence/c970/evidence/c970induction of labourfailguideline2.
4. http://www.babycentre.co. ok> precipitatelabour
5. http://www.tandfonlone.com>doi>pdf
6. http://www sweethaveen02.com/PDF_Health 922/ess0.3pdf
7. Mahon TR. Chazotte C, Cohen WR. Short labor: characteristics and outcome. Obstet gynecol. 1994:84(1):47-51.
8. Sheiner E, Levy A, Mazor M. Precipitate labor: higher rates of maternal complication. Eyr J obstet Gynecol Reprod Biol. 2004; 116(1):43-7.
9. Silver DW, sabatino F. Precipitous and difficult deliveries. Emerg Med Clin North Am. 2012;30(4):961-75.

CHAPTER

17

Forceps and Vacuum Delivery

Shaheen Anjum, Nazia Ishrat, Narendra Malhotra

▪ FORCEPS DELIVERY

Definition

It is a pair of instruments that help in the delivery of fetal head. It is applied to fetal head and traction generates forces that augment the delivery of fetal head.[1,2]

The criteria for types of forceps deliveries are described in **Table 1**. The indications for forceps delivery are given in **Table 2**.

The types and parts of forceps are described in **Tables 3 and 4**, respectively.

Prerequisite of Forceps Delivery

- **F**—Fully dilated cervix, favorable head position (occipitoanterior)
- **O**—Obstruction (pelvis) ruled out
- **R**—Ruptured membrane, rotation is <45° in case of outlet forceps

TABLE 1: Criteria for types of forceps deliveries.	
Types	*Delivery*
Outlet forceps	• Fetal scalp is visible at introitus without separating the labia • Fetal skull reached at pelvic floor • Fetal head is at on perineum • Sagittal suture is an anteroposterior diameter or right or left occipitoanterior or posterior position (rotation does not exceed 45°)
Low forceps	• Leading point of fetal skull is at station +2 cm or more not on pelvic floor • *Without rotation*: Rotation is 45° or less – Left or right occipitoanterior to direct occipitoanterior position – Left or right occipitoposterior to direct occipitoposterior position
Mid forceps	• Fetal head is not >1/5 palpable per abdomen • Leading point of fetal skull is above station +2 cm but not above ischial spine
High forceps	Not recommended
Mostly outlet forceps deliveries are performed in modern obstetrics	

TABLE 2: Indications for forceps delivery.	
Fetal	• Fetal distress in late second stage of labor including cord prolapse • Nonreassuring fetal CTG in second stage of labor
Maternal	• Maternal distress/exhaustion/poor bearing down efforts • To shorten or cut short the second stage of labor on medical conditions (eclampsia, severe pre-eclampsia, cardiac disease, pulmonary disease, severe anemia) • Maternal distress need to be avoided (e.g., ocular disease, proliferative retinopathy, cardiac disease, hypertensive crisis, cerebrovascular disease)
Labor dysfunction	Prolonged second stage of labor >3 hours in primi and more than 2 hours in multiparous woman and in case where epidural analgesia is given
When applying forceps, one should know that no indication is absolute and clinical judgment is required in all cases[3]	

- **C**—Contractions are good, consent (patient being informed about risks and benefits of procedure and ready for instrumental delivery)
- **E**—Empty bladder, engaged head <1/5th head palpable per abdomen, episiotomy if needed
- **P**—Preparedness for C-section, pudendal block, pediatrician should be available.
- **S**—Sagittal suture in anteroposterior diameter of outlet, stirrups

Procedure

Preprocedure Preparations

- Ensure that application of forceps is indicated in this case.
- Explain the procedure to the woman and take written consent. Arrange for assistant.

- Review for fulfillments of the prerequisites.
- Give emotional support and encourage the woman.
- Place the woman in lithotomy/dorsal position after emptying the bladder.
- Prepare yourself with personal protective equipment.
- Prepare the part with antiseptic solution and sterile drapings.
- Pelvic examination to confirm position, presentation and rule out cephalopelvic disproportion (CPD).
- Prepare all necessary equipment.
- *Instruments* (**Fig. 5**):
  - Sponge holder
  - Wrigley's forceps

TABLE 3: Types of forceps.	
Outlet forceps	Wrigley's forceps (**Fig. 1**)
Outlet or low cavity forceps	Simpson's/Elliot forceps (**Fig. 2**)
Mid-cavity forceps	Tucker-Mclane forceps
Mid-cavity or rotational forceps	Kielland's forceps (**Fig. 3**)
After coming head in breech	Piper forceps

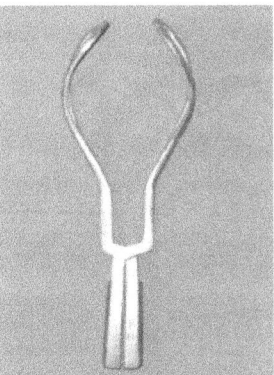

Fig. 1: Wrigley's forceps.

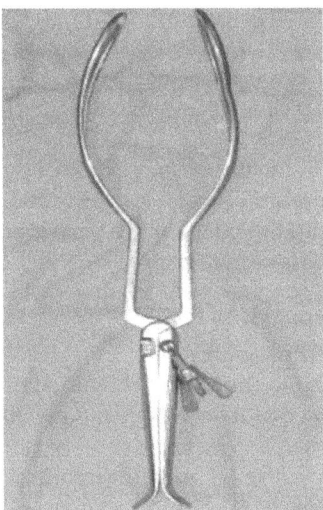

Fig. 2: Simpson's forceps.

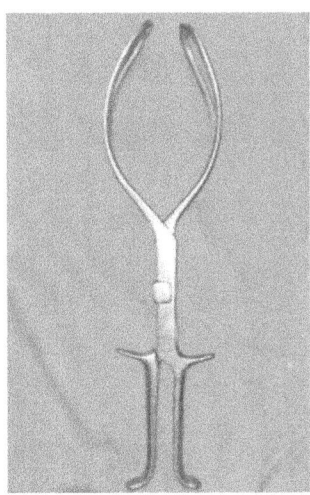

Fig. 3: Kielland's forceps.

TABLE 4: Parts of forceps **(Fig. 4)**.	
Handle	To grip the fetal head
Lock	To hold the two blades together
Shank	It is the connection between handle and blade
Blade	There are two blades: Right and left blade are applied on baby's/fetal head
Each blade has two curves	
Cephalic curve	Fits over fetal head
Pelvic curve	Follows direction of birth canal[2]

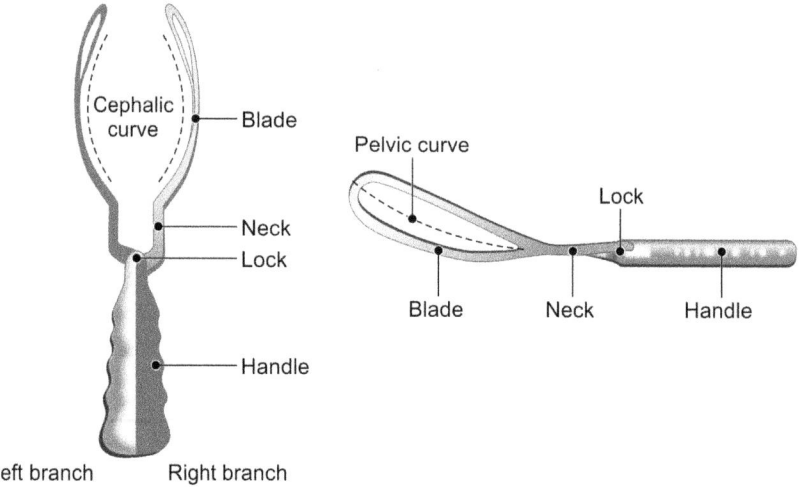

Fig. 4: Parts of forceps.

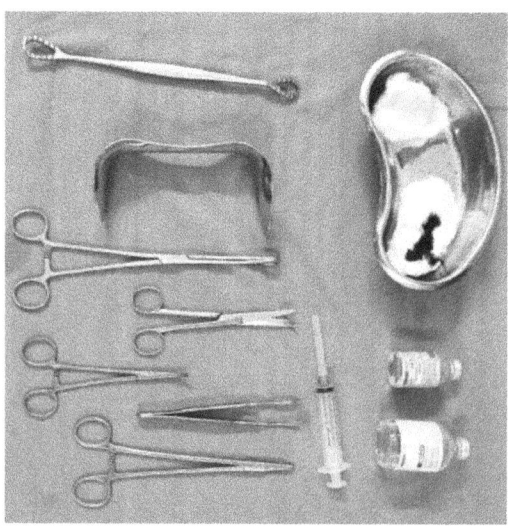

Fig. 5: Instruments tray.

- Sims speculums
- Anterior vaginal wall retractor
- Curved artery forceps
- Episiotomy and suture cutting scissor
- Needle holder
- Toothed and Nontoothed forceps
- *Materials:*
  - 10-mL syringe with 22-gauge needle
  - Irrigation solution
  - Local anesthetic solution (Xylocaine 2%)
  - Sponges
  - Sterile gloves
- Assemble the forceps before application to ensure that it locks well and identification of blades.
- Ensure uterus must be contracting and relaxing.
- Perform mediolateral episiotomy, if needed[3,4]

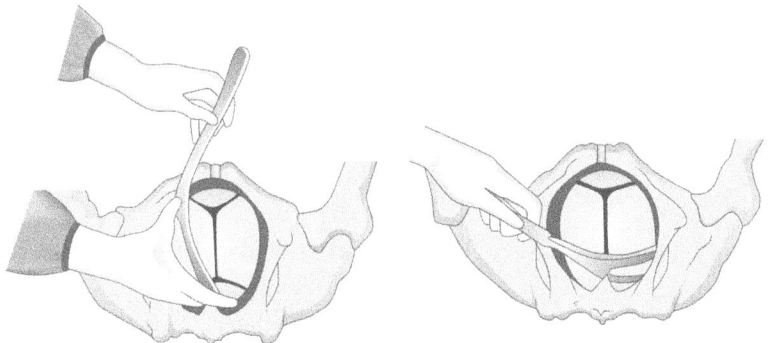

Fig. 6: Application of left blade.

Application of Forceps

Forceps are applied after checking for all the prerequisites for forceps delivery.

Step I: Identification and application of left blade
- For identification, hold-locked forceps with the pelvic curve pointing upward. Place the forceps toward pelvis of the woman. The blade that is placed against left side of woman's pelvis is left blade. Also, the handle of left blade is grasped by operator's left hand and vice versa.
- Lubricate the blades
- Left or lower blade is introduced first, handle of the blade is gripped by left hand in pen-holding manner, fenestrated portion of blade is guided gently with palmer surface of two fingers of right hand between fetal head and left pelvic wall **(Fig. 6)**.
- As the blade is advanced into vagina it rests on the side of fetal head and handle rest on perineum.

Step II: Application of right blade
- Ask the assistant to hold left blade and repeat the same procedure to apply right blade over left blade **(Fig. 7)**.
- Depress the handle and lock the forceps.
- Difficulty in locking indicates incorrect application. In this case, remove the blades and recheck the presentation. Reapply if rotation is confirmed.

Step III: Traction
- Before traction ensure correct application, which is evident by:
  - Easy locking

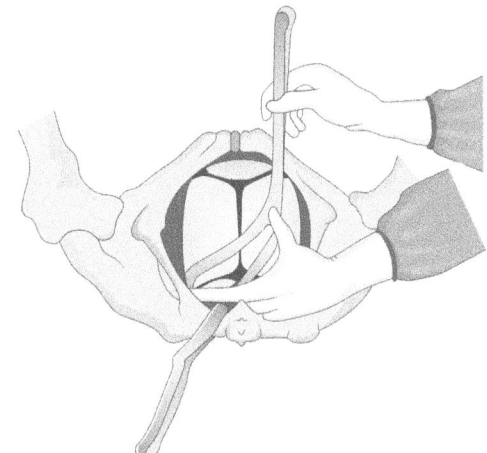

Fig. 7: Application of right blade.

  - Blades are equidistant from lambdoid suture
  - Firm grip of the head
- Steady traction is applied during contraction by gripping the handle, placing the fingers in between shank and the thumb on the under surface of handles. Descent of head is noted with each pull. Apply only 2–3 pulls and check the fetal heart rate in between contractions.
- Direction of pull is downward and forward till crowning (nape of neck is visible), then gradually upward and forward toward mother's abdomen **(Fig. 8)**.
- Traction force should be applied only by forearms. Episiotomy can be given during crowning *if needed.*
- Deliver the head slowly and protect the perineum **(Fig. 9)**.

Step IV: Removal of blades
- The blades are removed when head is visible outside the vulva.
- Right blade is removed first then left blade. Proceed for the delivery of baby as done normally.

Postprocedure Tasks
- Active management of third stage of labor to be done as in all cases.
- Inspection of vagina, perineum and cervix should be done for tears and repair immediately.

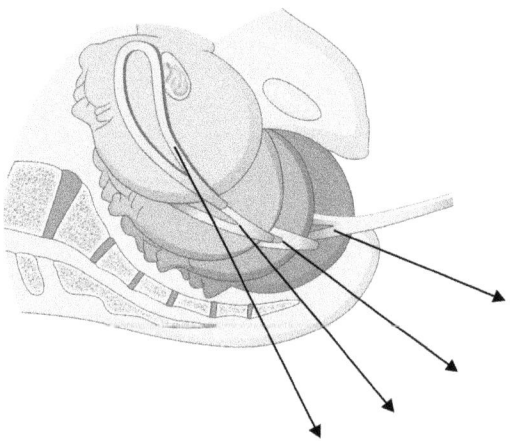

Fig. 8: Direction of traction.

- Examine the baby for possible injuries.
- Routine antibiotic is not recommended.
- Waste material should be disposed-off in appropriate plastic bags.
- Place instruments and gloves in chlorine solution for decontamination.
- Record the procedure and the findings.

Contraindications or Forceps Delivery Failure
- Maternal body mass index over 30
- Estimated fetal weight over 4,000 g or clinically big baby (macrosomia)
- Mid-cavity delivery or when 1/5th of the head palpable per abdomen
- Occipitoposterior position
- Evidence of CPD
- Constriction ring
- Unrecognized malpresentation or hydrocephalus

Failed Forceps
- Fetal head does not advance with each pull.
- There is no head descent after three pulls.
- If forceps fails, patient to be taken up for cesarean section.

Complications of Forceps Delivery
The complications of forceps delivery are given in **Table 5.**

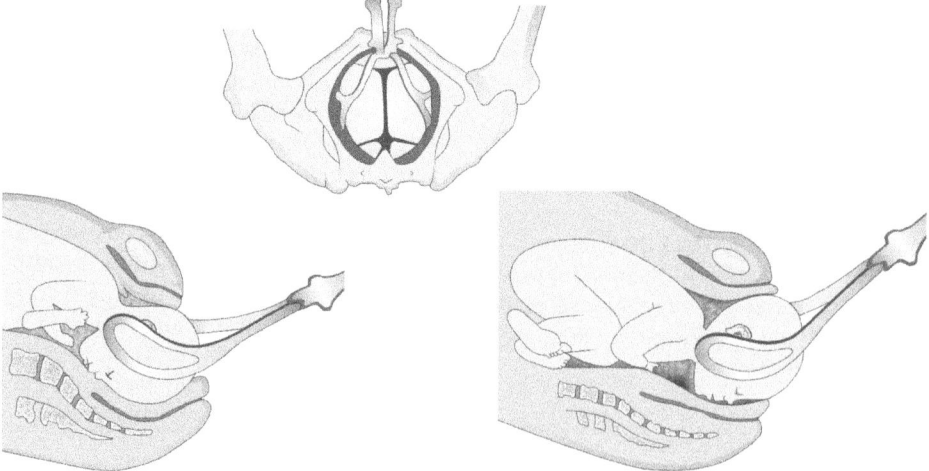

Fig. 9: Delivery of head by forceps.

TABLE 5: Complications of forceps delivery.

Maternal	• Perineal tears (sometime third- and fourth-degree tear) • Vaginal laceration • Cervical tear • Extension of episiotomy • Traumatic and atonic postpartum hemorrhage (PPH) • Retention of urine • Sphincter dysfunction • Painful perineal scars • Dyspareunia
Fetal	• Asphyxia • Intracranial hemorrhage • Facial palsy • Skull fracture • Cephalhematoma

TABLE 6: Components of a vacuum.

Suction cup	• Cup can be made of **(Fig. 10)**:
	  – *Silicone or Silastic cup*: Silastic cup causes lesser trauma than metallic cups **(Fig. 10A)**
	  – Disposable plastic (Kiwi Omnicup) **(Fig. 10B)**
	• Metal **(Fig. 10C)**
	Cups are of different sizes (30, 40, 50 and 60 mm)

Vacuum generator	Vacuum generator with manometer showing negative pressure generated **(Fig. 11)**
Traction tubings	Cup is connected to vacuum pump through a thick wall tube by which air is evacuated and traction given **(Fig. 11)**

VACUUM DELIVERY

Definition

Vacuum or Ventouse is an instrument designed to assist delivery of fetal head by creating a vacuum between cup and fetal head.

Indications of Vacuum Delivery

Indications of vacuum delivery are same as for forceps application except where vacuum cannot be applied. Vacuum cannot be applied on face presentation, after coming head of breech.

Components of Vacuum

The important components of a vacuum are described in **Table 6**.

Prerequisites for Vacuum Delivery

• Vertex presentation
• Term fetus (gestational age should be >34 weeks according to ACOG 2020 and >36 weeks according to RCOG 2020)
• Fully dilated cervix
• Membrane ruptured
• Bladder and bowel empty
• No outlet obstruction
• Adequate uterine contractions
• No caput succedaneum
• Fetal head should not be palpable abdominally.

Preprocedure Preparation

• Informed written consent should be taken from woman.

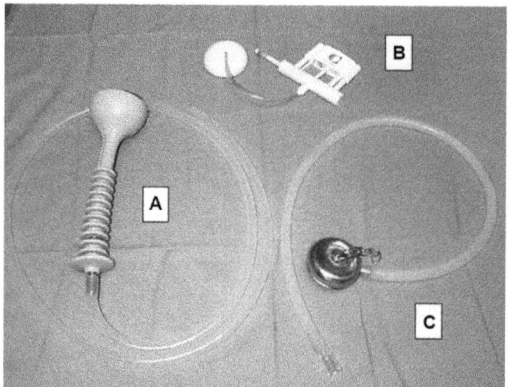

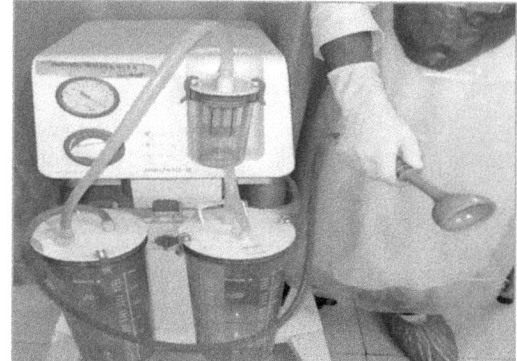

Fig. 10A to C: (A) Silicon cup; (B) Kiwi cup; (C) Metal cup.

Fig. 11: Vacuum generator and traction tubings.

- Explain the procedure and give emotional support and encouragement.
- Prerequisites are checked before application.
- Prepare vacuum and assemble all other necessary equipment as in case of forceps.
- Vacuum should be checked prior to application.
- Select the largest cup size to fit on fetal head.
- Arrange for assistant.
- Wear personal protective equipment (shoe cover, cap, mask, sterile gown, goggles)
- Wash hands and put sterile gloves
- Clean vulva with antiseptic solution
- Check tubings and test vacuum on gloved hand
- Infiltrate local anesthetic agent at episiotomy site, if needed

Procedure

Steps

1. *Application of the cup*: The largest size cup is to be selected and introduced into vagina and placed against the flexion point (3 cm anterior to posterior fontanel) with knob pointing towards occiput **(Fig. 12)**.
2. *Vacuum generation*: Before creating vacuum, ensure no vaginal or cervical tissue is trapped inside the cup. Create vacuum of 0.2 kg/cm². Pressure is gradually increased until 0.8 kg/cm². Fetal scalp is sucked into the cup and an artificial caput (Chignon) is formed.
3. *Traction*:
   - Traction is given with uterine contraction at right angle to cup with one hand

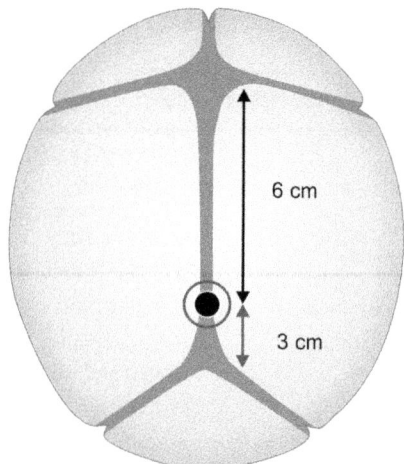

Fig. 12: Flexion point 3 cm anterior to posterior fontanel.

- Other hand is placed against the cup to check correct angle of traction, rotation and advancement of hand **(Fig. 13)**
- Do not apply traction during uterine relaxation.
- Direction of traction is along the axis of birth canal.
- Do not try to actively rotate fetal head. Rotation of head will occur with traction.
- In between contractions check for fetal heart sounds and application of cup.
- Encourage the woman to assist descent with expulsive efforts
- Deliver the head slowly and protect the perineum **(Figs. 14A to C)**

4. *Removal of cup*: Release the vacuum as soon as the head is delivered, gently remove the cup and complete the delivery of baby.

Postprocedure Tasks

• Active management of third stage of labor to be done as in all cases.

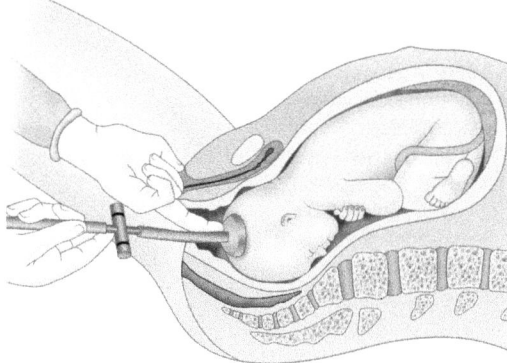

Fig. 13: Traction is given with uterine contraction at right angle to cup with one hand and other hand is placed against the cup to check correct angle of traction, rotation and advancement of hand.

• After delivery inspection vagina, cervix and perineum should be done for tears and repair immediately.
• Give newborn care and postpartum care as required.
• Waste material should be disposed-off in appropriate plastic bags.
• Place instruments and gloves in chlorine solution for decontamination.
• Record the procedure and the findings.

Failure of Vacuum Delivery

• Traction should be stopped if:
    – No progress/descent of head with 3 traction aided contractions.
    – Cup pops off 2 times[3]
    – Failure of delivery after 30 minutes of attempting vacuum.
• If vacuum delivery fails, proceed to cesarean section.

Contraindications of Vacuum Delivery

• Nonvertex presentation
• Preterm fetus—gestational age <34 weeks
• Fetal coagulopathies
• Intrauterine death
• Known fetal macrosomia >4 kg baby weight

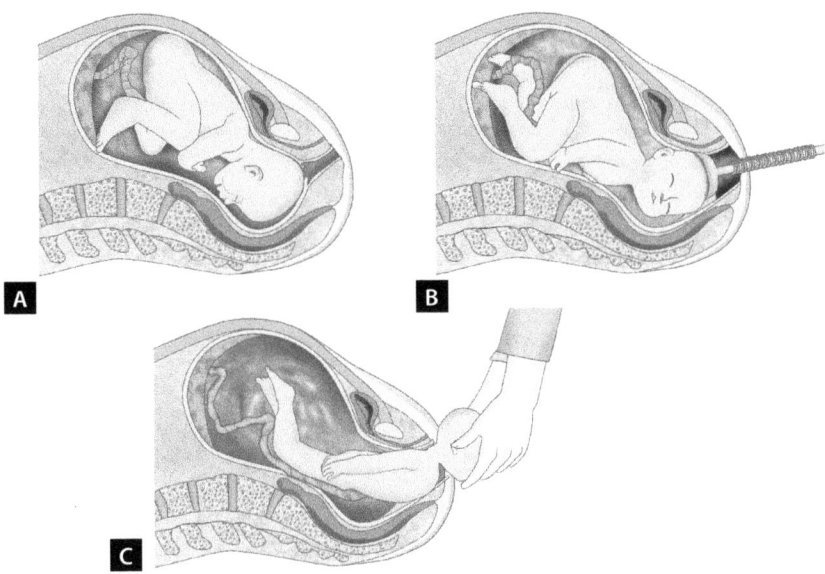

Figs. 14A to C: Placement of vacuum cup and delivery of baby.

TABLE 7: Complications of vacuum delivery.

Maternal	Genital lacerations and tears are usually uncommon
Fetal	• Localized scalp edema (chignon) usually harmless and disappears in few hours • Cephalhematoma • Scalp lacerations • Intracranial or subgaleal hemorrhage (rare) • Jaundice

Sequential use of forceps and vacuum put both mother and neonate to more risk of complication therefore not recommended.[4]

TABLE 8: Forceps delivery versus vacuum delivery.

Benefits of forceps over vacuum delivery	Benefit of vacuum over forceps delivery
• Faster • Higher success rate • Less chance of cephalhematoma or subgaleal hematoma • Safer in preterm, assisted breech delivery, face presentation • If fetal coagulopathy or thrombocytopenia is present • It can be used under epidural anesthesia, which could inhibit maternal expulsive efforts[2]	• Less incidence of severe perineal laceration • It does not need pudendal block • Less perineal pain • Less chance of cesarean section[2]

Complications of Vacuum Delivery

Complications occur usually if prerequisites are not met and continuing efforts for ventouse delivery beyond the limits mentioned **(Table 7)**.

The comparison of forceps delivery and vacuum delivery are given in **Table 8**.

CONCLUSION

Timely and skilled use of instrumental vaginal birth has the potential to decrease the rate of cesarean section and exposure of fetus to intrauterine insult leading to birth asphyxia and its related complications.

REFERENCES

1. Cunningham FG, Leveno KJ, Bloom SL, Dashe JS, Hoffman BL, Casey BM, et al. Williams Obstetrics, 25th edition. New York: McGraw Hill Education; 2018. pp. 1215-42.
2. Konar H. DC Dutta's Textbook of Obstetrics, Operative Obstetrics, 9th edition. New Delhi: Jaypee Brothers Medical Publishers; 2020. pp. 652-60.
3. Murphy DJ, Strachan BK, Bahl R. Assisted Vaginal Birth. Green Top guideline No. 26. BJOG. 2020;127(9):e70-e112.
4. American College of Obstetricians and Gynecologists. Operative vaginal birth. Practice Bulletin No. 219. Obstet Gynecol. 2020;135(4):982-4.

CHAPTER

18

Cesarean Section

Vidya A Thobbi, Bhagyashree Bijjaragi

INTRODUCTION

Cesarean section (CS) is now the most commonly performed operation around the world, with >1 million procedures performed each year in the United States alone. It has become such a common procedure that it is one of the first surgical procedures performed independently by residents/trainees in obstetrics/gynecology. In most of the world, the rise in the frequency of cesarean is relatively recent occurrence.

A CS is done when delivering by vaginal route is difficult or if there is risk to the life of mother and/or child. The incidence of CS is continuously increasing giving women the tile "previous lower segment cesarean section (LSCS)". The advent of better anesthesia, availability of improved surgical techniques and prophylactic antibiotics, has made CS a relatively safer and common procedure.

Asian countries remain lower in the incidence of cesarean. However, the World Health Organization (WHO) proposed ideal rates of cesarean should be 10–15% to optimize the maternal and perinatal health.

Increased international awareness of the need to provide accessible essential or emergency obstetrics and newborn care in developing countries has resulted in the recognition of new training needs and in a number of new initiatives to meet those needs. In some cases, educational programs have been implemented to train general practitioners and nurses in performing emergency CS in rural areas of India and sub-Saharan Africa.

New knowledge of human anatomy in the eighteenth century led to the first modern CS by Henry Thomson and John Hunter in London in 1769.

A planned (elective) CS carries an overall risk of complications that is only slightly higher than that of a vaginal delivery when performed at full term by an experienced team with adequate resources. Nevertheless, CS and in particular emergency CS is associated with increased risk of adhesion, hemorrhage, infection, hysterectomy, thrombotic diseases, and bladder injury.

HISTORY OF CESAREAN SECTION

Etymologically, the word "Caesar" originates from the Latin word—"caedare" meaning "to cut". So, cutting remains the core point. But little is known about the history of CS. It is still a riddle wrapped in mystery inside enigma of myth, mythology, fanciful fantasies, and spurious speculations.

According to the Roman Scholar Pliny (The Elder), the procedure takes its name from branch of ancient Roman family of the "The Julii" whose family name—CAESAR (Latin "caedere"—to cut) originated from a birth of a baby by this means in that family.

Some modern historians, however, have suggested that the procedure and its name derived from Roman "LEX REGIA"—a decree issued during the reign of Numa Pompilius, King of Rome which continued to be enforced under the rule of Caesars (LEX CAESAREA) that required abdominal section to be performed before the burial of a woman who had died in an advanced stage of pregnancy.

There is a mythical belief, probably false, that Roman Emperor, Gaius Julius Caesar was born by this procedure. It is highly unlikely because the mother of Julius Caesar, Aurelia, was alive when he invaded Britain in 55 BC and again in 54 BC and in early times no woman delivered in this way was at all likely to survive (**Figs. 1A to C**).

MILESTONES IN HISTORY OF CESAREAN SECTION

Milestones in history of cesarean section are given in **Table 1**.

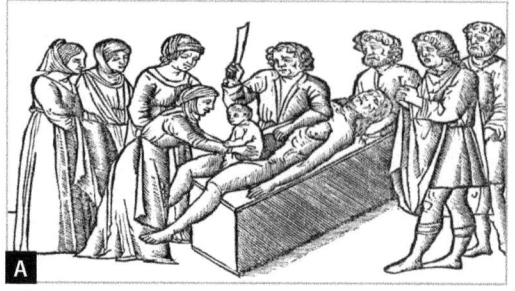

1A: An early printed illustration of cesarean section. A LIVE BIRTH OF Julius Caesar being surgically removed from a dead women. From Suetonius' lives of the Twelve Caesars, 1506 woodcut

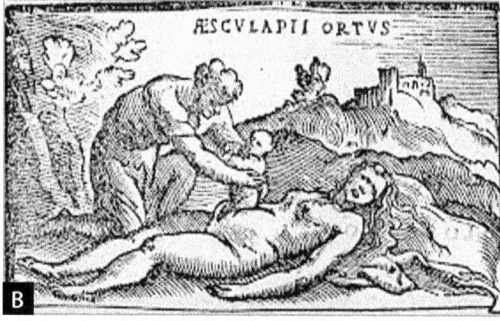

1B: The extraction of Asclepius from the abdomen of his mother Coronis by his father Apollo. Woodcut from the 1549 edition of Alessandro Beneditti's De Re Medica

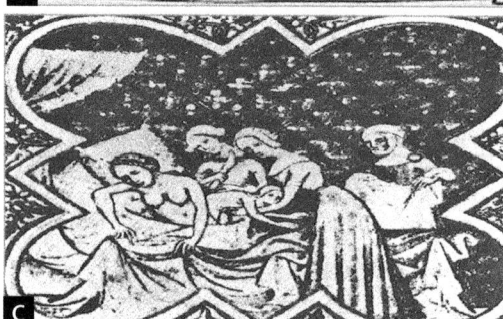

1C: Cesarean section performed on living women by a female practitioners. Miniature from a fourteenth-century "Histoire Ancienne"

Figs. 1A to C: Illustrations of historical evolution of cesarean section.
Courtesy: National Library of Medicine.

TABLE 1: Milestones in history of cesarean section.	
563 BC	• Gautam Buddha was said to have been born from his mother's right flank • Rustam—a hero in Persian mythology was born to Rudaba, after his mother's body was cut open
1581	F Rousset—described cesarean section performed on living women in hysterotomotokia
1610	J Trautmann—first authenticated cesarean with survival of mother
1769	J Lebas—first closure of uterus after cesarean
1786	S Johnson—first description of lower segment uterine incision
1882	F Kehrer and M Sanger—transverse incision of lower segment and uterine closure using silver wire
1900	H Pfannenstiel—described suprapubic skin incision
1908	M Munro Kerr—first series of suprapubic skin incision and transperitoneal lower segment cesarean

EPIDEMIOLOGY AND INCIDENCE OF CESAREAN SECTION

On the basis from 169 countries that include 98.4% of world's births, there are 29.7 million (21.1%) birth occurred through CS in 2015, which was almost double the number of births by this method in 2000 (16 million, i.e., 12.1%) **(Figs. 2A and B)**. CS use in 2015 was up to 10 times more frequent in the Latin America and Caribbean region, where it was used in 44.3% of births, than in west and central Africa region, where it was used in 4.1% of births. The global and regional increase in CS use were driven by both by an increasing proportion of births occurring in health facilities and increasing CS use within health facilities with considerable variation between regions. National CS use varied from 0.6% in south Sudan to 58.1% in Dominican Republic. Within country disparities in CS use were also very large: CS use was almost five times more frequent in births in the richest versus the poorest quintiles in low income and middle-income countries. Markedly high CS use was observed among low obstetric risk births, especially among more educated women in, for example Brazil and China: and CS use was 1.6 times more frequent in private facilities than in public facilities **(Fig. 3)**.

INDICATIONS AND CLASSIFICATION OF CESAREAN SECTION

Indications

The indications for CS are generally applicable in both developed and developing country setting and can be classified into absolute and relative indications. While absolute indications mandatory need cesarean delivery and therefore it will always contribute to baseline cesarean rate and are uncommon. Relative indications represent potentially modifiable conditions that may or may not always lead to a CS. Such relative indications can be subdivided into maternal, obstetric, and fetal categories **(Flowchart 1)**.

Classification

Classification of CS is important for monitoring and comparing CS rates in a standardized, reliable and consistent and action-oriented manner across the world and should be useful for clinicians and public health authorities. The traditional classification of CS as elective and emergency is not of much help as it gives not much clues regarding need for CS. Among existing classification the women-based classification in general and Robson's classifications in particular are the best available classification system for CS.

Robson's Classification

This classification is simple, reproducible, clinically relevant, and prospective classification method, which means that every woman admitted for delivery can be immediately classified into one of the 10 groups based on these few basic characteristics. This allows a comparisons and analysis of CS rates within and across these groups **(Fig. 4)**.

Classification Based on Urgency

Royal College of Obstetricians and Gynaecologists (RCOG) classification of urgency of CS, it is categorized into four categories and is a modification of classification proposed by Lucas et al. The color scale reinforces the need to recognize that the continuum of urgency applies to CS, rather than discrete categories **(Fig. 5)**.

Based on timing: Lucas et al. classified CS into following types:
- *Emergency*: Immediate threat to life of woman or fetus. Decision delivery interval 30 minutes
- *Urgent*: Maternal or fetal compromise which is not immediately life threatening. Done within 75 minutes of decision making.
- *Scheduled*: Needing early delivery but no maternal or fetal compromise.
- *Elective*: At the time to suit the woman and maternity team.

MODERN CESAREAN SECTION

Over the past few decades, there have been several changes in the method and techniques of CS. The classical upper segment cesarean is being replaced by classic Pfannenstiel which is again being replaced by Joel-Cohen firstly and now by gentle Misgav Ladach technique. These changes in techniques have resulted in lesser operating time, less blood loss, less tissue trauma,

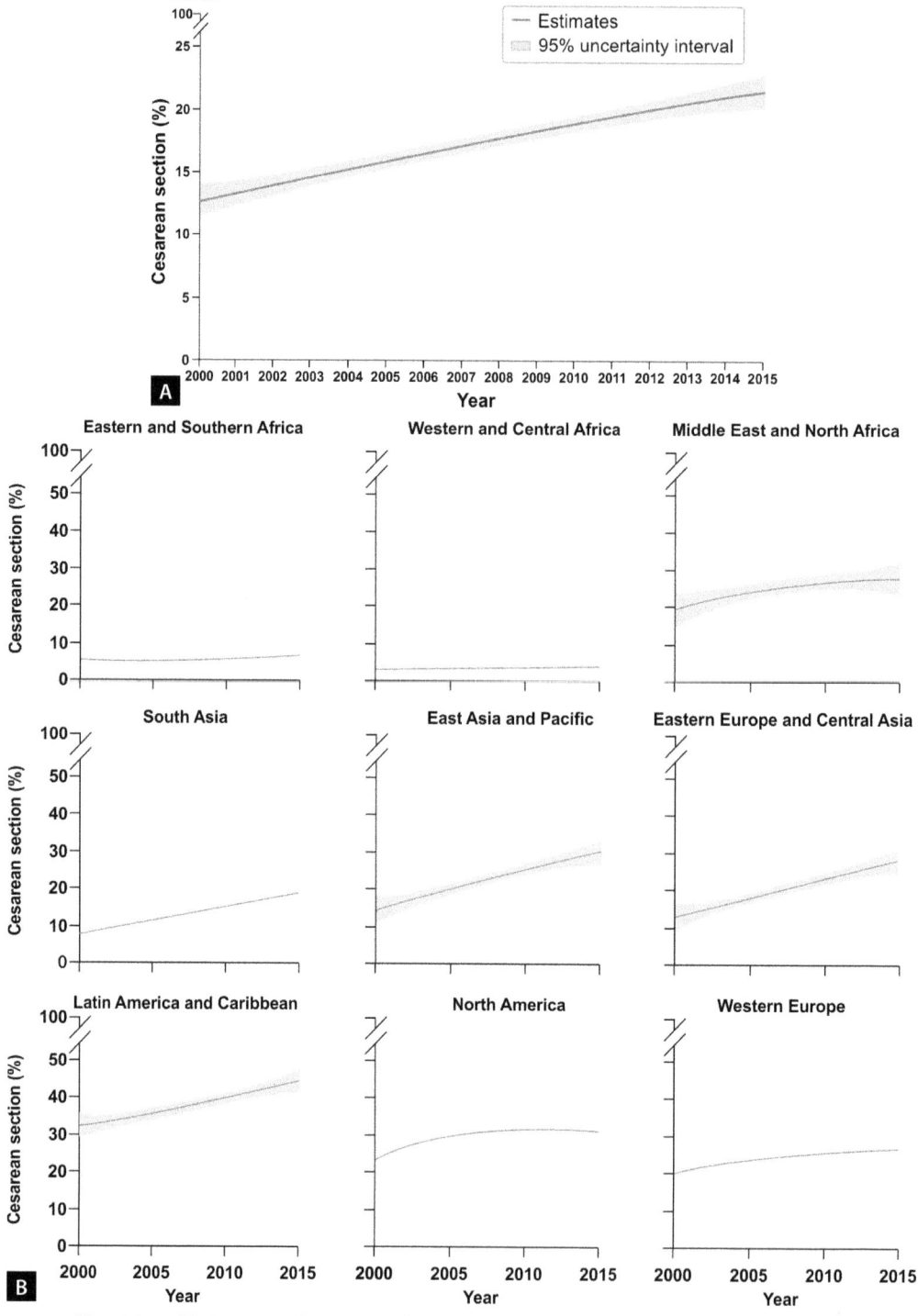

Figs. 2A and B: Estimated frequency of and trends in cesarean section use, as a proportion of live births between 2000 and 2015—(A) Global data; (B) Regional data.

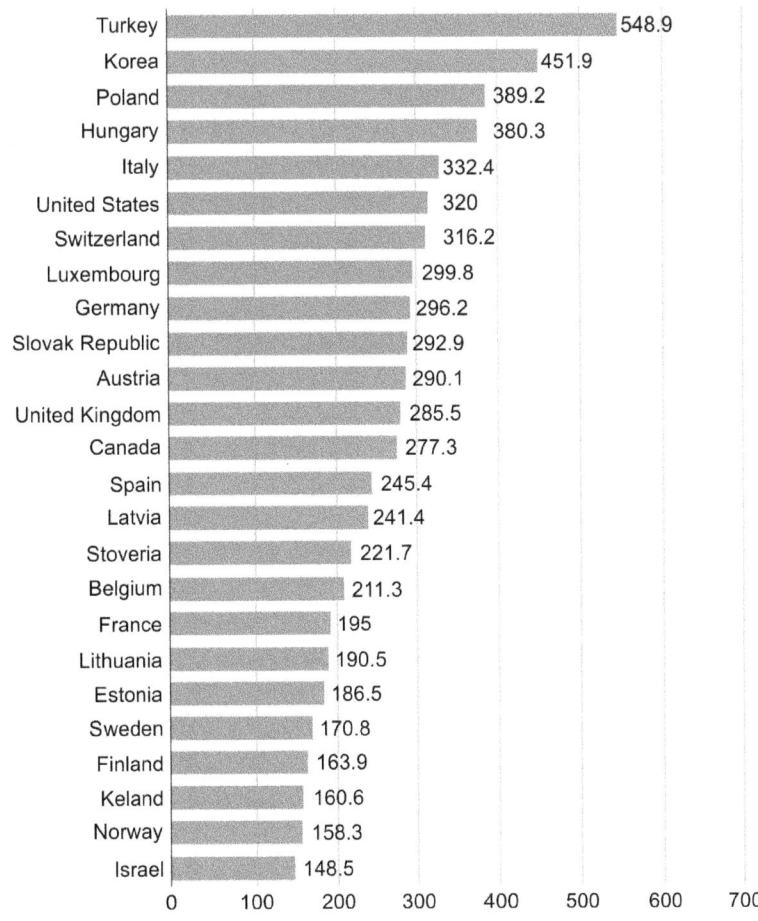

Fig. 3: Cesarean section rate per 1,000 live births [2019 data of Organization for Economic Co-operation and Development (OECD)].

Flowchart 1: Indications for cesarean section (CS).

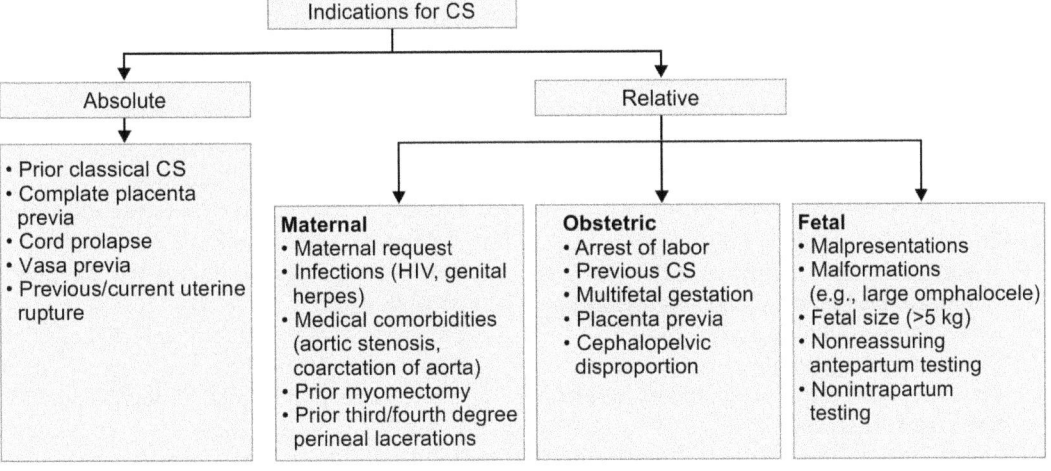

Group 1	• Nulliparous women with single cephalic pregnancy, >37 weeks of gestation in spontaneous labor	Group 6	• All nulliparous women with single breech pregnancy
Group 2	• Nulliparous women with single cephalic pregnancy, >37 weeks who either had labor induced or were delivered by cesarean section before labor	Group 7	• All multiparous women with single breech pregnancy, including women with previous uterine scar
Group 3	• Multiparous women without a previous uterine scar, with single cephalic pregnancy, >37 weeks gestation in spontaneous labor	Group 8	• All women with multiple pregnancies, including women with previous uterine scar
Group 4	• Multiparous women without a previous uterine scar, with single cephalic pregnancy, ≥37 weeks gestation who either had labour induced or were delivered by cesarean section before labor	Group 9	• All women with single pregnancy with a transverse or oblique lie, including women with previous uterine scar
Group 5	• All multiparous women with atleast one previous uterine scar, with single cephalic pregnancy >37 weeks gestation	Group 10	• All women with single cephalic pregnancy <37 weeks gestation, including women with previus scar

Fig. 4: Robson's classification.

Urgency	Definition	Category
Maternal or fetal compromise	Immediate threat to life of woman or fetus	1
	No immediate threat to life of woman or fetus	2
No maternal or fetal compromise	Requires early delivery	3
	At a time to suit the woman and maternity services	4

Fig. 5: A classification relating the degree of urgency to the presence or absence of maternal or fetal compromise.

less postoperative pain, and greater patient satisfaction.

PREOPERATIVE PREPARATION FOR CESAREAN SECTION

Preparation for CS depends on the urgency of CS. If there is need for emergency CS then procedure should be done as soon as possible to safeguard the health of other and unborn child in presence of expert team including gynecologist, anesthetist, pediatrician, staff nurse, and technicians.

Clinical Assessment Prior to CS

- Ensure the indication for CS
- Through history taking to rule out any significant past medical and surgical history which interfere with current procedure.
- Checking maternal vitals
- Fetal lie, position and presentation, and fetal heart rate (FHR) check

Preoperative Preparation

- Fasting for the period of 6 hours for solids and 2 hours for liquids
- Informed written consent in patients own understandable language
- Blood tests—complete blood count (CBC), blood group and Rh typing, human immunodeficiency virus (HIV), hepatitis B surface antigen (HBsAg), hepatitis C virus (HCV), BT, CT, etc.
- Arrange cross matched blood
- Secure intravenous (IV) cannula
- Preparation of operative site—clipping/shaving of operative area
- Bowel preparation—enema to be given previous night.
- Prophylactic antiemetic and antacid (injection pantoprazole 40 mg given prior night or 1 hour before surgery and injection metoclopramide 10 mg IV)

Surgical safety checklist (first edition)

Before induction of anesthesia	Before skin incision	Before patient leaves operating room
Sign in	**Time out**	**Sign out**
☐ **Patient has confirmed** • Identity • Site • Procedure • Consent	☐ **Confirm all team members have introduced themselves by name and role**	Nurse verbally confirms with the team:
☐ **Site marked/not applicable**	☐ **Surgeon, anesthesia professional and nurse verbally confirm** • Patient • Site • Procedure	☐ **The name of the procedure recorded**
☐ **Anesthesia safety check completed**		☐ **That instrument, sponge and needle counts (or not applicable)**
☐ **Pulse oximeter on patient and functioning**	**Anticipated critical events** ☐ **Surgeon reviews:** What are the critical or unexpected steps, operative duration, anticipated blood loss?	☐ **How the specimen is labeled** (including patient name)
Does patient have a: **Known allergy?** ☐ No ☐ Yes	☐ **Anaesthesia team reviews:** Are there any patient-specific concerns?	☐ **Whether there are any equipment problems to be addressed**
Difficult airway/aspiration risk? ☐ No ☐ Yes, and equipment/assistance available	☐ **Nursing team reviews:** Has sterility (including indicator results) been confirmed? are there equipment issues or any concerns?	☐ **Surgeon, anesthesia professional and nurse review the key concerns for recovery and management of this patient**
Risk of >500 mL blood loss (7 mL/kg in children)? ☐ No ☐ Yes, and adequate intravenous access and fluids planned	**Has antibiotic prophylaxis been given within the last 60 minutes?** ☐ Yes ☐ Not applicable **Is essential imaging displayed?** ☐ Yes ☐ Not applicable	

This checklist is not intended to be comprehensive. Additions and modifications to fit local practice are encouraged.

Fig. 6: Surgical safety checklist.

- Prophylactic antibiotics before skin incision (ampicillin first-generation cephalosporin)
- Preloading with 1,000 mL of in vitro fertilization (IVF)
- Catheterization of bladder (optional)
- Most importantly WHO checklist **(Fig. 6)**

During the Operation:
- Regional anesthesia is preferred unless there is a contraindication for the same.
- Mother is put in supine position with left lateral tilt of 30 degree.
- Paint the abdomen with antiseptic solution and drape with sterile drape.
- *Skin incision*: The commonly taken skin incision is Pfannenstiel incision, is a curvilinear incision 2 cm above the pubic symphysis **(Fig. 7 and Table 2)**.
- Another incision is Joel-Cohen incision (less common) which is higher than Pfannenstiel which is 3 cm below the line joining two anterior superior iliac spines.

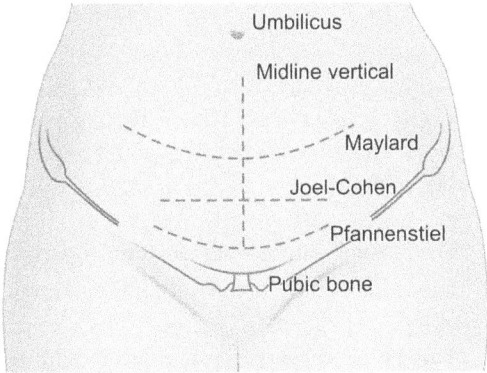

Fig. 7: Different skin incision in cesarean.

- The subcutaneous tissue is incised bluntly, sharply, or by cautery. The bleeding vessels, particularly epigastric vessels are ligated or cauterized.
- Once the rectus sheath is exposed an incision is taken in the center and is extended laterally on both sides sharply with Mayo scissors or bluntly with fingers.

TABLE 2: Advantages and disadvantages of transverse skin incision.	
Advantages	**Disadvantages**
Postoperative comfort is more	Not suitable in acute emergencies
Less chance of wound dehiscence	Slightly more blood loss
Less chance of incisional hernia	Requires competency during repeat section
Cosmetic value	Unsuitable for classical operation

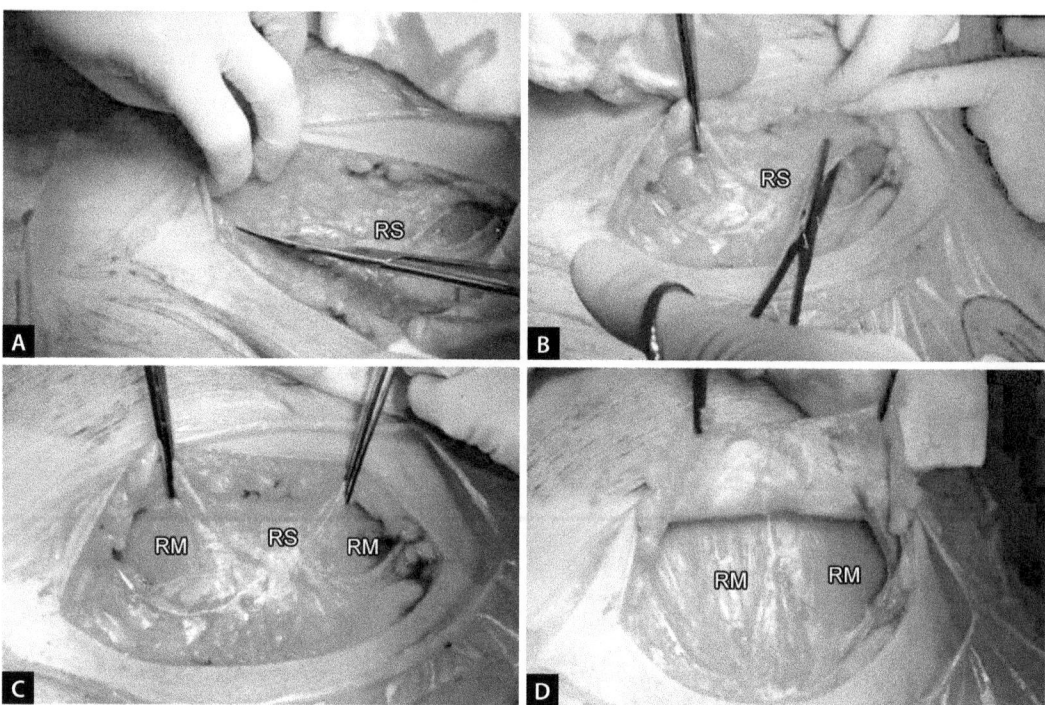

Figs. 8A to D: (A) Rectus sheath (RS) incised in the midline, (B) incision extended on either side using Mayo's scissor, (C) rectus muscle (RM) is exposed, and (D) rectus sheath freed vertically and transversely and rectus muscle is exposed.

- The rectus sheath is separated from underlying muscle by blunt and sharp dissection **(Figs. 8A to D)**.
- The rectus muscle is separated and the peritoneum is approached.
- The peritoneum is opened as high as possible in craniocaudal direction to prevent bowel and bladder injury, either by blunt dissection using fingers or by sharp dissection.
- To open the peritoneum by sharp dissection the peritoneum is held with two artery forceps and is cut open using scissors making sure

that there is no bowel or bladder immediately below the peritoneum.
- All the layers of abdomen are now stretched manually to extend the skin incision and improve access to the uterus and abdominal cavity **(Figs. 9A and B)**.
- The uterovesical fold of peritoneum is identified and the visceral peritoneum is held with allies forceps and UV fold of peritoneum is opened by Mayo scissors.
- The bladder is separated from lower uterine segment (LUS) and retracted downward by Doyen Retractor.

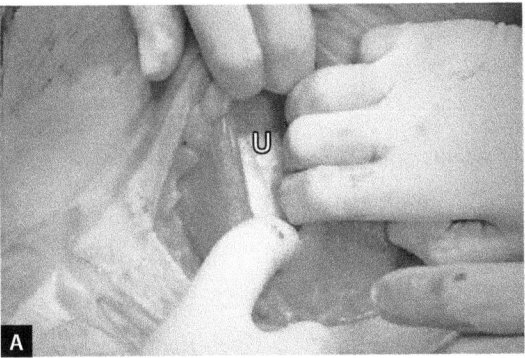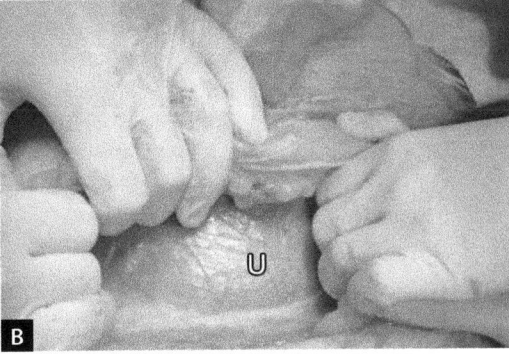

Figs. 9A and B: (A) Opening of the peritoneum; (B) Stretching the layers of abdomen with 8-finger pull technique.

TABLE 3: Comparison of lower segment and classical cesarean section.		
	Lower segment transverse	*Classical*
Techniques	• Slight difficult • Less blood loss • Perfect apposition • Perfect peritonization • Technically difficult in placenta previa and transverse lie	• Technically easy • More blood loss • Imperfect apposition of walls • No perfect peritonization • Comparatively safer
Postoperative	• Less hemorrhage and shock • Less peritonitis • Less adhesions • Lower morbidity and mortality • Better healing	• More hemorrhage and shock • More peritonitis • More adhesions • More morbidity and mortality • Delayed healing

Opening of the Uterus

- Once the LUS is identified and bladder is retracted downward, a transverse nick is taken over the LUS and is extended on either side by sharp dissection using scissors or by bluntly extending the incision using fingers.
- The incision can be extended bluntly by stretching the nick over LUS transversely or stretching in craniocaudal direction. Stretching the incision craniocaudally reduces the incidence of angle extension.
- The excess liquor is allowed to drain and right hand of the surgeon is inserted into the uterus below the presenting part and the baby will be extracted by gentle traction and with minimal fundal pressure by assistant if necessary.
- Once the baby is delivered out delayed cord clamping is employed if there are no contraindications for the same.

- The suctioning of the mouth followed by nose is done and baby is handed over to the pediatrician.
- Placenta is extracted once there is evidence of placental separation.
- The placenta is examined for its completeness and for any abnormality.
- However, in cases in which it is difficult to access the lower uterine segment, a vertical Hysterectomy (classical cesarean section) may be needed. Comparison of classical and lower segment cesarean section is shown in **Tables 3 and 4**.

Closure of the Uterus

- Uterus is closed in two layers by continuous interlocking sutures using Vicryl no 1 or catgut no 1.
- Two layer closure increases the myometrial thickness at the incision and there is less

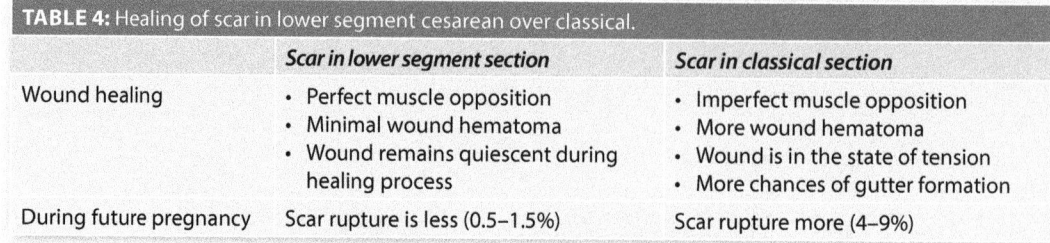

	Scar in lower segment section	Scar in classical section
Wound healing	• Perfect muscle opposition • Minimal wound hematoma • Wound remains quiescent during healing process	• Imperfect muscle opposition • More wound hematoma • Wound is in the state of tension • More chances of gutter formation
During future pregnancy	Scar rupture is less (0.5–1.5%)	Scar rupture more (4–9%)

TABLE 4: Healing of scar in lower segment cesarean over classical.

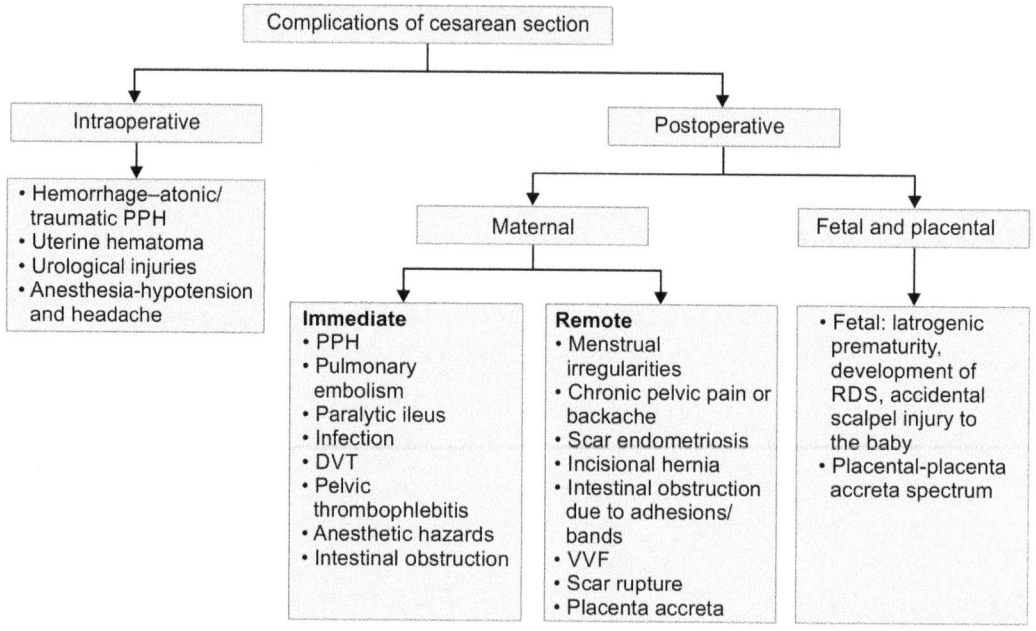

Flowchart 2: Complications of cesarean section.

(DVT: deep vein thrombosis; PPH: postpartum hemorrhage; VVF: vesicovaginal fold)

chance of niche formation and scar rupture in future pregnancy.

Closure of the Abdominal Wall in Layers

- Before closure make suture there are no bleeders. Hemostasis should be achieved.
- The mops and instrument counts are noted and ensured.
- Peritoneal nonclosure is highly recommended as it decreases operative time and reduces the postoperative pain.
- There are two schools of thoughts regarding closure versus nonclosure in reduction of adhesion. There is no definitive consensus for the same.

- Rectus muscle approximation is recommended.
- Rectus sheath is closed using polyglactin-1 or prolene-1 by continuous sutures.
- If the subcutaneous fat thickness is >2 cm then dead space closure is recommended before closing the skin.
- The skin is closed with ethilon no 2-0 or with monocryl no 3-0. Skin can be closed by matters sutures or by subcuticular sutures.

COMPLICATIONS DURING CESAREAN SECTION

Complications of CS can be divided into intraoperative and postoperative **(Flowchart 2)**.

Most common intraoperative complications are:

- *Hemorrhage*:
  - Atonic postpartum hemorrhage (PPH) or traumatic PPH
  - Managed using PPH bundle, uterotonic agents, prompt surgical repair, massive blood transfusion protocol, balloon tamponade, compression sutures, uterine devascularization, and hysterectomy as an end approach
- *Uterine hematoma*: Avoided by giving incision in curvilinear fashion, and correction of dextrorotation of uterus and treated with bilateral uterine artery compression sutures
- *Urological injury*:
  - Bladder injury is the most common lesion in urinary organs. Bladder injury can occur, when the peritoneum is opened if care is not taken to empty it adequately through a catheter, during blunt/sharp dissection in the vesicouterine space to create bladder flap or in cases of previous surgeries that firmly attach the bladder to the anterior side of the uterus.
  - Treatment:
    - Surgical repair with 2–0 Vicryl.
    - Consider possibility of ureteric damage
    - Bladder drainage
    - Cystogram 10–14 days later
- *Intestinal injuries*:
  - Extremely rare occurring only in previous nonobstetric surgical history and in urgent abdominal approach.
  - Treatment includes general surgical assistance, primary repair, resection, and stoma formation.
- *Anesthesia complications*: Hypotension and headache

Postoperative Complications: Maternal, Fetal, and Placental

- *Maternal*:
  - Immediate:
    - Postpartum hemorrhage
    - Shock
    - Pulmonary embolism
    - Anesthetic hazard
    - Paralytic ileus
    - Infection [urinary tract infection (UTI), wound, peritonitis, foreign body, and pelvic abscess]
    - Intestinal obstruction
    - Deep vein thrombosis (DVT)/pelvic thrombophlebitis
  - Remote:
    - Menstrual irregularities
    - Chronic pelvic pain or backache
    - Scar endometriosis
    - Incisional hernia
    - intestinal obstruction due to adhesions/bands
    - Vesicovaginal fold (VVF)
    - Scar rupture
    - Placenta accreta spectrum (PAS)
- *Fetal*:
  - Iatrogenic prematurity
  - Development of respiratory distress syndrome (RDS)
  - Accidental scalpel injury to the baby
- *Placental*: Due to increasing rate of cesarean sections, the incidence of placenta accrete spectrum is increased.

POSTOPERATIVE MONITORING

- First 24 hours
  - *Observation and monitoring*: Blood pressure (BP), pulse rate (PR), urine output, abdominal girth, and local examination for bleeding every 15 minutes for first 2 hours and every 30 minutes for next 4 hours
  - Fluid maintenance
  - Oxytocin infusion
  - Antibiotic administration
  - Analgesics
  - Ambulation
  - Breast feeding of the baby
- *Day 1*: Oral feeding in the form of plain clear fluids
- *Day 2*:
  - Semisolid diet
  - Bowel care with syrup lactulose if the bowels do not move spontaneously.

Misgav Ladach Cesarean Section

The Misgav Ladach method: This is the name of the hospital in Jerusalem where the method has evolved, beginning in 1983.

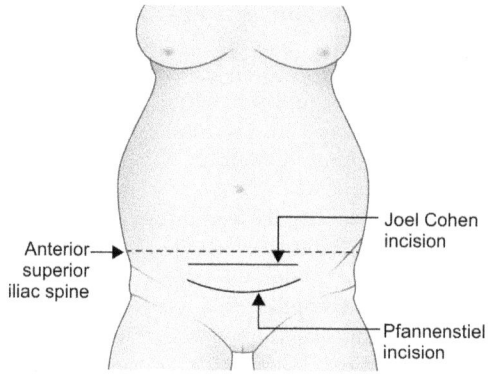

Fig. 10: Skin incision.

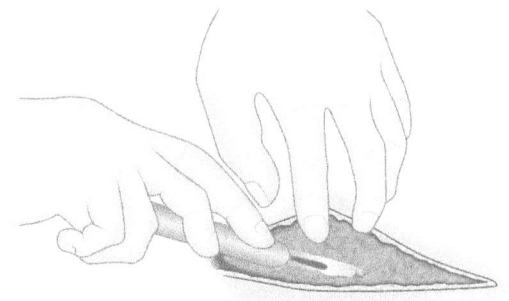

Fig. 11: Rectus sheath incision.

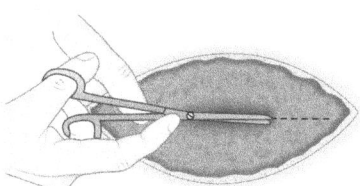

Fig. 12: Splitting the rectus sheath.

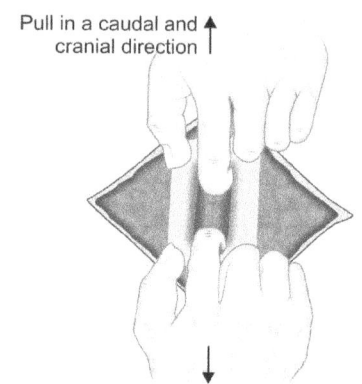

Pull in a caudal and cranial direction

Fig. 13: Open up the rectus sheath.

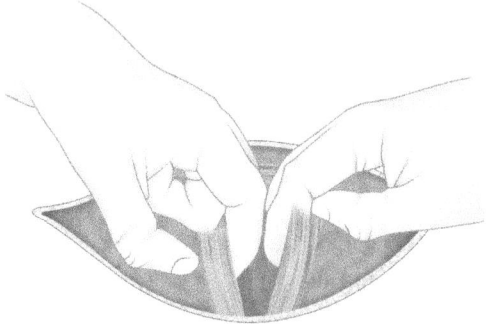

Fig. 14: Separate the rectus muscle.

Method of Misgav Ladach Cesarean Section (Figs. 10 to 16)

- Skin incision is straight transverse incision 3 cm below the line joining anterior superior iliac spines.
- Cut through the skin only not into the subcutaneous tissue, this makes the incision virtually blood less.

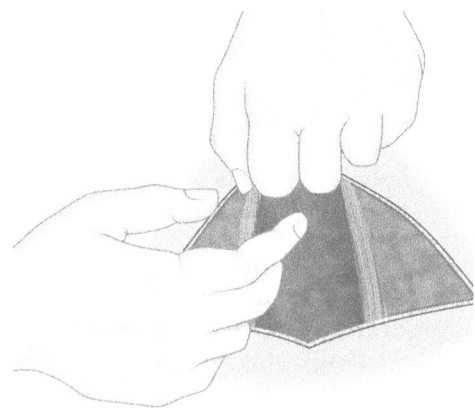

Fig. 15: Opening up of parietal peritoneum.

- Deepen the incision in the midline for 2–3 cm through knife till rectus sheath. Do not try to free any subcutaneous tissue.

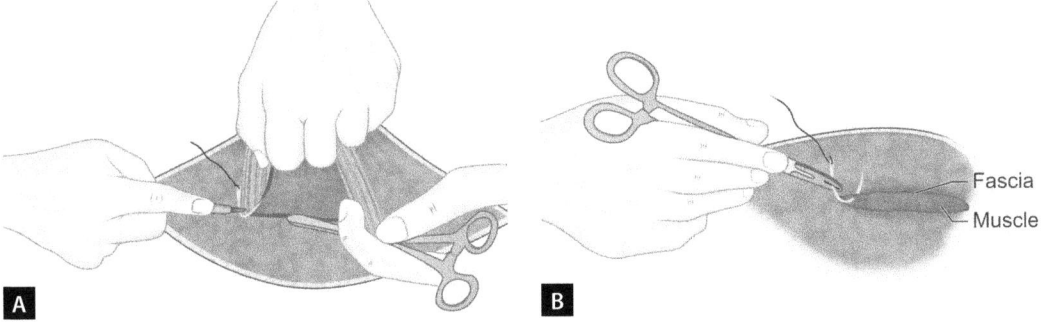

Figs. 16A and B: Suturing the uterus and rectus sheath.

- Make a small transverse incision in the rectus sheath and enlarge the transverse incision bilaterally underneath the fat and subcutaneous tissue without disturbing them.
- Place the tip of a partly open pair of scissors (supported underneath by your left index finger) with one blade under the cut sheath and one blade above.
- Push the scissors along the direction of the fibers in a transverse direction following the curvature of the body as you go further out.
- Gently separate the rectus sheath and muscle by pulling the rectus sheath with two index fingers in craniocaudal direction.
- Pull the rectus muscle apart with index and middle fingers in the midline between rectus muscles encircling the whole muscle bellies and then pull with balanced, smooth and increasing force.
- Open the parietal peritoneum using fingers as high as possible. Identify LUS and make nick on parietal peritoneum 1 cm above the bladder reflection and bladder is pushed down with retractor.
- A transverse nick is made on LUS and incision is extended with right thumb and left index finger.
- Place your right hand below the head and release the head. Deliver the head with minimal fundal pressure.
- Manually remove the placenta and oxytocin 10 units given at this stage.
- Exteriorize the uterus.
- Grasp the angle of the uterus with nontraumatic clamps such as Green Armytage forceps.
- Close the uterine wound in one layer with continuous locked stitches.
- Achieve hemostasis.

- Remove clots but not to pack peritoneal cavity.
- Leave the visceral and parietal peritoneum unstitched.
- Rectus sheath closed by continuous sutures which need not be locked using Vicryl no 1 or similar delayed absorbable material.
- Close the skin with 2 or maximum 3 mattress sutures.

Advantages of Misgav Ladach Technique

- Less traumatic for the mother with quicker postoperative recovery
- Less febrile reactions
- Less need for antibiotics
- A shorter period before normal bowel function returns
- Less peritoneal adhesions and less scarring in the abdominal layers
- Less bleeding in the abdominal wall
- It is so quick that it can be used for both planned and emergency sections.
- Also a method that is easy to learn

▦ SUMMARY

- Cesarean section is one of the most commonly done major surgical procedures worldwide, with an estimated 18.5 million cases performed annually.
- Multiple factors, contribute to significant variation in the rates of CS between developed and developing nations.
- Risk factors for CS include a history of previous CS, nulliparity, and increasing mater
- Maternal age, maternal medical comorbidities, prematurity, malpresentation, suspected

macrosomia, and abnormal cardiotocograph (CTG) tracings

- Recent health initiatives have established guidelines regarding the absolute and relative indications for cesarean section; these guidelines are applicable globally.
- Efforts to reduce rates of cesarean delivery emphasize decreasing the number of primary cesarean section performed for relative indications, and altering public perception of the procedure.
- The WHO recommends the 10-group (Robson) classification as the global standard for comparing varying CS rates across facilities.
- Parenteral antibiotic given 30–60 minutes before the skin incision reduces the risk of maternal infection by half, with no significant effect on neonatal sepsis or admission to intensive care unit.
- Skin preparation with 0.5% chlorhexidine in methylated spirits is associated with lower rates of site infection than alcohol-based povidone–iodine paint is.
- Omission of the bladder flap step at CS reduces the skin incision–delivery interval and is not associated with differences in the risks of bladder injury, total operating time, blood loss, or duration of hospitalization.
- Oxytocin infusion (10–40 IU in 500–1,000 mL crystalloid over 2–8 hours) is the most effective pharmacologic prophylaxis in uterine atony prevention at cesarean delivery.
- Spontaneous delivery of the placenta at CS is associated with less endometritis, less blood loss, and a shorter duration of hospital stay than manual removal is.
- Uterine exteriorization is particularly useful when visualization of the incision is difficult.
- Single-layer closure of the uterine incision is associated with shorter operative procedure time than double-layer closure in women attempting vaginal birth after caesarean section, and locked (but not unlocked single-layer) closure is associated with a higher risk of uterine rupture.

- Short-term postoperative outcome is improved when the peritoneum is not closed at cesarean section.
- Closure of the subcutaneous layer at cesarean section is recommended in all women with a subcutaneous tissue of ≥2 cm.
- Staples and sutures are associated with similar outcomes in terms of wound infection, pain, and cosmetic effects; however, compared to sutures, staples are associated with an increased incidence of skin separation and the need for reclosure if removed on day 3, particularly in obese women
- There is increasing evidence that for many techniques, short-term maternal outcomes are equivalent. Until long-term health effects are known, surgeons should continue to use the techniques they prefer and currently use.

▓ BIBLIOGRAPHY

1. Boerma T, Ronsmans C, Melesse DY, Barros AJD, Barros FC, Juan L, et al. Global epidemiology of use of and disparities in caesarean sections. Lancet. 2018;392:1341-8.
2. Holmgren G, Sjöholm L, Stark M. The Misgav Ladach method for cesarean section: method description. Acta Obstet Gynecol Scand. 1999;78:615-21.
3. Sarmiento A. (2018). Trends in Cesarean Section. [online] Available from https://www.researchgate.net/publication/327984618_Trends_in_Cesarean_Section [Last accessed December, 2021].
4. Torloni MR, Betran AP, Souza JP, Widmer M, Allen T, Gulmezoglu M, et al. Classifications for cesarean section: A systematic Review. PLoS One. 2011;6(1):e14566. doi:10.1371/journal.pone.0014566
5. WHO. (2015). WHO Statement on Caesarean Section Rates. [online] Available from https://www.who.int/reproductivehealth/publications/maternal_perinatal_health/cs-statement/en/ [Last accessed December, 2021].

Anesthesia for Cesarean Section

Rajesh Kumar Verma, Kartik Syal, Rohini Rao

INTRODUCTION

Anesthesia technique for cesarean section is dependent on various factors like:

- Whether elective, semiurgent, or urgent
- Indication
- Fasting status of the mother
- Comorbidities
- Maternal demand for type of anesthesia

TYPES OF ANESTHESIA (TABLE 1)

Spinal Anesthesia for Cesarean Section

Technique

- Injection of local anesthetic agents (bupivacaine or ropivacaine generally) with or without adjuncts (opioids like fentanyl mostly) into subarachnoid space.
- Spinal anesthesia is the most used technique for cesarean section due to following reasons:
  - Quick onset (around 5–10 minutes)

- Simple to perform with easily identifiable target [cerebrospinal fluid (CSF)]
- Reliable with good quality regional anesthesia
- With small manipulation in dose and head tilt, anesthetist can vary the spread of block
- No direct effect of drug on the fetus
- Good intraoperative conditions

Complications Associated with Spinal Anesthesia

- *Hypotension*:
  - Most common side effect
  - Necessitates fluid bolus
  - May require intermittent vasoconstrictors
  - Preloading with 10-15 mL/kg of Ringer lactate or normal saline, left lateral position, and elevated legs can help in decreasing the incidence and severity of hypotension.

TABLE 1: Types of anesthesia.

Spinal anesthesia	• Most common technique • Quick onset (around 5–10 minutes) • Simple to perform • Reliable with good quality regional anesthesia • No direct effect of drug on fetus • Good intraoperative conditions
Epidural anesthesia	• Time consuming • Difficult to perform as compared to spinal anesthesia • Restricted use in emergency cases, like fetal distress • Can be extended from providing labor analgesia to operative anesthesia to postoperative analgesia in elective surgeries
General anesthesia	• Reserved only for dire maternal and fetal emergencies • Airway problems • Risk of aspiration • Drugs may cross placenta

Ephedrine and phenylephrine are the preferred vasoconstrictors.

- *High spinal*:
  - Hormonal and mechanical factors in pregnancy decrease the need of local anesthetic agents.
  - Higher doses can cause hypotension, bradycardia, and even loss of consciousness.
- *Postdural-puncture headache (PDPH)*:
  - Due to dural breach and continuous leak of CSF
  - Caused by larger gauged spinal needle or less frequently but more drastically by larger epidural needle.
  - Pain typically occurs in fronto-occipital region, within 24–48 hours of regional anesthesia, increases with sitting or standing and is usually of thumping type.
  - Its incidence has decreased from over 50% (20 gauge cutting spinal needle) to <10% with the use of smaller diameter non-traumatic (26 gauge splitting needles).[1]
  - In cases of inadvertent dural puncture with 16 gauge or 18 gauge epidural needle, the incidence goes up to even 70%, warranting prophylactic steps, like proper hydration, analgesics, caffeine, bed rest, and even epidural fluids and blood patch to be considered.
- *Persistent neurological symptoms*: These were related to use of chloroprocaine and continuous lignocaine anesthesia which are rarely used these days.

Epidural Anesthesia for Cesarean Section

- Epidural anesthesia involves injection of local anesthetic agents into epidural space.
- The space is further from nerves, thus the dose of drug injected is higher and time taken to effect is also longer.
- This restricts its usefulness in emergency cases, like fetal distress.
- The greatest advantage of this technique is that it can be extended from providing labor analgesia to operative anesthesia to postoperative analgesia.[2]
- Around 15–18 mL of 2% lignocaine or bupivacaine (concentration > 0.25%) is needed for operative procedures (T4 level needed).

Complications Associated with Epidural Anesthesia

- As there is no clear endpoint other than loss of resistance through ligamentum flavum, which itself is edematous and lax in pregnancy, a good "feel" of reaching epidural space is not appreciated.
- This can cause failure and dural puncture leading to PDPH.
- Intraspinal injection of epidural dose will cause high spinal and will require intensive care unit care.
- Hypotension can occur but less in severity and incidence compared from spinal anesthesia due to slow onset of effect.
- Patchiness of effect is common with plain epidural technique due.

General Anesthesia

The use of this technique for routine cesarean section is declining with time due to following reasons:

- *Airway problems*:
  - Difficulty in intubation and ventilation is the most dreaded complication in general anesthesia.
  - Enlarged breasts, buccal fat depositions, mucosal edema, and capillary engorgement make ventilation, laryngoscopy, and intubation difficult in obstetrics cases.
  - In addition, patients are prone to sudden desaturation due to higher demand and decreased reserve.
  - This makes it the most significant cause of anesthesia-related obstetric mortality.
- *Aspiration*:
  - There is high incidence of aspiration in pregnant patients, going even up to 15%.[3]
  - Difficult intubation and laryngoscopy, delayed gastric emptying, acidic and particulate gastric contents, nonfasting emergent cases, and noneffective lower gastroesophageal sphincter (mechanical as well as hormonal) puts the parturient in higher risk of this complication.

As discussed above these two airway-related complications lead to more than half of anesthesia-related deaths in cesarean section. In one survey spreading over 5 years, it was found that general anesthesia was associated with 16 times more case fatality rate than regional anesthesia;[4] though this difference since then has decreased due to better airway management and aids to intubation.

- *Multiple drugs:*
  - General anesthesia involves addition of multiple drugs into maternal and fetal circulations.
  - In standard doses, the drugs rarely have significant effects, but chances of neonatal respiratory and central depression remain.
  - Also, unknown teratogenic and neurohormonal influence of drugs further complicates this choice of anesthesia.
- *Awareness:*
  - Tendency of keeping anesthetic drugs on the lower side in view of fetal safety increases the risk of awareness among these patients.[5]
  - This should be explained to the patient and should be included in the consent to avoid legal matters in the future.

Due to these reasons, especially morbidity and mortality increasing complications of airway and aspiration, regional anesthesia has become the favored approach in pregnant patients.

Indications for General Anesthesia

- Dire maternal and fetal emergency, like profound fetal bradycardia, cord prolapse with fetal compromise, uncontrolled eclampsia, etc.
- Coagulopathies and other contraindications to regional anesthesia
- Maternal wish
- Acute severe maternal hypovolemia
- Inadequate regional anesthesia

CONCLUSION

- Regional anesthesia is mostly used.
- Single shot spinal anesthesia is the most preferred technique.
- General anesthesia is reserved for extreme situations where regional anesthesia is contraindicated.

REFERENCES

1. Turnbull DK, Shepherd DB. Post-dural puncture headache: pathogenesis, prevention and treatment. Br J Anaesth. 2003;91(5): 718-29.
2. Segal S, Su M, Gilbert P. The effect of a rapid change in availability of epidural analgesia on the cesarean delivery rate: a meta-analysis. Am J Obstet Gynecol. 2000;183(4):974-8.
3. Mendelson CL. The aspiration of stomach contents into the lungs during obstetric anesthesia. Am J Obstet Gynecol. 1946;52: 191-205.
4. Chestnut DH. Anesthesia and maternal mortality. Anesthesiology. 1997;86(2):273-6.
5. Robins K, Lyons G. Intraoperative awareness during general anaesthesia for cesarean delivery. Anesth Analg. 2009;109(3):886-90.

Cesarean Section in Special Situation

Vidya A Thobbi, Vibhavaree Dandawate

INTRODUCTION

The incidence of cesarean section (CS) is being on rise. It is commonly perceived as simple and safe alternative to vaginal delivery. There are situations where in the CS is considered as difficult. These are the few special situations where in the technique of CS is bit different from routine CS. These special situations can be broadly categorized into:

- Special approach to lower uterine segment (LUS)
- Technique of fetal extraction in special situations
- Technique of CS in abnormal placentation

APPROACH TO LOWER UTERINE SEGMENT

Routine approach to LUS is considered quite easy. But it is difficult in some situations, e.g., in situations of adhesions in previous lower segment cesarean section (LSCS), extreme premature babies, and fibroid in LUS.

Adhesions

- Postoperative adhesions are a common complication of major abdominal surgery, including cesarean delivery (CD).
- Adhesions form during healing and consist of fibrous scar tissue that often abnormally connects internal organs or structures.
- Adhesions are result of abnormal wound healing.
- During healing process, the fibrinolytic activity prevents formation of fibrin deposits and abnormal tissue attachments.
- Infection, tissue ischemia, tissue desiccation, intraperitoneal blood, and reactive foreign bodies (such as talc powder from gloves and sutures) have been reported as being common risk factors.
- Surgical technique, genetic factors, white blood cells, and fibroblast activities are also proposed as risk factors in adhesion development.

Adhesion increases the duration of surgery and increases the incision to extraction time. The only treatment is surgical lysis of adhesion, but this results in formation adhesion again.

The best possible treatment is to prevent the formation of adhesion as much as possible.

The preventive strategies for adhesion formation:

- Modification of surgical technique
- *Adhesion preventive agents*: Currently, the most widely used adhesion-prevention agents in the labor and delivery setting that are approved by the US FDA are oxidized regenerated cellulose (ORC; Interceed; Ethicon Inc., NJ, USA) and sodium hyaluronate/carboxymethylcellulose (HA/CMC; Seprafilm; Genzyme Biosurgery, MA, USA).

These act as absorbable barriers that act as a mechanical barrier between adjacent tissues to attempt to reduce adhesion formation while healing takes place.

Premature Babies/Extreme Low Birth Weight Babies

- In these cases, the LUS is not well formed.
- LUS will be thick as the uterus is not well distended due to extreme prematurity or extreme low birth weight (LBW).
- In such cases, the incision on LUS should be big.
- The trick here will be to open the full incision on the uterus and do not have small incision

going down and down which will bleed due to thick LUS.

- Once the uterine cavity is entered with big bold incision the baby is extracted.
- When the extraction is difficult then uterine tocolysis is recommended or incision is converted to J shaped or inverted T-shaped incision.
- The dictum here will be "big baby big incision: small baby big incision".

Another method to deliver extreme preterm or LBW baby is to delivery "en caul".

- If the membranes are ruptured at the time of delivery, the preterm fetus will be trapped instantly by a so-called "hug-me-tight uterus".
- When baby is to be delivered by en caul make sure that while taking incision on uterus membranes are not incised.
- Once, the incision is extended then the surgeons fingers are introduced between membranes and uterine cavity and placenta is separated.
- The sac is delivered out with minimal fundal pressure and assistance help.
- The membrane is ruptured artificially and baby is removed and cord clamped.

When above-mentioned technique fails then ultimate procedure will be classical cesarean incision.

Cesarean in Fibroid Uterus at LUS

- It is very important to map the fibroid before CS.
- Always try to avoid taking incision over the fibroid.
- In very rare cases, there is a need for taking incision through fibroid, in such cases the procedure should be quick.
- In rare, instances myomectomy should be performed quickly before extracting the baby.
- If it is not at all possible to go through LUS then classical incision is taken.

CESAREAN SECTION DELIVERY: MALPRESENTATIONS

Transverse Lie

External cephalic version is an option if membranes intact:

- Transverse lie to be converted to longitudinal.

- Cephalic version is an option though conversion to breech by traction on feet preferred.
- Knowledge of position of fetal head is important. A liberal J-shaped incision in LUS is usually required if baby is term with or without premature rupture of membrane (PROM).
- Inverted "T" incision to be avoided.
- Neglected transverse lie is a dangerous situation and possibility of extension of the incision exists.
- Beware of sepsis in PROM

BREECH DELIVERY

Abdominal delivery no different from vaginal breech extraction with many of the risks:

- Limbs manipulated through natural range of movement
- Trunk supported by the pelvic girdle to encourage suitable rotation. The premature breech is more prone to injury as the lower segment is thick walled, narrow, and retractile delivery of after coming head.
- Avoid trapping of after coming head by the retracting
- Uterus especially in premature breech (head-trunk ratio)
- Mauriceau–Smellie–Veit maneuver
- Forceps application

Cesarean Section: Delivery of Multiple Pregnancies

- Planning delivery
- Identify placental location
- Assess the fetal lie and relationships
- Plan delivery of presenting fetus
- Adequate abdominal and uterine incision
- Care taken to deliver floating head or breech
- Orientation may be distorted
- Mobilize adequate neonatal support
- Prophylaxis for postpartum hemorrhage (PPH)

Fetal Extraction in Special Situation

- *Floating head*: Floating head is difficult to catch, control and to give traction during extraction, hence it is difficult to take out the fetus through uterine and abdominal incision.
  - The traditional fundal pressure at times won't help to deliver the baby safely as

fundal pressure do not push the head towards incision rather it pushes the head laterally or it might even change the presentation.

– To deliver the floating head uterine axis is corrected, amniotic fluid is allowed to drain slowly so that head is descended towards incision keeping the flexion of head.

– Once the adequate amniotic fluid is drained uterine incision is extended and then baby is delivered.

Other measures to deliver the floating head are instrumental delivery using:

- Vacuum cup
- Forceps
- Vectis
- *Vacuum-assisted delivery*: Once the head is stabilized after draining the adequate liquor and extending the uterine incision, the vacuum cup is applied to fetal vertex taking care not to include myometrium.
  – Then vacuum tube is connected. Negative pressure of 300–400 mm Hg is created and fetal head is extracted with gentle traction and if necessary with minimal fundal pressure **(Fig. 1)**.
- *Forceps-assisted delivery*: One forceps blade can be used as lever or both blades (short forceps) can be used to extract head through incision **(Fig. 2)**.
  – During forceps blade application, flexion of fetal head is maintained as far as possible with little fundal pressure to push head toward incision.
  – Lower blade is applied first followed by anterior blade.
  – The concavity of pelvic curve of blade should be toward fetal occiput.
  – Head is extracted with controlled traction.

In some cases, internal podalic version can be done and baby is extracted by footling breech.

Deeply-engaged Head

- In advanced labor the fetal head is deeply engaged into the pelvis.
- The true incidence of CS with a deeply engaged head is unknown but it probably accounts for 25% of all emergency sections.
- Failed instrumental delivery
- Deep transverse arrest
- Arrest in the opp is occipitoposterior position
- Unanticipated cephalopelvic disproportion (CPD) late in labor
- Different factors act for impaction of the fetal head in maternal pelvis.

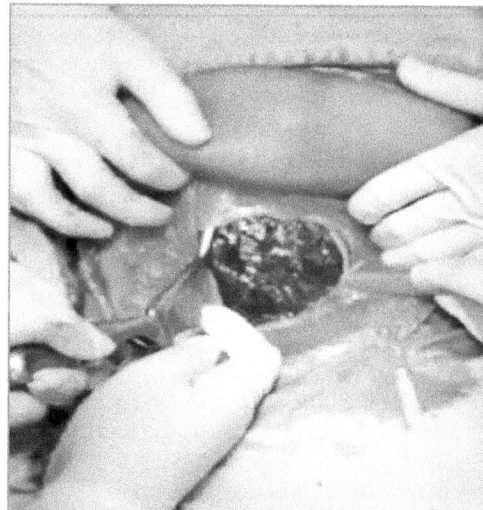

Fig. 2: Application of forceps—sagittal suture placed transversely, slight fundal pressure to push head toward the incision, concavity of the pelvic curve toward the fetal occiput, lower blade is applied first followed by the anterior, flex fetal head with traction aided by fundal pressure, crowning of the fetal head in abdominal incision, and delivery by controlled extension.

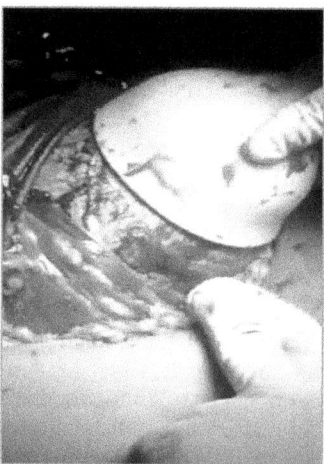

Fig. 1: Vacuum application at cesarean section.

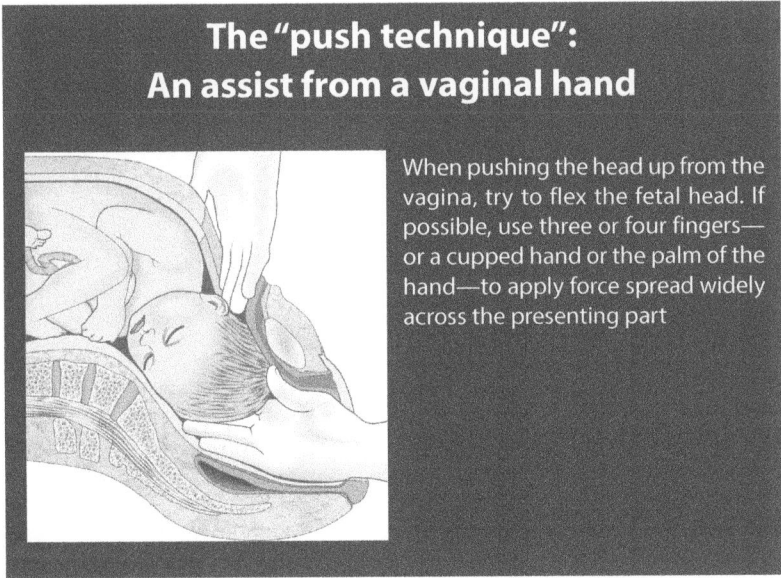

Fig. 3: The push technique.

- Performing CS in such situation is challenging.
- In advanced labor with deep impacted head the LUS will be stretched out and is indistinguishable from cervix and vagina.
- Therefore uterine incision is inadvertently taken too low or into the vagina.
- It may be difficult for the operating surgeon to maneuver his hand below the deeply engaged fetal head, which may be further compounded by the presence of molding and edema on the fetal head (caput succedaneum).
- Use of undue force to deliver the head may result in extension of the uterine incision into the broad ligament, cervix, or vagina.

Methods to Deliver the Deeply-engaged Head

- Assistant pushing the fetal head from the vagina and operating surgeon applying steady traction on fetal shoulder and disimpaction and extraction of the baby by vertex. The assistant needs to use 3–4 fingers or hand in the form of cup to push to maintain flexion. It is advisable not to use pressure with 1–2 fingers to push as it can cause skull fracture **(Fig. 3)**.
- *Reverse breech extraction*: Fetus is in occipitoposterior position. After uterine

incision, surgeon first extracts fetal arms **(Figs. 4A to D)**.
  - Then both feet are grasped by surgeon, which are present in fundus of uterus and with gentle traction legs are extracted.
  - The fetal body is extracted next by symmetrically pulling the legs with minimal fundal pressure if necessary.
  - Then the fetal head can be disengaged from maternal pelvis by unscrewing movement.
  - *Reverse breech extraction in occipito-anterior position*: Here surgeon first extracts both arms and then grasping the fetal back and shoulder with gentle traction trunk and legs are delivered **(Fig. 5)**.
- *Patwardhan method (shoulders first method)*: In cases of occipitotransverse or occipito-anterior positions with the head deeply impacted in the pelvis, an incision is made in the LUS, at the level of the anterior shoulder, which is then delivered out. The posterior shoulder is also delivered with gentle traction on this shoulder. Now, the fingers are hooked into both axilla and trunk and body is delivered out by gentle traction. Fetal head is then gently lifted out of pelvis **(Figs. 6A to D)**.

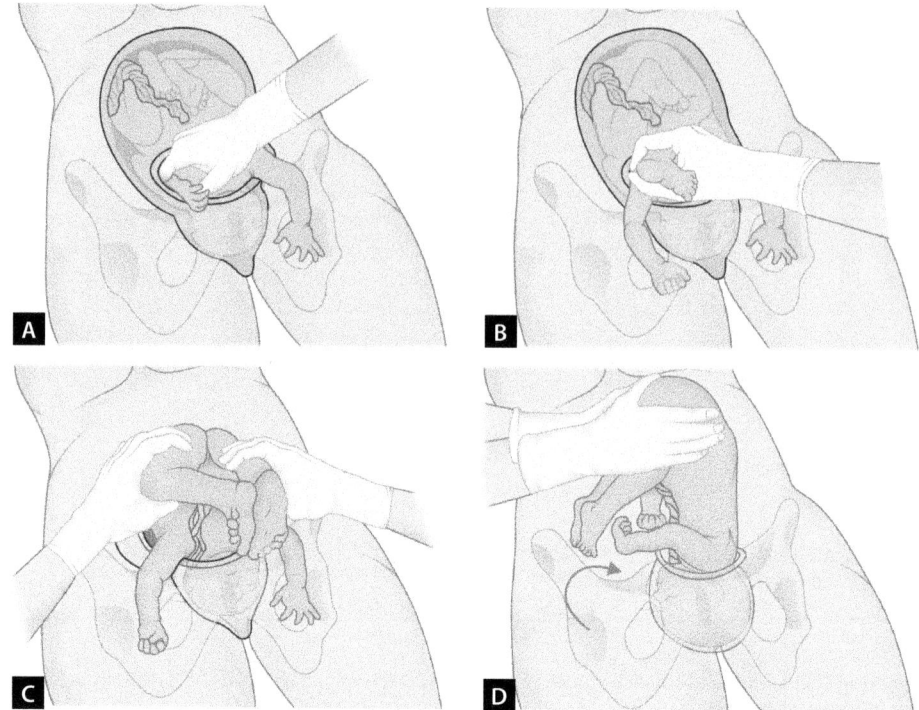

Figs. 4A to D: Reverse breech extraction in occipitoposterior position: (A) Extraction of arms; (B) Extraction of legs; (C) Extraction of trunk; (D) Unscrewing of head; (E) Delivery of head.

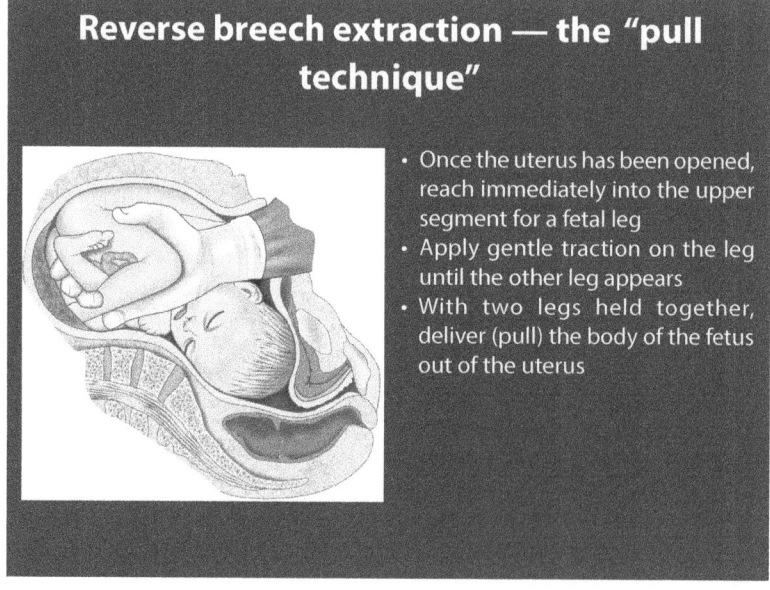

Reverse breech extraction — the "pull technique"

- Once the uterus has been opened, reach immediately into the upper segment for a fetal leg
- Apply gentle traction on the leg until the other leg appears
- With two legs held together, deliver (pull) the body of the fetus out of the uterus

Fig. 5: Reverse breech extraction—the "pull technique".

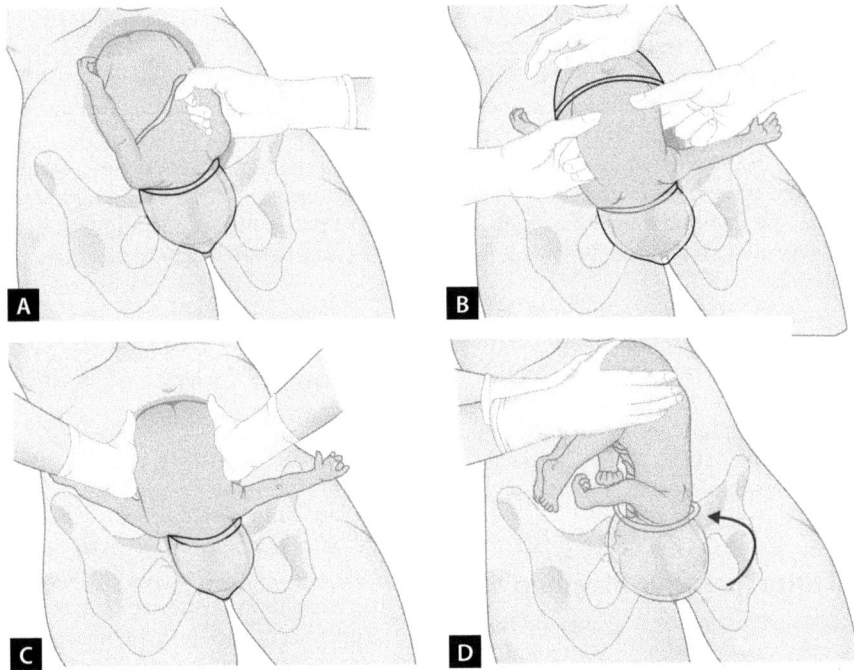

Figs. 6A to D: (A) Reverse breech extraction in occipitoanterior position; (B) Extraction of both arms; (C) Extraction of trunk; (D) Extraction of legs.

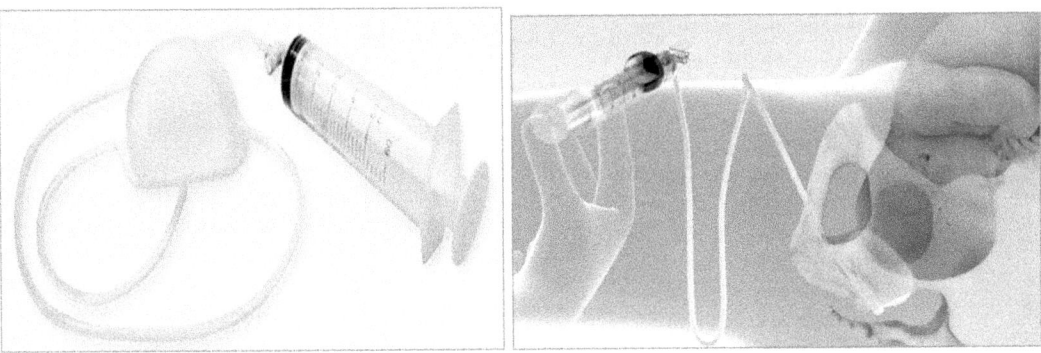

Fig. 7: Fetal pillow.

- *"Fetal disimpacting system" and "fetal pillow"*: It has a foldable base plate that is 11 cm long and 4.5 cm wide, with a balloon attached to it which is inserted below the fetal head vaginally, at the time of inserting a Foley's catheter before the cesarean. Just before making the uterine incision an assistant inflates the balloon with 180 mL of saline solution. This straightens the base plate which opens to become flat against the pelvic floor. The inflated balloon gently elevates the fetal head 3–4 cm from its original position, making it easier to deliver. The balloon is deflated once delivery is achieved, and the device is gently pulled out using the attached tubing or by hooking a finger into the base plate **(Fig. 7)**.
  - *Extraction of fetus in transverse lie*: This should be done by experienced surgeon. Always anticipate problems and be prepared for the same. It needs

experienced assistance as well. A liberal incision at LUS is taken and surgeon after inserting hand into the uterine cavity feels for the fetal back. Trace the back and reach out to fetal feet. Feet are grasped and internal podalic version is done and baby is extracted by breech. If in case baby's hand comes out reposit it into uterine cavity and trace back from shoulder.

- *Extraction of fetus in breech*: Limbs should be manipulated within natural range (movements); trunk should be supported by pelvic girdle to encourage rotation and after coming head of breech can be delivered by Burns Marshall or Mauriceau–Smellie–Veit method or with help of forceps

Control of Intraoperative Bleeding

- *Localized site*: Pressure by a sponge on holder or pack to isolate the bleeding site and then deep interrupted sutures to ligate bleeding preferably with chromic catgut No. 1 as with delayed absorbable sutures cutting through tissue is common.
- Bleeding from angles and suture line
- Step-wise devascularization of the uterus
  - Effective in controlling PPH in 80% of cases
  - Unilateral uterine artery ligation
  - Bilateral uterine artery ligation at the upper part of the LUS
  - Low uterine vessels ligation after mobilization of the bladder
  - Unilateral ovarian vessel ligation
  - Bilateral ovarian vessel ligation
  - B-Lynch suture bleeding
  - Simple, effective, relatively safe and requires minimal expertise.
  - A woman meets the criteria for the B-Lynch compression suture if bimanual compression decreases the amount of uterine bleeding by abdominal and perineal inspection.
  - *Modified technique*: Cho's square suture—Hayman's modification is equally effective to internal iliac artery ligation.
  - Experiments in the 1960s by Burchell ascertained that the effect of ligation of

the internal iliac (hypogastric) artery was to convert the affected pelvic circulation to a venous system, thereby allowing clotting to develop and persist resulting into control of PPH.

- Effective in uterine atony, midline perforation, large broad ligament or lateral pelvic hematoma, multiple cervical tears, and lower segment bleeding
- Less effective in placenta accreta
- Not useful for uterine laceration

Technique of CS in Abnormal Placentation

- Abnormal placentation means abnormal presence of placenta in LUS which is termed as low lying placenta (when placenta within 20 mm from internal os)/placenta previa (when placenta covering the internal os) based on its relation to internal os of cervix.
- There is increase in incidence of placenta previa due to increase in maternal age, increase incidence of CS, increased assisted reproductive technology (ART) pregnancies, and multiparity.
- Placenta previa in general and placenta previa in previous cesarean in particular is important as it increases the postpartum bleeding, increases maternal morbidity and perinatal morbidity and mortality.
- The incidence of PAS (placenta accreta spectrum) is increased due to previous uterine scar of any type (D&C, and CS, myomectomy).
- It is need of the hour to treat the placenta previa/placenta accreta spectrum (PAS) effectively to reduce morbidity and mortality of mother and the baby.
- In placenta previa, abundant blood flow enters the LUS and placenta not only from internal iliac artery but also from the anastomosis from other pelvic arteries.
- Therefore, it is difficult to control bleeding even after stepwise devascularization.
- So one should know the various hemostatic methods, resuscitation methods for massive hemorrhage and systemic management.

Once the mother is diagnosed with placenta previa delivery should be conducted in tertiary care hospital with senior doctors. It should be multidisciplinary approach involving senior obstetrician, senior anesthetist, and senior surgeon if required, pediatrician, interventional radiologist, and expert assistance. There should be availability of blood and blood products.

PREOPERATIVE PREPARATION

- Localization of placenta by transvaginal sonography/magnetic resonance imaging (TVS/MRI), fetal position, and presentation should be noted.
- Explaining the risk to family members and take consent for blood transfusion, cesarean hysterectomy, and high risk consent.
- Adequate blood and blood product should be arranged.
- Discussion with obstetrician, transfusion medicine specialist, anesthetist, urologist, and OT staff should be done in advance.

METHODS TO REDUCE INTRAOPERATIVE BLOOD LOSS

Intra-arterial balloon occlusion: Place the balloon catheter in common iliac artery or abdominal aorta. Occluding internal iliac artery is ineffective as there is abundant anastomosis between internal and external iliac artery branches **(Fig. 8)**.

Other measures to reduce bleeding are:
- The internal iliac arteries should be freed to allow clipping.

- Nelaton catheter/tourniquet should be passed through the bilateral broad ligament under the lower segment of the uterus to make the LUS ischemic by tying.
- Arterial ligation or local hemostasis such as U-shaped sutures, enclosing sutures, an interrupted circular suture, compression sutures, and balloon tamponade.

INCISION ON THE UTERUS

When there are engorged blood vessels in LUS in case of placenta previa, no attempt should be made to separate the bladder from LUS by taking incision on uterovesical (UV) fold of peritoneum. If we do so there will be massive hemorrhage and lead to bladder injury if it is PAS **(Fig. 9)**.

- *Transverse incision on the fundus*: It should be made to prevent incision reaching the placenta there by preventing placental separation and hence preventing massive hemorrhage **(Fig. 10)**.
- Inverted T incision
- J-shaped incision
- Classical CS
- *Lower segment transverse incision*: After taking incision on LUS, there are two methods to deliver the baby out.
  1. One is taking the incision through the placenta and entering amniotic cavity and delivering the fetus out.
  2. Second one being after uterine incision placenta is separated by inserting hand between placenta and uterus causing abruption and delivering the baby out.

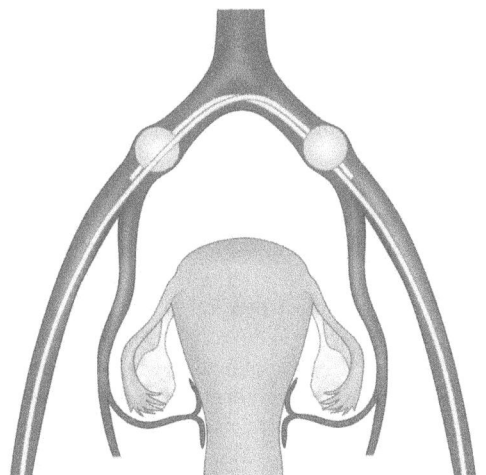

Fig. 8: Intra-arterial balloon occlusion.

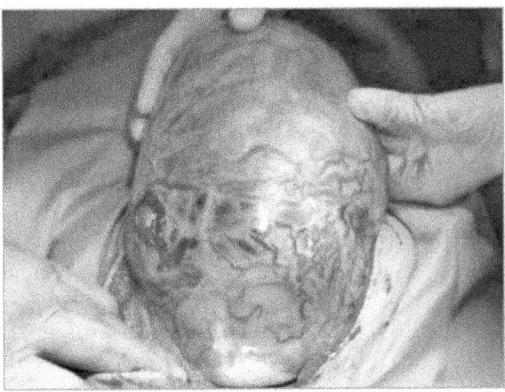

Fig. 9: Engorged blood vessels at LUS.

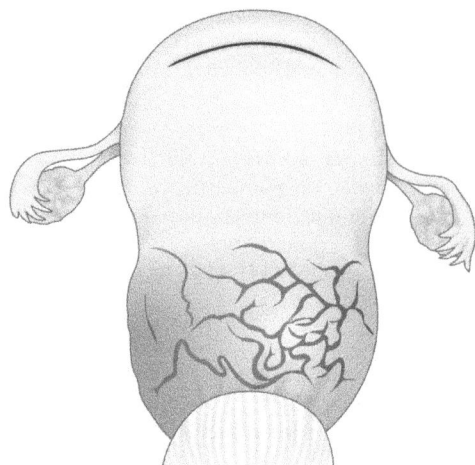

Fig. 10: Transverse incision over fundus to prevent incision reaching placenta.

These two methods are associated with increased bleeding and also neonatal anemia due to fetal blood loss during the procedure.

- *Placental delivery*:
  - If placenta is separated on its own then it can be taken out from the uterus.
  - If placenta is not separated, no attempt should be made to separate the placenta manually. It should be left in situ and uterus is closed. The postoperative monitoring should be done for bleeding and infection.
  - If placenta is let in situ, methotrexate does not help in decreasing the hemorrhage instead it causes harm.
- *Delayed hysterectomy (the two-stage hysterectomy)*:
  - In CS cases, if the placenta does not separate spontaneously, and there is no bleeding, the surgery can be completed with the placenta left in situ without trying vigorously to separate it.
  - The placenta may be separated at the second stage after blood flow into the placenta is reduced, or the amount of bleeding may be decreased by scheduled delayed hysterectomy.
  - In these cases, embolization of the internal iliac artery or the uterine artery prior to the two-stage operation reportedly leads to a decrease in the amount of bleeding.

- Delayed hysterectomy has a drawback since, even if scheduled, it cannot be performed in cases in which placenta is separated and hemorrhage has occurred during CS.
- *Triple P procedure*:
  - This is a conservative surgical approach in placenta previa with PAS.
  - It has three step surgical technique involving:
    1. *First P*: Preoperative localization of placental edge and delivery of the fetus above the upper border of the placenta.
    2. *Second P*: Pelvic devascularization
    3. *Third P*: Placental nonseparation with myometrial excision
  - *Advantages*: Reduction in operative time, reduction in intraoperative and postoperative bleeding, minimizes the complications associated with placental retention, i.e., sepsis, hemorrhage, and disseminated intravascular coagulation (DIC).

Cesarean Hysterectomy

Early recourse to hysterectomy is recommended if conservative medical and surgical intervention prove ineffective.

BIBLIOGRAPHY

1. Chopra S, Bagga R, Keepanasseril A, Jain V, Kalra J, Suri V. Disengagement of the deeply engaged fetal head during cesarean section in advanced labor: Conventional method versus reverse breech extraction. Acta Obstetriciaet Gynecologica. 2009; 88:1163-6.
2. Chopra S. Disengagement of the Deeply Engaged Fetal Head during Cesarean Section Conventional Method versus Reverse Breech Extraction-Review of Literature. Clin Mother Child Health: 2016;13(2).
3. Dalvi SA. Difficult deliveries in cesarean section. J Obstetr Gynecol India. 2018;68(5):344-8.
4. Högberg U, Håkansson S, Serenius F, Holmgren PA. Extremely preterm cesarean delivery: a clinical study. Acta Obstetriciaet Gynecologica. 2006;85:1442-7.
5. Hong DH, Kim E, Kyeong KS, Hong SH, Jeong EH. Safety of cesarean delivery through placental

incision in patients with anterior placenta previa. Obstet Gynecol Sci. 2016;59(2):103-9.

6. Lin CH, Lin CY, Yang YH, Shih JC, Shy MK, Lee CN, et al. Extremely preterm cesarean delivery "en caul". Taiwan J Obstet Gynecol. 2010;49(3): 254-9.

7. Lenz F, Kimmich N, Zimmermann R, Kreft M. Maternal and neonatal outcome of reverse breech extraction of an impacted fetal head during caesarean section in advanced stage of labour: a retrospective cohort study. BMC Pregnancy Childbirth. 2019;19:98.

8. Piñas-Carrillo A, Chandraharan E. Conservative surgical approach: The Triple P procedure. Best Prac Res Clin Obstetr Gynaecol 2021;72: 67-74.

9. Poole JH. Adhesions following cesarean delivery: a review of their occurrence, consequences and preventative management using adhesion barriers. Women's Health. 2013;9(5):467-77.

10. RCOG. (2018). Placenta Praevia and Placenta Accreta: Diagnosis and Management, Green top guidelines no 27a. [online] Available from https://www.rcog.org.uk/en/guidelines-research-services/guidelines/gtg27a/ [Last accessed December, 2021].

11. Takeda S, Takeda J, Makino S. Cesarean section for placenta previa and placenta previa accreta spectrum. Surg J. 2020;6(Suppl S2):S110-21.

12. Visconti F, Quaresima P, Rania E, Palumbo AR, Micieli M, Zullo F. Difficult caesarean section: a literature review. Euro J Obstetr Gynecol Reprod Biol. 2020;246:72-8.

CHAPTER

21

Retained Placenta

Poonam Goyal, Gunjan Kumari Bhagwat, Pallavi Goel

INTRODUCTION

The third stage of labor is defined as the period after delivery of the baby to complete delivery of the placenta. So basically the placenta is delivered in the third stage and a delay in delivery of the placenta after a normal vaginal delivery beyond the stipulated time is termed as *retained placenta*. This time limit after which we call it retained placenta varies according to how the third stage of labor has been managed and the gestational age at delivery.

When active management of the third stage of labor has been done, 98% of the placenta are delivered within 30 minutes and in contrast to this in physiological management of third stage, it takes 60 minutes for delivery of 98% of the placenta.[1] In preterm gestation it takes longer for the placenta to be delivered especially in the second trimester deliveries. For gestational age between 20 and 30 weeks it has been predicted that spontaneous delivery of placenta may take 180–210 minutes.[2]

DEFINITION

In a term pregnancy with active management of third stage of labor if the placenta is not delivered within 30 minutes of the delivery of the infant, it is termed as retained placenta, whereas in physiological management of the third stage one can wait for 60 minutes.[3] In second trimester deliveries one can wait for 120 minutes in the absence of bleeding before attempting manual removal of placenta. So World Health Organization (WHO) suggests that the time period after which we call it a case of retained placenta should be left to the "judgment of the clinician".[4]

INCIDENCE

It varies from 0.1 to 3%.[5,6] The incidence is more in physiological management of the third stage of labor

as compared to active management. The incidence also increases in preterm deliveries, being three times higher and in the second trimester the risk increases 21-fold.[2]

PHASES OF THIRD STAGE OF LABOR

Four phases of third stage of labor have been defined based on ultrasound (USG) findings:[7]
1. *Latent phase*: In this, after delivery of the baby, the myometrium contracts all over except the site of placental attachment.
2. *Contraction phase*: Myometrium at the site of placental attachment contracts.
3. *Detachment phase*: Because of the myometrial contraction, there is a shearing force on the placental surface, thus leading to its separation.
4. *Expulsion phase*: The separated placenta is pushed out through the open cervix because of the myometrial contractions.

PREREQUISITES FOR SPONTANEOUS DELIVERY OF THE PLACENTA[8]

- Adequate uterine contraction
- Cervix should be opened
- Placenta should be normally attached to the endometrium

TYPES OF RETAINED PLACENTA AND THEIR PATHOGENESIS (FIGS. 1A TO C)[1]

1. *Trapped or incarcerated placenta*: In this, a completely separated placenta is trapped behind a closed cervix as in case of administration of ergotamine derivative which causes tetanic contraction of the uterus and cervix,

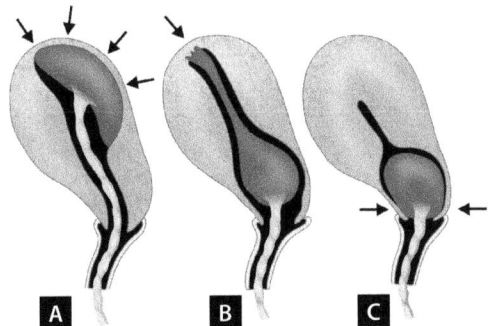

Figs. 1A to C: (A) Placenta adherens. The placenta is adherent to the uterine wall but is easily separated manually. Arrows indicate the lack of subplacental myometrial contraction; (B) Focal accreta—Arrow indicates the small portion of the placenta pathologically invading the myometrium; (C) Trapped or incarcerated placenta. The placenta has detached completely from the uterus but has not delivered spontaneously or with light cord traction because the cervix has begun to close (arrows).

so defect in expulsion phase. This accounts for approximately 13% of the entire retained placenta.[9]

2. *Placenta adherens*: In this, the placenta is adherent to the uterine wall but can be easily separated manually. In this, there is a defect in the contraction phase because of which the placenta does not separate. This accounts for nearly 81% of the cases.[9]

3. *Placenta accreta spectrum*: This is a structural defect in which there is invasion of the placenta into the myometrium in varying degrees and extent. This accounts for nearly 6% of all the cases.[9]

RISK FACTORS[5,10-14]

The important risk factors for retained placenta are mentioned in **Table 1.**

DIAGNOSIS

Diagnosis of retained placenta is made when the placenta is not delivered even after 30 minutes of the delivery of the baby after active management of third stage of labor in term gestation. The management of retained placenta depends on its type, so we need to define the type of retained placenta. The diagnosis is made on the basis of

clinical findings, which has been explained by **Flowchart 1.**

Ultrasound is rarely required to make the diagnosis, when physical examination is non-conclusive **(Figs. 2A to E)**. The USG findings are as follows:[7]

Trapped placenta: The entire myometrium is thickened and placenta can be seen separate from the uterine wall in the lower segment.

Adherent placenta: The myometrium at the site of placental attachment can be seen as thin in contrast to the rest of the myometrium which is thickened and placenta cannot be seen separate from the uterine wall.

COMPLICATIONS

1. *Postpartum hemorrhage:* Retained placenta increases the risk of hemorrhage and requires prompt intervention.

2. *Shock:* This can be either because of hemorrhage or because of too much abdominal or intrauterine manipulation.

3. *Postpartum endometritis:* Manual removal of the placenta increases the risk, so WHO recommends a dose of prophylactic broad-spectrum antibiotics, ampicillin or a first-generation cephalosporin.

4. *Uterine inversion:* It is a rare complication seen if adherent placenta is inadvertently pulled.

MANAGEMENT

1. *Trapped placenta:* Do active management of third stage of labor if not already done. Administer 10 units of oxytocin, do controlled cord traction (Brandt–Andrews technique) **(Flowchart 2).**

2. *Placenta adherens:* The basic pathology is defective myometrial contraction in the area of placental attachment. The management of placenta adherens has been explained in the **Flowchart 3.**

In various trials the intraumbilical injection of oxytocin has not been found effective, so now WHO recommends that this can be used only for the purpose of randomized trials in the absence of heavy bleeding.[16] There are few trials which show the effectiveness of intraumbilical misoprostol and carboprost but we need further studies to prove them.

TABLE 1: Risk factors for retained placenta.

Factors causing entrapment of separated placenta	• Use of ergotamines • *Mismanaged third stage of labor:* Attempts of cord traction before signs of placental separation • *Preterm deliveries:* Especially second trimester deliveries are the strongest risk factor • Velamentous cord insertion
Factors causing poor uterine contraction (placenta adherens)	• Maternal age >30 years • Multiparity • Prolonged use of oxytocin making the endometrium tired and losing its strength to contract
Factors causing abnormal placentation (placenta accreta spectrum)	• *Previous uterine surgeries:* Previous LSCS, curettage, myomectomy • Advanced maternal age • IVF conception
Other risk factors	• *Congenital uterine anomalies:* Incomplete uterine septum is seen in many cases of retained placenta • *History of retained placenta in previous pregnancies:* It increases the risk to 25% • *Placental hypoperfusion disorders:* As seen in pre-eclampsia, fetal growth restriction, stillbirths, etc. The pathophysiology in this is not known

(IVF: in vitro fertilization; LSCS: lower segment cesarean section)

Flowchart 1: Clinical findings for diagnosis of retained placenta.

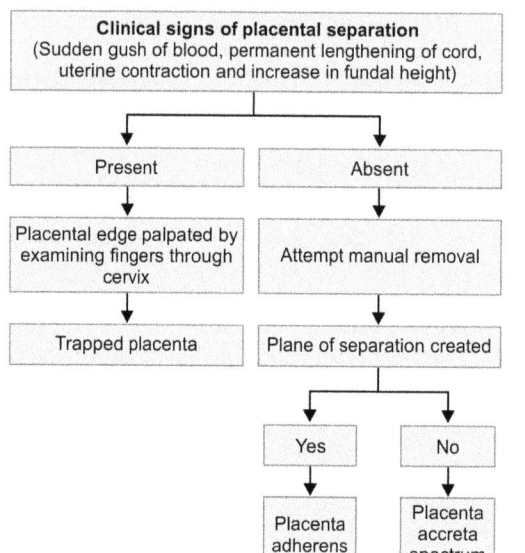

completed the family, hysterectomy is the best approach. Conservative approach can be undertaken if the patient is desirous to have further child bearing, but all the risks should be explained. Its management has been dealt in a separate chapter.

Special Circumstances

1. *Retained placenta with heavy bleeding:* In this case, all the measures should go hand in hand. Resuscitation should be started, oxytocics should be given, controlled cord traction tried and along with this the patient should be immediately shifted for manual removal of placenta. If the bleeding is still not controlled then immediate laparotomy followed by hysterectomy may have to be planned.

2. *Incomplete placental extraction:* During manual removal of the placenta, a small area may be very adherent to the uterus. In this case, one should try to dissect the area slowly with fingers which can cause the plane of separation through the placenta, so a small area of placenta may be left attached to the uterus. This usually does not cause bleeding if the uterus is well contracted. Curettage should

3. *Placenta accreta:* If the plane of separation is not found then the diagnosis is placenta accreta. In this case, in a female who has

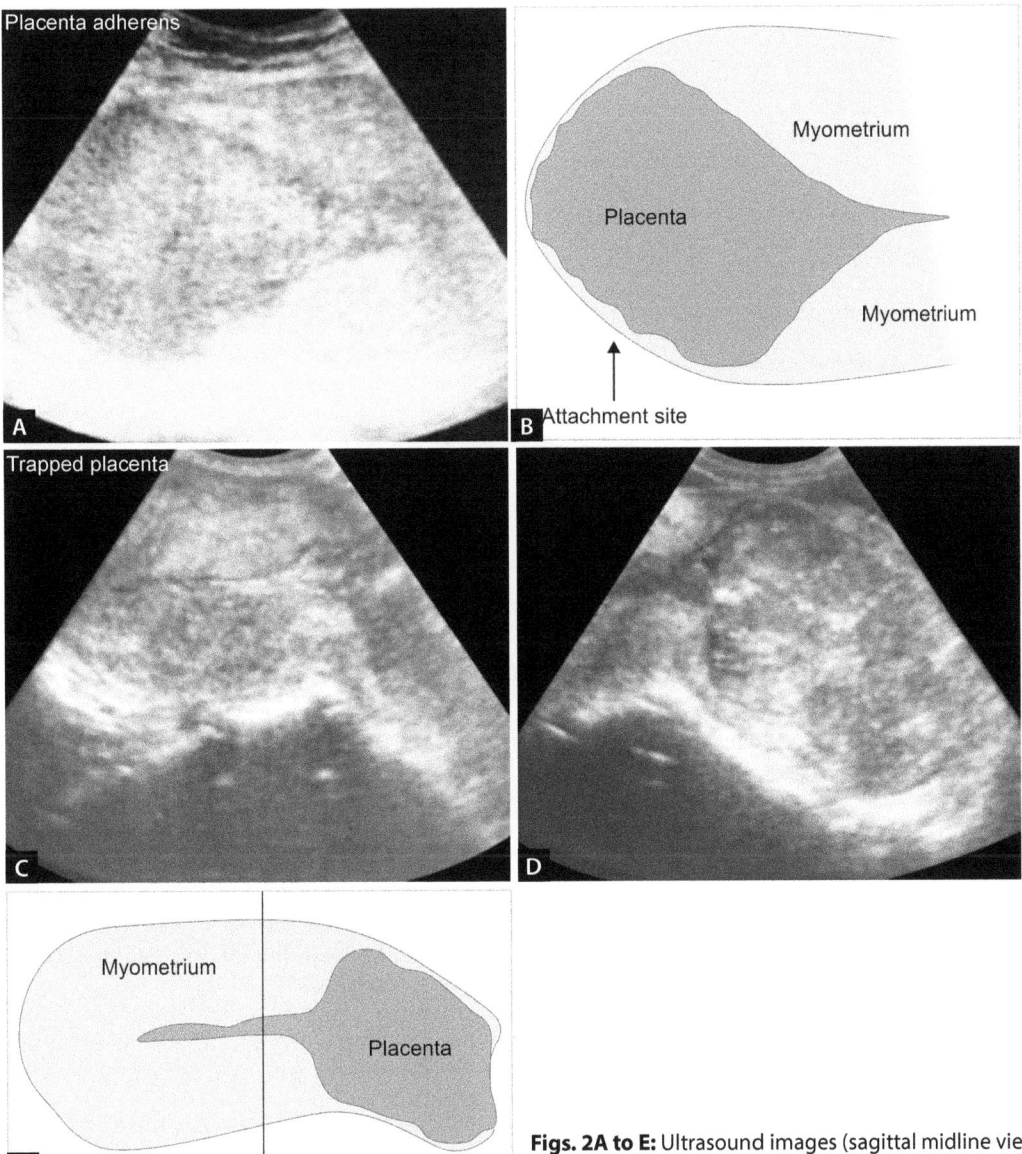

Figs. 2A to E: Ultrasound images (sagittal midline view) of placenta adherens and a trapped placenta.

not be done here as the area of myometrium here is thin and it increases the risk of perforation and it also increases the risk of intrauterine adhesions.

STEPS OF MANUAL REMOVAL OF THE PLACENTA

As already discussed one should wait for 30 minutes for expulsion of the placenta in a term gestation with active management of labor before planning for manual removal of placenta, whereas in second trimester pregnancies one should wait for 90–120 minutes before attempting manual removal.

- This is a painful process with intrauterine manipulation so it is always done in operation theater (OT) under anesthesia. General anesthesia is given with halothane for uterine relaxation.

Flowchart 2: Management of retained placenta.

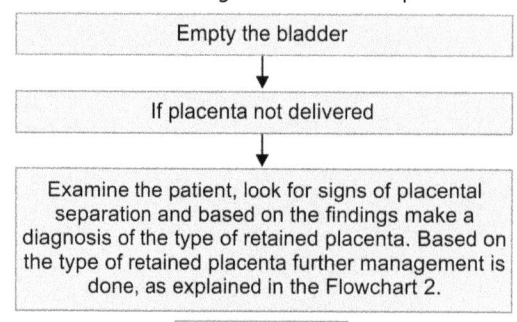

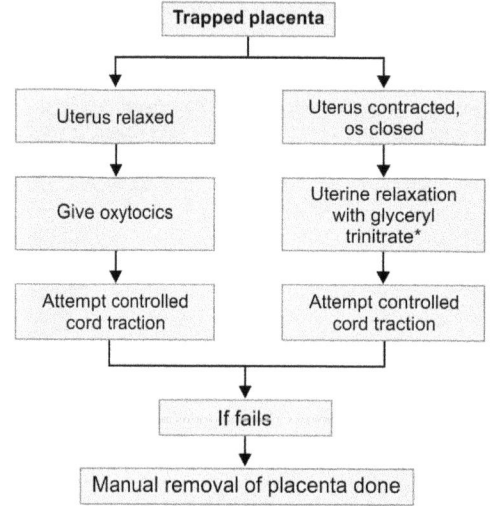

*Dose of Glyceryl trinitrate[1]
– *Spray*: 2 spray (400 µg/spray) onto/under the tongue
– *Sequential IV bolus*: 50 µg repeated at 1 minute interval (maximum 250 µg)
– *Sublingual tablets*: 0.6–1 mg
– Relaxation of the cervix and lower uterine segment occurs within 1 minute and lasts for 1–2 minutes.

- Prophylactic broad-spectrum antibiotics should be given, ampicillin or first-generation cephalosporin with metronidazole.
- Patient is placed in a lithotomy position, parts painted and draped, bladder catheterized.
- The umbilical cord is held with the left hand and stretched. The right hand is introduced through the vagina, cervix into the uterine cavity in a cone-shaped manner under aseptic precautions to reach for the margins of the placenta.
- Now the left hand is placed over the fundus to support it and guide the movement of intrauterine fingers.

Flowchart 3: Management of placenta adherens.

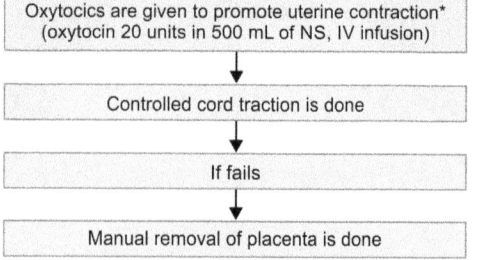

*1. *Systemic Oxytocics*:
  – Oxytocin 20 units in 500 mL of NS, IV infusion.
  – Carbetocin, a long acting oxytocin analog can be used instead of oxytocin.
  – It has been found to have a rapid onset of action (within 1–2 minutes) with a prolonged action (1 h). Studies have shown that use of additional uterotonic can be reduced by 50% with its use.[15]
  – If the uterus is still flabby and bleeding persists, prostaglandin (PG) F2-alpha (carboprost) should be given.
  – Ergometrine should be avoided as it causes tetanic contraction of the uterus and cervix and so will interfere with manual removal of placenta.
*2. *Intraumbilical vein injection of oxytocics*: This can be done through a nasogastric tube size 10 inserted into the umbilical vein.
  – PGF2-alpha (20 mg in 20 mL NS)
  – Misoprostol (800 µg in 30 mL NS)
  – Oxytocin (50 units in 30 mL NS)

- The right hand is inserted between the placenta and the uterine wall with the back of the hand toward the uterine wall to find the plane of separation.
- Once the plane of separation is found, the hand is further advanced in slicing manner by sideways movement to separate the whole placenta.
- The placenta is extracted with the left hand with the uterine hand still inside and the uterus is explored again to look for any placental tissue left behind.
- The left hand is again placed on the fundus and the fundus is massaged to promote uterine contraction.
- Oxytocin infusion is started (20 units in 500 mL of NS) to promote uterine contractions.
- Cervicovaginal canal is explored to exclude any injury.
- Inspection of the placenta and membranes is done to check whether it is complete or not.

CONCLUSION

- If active management of third stage of labor has been done in a term gestation, then if the placenta is not delivered within 30 minutes of delivery of the baby we call it retained placenta whereas in second trimester deliveries the wait time is 90–120 minutes
- The three types of retained placenta are—(1) trapped placenta (placenta separated but trapped behind closed cervix); (2) placenta adherens (placenta adherent to uterine wall due to poor uterine contraction especially behind the placenta, so can be separated); (3) placenta accreta spectrum (morbidly adherent placenta, which cannot be separated).
  - Trapped placenta is differentiated from adherent placenta by presence of signs of placental separation. Trapped placenta can be removed just by controlled cord traction and if the os is closed, glyceryl nitrate can be given for uterine relaxation. If this fails then manual removal of placenta is done.
  - Placenta adherens is managed by promoting uterine contraction by giving oxytocics and then trying controlled cord traction. If this fails, manual removal of placenta is done. Manual removal of placenta is done in OT under general anesthesia.
  - Placenta accreta spectrum, if not diagnosed in the intranatal period, can be differentiated from placenta adherens only at the time of manual removal. Placenta accreta spectrum is managed by hysterectomy in those who have completed the family.

REFERENCES

1. Weeks AD. The retained placenta. Best Pract Res Clin Obstet Gynaecol. 2008;22:1103.
2. Dombrowski MP, Bottoms SF, Saleh AA, Romero R. Third stage of labor: analysis of duration and clinical practice. Am J Obstet Gynecol. 1995;172:1279-84.
3. Deneux-Tharaux C, Macfarlane A, Winter C, Zhang WH, Alexander S, Bouvier-Colle MH. Policies for manual removal of placenta at vaginal delivery: variations in timing within Europe. BJOG. 2009;116:119-24.
4. World Health Organization. (2012). WHO recommendations for the prevention and treatment of postpartum hemorrhage. [online] Available from: http://www.who.int/reproductivehealth/publications/maternal_perinatal_health/9789241548502/en/. [Last Accessed December, 2021].
5. Endler M, Grünewald C, Saltvedt S. Epidemiology of retained placenta: oxytocin as an independent risk factor. Obstet Gynecol. 2012;119(4):801-9.
6. Urner F, Zimmermann R, Krafft A. Manual removal of the placenta after vaginal delivery: an unsolved problem in obstetrics. J Pregnancy. 2014;2014:274651.
7. Herman A, Weinraub Z, Bukovsky I, Arieli S, Zabow P, Caspi E, et al. Dynamic ultrasonographic imaging of the third stage of labor: new perspectives into third-stage mechanisms. Am J Obstet Gynecol. 1993;168:1496-9.
8. Perlman NC, Carusi DA. Retained placenta after vaginal delivery: Risk factors and management. International J Women Health. 2019:11 527-34.
9. Khan N, Weeks AD. Liverpool Women's Hospital local audit data. 2006.
10. Adelusi B, Soltan MH, Chowdhury N, Kangave D. Risk of retained placenta: multivariate approach. Acta Obstet Gynecol Scand, 1997; 76:414.
11. Coviello EM, Grantz KL, Huang CC, Kelly TE, Landy HJ. Risk factors for retained placenta. Am J Obstet Gynecol. 2015; 213:864.e1-864.e11.
12. Favilli A, Tosto V, Ceccobelli M, Parazzini F, Franchi M, Bini V, et al. Risk factors for nonadherent retained placenta after vaginal delivery: a systematic review. BMC Pregnancy Childbirth. 2021;21:268.
13. Nikolajsen S, Løkkegaard ECL, Bergholt T. Reoccurrence of retained placenta at vaginal delivery: an observational study. Acta Obstet Gynecol Scand. 2013;92(4):421-5.
14. Endler M, Saltvedt S, Cnattingius S, Stephansson O, Wikström AK. Retained placenta is associated with pre-eclampsia, stillbirth, giving birth to a small-for-gestational-age infant, and spontaneous preterm birth: a national register-based study. BJOG. 2014;121(12):1462-70.
15. Holleboom CAG, Eyck JV, Koenen SV, Kreuwel IA, Bergwerff F, Creutzberg EC, et al. Carbetocin in comparison with oxytocin in several dosing regimens for the prevention of uterine atony after elective caesarean section. Arch Gynecol Obstet. 2013;287(6):1111-7.
16. WHO recommendation on umbilical vein injection of oxytocin for the treatment of retained placenta. Geneva: World Health Organization; 2020.

Kavita Mandrelle Bhatti, Sahir Bhatti

DEFINITION AND TYPES

Placenta accreta spectrum (PAS) is a term used to describe abnormal trophoblastic invasion into the myometrium of the uterine wall and includes placenta accreta, increta, and percreta. Also known as morbidly adherent placenta, it is characterized by abnormally implanted or invasive placenta. As the plane of cleavage is absent, the placenta does not separate spontaneously and any attempt of manual removal results in hemorrhage. This can be life-threatening and usually requires a hysterectomy at the time of delivery.

Placenta accreta spectrum also called morbidly adherent placenta can be of three types:
1. Placenta accreta when the placental villi are attached to the myometrium instead of the decidua.
2. Placenta increta when the placental villi penetrate into the myometrium.
3. Placenta percreta when the placental villi penetrate through the myometrium to the uterine serosa or adjacent organs.

According to the International Federation of Gynaecology and Obstetrics (FIGO) Placenta Accreta Spectrum Disorders Diagnosis and Management Expert Consensus Panel, PAS is classified as follows:
- *Grade 1*: Abnormally adherent placenta—placenta accreta
- *Grade 2*: Abnormally invasive placenta—placenta increta
- *Grade 3*: Abnormally invasive placenta—placenta percreta
  - Subtype 3a—limited to the uterine serosa
  - Subtype 3b—urinary bladder invasion
  - Subtype 3c—invasion of other pelvic tissue/organs

Placenta accreta is more common than placenta increta and percreta.

PATHOGENESIS

Defective decidualization due to scarring caused by previous surgery involving endometrial-myometrial interface is one of the etiological factors which allows the placental villi to attach directly or invade the myometrium. Partial or total absence of decidua basalis or imperfect development of the Nitabuch layer or fibrinoid layer can cause abnormal placental adherence. Absence of decidual spongy layer results in the defective physiological plane of cleavage.

Previous cesarean delivery, curettage, and myomectomy can lead to scarring of uterine cavity, and hence predispose to placenta accreta. Uterine pathology, such as bicornuate uterus, adenomyosis, or submucous fibroids may be associated with microscopic endometrial defects that may cause abnormal placental attachment.

RISK FACTORS

The most common risk factor for development of PAS is placenta previa after a prior cesarean delivery.

The frequency of PAS increases with an increasing number of cesarean deliveries and associated placenta previa as follows:
- First cesarean birth—3%
- Second cesarean birth—11%
- Third cesarean birth—40%
- Fourth cesarean birth—61%

In the absence of placenta previa, the frequency of placenta accrete spectrum in women undergoing cesarean delivery is much lower.
- First (primary) cesarean birth—0.03%
- Second cesarean birth—0.2%
- Third cesarean birth—0.1%
- Fourth or fifth cesarean birth—0.8%
- Sixth or greater cesarean birth—4.7%

Other risk factors include:
- Previous uterine surgery
- Myomectomy disrupting the endometrial lining
- Hysteroscopic removal of intrauterine adhesions
- Cornual resection of ectopic pregnancy
- Dilation and curettage
- Endometrial ablation
- Maternal age >35 years
- Multiparity
- Manual removal of the placenta
- Postpartum endometritis
- Infertility and procedures related to infertility treatment

CLINICAL PRESENTATION
- Patient may be asymptomatic.
- It may be an incidental finding during routine ultrasound examination.
- Sometimes the diagnosis is made during delivery of the placenta when there is usually profuse, life-threatening hemorrhage that occurs at the time of attempted manual removal of placenta. Placental separation is not achieved and no plane of separation can be developed.
- Placenta percreta with bladder invasion can cause hematuria during pregnancy.

CONSEQUENCES
- Massive hemorrhage leading to disseminated intravascular coagulopathy
- Respiratory distress syndrome
- Renal failure
- Emergency laparotomy
- Peripartum hysterectomy
- Transfusion-related morbidity and complications related to surgery
- Increased maternal morbidity and mortality
- Preterm birth and small for gestational age infants

PRENATAL SCREENING AND DIAGNOSIS

Placenta accreta spectrum is likely to be present in patients with placenta previa or a low-lying placenta after one or more previous cesarean deliveries.

Prenatal screening and diagnosis are important so that the patient can be counseled and an appropriate plan for delivery can be made. Women with a placenta previa or a low anterior placenta and prior uterine surgery should have a detailed transabdominal and transvaginal sonographic evaluation of the interface between the placenta and myometrium between 18 and 24 weeks of gestation. At this gestational age, the prenatal diagnosis of PAS can be made or ruled out with 90% accuracy.

Ultrasound Findings

First-trimester ultrasound examination: PAS should be suspected, if first-trimester ultrasound examination reveals implantation of the gestational sac in the lower anterior segment of the uterus, particularly in the niche of the prior cesarean delivery scar.

In the second and third trimesters, the following transabdominal and transvaginal sonographic findings suggest PAS.
- *Multiple placental, lacunae*: Multiple large, irregular intraplacental sonolucent spaces (i.e., placental lacunae) that give the placenta a "moth-eaten" appearance.

The placental lacunae in PAS are numerous and irregular in shape, and the underlying myometrium may be thinned out.
- *Disruption of the bladder line*: Loss or disruption of the normally continuous white line representing the bladder wall-uterine serosa interface is suggestive of PAS.
- *Loss of the clear zone*: The normal hypoechoic area behind the placenta termed the "clear space" or "clear zone" will be absent.
- *Myometrial thinning*: The retroplacental myometrium can be thin due to a prior hysterotomy scar or placental invasion.
- *Abnormal vascularity*: Vessels that extend from the placenta through the myometrium either into the bladder or through the serosa are suggestive of placenta percreta.
- *Placental bulge*: A portion of the uterus attached to the abnormally adherent placenta can balloon into the bladder.
- *Exophytic mass*: A focal mass that breaks through the uterine serosa may be seen usually extending into the bladder.
- *Color Doppler*: Color Doppler is useful for confirming the diagnosis of PAS when used in conjunction with the other ultrasound findings described above.

Specific findings on color Doppler ultrasonography include:

- Turbulent lacunar blood flow
- Bridging vessels which are placental vessels that extend through the myometrium and beyond the serosa into the bladder or other organs. These should not be mistaken for bladder varices, which are enlarged maternal bladder veins, often seen in normal pregnancy.
- Diffuse or focal intraparenchymal flow
- Hypervascularity of serosa-bladder interface
- Prominent sub-placental venous complex

Magnetic Resonance Imaging

Magnetic resonance imaging (MRI) may be more useful than ultrasound for evaluation of a possible posterior PAS, assessment of the depth of myometrial and parametrial involvement, and evaluation of the myometrium and placenta at the most lateral portions of the hysterotomy as this area is not well visualized by transvaginal ultrasound.

Magnetic resonance imaging is an adjunctive tool for diagnosing PAS though its increased accuracy beyond that noted with ultrasound is unproven. Magnetic resonance imaging is safe for the fetus, although the use of gadolinium, which may improve diagnostic performance, is generally avoided in pregnancy due to neurologic, inflammatory, and dermatologic complications to the fetus.

Magnetic resonance imaging findings which are the most accurate predictors of placenta accreta include the following:

- Uterine bulging into the bladder ("placental/uterine bulge")
- Interruption of the bladder wall
- Loss of retroplacental hypointense line on T2-weighted (T2W) images
- Abnormal vascularization of the placental bed
- Dark intraplacental bands on T2W imaging ("T2-dark bands")
- Myometrial thinning
- Focal exophytic mass

▓ MANAGEMENT

Prenatal Care

- All patients with suspected PAS should be counseled about the diagnosis, complications, and potential sequelae such as hemorrhage, blood transfusion, cesarean hysterectomy, and intensive care unit admission.
- Iron deficiency anemia if present should be corrected prenatally.
- Antenatal steroids should be given for antenatal mothers who are at increased risk of delivery within 7 days such as in those presenting with antepartum hemorrhage.
- If the patient has vaginal bleeding and is RhD negative, anti-D immunoglobulin should be administered. Advice the women against strenuous physical activity and sexual intercourse. Pelvic examination should be avoided.
- As the risk of bleeding and complications increase in the third trimester one should consider hospitalization. Asymptomatic women can be followed in outpatient department if they stay close by, are compliant with follow-up visits and can reach the hospital soon if symptoms develop.
- Routine tests for antepartum fetal surveillance such as nonstress tests and biophysical profile are done only if indicated such as in associated fetal growth restriction or preeclampsia.
- Serial sonographic assessment of the placenta is generally not useful after the diagnosis of PAS has been made. However, a sonogram at 32–34 weeks can precisely locate the placenta and help to assess the likelihood of bladder involvement. This information is useful for surgical planning and delivery.

Preparation for Delivery

Preoperative planning: Preoperative planning is important in PAS. One must provide information about the management and plan interventions that will reduce the risk of massive postpartum hemorrhage, as well as its substantial morbidity and potential mortality. Cesarean hysterectomy is usually performed because the placenta cannot be removed in any other way and, if left in situ, complications such as subinvolution often result in postpartum hemorrhage.

Preoperative planning should include:
Informed consent for interventions such as blood transfusion, hysterectomy, and surgical interventions to deal with bowel and bladder injuries.

Management by a multidisciplinary team and delivery in a tertiary care facility is essential to reduce chances of complications and maternal morbidity and mortality. The multidisciplinary team should include a maternal-fetal medicine specialist, anesthesiologists, urologists, neonatologists, interventional radiologists, pathologists, and blood bank and nursing personnel. It is desirable to have surgeons, urologists, and vascular surgeons as part of the team. If proper facility is lacking the patient should be referred to a higher center.

Delivery should be scheduled at a time with optimal availability of necessary personnel and facilities. An elective delivery has better outcomes than an emergency delivery.

Delivery in an operating room with facility for fluoroscopy is convenient if interventional radiological procedure is required.

Patent intravenous access has to be maintained. At least two large bore intravenous catheters should be placed peripherally. Rapid infusion of warmed blood products and fluids may be required in almost all cases. Strict monitoring of fluid infusion should be done. Also, cardiac monitoring is essential in many of the cases.

Thromboembolism prophylaxis in the form of pneumatic compression devices should be placed.

Blood products should be available and the blood bank should be notified. Adequate red blood cells, fresh-frozen plasma, cryoprecipitate, and platelets should be available at the time of delivery. A massive hemorrhage protocol is useful for managing laboratory evaluation and transfusion.

The woman should be catheterized with an indwelling urinary catheter and ureteral stents should be available. This is particularly needed in cases in which bladder resection is required. Preoperative placement of ureteric stents can be opted for in women with PAS, especially those with a percreta.

General anesthesia is most commonly administered for cesarean delivery in a case of PAS. Regional anesthesia in the form of continuous epidural is successful in scheduled and planned deliveries. Conversion to general anesthesia can be done if necessary. An intensive care unit bed should be available for postoperative care.

Prophylactic endovascular intervention with a balloon catheter in both internal iliac arteries, uterine artery embolization, or a combination of the two may be used to reduce bleeding during or after delivery. If prophylactic endovascular intervention is planned, the patient should undergo delivery on a fluoroscopy table so that the procedure can be performed intraoperatively immediately after delivery of the baby.

Delivery

- The optimum gestational age for scheduled delivery is controversial. The risks of preterm birth must be weighed against the risks of complications, such as bleeding, leading to emergency delivery under suboptimal circumstances.
- For stable patients, planned delivery between 34+0 and 35+6 weeks of gestation is advisable, in agreement with the American College of Obstetricians and Gynecologists.
- The Society for Maternal-Fetal Medicine recommends delivery between 34 and 37 weeks of gestation for stable women with placenta accreta.

Procedure

A vertical midline skin incision is made. A vertical hysterotomy at least two finger breadths above the placental edge leaving a myometrial margin between the placenta and incision helps to prevent disruption of the placenta during opening or closing of the uterus.

After delivery of the baby, the cord is cut, the uterine incision is rapidly closed to decrease blood loss, and hysterectomy is performed. Cesarean hysterectomy is recommended leaving the placenta undisturbed in situ. This decreases blood loss and associated complications. Even in the absence of extrauterine involvement by a percreta, the procedure is often difficult because of extensive parametrial vascular engorgement and friable tissues.

Prophylactic oxytocin is not routinely administered after delivery of the baby in PAS because it may lead to partial placental separation and, in turn, increase bleeding. If the placenta has separated partially or has been completely removed, then uterotonic drugs should be given.

Placenta percreta with bladder invasion may require partial cystectomy.

Conservative Management of Placenta Accreta

Uterine conservation may be considered in: Patients who want to preserve fertility. These patients should be counseled extensively regarding the risks of hemorrhage, infection, possible need for intra- or postoperative lifesaving hysterectomy, and even death, as well as suboptimal outcomes in future pregnancies.

Uterine conservation interventions can be done when placental resection is thought to be possible because of focal accreta or a fundal or posterior placenta.

In this approach, the placenta is left in situ after delivery of the baby. The umbilical cord is ligated at its placental insertion site. The hysterotomy incision is closed in the standard way and uterotonic drugs, compression sutures, intrauterine balloon tamponade, uterine artery embolization, and/or uterine artery ligation are variably used.

Delayed interval hysterectomy is another option, particularly for patients with placenta percreta, but experience is limited and experts have recommended against it. Clinicians experienced with the technique have suggested it as an option for only the most severe, potentially life-threatening cases of placenta percreta or when immediate hysterectomy is too dangerous because of the extent of placental invasion.

Adjunctive therapy with methotrexate therapy should not be used: There is no convincing evidence that it improves any outcome when the placenta is left in situ, and there is clear evidence of drug-related harms.

Complications of uterine conservation with placenta in situ include severe vaginal bleeding, sepsis, secondary hysterectomy, and death.

Uterine conservation with placental resection may be successful in focal accreta and fundal or posterior accreta.

Focal accreta may be suspected based on imaging findings or detected intrapartum because of hemorrhage and partially retained placenta at delivery. Management involves oversewing the bleeding sites or removing a small wedge of uterine tissue containing the focally adherent placenta. In fundal or posterior placenta accreta, uterine conservation may be possible since bleeding after removal of placenta accreta in these locations is more readily controlled medically, with interventional radiology, and with conservative surgery. In case of excessive bleeding, hysterectomy should be performed.

Unexpected Placenta Accreta Encountered during Delivery

Some cases of placenta accreta are first recognized at cesarean delivery, typically in a repeat cesarean delivery. The surgeon may make the diagnosis of PAS if one or more of the following are seen:

- Placental tissue invading the lower uterine segment, serosa, or bladder.
- Increased and tortuous vascularity along the serosa of the lower uterine segment. Vessels may run cranio caudally in the peritoneum.
- A bluish/purple and markedly distended lower uterine segment bulging toward the pelvic sidewalls.
- After delivery of the baby, PAS is suggested if light traction on the umbilical cord pulls the uterine wall inward, without placental separation. Gentle digital exploration for plane of cleavage can be attempted and the absence of a plane is diagnostic.
- If the patient is not bleeding heavily, mother and fetus are stable, and resources for managing complications are not possible locally, the abdomen should be closed and the patient transferred to a facility that can manage these patients, although the risk of massive hemorrhage in transit must be considered.
- If the mother is bleeding heavily and/or the fetus is compromised, the best option is delivery through a hysterotomy far from the placenta, followed by closure of the hysterotomy with the placenta left undisturbed until appropriate personnel and resources for maternal care are available.
- Rarely, a focal or complete placenta accreta is first recognized at the time of manual removal of a retained placenta after vaginal delivery. In these cases, there is no plane of cleavage between the myometrium and either the entire placenta or focal areas of the placenta. Life-threatening hemorrhage may occur. These patients should receive fluids and transfusion, as appropriate, while being prepared for laparotomy and surgical management.

Postoperative Care

An intensive care unit bed should be available for postoperative care, if needed. These patients may require ventilator support. Some patients need vasopressor support and invasive hemodynamic monitoring. Postoperative bleeding may occur, and the availability of interventional radiology to provide angiographic embolization of deep pelvic vessels, thus avoiding reoperation may be required.

BIBLIOGRAPHY

1. American College of Obstetricians and Gynecologists, Society for Maternal-Fetal Medicine. Obstetric Care Consensus No. 7: Placenta Accreta Spectrum. Obstet Gynecol. 2018;132:e259.
2. Jauniaux E, Chantraine F, Silver RM, Langhoff-Roos J, FIGO Placenta Accreta Diagnosis and Management Expert Consensus Pane. FIGO Consensus guidelines on placenta accreta spectrum disorders: Epidemiology. 2018;140(3): 265-73.
3. Publications Committee, Society for Maternal-Fetal Medicine, Belfort MA. Placenta accreta. Am J Obstet Gynecol. 2010;203:430.
4. Silver MD. Placenta accreta spectrum: Management. [online] Available from https://www.uptodate.com/contents/placenta-accreta-spectrum-management [Last accessed December, 2021].

23 Intrapartum Hemorrhage

Mahesh Koregol, Soumya Mahesh Koregol, Arati C Koregol

INTRODUCTION

Intrapartum hemorrhage is one of most dreaded complications, in obstetrics which is serious enough to be catastrophic and may lead to loss of life, if not treated promptly. Excessive blood loss associated with labor and delivery is associated with intrapartum hemorrhage. Around 5% of pregnancies are estimated to be complicated by intrapartum hemorrhage. Multiple etiologies are known to cause this condition and include atonic uterus, abruption of placenta, placenta accreta, and lacerations of genital tract.

Early recognition of underlying source of hemorrhage, amount of blood loss, and immediate replacement of blood volume by blood products and volume resuscitation often result in excellent outcome and save lives.

INTRAPARTUM HEMORRHAGE—CAUSES

There are various causative factors for intrapartum hemorrhage namely abruptio placentae, placenta previa, atonic uterus postdelivery, uterine rupture, laceration and uterine injury, cervical or vaginal laceration, and hematoma of vagina.

Placenta previa starts as antepartum hemorrhage and hence not covered in detail here.

Abruptio Placenta

Separation of placenta from uterus before the onset of labor constitutes abruptio placenta. Blood lost is stuck between placenta and uterine wall without revealing the magnitude of blood loss outside which might result in massive blood loss without revealing. Concealed blood tracking between placental membranes and uterus constitutes a great loss leading to life-threatening complications before actual assessment of blood loss is made. This volume of blood loss and resulting coagulopathy are responsible for the complications associated with abruption.

Massive fibrinolysis is followed by abnormal activation of extrinsic intravascular coagulation cascade. Thrombocytopenia might ensue and fibrinogen-fibrin degradation products and d-dimers are seen. Fetal delivery is known to stop this catastrophic cascade of abnormal coagulation and vaginal route is the preferred way of delivering in cases of placental abruption. Cesarean delivery is advisable in case of fetal indications only.

Risk factors for abruptio placenta include:
- Hypertension in pregnancy
- Abdominal trauma in pregnancy
- Previous history of abruption
- Polyhydramnios
- Fibroid uterus
- Elderly maternal age
- African American or Caucasian race
- Premature rupture of membranes

It is important to arrange adequate amount of crystalloid and blood products like platelets, plasma, and red blood cells (RBCs). It is possible that pregnant woman may deteriorate fast within short span of time, and hence need to keep hospitalized and also need to be prepared for any eventuality.

Atony of Uterus

Physiologic contraction of uterus after delivery is the ideal scenario but any factors related to abnormal contraction leads to atony of uterus and the sequelae of events leading to massive blood loss.

Risk factors for atony of uterus include:

- Prolonged duration of rupture of membranes
- Multiparity
- Prolonged labor—inductions and augmentations
- Uterine distention—multiple gestation, polyhydramnios, and macrosomia
- Retained placenta

Medical management of atony of uterus involves administration of oxytocic or prostaglandin derivatives.

Drugs used frequently in atony of uterus are listed in **Table 1**.

Steps to be taken for control and management of uterine atony:

1. Call out for all available helping hands.
2. Bimanual uterine compression to be initiated.
3. Oxytocin administration to be confirmed.
4. Start another accessory large bore intravenous catheter for colloid/blood transfusions.
5. Vaginal/cervical lacerations to be checked.
6. Start resuscitation of lost volume till blood transfusion is started.
7. Urine output measurement using a Foley catheter.
8. Uterine cavity to be explored for retained placental lobes or fragments.

Uterine Rupture

Thought the incidence of uterine rupture has reduced in recent years, it remains challenging issue of intrapartum hemorrhage in many developing countries. This is more likely in the patient with scarred uterus and multigravida women with injudicious oxytocin use and women with prolonged labor.

TABLE 1: Drugs used for atony of uterus.

Drug name	Drug dose/route
Oxytocin	20–30 mg/L of fluid/ IV or IM
Ergot derivatives (methylergonovine)	0.20 mg/IM
Prostaglandin analogs—F2 alpha carboprost	0.25 mg/IM
Prostaglandin analogs—prostaglandin F2	0.20 mg/per rectum
(IM: intramuscular; IV: intravenous)	

Depending upon the stage of uterine rupture, hysterectomy may have to be performed in extreme cases.

Lacerations of Cervix and Vagina

Various degrees of tissue damage in form of lacerations is commonly seen in cases of spontaneous vaginal delivery. Extensive damage to the vagina and cervix might lead to serious complications. Extensions of vaginal lacerations are known to involve vital structures such as vaginal wall laterally, anal sphincter, and even ischiorectal fascia. It is of prime importance to identify the lacerated area as fast as possible and repair the same to avoid further hemorrhage.

Cervix is commonly lacerated in vaginal deliveries and heals faster without major morbidities. It might extend up in few cases to reach lower uterine segment and retroperitoneal spaces. Such injuries may warrant abdominal approach to surgically repair and may lead to hysterectomy in worst case scenarios.

Vaginal Hematomas

In certain situations, vaginal hematoma occurs secondary to damage the vaginal arteries especially branches of pudendal arteries. This could be secondary to episiotomy, instrumental vaginal delivery, and primiparous delivery. Many times, the hematoma is small, self-limiting and tamponade off itself. In few hematomas, fast expansion is observed with acute pain and spread to ischiorectal fascia and retroperitoneal space. Large hematomas need to be surgically evacuated and if small can be managed conservatively.

Resuscitation

Primary aim of the resuscitation is to restore the lost blood volume as quick as possible without much delay to prevent the further vicious events. First line of lifesaving transfusions are crystalloid solutions which suffice in cases of mild hemorrhage. Limitation of this treatment is that, only 20% of crystalloids remain in circulation after about 1 hour and these can also lead to volume overload **(Table 2)**.

However, colloids are not associated with extra benefit but lead to additional cost burden.

TABLE 2: Aspect and considerations.

Aspect	Considerations
Clinical presentation	• Give RBC in response to hemodynamic changes and estimated blood loss rather than Hb trigger—do not wait for blood results to treat – Oozing from puncture/cannulation/injection sites or surgical field – Hematuria – Petechial, subconjunctival, and mucosal hemorrhage – Blood that no longer clots – Uterine atonia secondary to increased fibrin degradation products – Temperature <35°C • Laboratory signs
Coagulopathy correction	• If blood-clotting analyzer available, correct in response to results for targeted replacement of blood and blood products • If blood-clotting analyzer not available transfuse (and repeat as necessary) guided by laboratory findings: – RBC four units – Fibrinogen concentrate or cryoprecipitate to maintain fibrinogen level >2.5 g/L – Fresh frozen plasma (FFP) two units – Platelets to maintain platelet level greater than 50×10^9/L – If no level available, one therapeutic adult dose of platelets after 8–10 units of RBC
Fibrinogen	Use fibrinogen concentrate or cryoprecipitate early and aim to maintain fibrinogen levels above 2.5 g/L • Fibrinogen falls earlier than other coagulation factors and may be low despite normal PT/APTT • Fibrinogen/fibrin deficiency (and not thrombin) is the major informative marker for the severity of hemorrhage • Level of 2 g/L or less is associated with progression of bleeding, increased RBC and blood component requirement, and need for invasive procedures

(APTT: activated partial thromboplastin time; PT: prothrombin time; RBC: red blood cell)

Maintaining hematocrit value between 18% and 25% is better if no further bleeding occurs. Prolonged blood loss would necessitate RBCs transfusion along with fresh frozen plasma and platelets to replenish the lost volume and control further bleeding. Transfusion of platelets might be required when platelets fall below 50,000/µL and also in those patients needing massive transfusion (defined as requiring transfusion of 10 units of packed RBCs or more). Single donor platelets are often more preferred. After blood donation, plasma is separated from whole blood immediately and it can be frozen to be used later. In situations like abruption with consumption coagulopathy where fibrinogen levels fall below 100 mg/dL, frozen plasma can be thawed in 30 minutes and used. If fibrinogen levels fall extremely low, and active oozing is seen, cryoprecipitate which is made from plasma can be used especially in those cases where massive transfusion and volume overload leading to transfusion-related acute lung injury (TRALI) is a concern.

INTRAPARTUM HEMORRHAGE—SURGICAL MANAGEMENT

If first-line measures of resuscitation and pharmacotherapy fail, surgical modalities shown in **Table 3** can be used to control hemorrhage.

TABLE 3: Surgical modalities to control hemorrhage.

Surgical/radiological technique	Limitation/associated complication
Uterine artery ligation	Training required for the technique
Uterine compression sutures (B-Lynch, Cho stitch)	Ischemic necrosis and peritonitis
Uterine packing	Concealed hemorrhage and infection
Intrauterine Bakri balloon and Foley catheter	Infection
Angiographic embolization of pelvic vessels	Logistically challenging and nonavailability of trained interventional radiologist and embolization laboratory
Prophylactic arterial catheter placements in expected cases of hemorrhage	Thrombosis and necrosis of embolized tissue leading to infection

BIBLIOGRAPHY

1. Alexander JM, Wortman A. Intrapartum Hemorrhage. Obstet Gynecol Clin N Am. 2013; 40:15-26.

2. Queensland Clinical Guidelines. Postpartum Haemorrhage Guideline No. MN18.1-V10-R23. Queensland Health; 2021.

Atonic Postpartum Hemorrhage

Sheela Mane, Ramya VM

INTRODUCTION

Postpartum hemorrhage (PPH) is the worldwide leading cause of preventable maternal mortality. The major cause of PPH is uterine atony. PPH complicates 5% of deliveries worldwide. A key priority under the Sustainable Development Goal (SDG) health goal is reduction of global maternal mortality levels to <70 per 100,000 live births by year 2030.[1]

In spite of a low spending of 1% of GDP on public health expenditure, India has managed to reduce maternal mortality ratio down to 122 per 100,000 live births by the year 2015–2017, largely attributed to reform such as institutionalization of deliveries, provisioning of free cashless services to pregnant women, and addressing social determinants of health.[2-4] Despite ongoing efforts, India still accounts for nearly one-tenth of all maternal deaths globally with hemorrhage as the leading cause.[5] PPH accounts for more than two-thirds of all global maternal deaths due to bleeding.[6,7]

DEFINITIONS

Postpartum hemorrhage is defined as a blood loss of 500 mL during or after vaginal birth and 1,000 mL in cesarean section.

Postpartum hemorrhage can be either *primary PPH* occurring within 24 hours of delivery or *secondary PPH* that occurs between 24 hours and 6 weeks postpartum.

Postpartum hemorrhage can also be classified as:
- Minor (500–1,000 mL)
- Moderate (1,000–2,000 mL)
- Severe (>2,000 mL)[8]

For clinical purposes, any blood loss that has the potential to produce hemodynamic instability should be considered PPH.

Massive obstetric hemorrhage is variably defined as blood loss from uterus or genital tract > 1,500 mL or a rate of blood loss of 150/mL/min or 50% blood volume loss within 3 hours or decrease in hemoglobin of >4 g/dL or acute loss requiring transfusion of >4 units of packed cell transfusion, or any hemorrhage associated with hemodynamic instability.

ETIOLOGY

The causes of PPH can be broadly classified into four categories or the 4 "T's", the most common being uterine atony.
1. *Tone*: Uterine atony (incidence—70%)
2. *Tissue*: Retained placenta and clots (20%)
3. *Trauma*: Vaginal, cervical, or uterine injury (10%)
4. *Thrombin*: Coagulopathy (preexisting or acquired) (1%)

PREDICTION OF POSTPARTUM HEMORRHAGE

The prediction and prevention of PPH are the two main pillars in triad of PPH management. Prevention of PPH is via the recognition of any risk factors present either antenatally or during the intrapartum period, and the subsequent implementation of preventative management/strategies. Although there are a host of risk factors, PPH often occurs in women with no identifiable predictors and therefore clinicians must be prepared for this eventuality at each and every delivery.[9,10]

TABLE 1: Etiology of postpartum hemorrhage (PPH).

Tone	Tissue	Trauma	Thrombin
• Previous PPH • Overdistension of uterus-multiple pregnancy, polyhydramnios, macrosomia • Placenta previa • Uterine inversion • Prolonged labor • Uterine relaxants • Grand multiparity	• Retained placenta or products of conception • Placenta accreta	Genital tract injury, surgical-episiotomy, cesarean sections, angular extensions	• Placental abruption • Preeclampsia and HELLP syndrome • Preexisting coagulation abnormalities • Sepsis • Drugs (anticoagulants)

TABLE 2: Causes of primary and secondary postpartum hemorrhage (PPH).

Primary PPH	Secondary PPH
• Uterine atony • Trauma • Retained products of conception coagulopathy • Abnormal placentation • Uterine inversion	• Abnormal placentation • Retained products of conception • Infection • Uterine pathology—fibroids and cervical cancer

TABLE 3: Predictors of postpartum hemorrhage (PPH).

Antenatal risk factors	Intrapartum risk factors
• Age >35 years • Asian ethnicity • Obesity BMI > 30 kg/m^2 • Anemia • Grand multiparity • Overdistension of uterus—macrosomia, polyhydramnios, multiple pregnancy • APH • Uterine fibroids • Previous history of PPH	• Induction of labor • Prolonged labor • Use of oxytocin • Precipitate labor • Operative vaginal deliveries • Cesarean sections • Chorioamnionitis • Epidural, general anesthesia

(APH: antepartum hemorrhage; BMI: body mass index)

PREVENTION OF POSTPARTUM HEMORRHAGE

- Preparedness by labor room, i.e., equipment and staff readiness
    - A hemorrhage cart should be readily available with medications, supplies, checklist, and instruction cards.
    - A response team should be preassigned, assign telephone code for alerting in times of emergency.
    - Establish massive and emergency release transfusion protocols
    - Repeated training and refresher course or drills in management of obstetric emergencies for all staff and doctors.
    - Institute unit education on protocols and run unit-based drill.
- Antenatal management
    - Screen for and treat anemia antenatally
    - Screen for hemoglobinopathies

- Obtain ultrasound scans for women at high risk of invasive placenta and formulate and document delivery plan during antenatal visits.
- Delivery of high-risk cases in facility with blood bank and in-house surgical services
- Identify Jehovah's witnesses and other patients who decline blood products
- Intrapartum management
  - Use of active management of the third stage of labor in every delivery.
  - Maintain partogram and timely referrals or delivery when indicated
  - Avoid routine episiotomy
  - Instrumental deliveries should be performed by experienced obstetricians.
  - If oxytocin not available other agents may be used for prophylaxis, e.g., 600 µg misoprostol orally [World Health Organization (WHO)]
  - Carbetocin is licensed for the prevention of PPH during cesarean section.
  - Uterine massaging is not recommended for prophylaxis of PPH (WHO and RCOG).
  - Consider the use of IV tranexamic acid (0.5–1.0 g), in addition to oxytocin, during cesarean section to reduce blood loss in women at increased risk of PPH.
  - Measure cumulative blood loss and track postpartum vital signs.
- Response for every hemorrhage
  - Provide support program for patients, families, and staff.
  - Reporting and systems learning for every unit
  - Establish a culture of postevent debriefs.

DIAGNOSIS

The effectiveness of the management and prevention of morbidity and mortality depends on timely diagnosis, establishment of cause of PPH, and treatment. The process of managing a case of PPH is largely a team effort consisting of the obstetric team, and anesthetic team, nursing staff and blood bank staff. Correct estimation of blood loss is essential. In most instances, estimation of blood loss is accomplished visually despite the fact that numerous studies show that this method is up to 50% less accurate than other methods.[11-14]

There could be a component of traumatic PPH too hence a routine examination of the genital tract is mandatory. With continued blood loss coagulation disorder can slowly creep in making the situation more complex. Early replacement of lost blood and arrest of continuing loss are the most important aspects of treatment.

INITIAL MANAGEMENT OF PPH

The initial management of PPH is given in **Flowchart 1**.

UTEROTONICS

Table 6 explains about uterotonics.

CONSERVATIVE MANAGEMENT FOR PPH

Bimanual Compression

Insert one gloved hand into the vagina and push up against the body of the uterus. Place the other hand above the uterine fundus on the abdomen and compress the uterus against the hand in the vagina. To be effective bimanual uterine compression has to be maintained effectively for 8–10 minutes till the blood clots in the uterine vessels. It is a temporary measure in the management of PPH caused by uterine atony after vaginal delivery. This procedure is painful to the woman and is only undertaken in cases of PPH if drugs are not available or if drug therapy fails **(Fig. 1)**.[15]

Balloon Tamponade

In women who have not responded to treatment with uterotonics or if uterotonics are not available, the use of an intrauterine balloon should be considered in the treatment of PPH due to uterine atony. However, this intervention does require training and there are risks associated with the procedure such as infection and perforation of the uterus. A Sengstaken tube, Rüsch balloon, Bakri balloon, and even an inflated condom or glove have been used with success.

Insert the balloon and instill warm sterile water/saline in increments of 50 mL while observing for bleeding from the cervix. When bleeding stops, instill an extra 50 mL. If bleeding continues despite the balloon herniating via the cervix, the treatment is unlikely to be effective and

TABLE 4: Blood loss and clinical signs and symptoms.

	Class I	Class II	Class III	Class IV
Blood loss (mL)	750 mL	750–1,500 mL	1500–2000 mL	>2000 mL
Blood loss (% blood volume)	<15%	15–30%	30–40%	>40%
Heart rate	<100	>100	>120	>140
SBP	No change	No change	Reduced	Very low
DBP	No change	Raised	Reduced	Unrecordable
Respiratory rate	<20	>20	>30	>40
Urine output (mL/h)	>30	20–30	10–20	<10
Extremities	Normal	Pale	Pale	Cold
Capillary refill	Normal	Slow >2s	Slow >2 s	Minimal or absent
Mental state	Alert	Anxious	Aggressive/drowsy	Confused/unconscious

(DBP: diastolic blood pressure; SBP: systolic blood pressure)

Flowchart 1: Initial management of PPH.

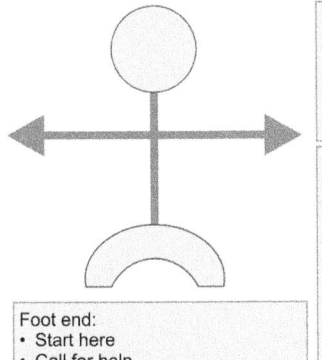

Head end:
- Check airway
- Check breathing
- Administer oxygen
- Record events

Arms:
- Check pulse and BP
- Secure two large bore IV cannulas 16 g
- Collect blood samples, send for CBC, LFT, RFT, coagulation profile cross match for blood and blood products
- If bleeding is excessive, activate MTP
- Start fluid resuscitation
- Two liters crystalloid
- *Drugs:* Oxytocin, ergometrine, carboprost, and tranexamic acid

Foot end:
- Start here
- Call for help
- Assess uterine tone, uterine massage
- Coordinate with assistants at head and foot end
- Deliver placenta
- Evaluate for cause for PPH, i.e., 4Ts
- Catheterize bladder
- Conservative management of PPH—bimanual compression, aortic compression
- If medical management fails, shift to OT

TABLE 5: Parameters to be assessed.

Method	Parameters to be assessed
Vital parameters	PR, BP, RR, and SBP of <80 mm Hg is associated with worsening tachycardia, tachypnea, and altered mental status and indicated a PPH of >1,500 mL
Rule of 30	Fall of SBP > 30 mm Hg, PR increases by 30 bpm and urine output <30 mL/h, Hct <30% the amount of blood loss is >30% of whole blood volume
Shock index	Pulse rate/SBP, if >1 it indicates patient is in shock

(BP: blood pressure; Hct: hematocrit; PR: pulse rate; RR: respiratory rate; SBP: systolic blood pressure)

the balloon will be expelled. The next step should be compression sutures. The fundal height should be marked and the height monitored with vaginal bleeding, pulse, blood pressure, and urinary output to identify signs of continued bleeding. Prophylactic antibiotics and slow IV oxytocin infusion are advised. The balloon tamponade can be removed after 4-6 hours, although it is usually left overnight to stabilize the patient. Once the fluid in the balloon is withdrawn, check for bleeding. If there is no further bleeding for 30 minutes, remove the balloon.

Condom Tamponade

Open the condom, insert the end of a piece of tubing from an IV set into the condom, tie securely with sterile string, insert the condom into the uterus via the cervix, release fluid from the IV bottle down the tubing and into the condom (or glove) until it has expanded fully between the walls of the uterus.

TABLE 6: Uterotonics.

Drugs	Dose	Frequency	Action	Maximum doses	Side effects	Caution	Storage
Oxytocin	5–10 unit IV/IM stat and IV infusion	125 mL/h of 20–40 units in 500 mL NS/RL	Onset 2–3 minutes Lasts up to 15–20 minutes	80 units	None or minimal	Direct IV oxytocin contraindicated in cases of heart diseases or failure	2–8° C
Methylergo-metrine	0.2 mg IV or IM if no contraindica-tions	Second dose repeated after 15 minutes rest 2–4 hourly	Onset 2–7 minutes Lasts up to 2–4 hours	5 doses	Nausea, vomiting, headache, hypertension, increased risk of retainer placenta	Avoid in heart disease, hypertension, Rh- negative mothers	2–8° C No freezing, protect from direct sunlight
Prostaglandin F2 alpha (PGF2 alpha)	250 μg IM or intramyometrial	15 minutes once	Onset 1–2 minutes Lasts up to 15–20 minutes	8 doses	Vomiting, diarrhea, bronchospasm		
Misoprostol	600–1,000 μg sublingual/oral/rectal	Single dose	Onset 3–5 minutes Lasts up to 75 minutes		Shivering, slight rise of temperature		Store at room temperature
Tranexamic acid	0.5–1 g slow IV	1 g, once in 8 hours			Gastrointestinal (GI) side effects, rarely visual disturbances	Use cautiously in patient with thrombotic events or family history of thrombosis	Store at room temperature
Carbetocin	100 μg IV or IM	One dose only	Sustained uterine contraction for 6 minutes followed by contraction for 60 minutes		Abdominal pain, nausea, flushing	Under study	Room temperature

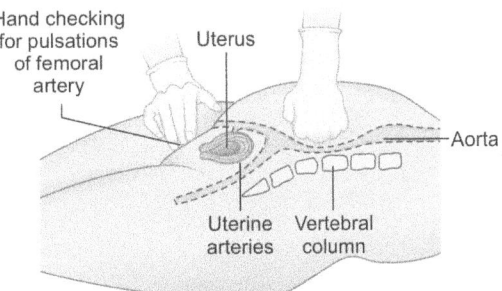

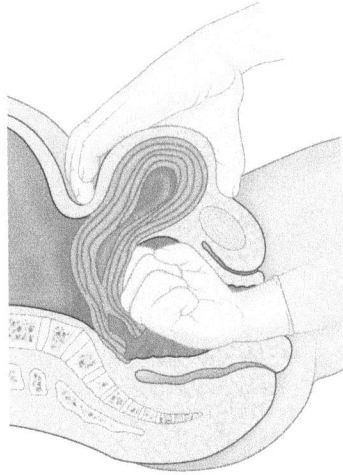

Fig. 1: Bimanual compression.

A balloon tamponade may arrest or stop bleeding in 77.5–88.8% or more cases without any further need for surgical treatment.[16]

Fig. 2: Aortic compression.

AORTIC COMPRESSION (FIG. 2)

If bleeding is severe and if initial measures are not successful, then external aortic compression should be considered.

Stand on the right side of the woman. Place left fist just above and to the left of the woman's umbilicus [the abdominal aorta passes slightly to the left of the midline (umbilicus)]. You should be able to feel the aorta against your knuckles. Before exerting aortic compression, feel the femoral artery for a pulse using the index and third fingers of the right hand.[6] Once the aorta and femoral pulse have been identified, slowly lean over the woman and increase the pressure over the aorta to seal it off.

Successful aortic compression is achieved when the femoral pulse ceases and when blood pressure in the lower limit is unrecordable; it may be of benefit as a temporary measure in the management of PPH whilst resuscitation and other management plans are made.

ANTISHOCK GARMENT (FIG. 3)

The best method of keeping a woman stable while transferring her is to use a noninflatable antishock garment (NASG) if available. This in itself may stop bleeding in many cases. The NASG is a simple

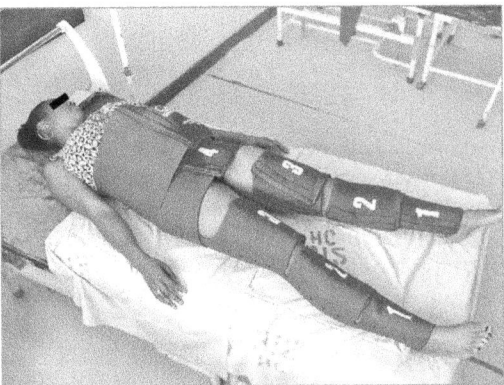

Fig. 3: Antishock garment.

neoprene and Velcro device made of articulated segments that are wrapped tightly around the legs, pelvis, and abdomen. It can be used to treat shock, resuscitate, stabilize, and prevent further bleeding in woman with obstetric hemorrhage. The NASG is not a definitive treatment—the woman will still need to have the source of bleeding found and definitive therapy performed. It has been designed to allow perineal access so that examinations and vaginal procedures can be performed without it being removed. Steps of application—place the NASG under the woman with the top edge at the level of her lowest rib (on her side). Close segment 1 (or 2, for short women) tightly around each ankle and make sure that when snapped, a sharp sound is heard. Close segment 2 tightly around calf. Check for snap sound. Leave the knee free so that the leg can be bent. Close segment 3 tightly around the thigh. Check for snap sound. Place segment 4 so it goes around the woman with its lower edge at the level of her pubic bone. Place segment 5 with

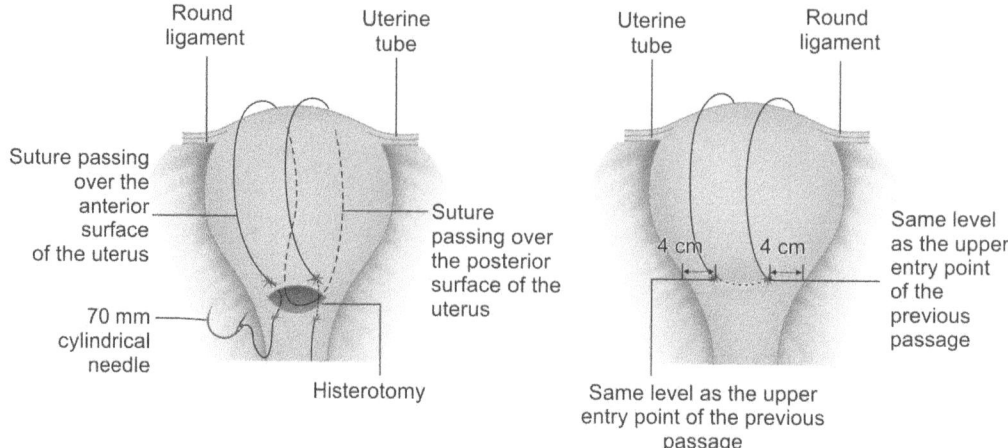

Round ligament   Uterine tube   Uterine tube   Round ligament

Suture passing over the anterior surface of the uterus

Suture passing over the posterior surface of the uterus

70 mm cylindrical needle

Histerotomy

4 cm   4 cm

Same level as the upper entry point of the previous passage

Same level as the upper entry point of the previous passage

Fig. 4: B-Lynch suture.

pressure ball directly over the umbilicus. Close the NASG using segment 6. Make sure the woman can breathe normally with segment 6 in place.

Removal of the NASG occurs only when the source of bleeding is treated, the woman has been hemodynamically stable for at least 2 hours, and blood loss is <50 mL/h. Removal begins at the ankle and proceeds slowly, waiting 15 minutes between opening each segment and taking vital signs (blood pressure and pulse) before opening the next segment.[17]

COMPRESSION SUTURES

B-Lynch Sutures (Fig. 4)

The B-Lynch suture (named for Christopher Balogun-Lynch) envelops and compresses the uterus, similar to the result achieved with manual uterine compression. The technique is relatively simple to learn, appears safe, preserves future reproductive potential, and does increase the risk of placentation-related adverse outcomes in a subsequent pregnancy. It should only be used in cases of uterine atony; it will not control hemorrhage from placenta accreta spectrum.

A large Mayo needle with number #1 or #2 chromic catgut (or any absorbable suture if catgut is unavailable) is used to enter and exit the uterine cavity laterally in the lower uterine segment.

The suture is looped over the fundus and reenters the lower uterine cavity through the posterior wall. The suture then crosses to the other side of the lower uterine segment, exits through the

posterior wall, and is looped back over the fundus to enter the anterior lateral lower uterine segment opposite and parallel to the initial bites. The free ends are pulled tightly and tied down securely to compress the uterus, assisted by bimanual compression.

This suture has success rates above 90% due to atony, and controls bleeding by compressing the uterine body's anterior wall against its posterior wall.

The technique has been used alone and in combination with balloon tamponade. This combination has been called the "uterine sandwich".

Other Uterine Compression Suture Techniques

- *Hayman* described placement of two to four vertical compression sutures from the anterior to posterior uterine wall without hysterotomy. A transverse cervicoisthmic suture can also be placed if needed to control bleeding from the lower uterine segment.[18]
- *Pereira* described a technique in which a series of transverse and longitudinal sutures of a delayed absorbable multifilament suture are placed around the uterus via a series of bites into the subserosal myometrium, without entering the uterine cavity.
- *Cho* described a technique using multiple squares/rectangles. It is useful for bleeding sites located in the body and lower segments of the uterus.[19] Some authors, when applying

Cho's sutures in S2 area dilate the cervix so as to avoid hematometra.[11] In an atonic uterus, 4-5 square sutures should be made (from the fundus to the uterine segment).

STEP WISE PELVIC VASCULATURE LIGATION

Pelvic vascular sutures (PVS) consist of selective ligatures of major pelvic vessels that nourish the pelvis, in order to reduce blood supply in a bleeding area. It usually does not treat the cause of PPH, instead of this, it reduces the perfusion pressure while definitive treatment is being performed. In some situations, it may be sufficient to control hemorrhage. The vessels most commonly addressed are the uterine arteries, the ovarian arteries, the round ligaments arteries, and the internal iliac arteries. If bleeding persists, the healthcare provider should move to next step of PPH treatment (frequently hysterectomy).

The uterine artery ligation has showed a success rate of 80-96% for controlling uterine bleeding. And the internal iliac arteries efficacy, usually, varies from 42 to 93%.[19,20]

Pelvic vascular sutures complications are not very frequent. They usually are related to devascularization of nontarget areas (that may complicate with necrosis, infertility, and so on) and lesions of surrounding structures, such as nerves, vessels, ureters, and bladder.[19,20]

Bilateral Uterine Artery Ligature (Fig. 5)

The first cases of bilateral uterine artery ligature (BUAL) were published by Waters in 1952 and O'Leary in 1966.

Uterine artery ligation is a relatively simple procedure and can be highly effective in controlling bleeding from uterine sources. These arteries provide approximately 90% of uterine blood flow. The uterus is grasped and tilted to expose the vessels coursing through the broad ligament immediately adjacent to the uterus. Ideally, place the stitch 2 cm below the level of a transverse lower uterine incision site. A large atraumatic (round) needle is used with a heavy absorbable suture. Include almost the full thickness of the myometrium to anchor the stitch and to ensure that the uterine artery and veins are completely included. The needle is then

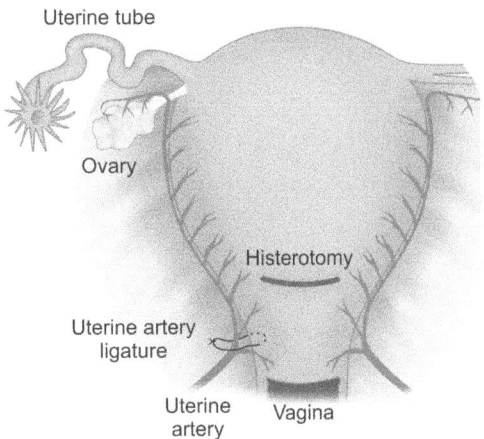

Fig. 5: Bilateral uterine artery ligature.

passed through an avascular portion of the broad ligament and tied anteriorly. Opening the broad ligament is unnecessary. Perform bilateral uterine artery ligation. While the uterus may remain atonic, blanching is usually noted and blood flow is greatly diminished or arrested.

The BUAL optionally may be performed vaginally, through a 2-cm horizontal incision that is made in the anterior cervix, 1 cm beneath the vaginal cervical fold, and the bladder re/ected in the natural plane. After it, the uterine arteries are bilaterally accessed and ligated.[21,22]

The main complication is ureteral injury, besides being rare; it is related to a technical mistake by placing the sutures too low.

LIGATIONS OF THE OVARIAN ARTERIES (FIG. 6)

The ovarian artery is usually performed when BUAL has failed to control the bleeding or in association with it. They are also useful for the treatment of bleeding from the uterine fundus and/or the upper portions of the uterine body. The ovarian artery has an anastomosis with the ascending branch of uterine artery, and corresponds to the other 10% of vascular irrigation of the uterine body. The ovarian arteries ligatures should be performed close to the level of the uterine-ovarian ligament (below or above it). Its complications are usually related to accidental ureter ligature, lesions of surrounding structures, or even ovarian failure.[23,24]

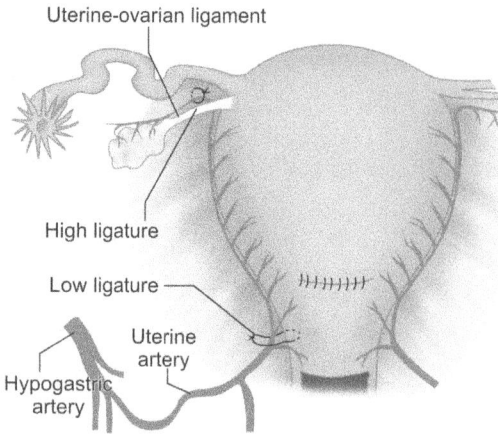

Fig. 6: Ligations of the ovarian arteries.

LIGATIONS OF THE INTERNAL ILIAC ARTERIES (HYPOGASTRIC ARTERY LIGATION)

Internal iliac artery ligation (IIAL) is indicated when there is an intractable hemorrhage, in an effort to reduce it. IIAL is more complex and so requires more surgical skills when compared to the other ligations.

Internal iliac artery ligation requires an abdominal approach. The uterus must be externalized and the broad ligament should be opened under the infundibulopelvic ligament. The bifurcation of the iliac trunk is identified and the hypogastric artery (internal iliac) is dissected over a distance of 3 cm, widely opening the vascular sheath to limit the risk of venous injury. After systematic identification of the ureter, a ligature is placed using a ligature passer about 2–3 cm below the bifurcation, taking care not to injure the vein. At the end of the procedure, we check the pulsations of the external iliac artery. The complications related to it can be infertility, buttock and thigh claudication, damage to the ureter, ischemic limb from damage to common or external iliac artery, damage to other pelvic vessels, and damage to pelvic nerves, including the hypogastric plexus.[25]

HYSTERECTOMY

Postpartum hysterectomy constitutes the final step to control PPH, as it can result in an additional blood loss of >2 L. However, it can be a lifesaving procedure when it is indicated and so it should not be postponed. Hysterectomy will take place when all conservative measures (pharmacological, mechanical, or other more conservative surgical strategies) have failed (or are not indicated) to achieve bleeding control in the setting of life-threatening hemorrhage.[26] Emergency postpartum hysterectomy has an incidence between 0.24 and 0.78 per 1,000 deliveries[27,28] and its most common indications are placenta accreta, uterine atony, and uterine rupture.[26,29]

Oophorectomy must be avoided, considering the fact that a hysterectomy already has a great impact on patient's emotional sphere.

The advantages of performing a subtotal versus total hysterectomy are not clear. Those who defend the subtotal technique sustain the arguments that surgical time is shortened; this procedure has less probability of ureteric or vesical lesions; it requires less surgical abilities; and it is better to preserve the sustaining elements of the pelvic floor. The authors who support total hysterectomy manifest that there may be some remaining vessels or tissue on the cervical stump which are responsible for bleeding; and that by performing a total hysterectomy, in countries with high prevalence of cervical cancer, it would be a measure to prevent these types of neoplasia.[21,30]

REFERENCES

1. WHO. (2018). WHO recommendations: Uterotonics for the prevention of postpartum haemorrhage. [online] Available from https://apps.who.int/iris/bitstream/handle/10665/277276/9789241550420-eng.pdf [Last accessed December, 2021].
2. Registrar General of India. (2019). Special BULLETIN on maternal mortality in India 2015-17. [online] Available from https://censusindia.gov.in/vital_statistics/SRS_Bulletins/MMR_Bulletin-2015-17.pdf [Last accessed December, 2021].
3. Singh PK. (2018). India has achieved groundbreaking success in reducing maternal mortality. [online] Available from https://www.who.int/southeastasia/news/detail/10-06-2018-india-has-achieved-ground breaking-success-in-reducing-maternal-mortality#:~:text=By%20Dr%20Poonam%20Khetrapal%20Singh,000%20live%20births%20in%202016].

4. DGHS. (2018). National health profile 2018, 13th issue. [online] Available from http://www.cbhidghs.nic.in/WriteReadData/l892s/Cover.pdf [Last accessed December, 2021].

5. The World Bank. (2015). Number of maternal deaths. [online] Available from https://data.worldbank.org/indicator/SH.MMR.DTHS [Last accessed, 2021].

6. India Ministry of Health and Family Welfare, Government of India. (2017). Health and family welfare statistics in India 2017. [online] Available from https://main.mohfw.gov.in/sit2es/default/files/ HealthandFamilyWelfare statisticsin India 201920.pdf [Last accessed December, 2021].

7. Say L, Chou D, Gemmill A, Tunçalp O, Moller AB, Daniels J, et al. Global causes of maternal death: A who systematic analysis. Lancet Glob Health. 2014;2:e323-33.

8. Mousa HA, Alfirevic Z. Treatment for primary postpartum haemorrhage. Cochrane Database Syst Rev. 2007;(1):CD003249.

9. American College of Obstetricians and Gynecologists. ACOG practice bulletin: clinical management guidelines for obstetrician-gyne-cologists number 76, October 2006: postpartum hemorrhage. Obstet Gynecol. 2006;108:1039-47.

10. Akins S. Postpartum hemorrhage. A 90s approach to an age-old problem. J Nurse Midwifery. 1994;39(Suppl 2):123S-34S.

11. Chua S, Ho LM, Vanaja K, Nordstrom L, Roy AC, Arulkumaran S. Validation of a laboratory method of measuring postpartum blood loss. Gynecol Obstet Invest. 1998;46:31-3.

12. Duthie SJ, Ven D, Yung GL, Guang DZ, Chan SY, Ma HK. Discrepancy between laboratory determination and visual estimation of blood loss during normal delivery. Eur J Obstet Gynecol Reprod Biol. 1991;38:119-24.

13. Pritchard JA. Blood volume changes in pregnancy and puerperium. Am J Obstet Gynecol. 1962;84:1271.

14. Bose P, Regan F, Paterson-Brown S. Improving the accuracy of estimated blood loss at obstetric haemorrhage using clinical reconstructions. Br J Obstet Gynaecol. 2006;113:919-24.

15. Crafter H. Intrapartum and Primary Postpartum Haemorrhage. In: Boyle M (Ed). Emergencies around Childbirth: a Handbook for Midwives. Oxford: Radcliffe Medical Press; 2002. pp. 149-68.

16. Lalonde A, Daviss BA, Acosta A, Herschderfer K. Postpartum hemorrhage today: ICM/FIGO initiative 2004-2006. Int J Gynecol Obstet. 2006;94(3):243-53.

17. Miller S, Hensleigh P. Postpartum Hemorrhage: New Thoughts, New Approaches. In: B-Lynch C, Lalonde A, West L (Eds). Non-pneumatic Anti-shock Garment for Obstetric Hemorrhage. London: Sapiens; 2006. pp. 136-45.

18. Matsubara S, Yano H, Ohkuchi A. Kuwata T, Usui R, Suzuki M. Uterine compression sutures for postpartum hemorrhage: an overview. Acta Obstet Gynecol Scand. 2013;92:378-85.

19. Cho JH, Jun HS, Lee CN. Hemostatic suturing technique for uterine bleeding during cesarean delivery. Obstet Gynecol. 2000;96(1):129-31.

20. Morel O, Malartic CJ, Muhlstein JE, Gayat E, Judlin P, Soyer P, Barranger E. Pelvic arterial ligations for severe post-partum hemorrhage. Indications and techniques. J Visc Surg. 2011; 148:95-102.

21. Rath W, Hackethal A, Bohlmann MK. Second-line treatment of postpartum haemorrhage (PPH). Arch Gynecol Obstet. 2012;286:549-61.

22. Hebisch G, Huch A. Vaginal uterine artery ligation avoids high blood loss and puerperal hysterectomy in postpartum hemorrhage. Obstet Gynecol. 2002;100(3):574-8.

23. Moise Jr KJ, Belfort MA. Damage control for the obstetric patient. Surg Clin North Am. 1997;77(4):835-52.

24. Roman H, Sentilhes L, Cingotti M, Verspyck E, Marpeau L. Uterine devascularization and subsequent major intrauterine synechiae and ovarian failure. Fertil Steril. 2005;83(3):755-7.

25. Sziller I, Hupuczi P, Papp Z. Hypogastric artery ligation for severe hemorrhage in obstetric patients. J Perinat Med. 2007;35(3):187-92.

26. Zhang Y, Yan J, Han Q, Yang T, Cai L, Fu Y, et al. Emergency obstetric hysterectomy for life threatening postpartum hemorrhage: A 12-year review. Medicine (Baltimore). 2017;96(45): e8443.

27. Imudia AN, Awonuga AO, Dbouk T, Kumar S, Cordoba MI, Diamond MP, et al. Incidence, trends, risk factors, indications for, and complications associated with cesarean hysterectomy: a 17-year experience from a single institution. Arch Gynecol Obstet. 2009; 280:619-23.

28. Demirci O, Tugrul AS, Yilmaz E, Tosun Ö, Demirci E, Eren YS. Emergency peripartum hysterectomy in a tertiary obstetric center: nine years' evaluation. J Obstet Gynaecol Res. 2011;37:1054-60.

29. Rath W, Hackethal A, Bohlmann MK. Second-line treatment of postpartum haemorrhage (PPH). Arch Gynecol Obstet. 2012;286:549-61.

30. Jacoby VL. Hysterectomy controversies: Ovarian and cervical preservation. Clin Obstet Gynecol. 2014;57(1):95-105.

Traumatic Postpartum Hemorrhage

Komal Chavan, Anusha Devalla

INTRODUCTION

Postpartum hemorrhage is essentially a life-threatening obstetric emergency and an obstetrician's nightmare. It also can be a frightening experience for some women who may eventually develop post-traumatic stress disorder.[1]

Although ACOG in 2017 has further redefined PPH as a cumulative blood loss >1,000 mL with signs and symptoms of hypovolemia within 24 hours of the birth process, regardless of the route of delivery;[2] nonetheless blood loss at vaginal delivery >500 mL should be considered abnormal that may necessitate intervention.[3]

DEFINITION

Postpartum hemorrhage (PPH) can be defined as any blood loss from the genital tract of >500 mL after a vaginal delivery or 1,000 mL after a cesarean section (RCOG Green top Guideline 2016).

EPIDEMIOLOGY

World: About 295,000 women died during and following pregnancy and childbirth in 2017. PPH accounts for 6% of all deliveries and 25% of the deaths worldwide.[4]

India: The reported incidence of PPH in India is 2–4% after vaginal delivery and 6% after cesarean section.[5] Indian statistics from SRS 2001–2003 state that PPH contributes to 38% of all maternal deaths (RGI-SRS 2001–2003).

ETIOLOGY

Trauma to the uterus, cervix, and/or vagina is the second most frequent cause, responsible for approximately 8–11% of PPH, which usually manifests within 24 hours.[6]

Traumatic PPH can be encountered both after vaginal or cesarean delivery. It usually results from:
- *Vaginal delivery*:
  - Precipitate labor
  - Injudicious instrumental delivery—applying on high head/incompletely dilated cervix
  - Imprudent applications of prostaglandins for induction of labor
  - Overzealous use of oxytocin for induction/augmentation of labor
  - Malpresentations
  - Macrosomia
  - Shoulder dystocia
  - Preterm delivery[7]
- The bleeding is predominantly venous in nature after a vaginal delivery.
  - *Cesarean section*: Trauma to the uterine angles while extending the incision (especially after prolonged labor causing thinned out lower segment, poorly healed previous lower uterine segment scar).

Other Predisposing Conditions

- Continued preference for home deliveries (conducted by unskilled birth attendants) for sociocultural and economic reasons
- Complications are not recognized as problems.
- Women lack decision-making power
- Transportation not available
- Delays even if they make it to the health facility.
- Supplies lacking for emergency obstetric care

MANAGEMENT (FLOWCHART 1)

Atonic uterus manifests as a "revealed" PPH unlike genital tract trauma that *may go unrecognized* and hence quantification of blood loss and ascertainment of PPH can be really challenging

Flowchart 1: Approach to a patient with traumatic PPH following vaginal delivery.

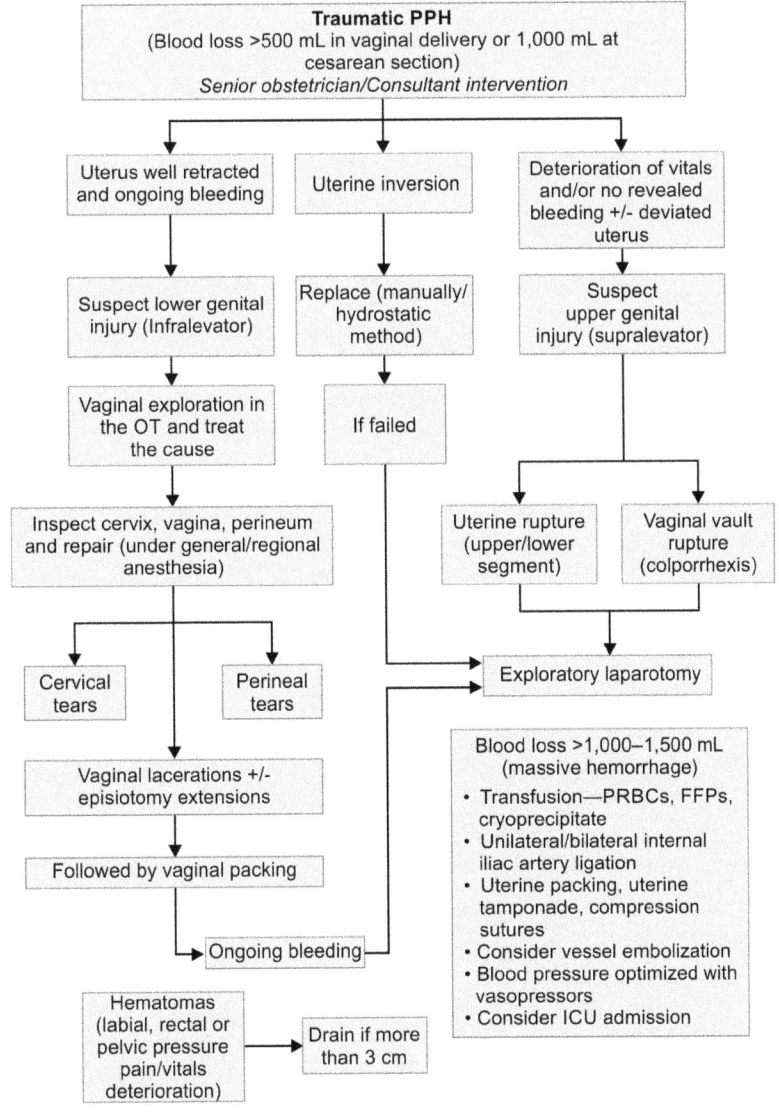

(FFP: fresh frozen plasma; PPH: postpartum hemorrhage; PRBC: packed red blood cell)

for the clinician. Traumatic PPH should always be strongly suspected with the retracted uterus and ongoing bleeding.[2]

Some degree of perineal trauma is seen in majority of the women delivering vaginally but rarely require extensive repair. Careful exploration of the cervix, vagina, and perineum is essential to exclude tears and lacerations.[6,8]

▉ TREATMENT

The patient is to be treated on the lines of standard PPH protocol starting with general measures as highlighted in the following algorithm as provided by FOGSI prevention of PPH guideline **(Fig. 1)**. An important point to note here is that the visual estimation of blood loss after delivery is unreliable as almost 16–41% blood loss

Safe Motherhood Committee

PPH

| Step 1: General management |

- Shout for help
- Rapid evaluation of vitals
- Oxygen by mask
- Uterine massage
- Oxytocin 10 U IM
- Site 2 large bore (16G-gray color) IV cannula
- Infuse IV fluid: NS/RL-run it fast
- Catheterize bladder
- Check the placenta:
  - Is it expelled
  - If it is expelled, re-examine and make sure it is complete
- Examine vagina, perineum and cervix for tears

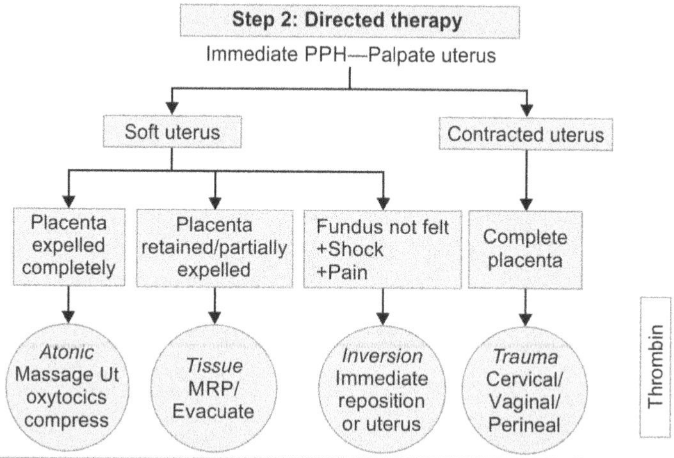

| Step 2: Directed therapy |

Immediate PPH—Palpate uterus

Soft uterus | **Contracted uterus**

| Placenta expelled completely | Placenta retained/partially expelled | Fundus not felt +Shock +Pain | Complete placenta |

(Atonic Massage Ut oxytocics compress) (Tissue MRP/ Evacuate) (Inversion Immediate reposition or uterus) (Trauma Cervical/ Vaginal/ Perineal)

Thrombin

Oxytocics

Drugs	Dose and route	Maintenance dose	Max dose	Frequency	Precaution/ CI
Oxytocin	IV infusion 10 U/500 mL 60 dpm	IV infuse 10 U/500 mL 40 dpm	Not more than 3 L	–	
Ergometrine/ Methergine	IM/Slow IV of 0.2 mg	0.2 mg after 15 minutes	5 doses (1 mg)	4th hourly	PIH, HT, heart disease
15-methyl PGFα	IM 250 ug	250 ug after 15 minutes	5 doses (2 mg)	15–90 minutes	Asthma, heart disease

Fig. 1: Management algorithm of PPH.
(*Source:* FOGSI prevention of PPH guideline)

is underestimated, the latter if the blood loss reached 2,000 mL.[9]

Traumatic PPH can be tackled once the bleeding point is identified. However, underlying conditions such as pre-eclampsia and hepatic disorders may worse the condition.

Additionally, the traumatic PPH management can be summarized using the **Flowchart 1**.

The specific treatment depends upon the immediate inciting event and is essentially managed surgically. Medical therapy needs to go hand-in-hand to further facilitate and speed up the recovery.

▦ MEDICAL MANAGEMENT

Use of Tranexamic Acid

World Health Organization (WHO), in its recent recommendations, has highlighted the use of injection Tranexamic acid for prevention and treatment of PPH issued in 2017. Additionally, traumatic PPH could be managed when uterotonics fail to control the bleeding.[10,11]

Blood Transfusion

An obstetric shock index >1 has been reported to be associated with increase in the likelihood of requiring a blood transfusion following PPH. Therefore, OSI, when compared to visual estimation of blood loss, may be a simple test to assess clinically and is relatively accurate.[8]

▦ SURGICAL MANAGEMENT

It is directed to treat the cause. Traumatic PPH following vaginal delivery:

- *Vaginal tears/lacerations*: It may occur spontaneously due to stretching the vagina especially in primipara. However, that encountered iatrogenically is more problematic especially involving the periurethral and clitoral region. Lacerations may occur during manipulations to resolve shoulder dystocia.[12]

- *Vulvovaginal hematomas*:
  - Space lies within the pelvic connective tissue extending from the vagina to the obturator fascia and is continuous with the adjacent spaces which readily accommodate any fluid or blood from either compartment. In pregnancy, a rich vulvovaginal plexus becomes very prominent near the upper and lateral walls of the vagina. The levator ani divides the paravaginal space into supra and infralevator spaces as shown in **Figures 2 and 3**.
  - Pain, swelling, ecchymosis, and urinary retention are the symptoms that prompt an infralevator hematoma and sometimes the vital signs are disproportionate to the estimated blood loss. Episiotomy hematomas also present the same way and such complaints should never be dismissed as it may appear small whereas a hematoma in the supralevator region can only be picked up by digital examination of the pelvis (painless rubbery mass) pushing in the vaginal wall **(Fig. 4)**.[13]
  - *Episiotomy extensions*: Many a times during difficult deliveries, one may encounter an episiotomy extension which exposes the ischiorectal fossa, a potential

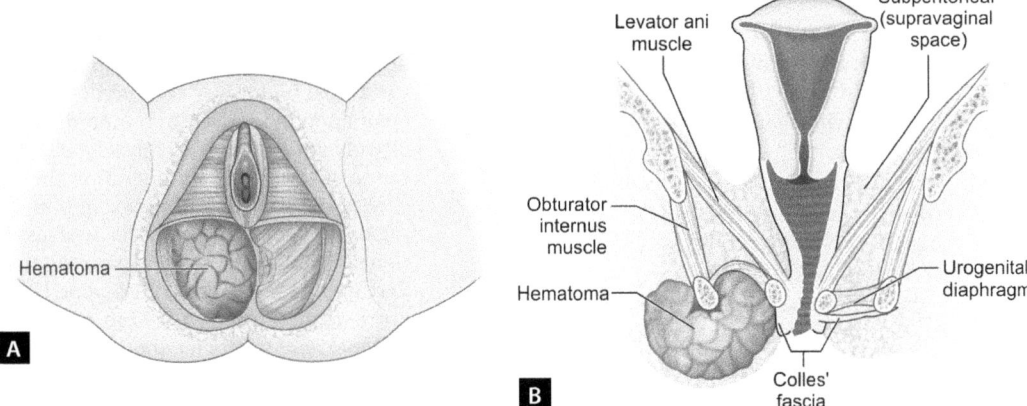

Figs. 2A and B: Infralevator hematoma.
(*Source:* Obgyn Key. (2021). Fastest Obstetric, Gynecology, and Pediatric Insight Engine. [online] Available from https://obgynkey.com/ [Last accessed December, 2021].)

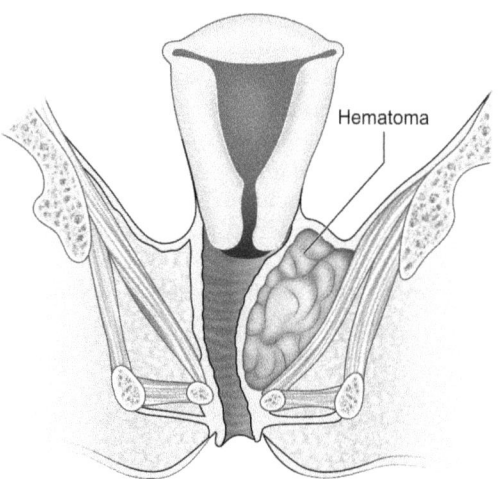

Fig. 3: Supralevator hematoma.
(*Source*: Obgyn Key. (2021). Fastest Obstetric, Gynecology and Pediatric Insight Engine. [online] Available from https://obgynkey.com/ [Last accessed December, 2021].)

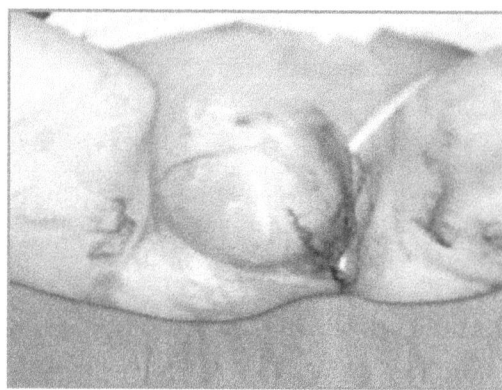

Fig. 4: Clinical presentation of vulvovaginal hematoma (infralevator).
(*Source*: Shilpa N, Thakur R, Verma A. Vulvar Haematoma following precipitate delivery: A case report. J Cases Obstet Gynecol. 2017;4(3):64-7.)

space for accommodating a huge amount of blood and cause vulvar hematoma even leading to severe anemia and shock. Suturing this space first is very important with interrupted sutures after securing the apex as it will be difficult later after suturing the vaginal mucosa.[7]

– Hematomas in this region <3 cm need conservative measures such as ice packs and analgesics. Larger hematomas need incision and evacuation followed by thorough irrigation. The bleeding vessel should be meticulously identified and ligated placing figure-of-eight sutures.[14]

• *Cervical tears*:
– Tears are more frequent on application of the instrument in the absence of a fully dilated cervix. The frequent practice of stretching the cervix just to expedite, the delivery can also lead to such tears, which may go unnoticed till late. Although a rare phenomenon now, deliberate lateral incisions on the cervix (Duhrssen incision is also a cause). Cervical exploration/tracing clockwise or counter-clockwise in lithotomy/dorsal lithotomy position is a must for all instrumental deliveries and

should be a part of the resident teaching curriculum.[12]

– While suturing the tear, the first stitch should start beyond the apex and then complete in continuous interlocking/noninterlocking fashion followed by the repair of the episiotomy **(Fig. 5A)**. If the apex is still not visualized, a stitch can be taken as high as possible and apply gentle traction to the suture material (stay-suture) as shown in **Figure 5B** and suturing continued above this point.[7]

– *Third and fourth degree perineal tears*: Although not a very important cause of obvious traumatic PPH, continuous trickling from these tears may underestimate the actual blood loss and might be sufficient enough to produce symptoms in an already anemic patient. It is advocated to repair such tears in an operation theater with good lighting and performed under regional or general anesthesia by an experienced clinician. Anal mucosa is repaired first in the case of a fourth degree laceration with running 4-0 Monocryl. The internal anal sphincter should be identified, if possible, and repaired via end-to-end anastomosis with running 3-0 or 4-0 PDS. The external anal sphincter may be repaired using either an overlapping or end-to-end anastomosis using a monofilament suture.[16]

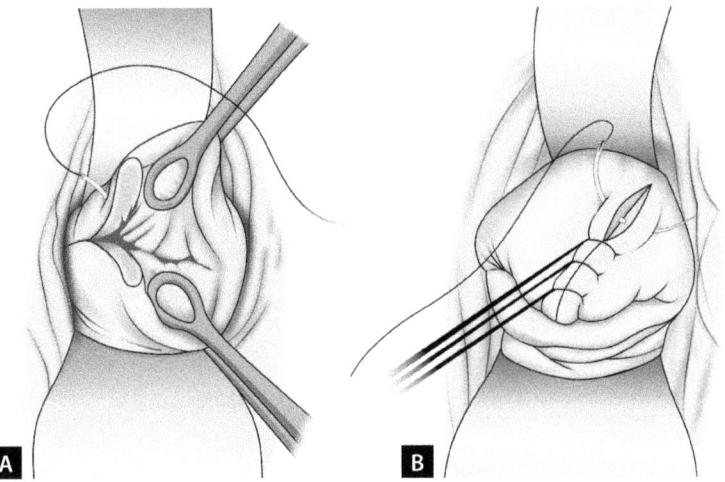

Figs. 5A and B: (A) Suturing of a cervical tear, (B) exposing the apex of the cervical tear by dragging the stay suture in case of a deep laceration.
(*Source*: Obgyn Key. (2021). Fastest Obstetric, Gynecology and Pediatric Insight Engine: [online] Available from https://obgynkey.com/ [Last accessed December, 2021].)[15]

SPECIAL CLINICAL SITUATIONS

Uterine Inversion

It is a rare life-threatening complication of vaginal or cesarean delivery, where uterine fundus collapses into the endometrial cavity partially or completely, protruding through the vaginal introitus. Severe hemorrhage, shock and even death may ensue if not promptly recognized **(Fig. 6)**.

In a series of 2,427 cases of puerperal uterine inversion in the United States, PPH was noted in 37.7%; those requiring blood transfusion were 22.4% and need for laparotomy was observed in 6.0%.[17]

Uterine inversion when diagnosed as a cause of PPH should be reposited using Johnson method **(Figs. 7A to C)**. Uterine relaxants such as a halogenated anesthetic, terbutaline, magnesium sulfate, or nitroglycerine can be used during uterine repositioning if contraction ring of lower segment forms, with oxytocin and other uterotonics upon reposition into the anatomical position. Rarely, surgical correction is required by laparotomy.[3]

Uterine Rupture

This should always be suspected in any patient with scarred uterus undergoing a prolonged

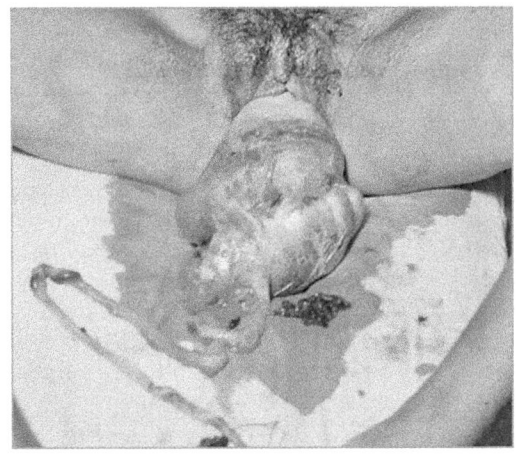

Fig. 6: Maternal death from exsanguination caused by uterine inversion associated with a fundal placenta accreta during a home delivery.
(*Source*: Pritchard J. Chapter-41: Obstetrical Hemorrhage. In: Cunningham FG; Williams JW (Eds). Williams obstetrics, 24th edition. New York, N.Y.: McGraw-Hill Education LLC; 2010.)[18]

trial. Trauma also may occur following extrauterine or intrauterine manipulation of the fetus. As was accepted before, routine transvaginal palpation of such scars is no longer recommended. Finally, trauma may result secondary to attempt

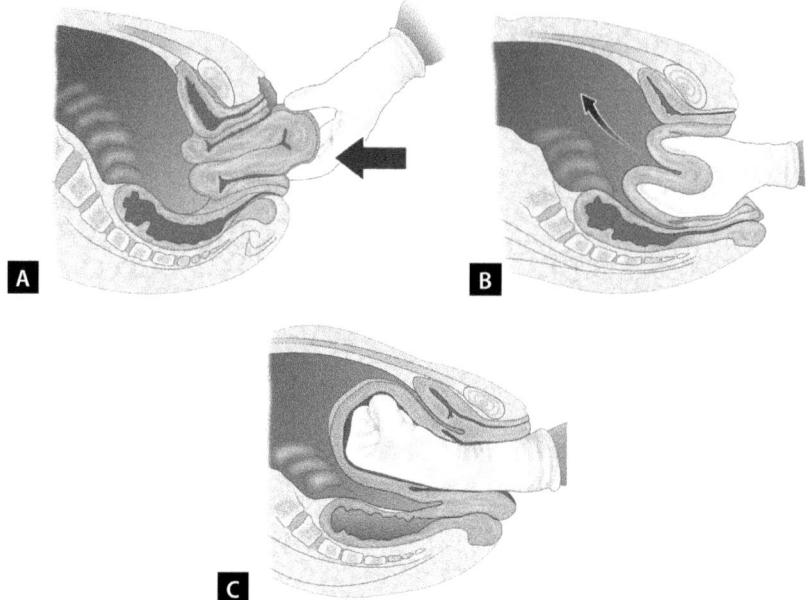

Figs. 7A to C: Reduction of uterine inversion (Johnson method). (A) The protruding fundus is grasped with fingers directed toward the posterior fornix; (B) The uterus is returned to position by pushing it through the pelvis and; (C) Into the abdomen with steady pressure toward the umbilicus.
(*Source*: Anderson JM, Etches D. Prevention and management of postpartum hemorrhage. Am Fam Physician. 2007;75(6):88.).[14]

to remove a retained placenta manually or with instrumentation. This should be accompanied by gentle handling of the uterus. An intraumbilical vein saline/oxytocin or saline/misoprostol injection may reduce the need for more invasive removal techniques. This condition obviously leads to massive hemorrhage and needs urgent surgical intervention through laparotomy.[12]

Colporrhexis

It is the rupture of vaginal vault or upper one-third of the vaginal wall as shown in **Figure 8**. An unusual but a dreaded complication which occurs spontaneously or due to instrumental delivery. Colporrhexis is usually associated with uterine rupture (secondary colporrhexis) and incidence reported in 7.5% of deliveries. High degree of suspicion is warranted when a large pool of blood is seen on vaginal exploration during PPH. On diagnosis, it usually requires exploratory laparotomy for the repair of the vaginal vault tear.[19]

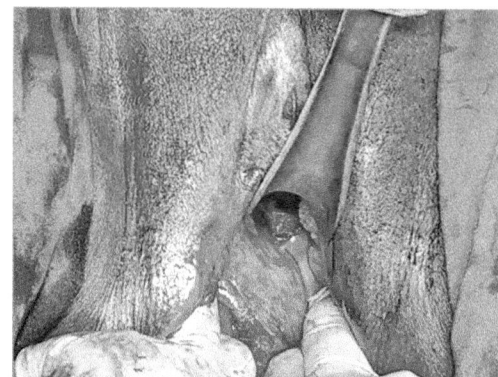

Fig. 8: Tear of the vaginal vault after a full-term vaginal delivery.
(*Source*: Maran C, Swapnaja M. Primary complete colporrhexis. Indian J Obstet Gynecol Res. 2020; 7(3):451-4.)[19]

Traumatic PPH during Cesarean Section

Lower segment cesarean section (LSCS) uterine incision extensions are uncommon but can be encountered in a cesarean done for deep transverse arrest as well as in a patient with prior LSCS, where the lower segment is usually thinned out.

Lateral extensions: Difficult baby delivery may lead to laceration of uterine arteries through the extension of the transverse uterine incisions sometimes extending to form broad ligament hematomas.

Exteriorization and quickly securing the angles of the uterine incision along with uterine artery ligation may help in mitigating further blood loss.

Downward extension: Thinned out slower segment in a previous LSCS is more prone to such extensions. Suturing the two edges of the uterine incision should be separately dealt for the extensions and main incision itself with each angle taken separately. Tracing the bladder folds and ureter may become necessary if there are deep-down/lateral extensions requiring the assistance from an urologist.

FAILURE TO CONTROL THE BLEEDING/UNCONTROLLED MASSIVE PPH

- *Unilateral/bilateral internal iliac artery ligation*: Timely decision can help save the patient from life-threatening hemorrhage as the arterial pressures are converted into venous flow pressures by ligating the internal iliac arteries.
- *Embolization of arteries*: A retrospective analysis performed in 60 patients undergoing transarterial embolization with a detection rate of 93% concluded that it is safe and effective treatment for PPH related to genital tract injury using angiographic embolization of uterine, cervical, and vaginal arteries. However, presence of paravaginal hematomas decreased the chances of success.[6]
- Cesarean hysterectomy

PREVENTION

However, advanced can be the treatment procedures but preventive measures can never get outdated.
- Careful assessment of the pelvis for all the patients to be given a trial of labor must be performed by a senior obstetrician to assess for cephalopelvic disproportion.
- Close watch on the labor progress and fetal status throughout is important as signs such as meconium, fetal distress and increasing caput are ominous.
- Arrest of the descent of the head in the second stage of labor should raise a suspicion of cord around the neck, occipitoposterior position and in such instances the decision for LSCS should be taken timely.
- Avoid routine episiotomy unless urgent delivery is necessary in an unfavorably tight perineum to avoid unnecessary blood loss and tears.[14]

CONCLUSION

The concept of "birth preparedness" might help go a long way in preventing maternal mortality by encouraging the pregnant women, their families and the wider community as a whole to anticipate the possible complications and cater to her transport facilities, if the need arises. Comprehensive obstetric care is particularly essential and to be provided by the healthcare systems along with the protocol-based management. Hence, a broad scope of improvement is essential at individual, community, and political levels.

REFERENCES

1. Zaat TR, van Steijn ME, de Haan-Jebbink JM, Olff M, Stramrood CAI, van Pampus MG. Posttraumatic stress disorder related to postpartum haemorrhage: A systematic review. Eur J Obstet Gynecol Reprod Biol. 2018; 225:214-20.
2. ACOG. (2017). Postpartum Hemorrhage. [online] Available from https://www.acog.org/en/clinical/clinical-guidance/practice-bulletin/articles/2017/10/postpartum-hemorrhage [Last accessed December, 2021].
3. Wormer KC, Jamil RT, Bryant SB. Acute Postpartum Hemorrhage. StatPearls Publishing. 2021.
4. WHO. (2019). Maternal mortality. [online] Available from https://www.who.int/news-room/fact-sheets/detail/maternal-mortality [Last accessed December, 2021].
5. Kumar N. Postpartum Hemorrhage; a Major Killer of Woman: Review of Current Scenario. Obstet Gynecol Int J. 2016;4(4):00116.

6. Lee SM, Shin JH, Shim JJ, Yoon KW, Cho YJ, Kim JW, et al. Postpartum haemorrhage due to genital tract injury after vaginal delivery: safety and efficacy of transcatheter arterial embolisation. Eur Radiol. 2018;28(11):4800-9.

7. Podder AR, Seshadri JG. Traumatic postpartum hemorrhage: How to Avoid and how to manage. In: Podder AR, Seshadri JG (Eds). Atlas of Difficult Gynecological Surgery. Singapore: Springer; 2020. pp. 169-93.

8. Sebghati M, Chandraharan E. An update on the risk factors for and management of obstetric haemorrhage. Womens Health. 2017; 13(2):34-40.

9. Toledo P, McCarthy RJ, Hewlett BJ, Fitzgerald PC, Wong CA. The accuracy of blood loss estimation after simulated vaginal delivery. Anesth Analg. 200;105(6):1736-40

10. The Federation of Obstetric & Gynecological Societies of India. (2015). Emergency Obstetric Kit. [online] Available from https://www.fogsi.org/emergency-obstetric-kit/ [Last accessed December, 2021].

11. WHO. (2017). WHO updates recommendation on intravenous tranexamic acid for the treatment of postpartum haemorrhage. [online]. Available from http://www.who.int/reproductivehealth/tranexamic-acid-pph-treatment/en/ [Last accessed December, 2019].

12. Medsape. (2018). What is the role of trauma in the etiology of postpartum hemorrhage (PPH)? [online] Available from https://www.medscape.com/answers/796785-122152/what-is-the-role-of-trauma-in-the-etiology-of-postpartum-hemorrhage-pph [Last accessed December, 2019].

13. Melody GF. Paravaginal hematomas—Their recognition and management postpartum. Calif Med. 1955;82(1):16-8.

14. Evensen A, Anderson JM, Fontaine P. Postpartum hemorrhage: Prevention and treatment. Am Fam Physician. 2017;95(7): 442-9.

15. Themes UFO. (2016). Genital Tract Lacerations and Puerperal Hematomas. [online] Available from https://obgynkey.com/genital-tract-lacerations-and-puerperal-hematomas/ [Last accessed December, 2019].

16. Meister MR, Rosenbloom JI, Lowder JL, Cahill AG. Techniques for Repair of Obstetric Anal Sphincter Injuries. Obstet Gynecol Surv. 2018;73(1):33-9.

17. Coad SL, Dahlgren LS, Hutcheon JA. Risks and consequences of puerperal uterine inversion in the United States, 2004 through 2013. Am J Obstet Gynecol. 2017;217(3):377.

18. Pritchard J. Obstetrical Hemorrhage. In: Cunningham FG; Williams JW (Eds) Williams Obstetrics, 24th edition. New York, N.Y.: McGraw-Hill Education LLC; 2010.

19. Maran C, Mohanapriya S. Primary complete colporrhexis. Indian J Obstet Gynecol Res. 2020;7(3):451-4.

Monisha Singh, Narendra Malhotra

DEFINITION

Uterine inversion is the folding of the fundus into the uterine cavity in varying degrees.

Acute uterine inversion is a potentially fatal complication of a mismanaged third stage of labor, leading to severe postpartum hemorrhage and shock; if not managed aggressively, it can prove lethal.

EXTENT OF INVERSION (FIGS. 1A TO D)

- *First degree (also called incomplete)*: The fundus is within the endometrial cavity.
- *Second degree (also called complete)*: The fundus protrudes through the cervical os.
- *Third degree (also called prolapsed)*: The fundus protrudes to or beyond the introitus

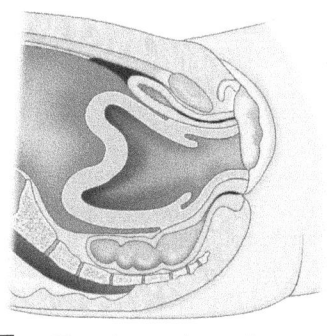
A First degree inversion

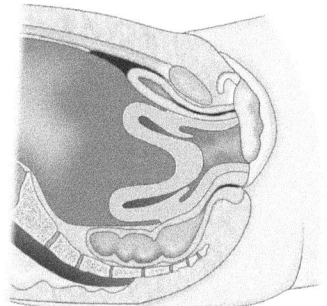
B Second degree inversion

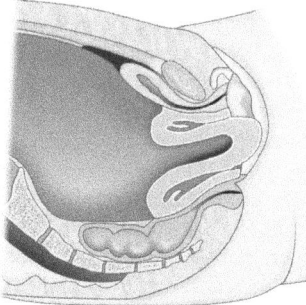
C Third degree inversion

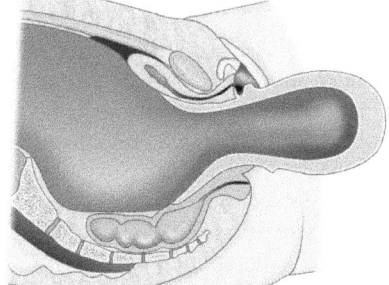
D Fourth degree inversion

Figs. 1A to D: Various degrees of uterine inversion.

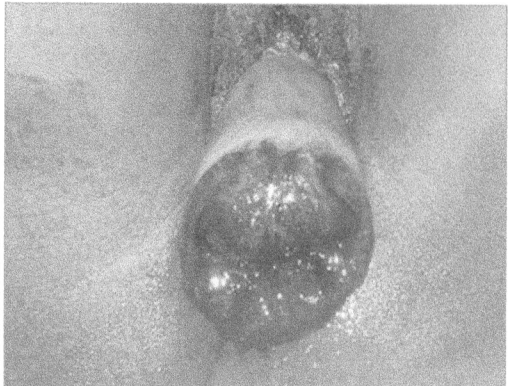

Fig. 2: Completely inverted uterus.

- *Fourth degree (also called total)*: Both the uterus and vagina are inverted.

TIME OF OCCURRENCE

- Acute inversion occurs within 24 hours of birth.
- Subacute inversion occurs between 24 hours and 30 days postpartum.
- Chronic inversion occurs after 30 days postpartum **(Fig. 2)** and is rare.

   It can be complete (if it passes through the cervix) or incomplete (if it does not pass through the cervix).

Incidence: 1 in 2,000–1 in 50,000 deliveries, as described in articles.[1]

CAUSES

- Deliveries conducted by untrained birth attendants ("dais")
- Aggressive fundal pressure in the second stage of labor due to insufficient bearing-down efforts. Short umbilical cord and excessive tug on the cord before the signs of placental separation
- Relaxed uterus, lower uterine segment and cervix; placenta accreta, particularly involving the uterine fundus; congenital weakness or anomalies of the uterus; and antepartum use of magnesium sulfate or oxytocin
- Rapid emptying of the uterus after prolonged distension as possible predisposing factors

DIAGNOSIS

Complete inversion: Palpate the inverted fundus at the cervical os or vaginal area

Incomplete inversion: Palpate the fundus in the lower uterine segment and cervix.

   It is associated with excessive bleeding, unable to palpate uterine fundus, or unable to palpate uterus abdominally, with picture of shock.

MANAGEMENT

Goals

- Replace the uterine fundus correctly
- Manage hemorrhage and shock
- Prevent recurrence

   Acute uterine inversion is an emergency, can be managed nonsurgically if detected early, uterine relaxation can be provided from tocolytic therapy (magnesium sulfate, terbutaline, and nitroglycerine), to general anesthesia. Chronic uterine inversion correction requires elective surgery.[1]

Prevention

Proper education and training should be imparted to traditional birth attendants, local village health practitioners, and over enthusiast residents about the management of labor, placental delivery, timely diagnosis, and proper management of uterine inversion to avoid this grave complication.

Clinical Picture

- *Acute*: Hypovolemic and neurogenic shock, which include pelvic pain and intense vaginal bleeding. The shock is thought to be due to the parasympathetic effect of traction on the ligaments supporting the uterus and may be associated with bradycardia.
- *Chronic*: History of progressively increasing painless vaginal mass along with blood-stained vaginal discharge for the last 6 months and dyspareunia, menometrorrhagia, foul-smelling discharge per vaginum, or a mass coming out of the vagina.

Clinical Features

- *General examination*: Acute may have symptoms/ signs suggestive of sudden shock; moderate pallor.

- *Vitals*: Stages of shock can be variable based on her blood loss.
- *Systemic examination*: Check saturation; breathlessness, pale sweaty skin, and sudden cardiovascular collapse
- *Abdominal examination*: Severe abdominal pain with tenderness, contracted uterus may not be felt giving picture of atonia.
- *Local examination*: A congested globular mass with smooth margins that may bleed upon manipulation.
- *Vaginal examination*: A congested, globular mass can be palpated, which can be felt originating from cervix and reaching into vagina. A thinned-out cervical rim can be palpated around the mass, forming a firm constriction ring, and uterine sound could not be passed around the mass. The uterine fundus cannot be appreciated.
- *Per rectal examination*: The uterus cannot be felt.

- *Ultrasonography (USG) (Fig. 3A)*: An inverted uterus with the fundus of the uterus within the vagina. Transverse images were seen as a hyperechoic mass in the vagina with a central hypoechoic H-shaped cavity. Longitudinal images displayed a U-shaped depressed longitudinal groove (representing from the uterine fundus to the center of the inverted part).[2]
- *Pelvis computed tomography (CT) pelvis (Figs. 3B to D)*: Complete uterine prolapse can be visualized; bladder with irregular contours and spaced walls, with an apparent low bladder component; no filling failure ureters, with low insertion ureteral meatus; absence of free fluid or lymph node enlargement in the pelvis; absence of adnexal masses; and bone structures without particularities and abdominal wall without abnormalities
- Laboratory investigations including hemoglobin, cross matches for blood transfusion, arterial blood gas (ABG)

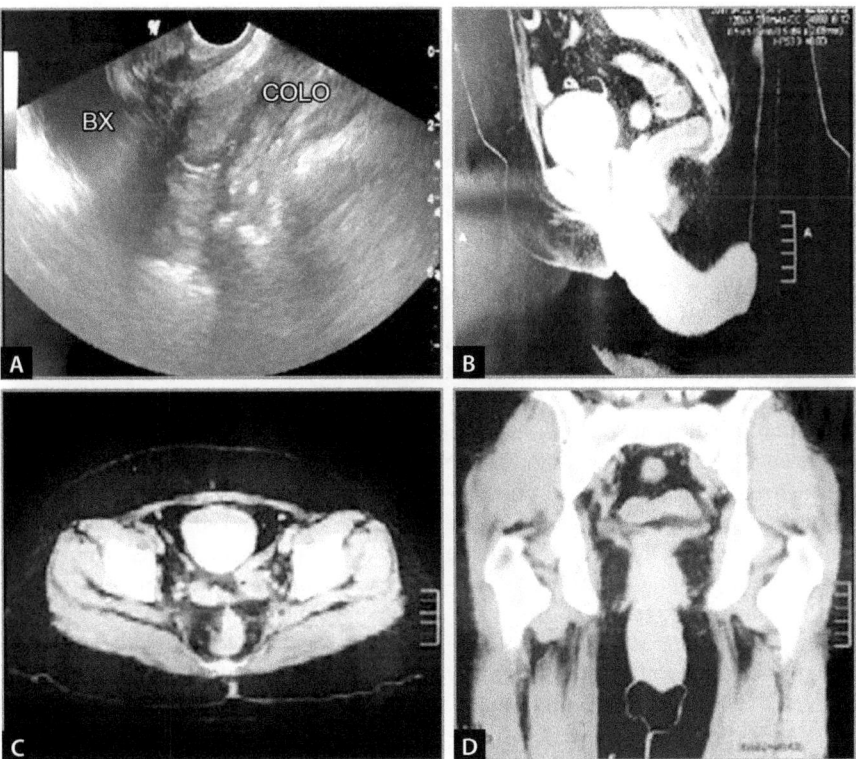

Figs. 3A to D: Imaging exams. (A) Transvaginal ultrasonography (TVUS) with uterine myoma in uterine prolapse; (B) Pelvic computed tomography (CT) sagittal cut; (C) Pelvic CT axial cut; and (D) Pelvic CT coronal cut.

Management

- *Acute uterine inversion*: It includes immediate treatment of hypovolemic shock and repositioning of the uterus, either manually or by hydrostatic pressure (Sullivan's method).
- *Chronic inversion*: It requires a surgical approach because uterine walls show resilience. The firmness of the constriction ring and its inelastic walls has to be divided along with the rigid myometrium obstructing it. The *abdominal methods* are Huntington's and Haultain's methods (mentioned below). The *vaginal surgeries* include Spinelli's and Kustner's techniques for repositioning the prolapsed fundus through the anterior and posterior transections (through cul-de-sac), respectively.
- The *abdominal route is preferred* due to better vision, precise incision of the constriction ring, easy repositioning with traction on the round and broad ligaments, adequate hemostasis, and flawless suturing over the vaginal route. In subsequent pregnancies, recurrence is rare if good obstetrical care is provided.
- *Initial interventions*: Interventions for the management of acute uterine inversion should begin promptly and simultaneously. A delay in diagnosis or in prompt initiation of treatment increases the risk of maternal morbidity and mortality. We suggest **Flowchart 1**:
  - Discontinue uterotonic drugs
  - Call for immediate assistance
  - Establish adequate intravenous access and aggressive fluid/blood product resuscitation
  - Do not remove the placenta
  - *Immediately attempt to manually replace the inverted uterus*: This is best accomplished by placing a hand inside the vagina and pushing the fundus along the long axis of the vagina toward the umbilicus (Johnson maneuver).

If a constriction ring is palpable, pressure should be applied to the part of the fundus nearest the ring to ease it through from bottom to top. This avoids attempting to push a wider diameter of the fundal mass through the ring, which is likely to fail. *Principle—"the part of the uterus which has come down last, should go back first".*[3]

- If the patient is hemodynamically unstable after an initial attempt at replacement, it is reasonable to proceed directly to laparotomy.
- In hemodynamically stable patients, *give uterine relaxants* (nitroglycerine, terbutaline, magnesium sulfate, inhalational methods such as sevoflurane, desflurane, and isoflurane) when immediate uterine replacement is unsuccessful. Manual replacement is then reattempted **(Figs. 4A to C)**.

Preferred Secondary Interventions

Indication: If the manual measures to replace the uterus fail, surgical methods are applied in operating theater.

At laparotomy, in place of the uterus, a constriction ring containing a dimple or cup or slit is often observed, and the adnexa (fallopian tubes, round ligaments, and possibly one or both ovaries) are typically pulled into this hole.

- *Huntington procedure (Fig. 5A)*:
  - Locate the cup formed by the inversion
  - Clamp the myometrium if the round ligaments cannot be identified.
  - Gently pull on the clamps to exert upward traction on the inverted fundus.

Repeatedly clamp in 2 cm increments along the ligament and exert traction until the inversion is corrected.

The assistant surgeon in meantime can place a hand in the vagina and apply upward pressure on the fundus to facilitate the procedure, or they can pull one of the clamps while the first operator pulls the other clamp.

- *Haultain procedure (Fig. 5B)*:
  - Make an incision (approximately 1.5″ in length) in the posterior surface of the uterus to transect the constriction ring.
  - Manual reduction can be performed through the vagina or by placing a finger abdominally through the myometrial incision to below the fundus and then exerting pressure on the fundus to reduce the inversion.
  - The incision is repaired when the uterus has been returned to a normal position.

Other options: Further investigation of safety and efficacy of these other options are needed before they can be recommended.

Flowchart 1: Management of puerperal uterine inversion with hemodynamic instability.

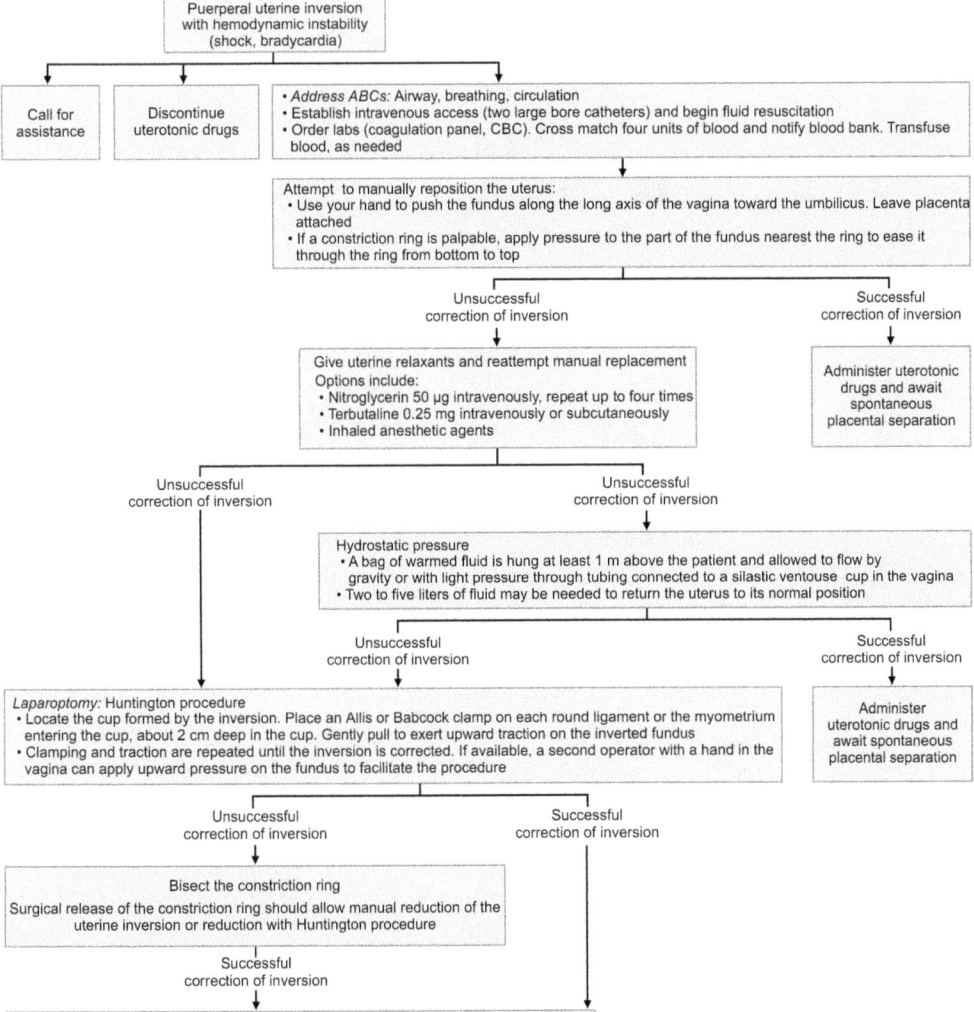

- *Hydrostatic reduction* is tried when initial nonsurgical interventions have failed and surgical intervention is not possible **(Fig. 6)**.
    - The patient is placed in reversed Trendelenburg lithotomy position.
    - A bag of warmed fluid is hung at least a meter above the patient's bed and allowed to flow by gravity or with light pressure through tubing connected to a silastic ventouse cup in the vagina; the seal between the perimeter of the cup and the vagina prevents significant leakage.

- *Procedures to avoid*: Vaginal surgical approaches are no longer performed and are potentially dangerous.
- *Management of the placenta*: Do not remove the placenta until the uterus has been replaced (may increases blood loss). After the uterus has been replaced, the most conservative approach is to await spontaneous separation of the placenta (reserving manual extraction for usual obstetric indications).
- *Management after correction of inversion*:
    - *Hold the uterus in place*: After the uterus has been replaced, the fundus should be

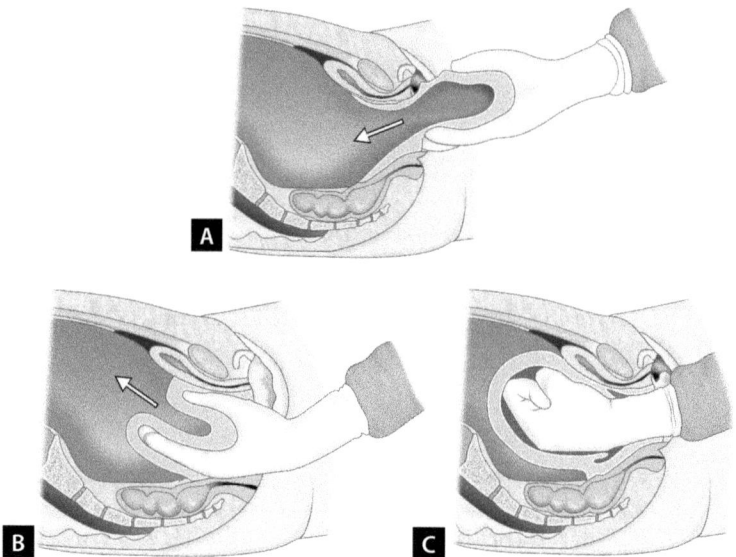

Figs. 4A to C: Reposition of uterus manual method.

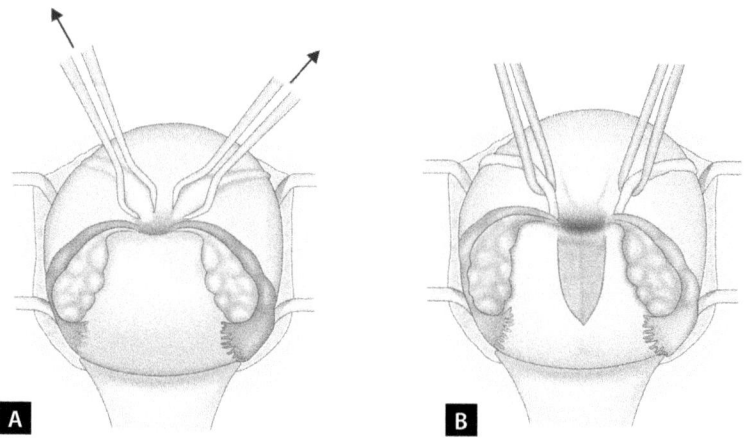

Figs. 5A and B: (A) Huntington procedure; (B) Haultain method.

held in place and then monitored until the surgeon is sure that the uterus is firm and its position is stable. The fundus can be held in place with the clinician's hand(s) placed internally, externally, or both.

– *Administer uterotonic drugs*: Atony is common after restoration of the normal uterine position. Uterotonic agents are administered to induce myometrial contraction and maintain uterine involution, thereby impeding reinversion and reducing the risk of hemorrhage.

• *Antibiotic prophylaxis*:

– *Reinversion*: The treatment of reinversion is similar to that for the initial inversion to prevent reinversions, procedures such as abdominal encerclage, intrauterine balloon, or uterine compression sutures have

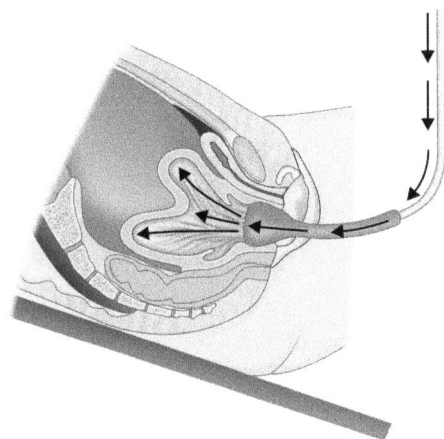

Fig. 6: Hydrostatic method.

also been tried to prevent hemorrhage and prevent reinversion.[4]

Complications were:
- Postpartum hemorrhage
- Blood transfusion
- Need for laparotomy
- Hysterectomy
- Hypotension
- Shock
- Death

DIFFERENTIAL DIAGNOSIS
- Uterine rupture
- Prolapse of uterine tumor (submucous fibroid)

- Large endometrial polyp
- Passage of succenturiate lobe of placenta

CONCLUSION
The classical presentation is of an obviously displaced uterus while delivering the placenta, usually in association with postpartum hemorrhage and clinical shock (hypotension and inadequate tissue perfusion), out of proportion to the blood loss. The most important aspect of treatment remains immediate recognition and prompt attention to its management.

REFERENCES
1. Irani S, Jordan J. Management of uterine inversion. Curr Obstetr Gynaecol. 1997;7(4): 232-5.
2. Medecins Sans Frontieres. (2019). 8.4 Uterine inversion—Essential obstetric and newborn care. [online] Available from https://medicalguidelines.msf.org/viewport/ONC/english/8-4-uterine-inversion-51417808.html [Last accessed December, 2021].
3. Garg p, Bansal R. Unusual and delayed presentation of chronic uterine inversion in a young woman as a result of negligence by an untrained birth attendant: a case report. J Med Case Rep. 2020;14:143.
4. Bhalla R, Wuntakal R, Odejinmi F, Khan RU. (2009). Acute inversion of the uterus. [online] Available from https://obgyn.onlinelibrary.wiley.com/doi/abs/10.1576/toag.11.1.13.27463.

Uterine Rupture

Mitra Saxena

INTRODUCTION

It is a life-threatening complication for both mother and fetus. It can occur during pregnancy and during labor. Rupture is defined as clinically significant uterine disruption of all the uterine layers, leading to changes to maternal and fetus status.

Dehiscence—clinically occults incomplete uterine disruption.

CAUSES

During Pregnancy

- Weak scar after previous operation on the uterus, e.g., history of cesarean section, myomectomy, previous perforation of the uterus (D and C, hysteroscopy), excision of uterine septum. External cephalic version
- Types—classical incisions and lower uterine incisions

During Labor

- Uterine hyperstimulation (oxytocin and prostaglandins)
- Obstructed labor [(macrosomia and cephalo-pelvic disproportion (CPD)]
- Intrauterine manipulation (internal version, MRP)
- Forcible dilatation (cervical tear—forceps)
- Congenital uterine anomalies
- Weak scar—cesarean section or any other uterine operation
- Destructive operations

RISK FACTORS

- Increased maternal age
- Gestational age >40 weeks
- Birth weight >4 kg
- Interdelivery interval < 18 months

- Single layer uterine closure if locked
- More than one cesarean delivery
- Previous second trimester cesarean delivery

There is no reliable method for predicting uterine rupture in woman with previous cesarean delivery.

CLINICAL MANIFESTATIONS

- Abnormal fetal heart rate (FHR)
- Category II or III FHR pattern
- Abdominal pain
- Vaginal bleeding
- Loss of station of fetal presenting part
- Hematuria
- Hemodynamic instability
- Changes in contraction pattern—staircase sign

Postpartum

- Occult rupture
- Pain and persistent vaginal bleeding

DIAGNOSIS

Women not in Labor—USG Findings

- Disruption of the myometrium
- Hematoma adjacent to the hysterotomy scar
- Extrauterine fluids
- Distended fetal membranes
- Free peritoneal fluid
- Anhydramnios
- Empty uterus
- Fetal parts outside the uterus
- Intrauterine device (IUD)

Computed Tomography

Peritoneal air ileus abscess.

Intraoperative

Hemoperitoneum, fetal parts, and membranes.

MANAGEMENT

Goals

- Intensive resuscitation
- Emergency laparotomy
- Broad-spectrum antibiotics
- Adequate postoperative care

Antepartum rupture suspected by sudden onset of abdominal pain FHR abnormality, and maternal hemodynamic instability—urgent delivery. Stabilize with fluid, blood transfusion, and prepare for cesarean section.

Uterine Rupture at Laparotomy

- *Repair versus hysterectomy*:
  - Goal of conservative surgery:
    - Repair of uterine defect
    - Control hemorrhage
    - Identify damage to other organs
    - Minimize early postsurgical morbidity
    - Reduce the risk of complications in future pregnancy
- Hysterectomy is indicated when the uterine defect is irreparable
- Setting of uncontrollable maternal hemorrhage

Management of Coexistent Complications

- Uterine atony managed by
  - Uterotonic agents
  - Hemostatic suture
  - Uterine balloon tamponade
- Bladder injury
- Injury to blood vessels and other pelvic organs

OUTCOME

- Obstetric hysterectomy 14–33%
- Perinatal mortality 20–30%

MANAGEMENT OF SUBSEQUENT PREGNANCY

Timing of delivery is 36–37 weeks with individualization.

BIBLIOGRAPHY

1. ACOG Practice Bulletin No. 205: Vaginal Birth After Cesarean Delivery. Obstet Gynecol. 2019;133:e110.
2. Aslan H, Unlu E, Agar M, Ceylan Y. Uterine rupture associated with misoprostol labor induction in women with previous cesarean delivery. Eur J Obstet Gynecol Reprod Biol. 2004;113:45.
3. Fox NS. Pregnancy outcomes in patients with prior uterine rupture or dehiscence: A 5-year update. Obstet Gynecol. 2020;135:211.
4. Guise JM, Eden K, Emeis C, Denman MA, Marshall N, Fu RR, et al. Vaginal birth after cesarean: new insights. Evid Rep Technol Assess (Full Rep). 2010;191:1-397.
5. Guise JM, Denman MA, Emeis C, Marshall N, Walker M, Fu R, et al. Vaginal birth after cesarean: new insights on maternal and neonatal outcomes. Obstet Gynecol. 2010; 115:1267-78.
6. Hamilton EF, Bujold E, McNamara H, Gauthier R, Platt RW. Dystocia among women with symptomatic uterine rupture. Am J Obstet Gynecol. 2001;184:620.
7. Harper LM, Cahill AG, Roehl KA, Odibo AO, Stamilio DM, Macones GA. The pattern of labor preceding uterine rupture. Am J Obstet Gynecol. 2012;207:210.e1.
8. Khan KS, Rizvi A. The partograph in the management of labor following cesarean section. Int J Gynaecol Obstet. 1995;50:151.
9. Landon MB, Lynch CD. Optimal timing and mode of delivery after cesarean with previous classical incision or myomectomy: a review of the data. Semin Perinatol. 2011;35:257.
10. Landon MB, Hauth JC, Leveno KJ, Spong CY, Leindecker S, Varner MW, et al. Maternal and perinatal outcomes associated with a trial of labor after prior cesarean delivery. N Engl J Med. 2004;351:2581.
11. Lin C, Raynor BD. Risk of uterine rupture in labor induction of patients with prior cesarean section: an inner city hospital experience. Am J Obstet Gynecol. 2004;190:1476.
12. Lydon-Rochelle M, Holt VL, Easterling TR, Martin DP. Risk of uterine rupture during labor among women with a prior cesarean delivery. N Engl J Med. 2001;345:3.
13. Macones GA, Peipert J, Nelson DB, Odibo A, Stevens EJ, Stamilio DM, et al. Maternal complications with vaginal birth after cesarean delivery: a multicenter study. Am J Obstet Gynecol. 2005;193:1656.
14. Naef RW 3rd, Ray MA, Chauhan SP, Roach H, Blake PG, Martin JN Jr, et al. Trial of labor after cesarean delivery with a lower-segment, vertical

uterine incision: is it safe? Am J Obstet Gynecol. 1995;172:1666.

15. National Institutes of Health Consensus Development Conference Panel. National Institutes of Health Consensus Development conference statement: vaginal birth after cesarean: new insights March 8-10, 2010. Obstet Gynecol. 2010;115:1279.

16. Plaut MM, Schwartz ML, Lubarsky SL. Uterine rupture associated with the use of misoprostol in the gravid patient with a previous cesarean section. Am J Obstet Gynecol. 1999;180:1535.

17. Rossi AC, Prefumo F. Pregnancy outcomes of induced labor in women with previous cesarean section: a systematic review and meta-analysis. Arch Gynecol Obstet. 2015;291:273.

18. Shipp TD, Zelop CM, Repke JT, Cohen A, Caughey AB, Lieberman E, et al. Intrapartum uterine rupture and dehiscence in patients with prior lower uterine segment vertical and transverse incisions. Obstet Gynecol. 1999;94:735.

19. Usta IM, Hamdi MA, Musa AA, Nassar AH. Pregnancy outcome in patients with previous uterine rupture. Acta Obstet Gynecol Scand. 2007;86:172.

20. Vachon-Marceau C, Demers S, Goyet M, Gauthier R, Roberge S, Chaillet N, et al. Labor Dystocia and the Risk of Uterine Rupture in Women with Prior Cesarean. Am J Perinatol. 2016;33:577.

Obstetric Hysterectomy

Mitra Saxena, Renu Yadav

INTRODUCTION

Obstetric hysterectomy is defined as removal of the uterus at the time of cesarean section or following vaginal delivery or within puerperium. It is a lifesaving procedure in the management of intractable hemorrhage unresponsive to conservative management. It is associated with increased intraoperative and postoperative maternal morbidity and mortality.

INDICATIONS

- Placenta accreta syndrome
- Uterine rupture
- Postpartum hemorrhage (PPH)
- Cervical and ovarian cancer
- Lacerations of uterine vessels
- Leiomyoma

SURGICAL PLANNING

Types of equipment for surgery and patient preparation are given in **Box 1**.
- Abdominal preparation (povidone-iodine or chlorhexidine)
- Pneumatic compression boots
- Laparotomy drapes and leg drapes if stirrups are used

Steps in management of postpartum hemorrhage are given in **Box 2**.

Patient Counseling

Patient should be counseled about the likelihood of the procedure and the decision to proceed, likely complications and outcome, need for blood transfusion, mechanical ventilation, and intensive care unit (ICU). Schedule and the need for high-risk anesthesiologist, interventional radiologist, gynecological oncologist, and urologist.

Preoperative Preparation

Prophylactic antibiotics, IV line, cross matched packed red blood cell (PRBC) and plasma, bladder catheter, pneumatic compression, and lithotomy position with preparedness for blood loss quantification.

Operative Procedure

Lower abdomen vertical incision or if transverse skin incision, prepare for Maylard incision. Uterine incision—low transverse hysterotomy but not over the placenta or a classical fundal incision. Avoiding the placenta or large bladder varicosities or adhesions.

Fetus is removed easily by breech. Oxytocin is given to maintain uterine tone; adherent placenta should be left in place. Insertion of balloon or packing for tamponade reduces bleeding. Hysterectomy to be performed rapidly by clamping and cutting the pedicles and ligating later on. Posterior leaf of the broad ligament is opened and uterine vessels skeletonized, clamp, cut, and ligated. Bladder is dissected and large blood vessels are coagulated or ligated. Supracervical hysterectomy can be done and cervical edges closed with a figure of eight suture. Examine bladder, rectum, and ureter for injuries. Hemostatic agents and pelvic packing may be used.

COMPLICATIONS

Fever, ileus, exploratory laparotomy, urinary tract infection (UTI), hospital readmission, abscess,

---

BOX 1: Surgical equipment and patient preparation steps.

Surgical equipment and supplies

- Heavy clamps for vascular pedicles (e.g., Heaney or Zeppelin; at least four clamps should be available)
- Kelly clamps (long and short), Kocher clamps for holding tissue
- Tonsil and right angle clamps for dissection
- Hand-held retractors
- Self-retaining retractor (e.g., Bookwalter)
- Electrocautery device with appropriate grounding
- Bipolar tissue sealing device, if available
- Suction cannula(s) with wall suction
- Laparotomy packs and surgical sponges
- Hemostatic agents (e.g., thrombin, gelatin products, and cellulose products)
- Fluids for irrigation
- Standard cesarean delivery equipment, if indicated
- Multiple sutures (e.g., #0-polyglactin 910, #2-0 polyglactin 910, polydioxanone for fascial closure)

Patient preparation

- Allen stirrups, if readily available (for access to vagina and bladder)
- Bladder catheter (3-way, if possible)
- Vaginal preparation with povidone-iodine
- Abdominal preparation (povidone-iodine or chlorhexidine)
- Pneumatic compression boots
- Laparotomy drapes and leg drapes if stirrups are used
- Broad-spectrum antibiotics (e.g., cefotetan, cefazolin, and gentamicin plus clindamycin)

Patient stabilization

- Blood products (activate massive transfusion protocol, if available)
- Uterotonic agents (use until uterine blood supply is disconnected)
- Multiple large-bore intravenous lines
- Arterial line
- Warming devices for patient and for blood products
- Rapid blood infuser, if available
- Intubation equipment

BOX 2: Steps in management of postpartum hemorrhage.

- *Assemble team and notify appropriate departments (obstetrics, nursing, anesthesiology, blood bank, and laboratory)*
- *Initiate uterine massage and/or manual compression and establish large-bore (two 16- or 18-gauge, ideally 14-gauge) intravenous access*
- *Tamponade bleeding from the uterine cavity:* Balloon tamponade should be initiated early if bleeding is brisk, particularly if the patient is not hemodynamically stable, and blood products are not readily available. Both balloon tamponade and packing can be performed prior to, or in conjunction with, preparations for laparotomy or transarterial embolization. Balloon tamponade may reduce blood loss while initiating carboprost or ergot drugs, if used after oxytocin has failed. Early use of a balloon tamponade with or after use of these agents may reduce the incidence of heavy blood loss and the need for blood products
- *Administer oxygen (10–15 L/min) by face mask. Anesthesia team should evaluate airway and breathing; intubate if indicated*
- *Fluid resuscitation:* Infuse isotonic crystalloid to prevent hypotension (target systolic pressure 90 mm Hg) and maintain urine output at >30 mL/h
- *Transfusion:* If hemodynamics do not improve with 2–3 L of crystalloid administration and bleeding continues, administer blood products, initially two units packed red blood cells

Contd...

Contd...

- Aggressive use of plasma replacement is also important to reverse dilutional coagulopathy. Coagulation factor concentrates may also be needed. For patients with massive hemorrhage, red blood cells, fresh frozen plasma, and apheresis platelets are best administered according to an established massive transfusion protocol
- *Administer uterotonic drugs to reverse atony:* It should bepossible to determine within 30 minutes whether uterotonic treatment will reverse atony. If it does not, prompt invasive intervention is usually warranted
- *Initiate oxytocin:*
  - Begin with oxytocin 40 units in 1 L of normal saline or Ringer's lactate. Using an intravenous infusion pump, start at 10–40 mL/min. Adjust rate to achieve and maintain uterine contraction; 15 units in 250 mL normal saline or Ringer's lactate may be given if a high concentration must be administered rapidly. Expect rapid response
  - Avoid rapid intravenous bolus injection of oxytocin
  - If no intravenous access, give 10 units intramuscularly; expect response within 3–5 minutes
  - There are no absolute contraindications to oxytocin for PPH; oxytocin is the uterotonic of choice, even if it was already given as prophylaxis
  - Carbetocin 100 µg slow intravenous injection as single dose. A long-acting analog of oxytocin, carbetocin is a potential alternative if titrable oxytocin intravenous infusion is not feasible
- *If oxytocin is not immediately available or does notcontrol PPH:*
  - *Add ergot:*
    - Methylergonovine (methylergometrine) 200 µg intramuscularly (including intramyometrial) every 2–4 hours up to a maximum of 1 mg (five doses). Expect response within 2–5 minutes
    - Do not give intravenously
    - Avoid in women with hypertension, Raynaud's phenomenon, or scleroderma
    - If the first dose is ineffective, quickly add a different uterotonic agent (e.g., carboprost tromethamine)
    - Ergonovine (ergometrine), where available, is an alternative to methylergonovine; its actions and contraindications are similar to methylergonovine
    - Ergonovine (ergometrine) 200 µg intramuscularly; may be repeated once in 15 minutes
    - If required, additional doses of 200 µg intramuscularly may be given every 4 hours up to a maximum of 1 mg (five doses)
  - *Add carboprost:*
    - Carboprost tromethamine (PGF2 alpha, hemabate) 250 µg intramuscularly every 15–90 minutes, as needed, to a maximum of 2 mg (eight doses). Peak plasma level is approximately 30 minutes after injection
    - Do not give intravenously
    - Avoid in women with asthma/bronchospasm or hypertension
    - Relatively contraindicated in renal or hepatic insufficiency or reduced cardiac output
    - Can cause tachycardia, pyrexia, and diarrhea
    - If no response after one or two doses, quickly move to a different uterotonic agent
- *Inspect the vagina and cervix for lacerations; repair as necessary. Evacuate any retained products of conception. Replace uterus if inverted. Use of balloon tamponade*
- *Perform transarterial embolization if the woman is stable and there is time for personnel and facilities to mobilize*
- *Perform laparotomy if the above measures fail:* Surgical approaches that are quick, relatively easy, and effective should be tried first. In utilizing these measures, the surgeon should be cognizant of the amount of blood loss and the stability of the patient, and should perform hysterectomy rather than resort to temporizing measures if her cardiovascular status is unstable or if it appears that the anesthesiologist will not be able to keep up with her fluid needs.
  Options include:
  - Ligate bleeding sites
  - Perform uterine artery ligation, including the utero-ovarian arcade

Contd...

Contd...

- Place a B-Lynch stitch or other uterine compression suture
- Perform hysterectomy—hysterectomy is the last resort for atony, but should not be delayed in women who have disseminated
- Intravascular coagulation and require prompt control of uterine hemorrhage to prevent death. Planned hysterectomy is often the appropriate first-line approach for placenta accreta
- Suture deep pelvic bleeders
- Tamponade pelvic bleeding with pelvic packing

bowel injury, wound dehiscence, and maternal death.

BIBLIOGRAPHY

1. Bodelon C, Bernabe-Ortiz A, Schiff MA, Reed SD. Factors associated with peripartum hysterectomy. Obstet Gynecol. 2009;114:115.
2. Campbell SM, Corcoran P, Manning E, Greene RA, Irish Maternal Morbidity Advisory Group. Peripartum hysterectomy incidence, risk factors and clinical characteristics in Ireland. Eur J Obstet Gynecol Reprod Biol. 2016;207:56.
3. Colmorn LB, Krebs L, Langhoff-Roos J, NOSS study group. Potentially Avoidable Peripartum Hysterectomies in Denmark: A Population Based Clinical Audit. PLoS One. 2016;11:e0161302.
4. Cromi A, Candeloro I, Marconi N, Casarin J, Serati M, Agosti M. Risk of peripartum hysterectomy in births after assisted reproductive technology. Fertil Steril. 2016;106:623.
5. Flood KM, Said S, Geary M, Robson M, Fitzpatrick C. Malone FD. Changing trends in peripartum hysterectomy over the last 4 decades. Am J Obstet Gynecol. 2009;200:632.e1.
6. Friedman AM, Wright JD, Ananth CV, Siddiq Z, D'Alton ME, Bateman BT. Population-based risk for peripartum hysterectomy during low- and moderate-risk delivery hospitalizations. Am J Obstet Gynecol. 2016;215:640.
7. Glaze S, Ekwalanga P, Roberts G, Lange I, Birch C, Rosengarten A, et al. Peripartum hysterectomy: 1999 to 2006. Obstet Gynecol. 2008;111:732-8.
8. Govindappagari S, Wright JD, Ananth CV, Huang Y, D'Alton ME, Friedman AM. Risk of Peripartum Hysterectomy and Center Hysterectomy and Delivery Volume. Obstet Gynecol. 2016;128:1215-24.
9. Huque S, Roberts I, Fawole B, Chaudhri R, Arulkumaran S, Shakur-Still H. Risk factors for peripartum hysterectomy among women with postpartum haemorrhage: analysis of data from the WOMAN trial. BMC Pregnancy Childbirth. 2018;18:186.
10. Imudia AN, Awonuga AO, Dbouk T, Kumar S, Cordoba MI, Diamond MP, et al. Incidence, trends, risk factors, indications for, and complications associated with cesarean hysterectomy: a 17-year experience from a single institution. Arch Gynecol Obstet. 2009;280: 619.
11. Jakobsson M, Tapper AM, Colmorn LB, Lindqvist PG, Klungsøyr KG, Krebs L, et al. Emergency peripartum hysterectomy: results from the prospective Nordic Obstetric Surveillance Study (NOSS). Acta Obstet Gynecol Scand. 2015;94:745.
12. Maraschini A, Lega I, D'Aloja P, Buoncristiano M, Dell'Oro S, Donati S, et al. Women undergoing peripartum hysterectomy due to obstetric hemorrhage: A prospective population-based study. Acta Obstet Gynecol Scand. 2020;99:274.
13. Rossi AC, Lee RH, Chmait RH. Emergency postpartum hysterectomy for uncontrolled postpartum bleeding: a systematic review. Obstet Gynecol. 2010;115:637.
14. Whiteman MK, Kuklina E, Hillis SD, Jamieson DJ, Meikle SF, Posner SF, et al. Incidence and determinants of peripartum hysterectomy. Obstet Gynecol . 2006;108:1486-92.

Perineal Injury

Jaideep Malhotra, Shaheen Anjum, Deeba Khanam

DEFINITION

Perineal injury or tear or laceration is a laceration of the skin and subcutaneous tissues, which separate the vagina from the anus **(Figs. 1 to 3)**. Lacerations can lead to chronic pain, anal dysfunctions, and anal and rectal fistulas.

CLASSIFICATION

Classification of perineal injury is given in **Table 1**.

RISK FACTORS

Risk factors are shown in **Box 1**.

PREVENTION

Prevention of perineal injury is given in **Table 2**.

MANAGEMENT
Preprocedural Task

Preprocedural task is given in **Table 3**.

Procedure

The procedure of perineal examination is given in **Table 4**.

Place of Performing Procedure

Lacerations can usually be repaired in the delivery room with the patient in the lithotomy position; however, third- and fourth-degree lacerations may require an operating room.

Anesthesia

Repair of first-degree tear requires adequate analgesia. Pudendal block or local anesthesia may be given to alleviate pain from minor surgical procedures involving the perineum.[6]

Local anesthesia—1% lignocaine 5 mL infiltrated with 10 mL syringe with 22-gauge needle in the tissues, wait for 2 minutes for the effect.

Pudendal block— transvaginal or transperineal approach to the ischial spine can be used, local

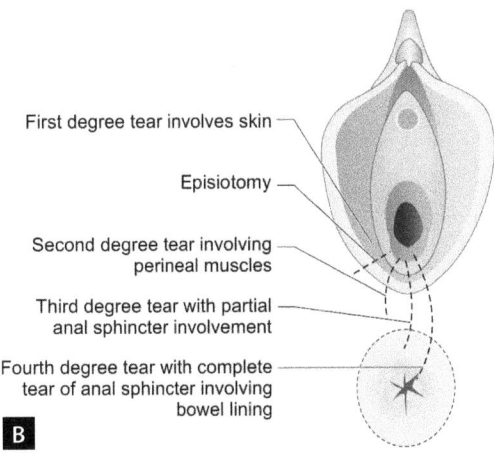

Hymen

Deep perineal muscles

Anus

Bulbospongiosus muscle

Transverse perineal muscle

Perineal body

External anal sphincter (internal anal sphincter not shown)

A

First degree tear involves skin

Episiotomy

Second degree tear involving perineal muscles

Third degree tear with partial anal sphincter involvement

Fourth degree tear with complete tear of anal sphincter involving bowel lining

B

Figs. 1A and B: (A) Showing the anatomy of perineum; (B) Diagrammatic representation of degrees of perineal injury.

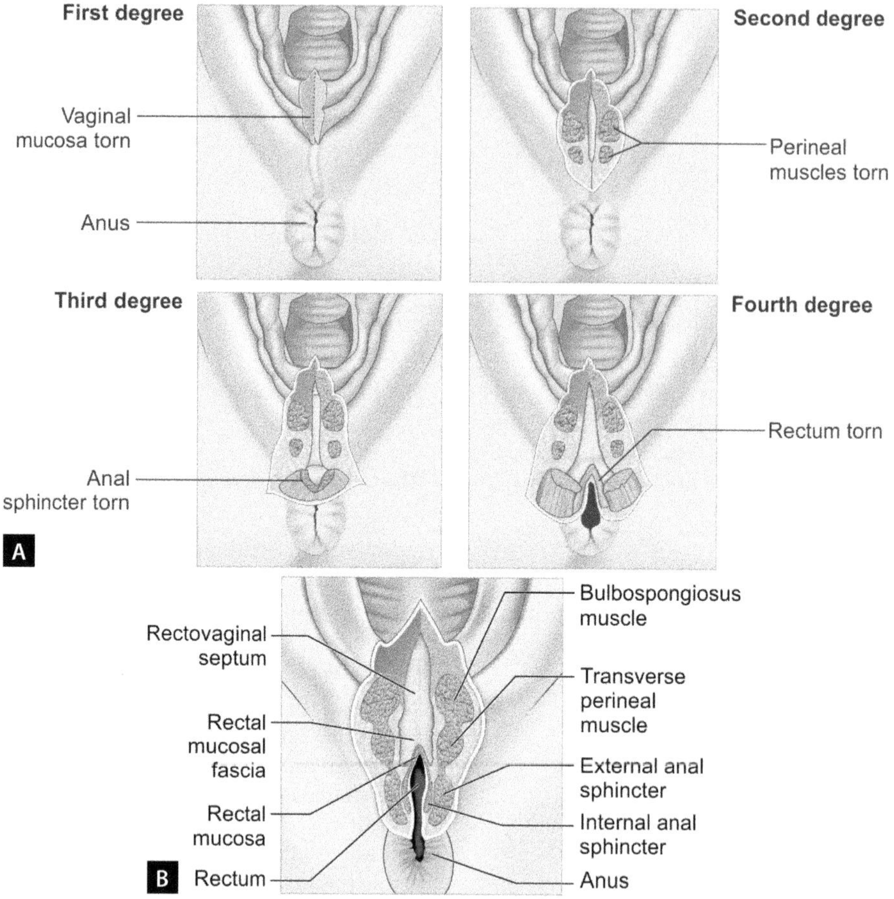

First degree

Vaginal
mucosa torn

Anus

Second degree

Perineal
muscles torn

Third degree

Anal
sphincter torn

A

Fourth degree

Rectum torn

Rectovaginal
septum

Rectal
mucosal
fascia

Rectal
mucosa

B Rectum

Bulbospongiosus
muscle

Transverse
perineal
muscle

External anal
sphincter

Internal anal
sphincter

Anus

Figs. 2A and B: (A) Diagrammatic representation of involvement of different structures in various degrees of perineal tear; (B) Diagrammatic representation of involvement of different structures and perineal muscles in fourth degrees of perineal tear.

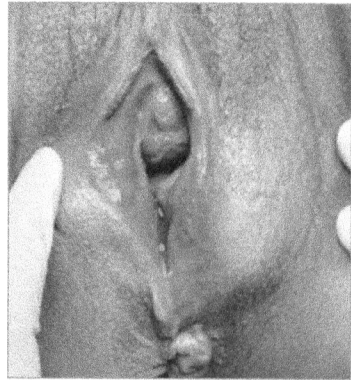

Fig. 3: First-degree perineal tear involving perineal skin.

anesthetic (1% lignocaine) is injected through the sacrospinous ligament into the pudendal nerve behind ischial spine. Maximal effect is obtained after 10–20 minutes.[7]

For third- and fourth-degree tears, bilateral pudendal block with or without a local field block, a saddle block, or general anesthesia is alternatives.[4]

Suture Material Required

Suture material required for perineal injury is given in **Table 5**.

Technique of Repair

Technique of repair is given in **Table 6**.

TABLE 1: Classification of perineal injury.	
First-degree lacerations	Involve injury to the skin and subcutaneous tissue of the perineum and vaginal epithelium only. The perineal muscles remain intact **(Fig. 4)**
Second-degree lacerations	Extends into the fascia and musculature of the perineal body, which includes the deep and superficial transverse perineal muscles and fibers of the pubococcygeus and bulbocavernosus muscles. The anal sphincter muscles remain intact **(Fig. 5)**
Third-degree lacerations	Involves some or all of the fibers of the external anal sphincter (EAS) and/or the internal anal sphincter (IAS) **(Fig. 6)** Third-degree lacerations are subclassified as follows: • *3a*: <50% of EAS thickness is torn • *3b*: >50% of EAS thickness is torn • *3c*: Both EAS and IAS are torn
Fourth-degree lacerations	Injury to the perineum that involves both the anal sphincter complex (EAS and IAS), and anal and rectal epithelium[1] **(Fig. 7)**

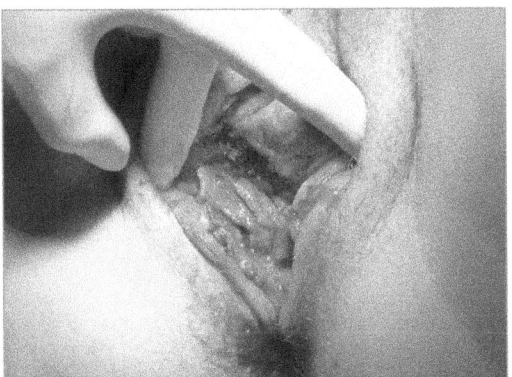

Fig. 4: Second-degree perineal tear involving perineal muscles.

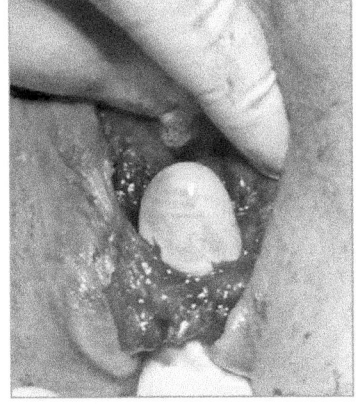

Fig. 6: Fourth-degree perineal tear involving anal and rectal mucosa.

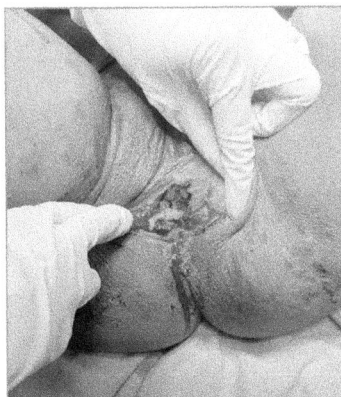

Fig. 5: Third-degree perineal tear with torn external anal sphincter.

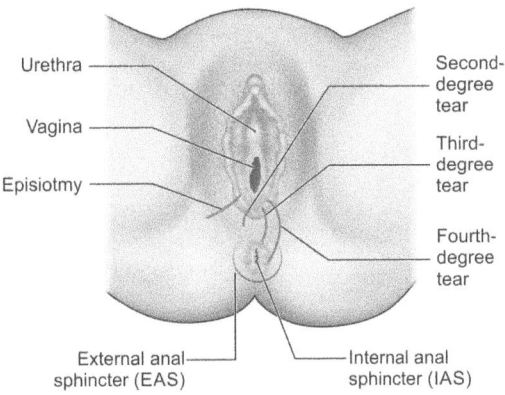

Fig. 7: Injury to the perineum involving both the anal sphincter complex and anal and rectal epithelium.

BOX 1: Risk factors of perineal injury.

Intrapartum:
- Instrumental delivery—forceps and vacuum-assisted delivery
- Midline episiotomy
- Delivery in lithotomy position
- Epidural analgesia/anesthesia
- Prolonged second stage of labor (>60 min)
- Augmentation of labor/oxytocin use
- Persistent occipitoposterior position
- Induction of labor

Maternal:
- 20 years or younger
- Vaginal birth after cesarean
- Primipara
- Asian ethnicity

Fetal:
- Increased fetal birth weight (≥4 kg)
- Familial factors

TABLE 2: Prevention of perineal injury.

Antepartum	
Perineal massage	Self-perineal massage starting at 35 weeks
Intrapartum	
Perineal massage	During second stage of labor, perineal massage is beneficial
Warm compresses	Application of a warm compress to the perineum are effective
Perineal support	During delivery of head, applying pressure to the lateral perineal tissue with the first and second fingers of right hand to lower the pressure in the middle posterior perineum while the left hand slows the delivery of the fetal head

Routine episiotomy does not reduce the chances of perineal lacerations

TABLE 3: Preprocedural task of management of perineal injury.

Consent	Verbal consent is required, explaining the patient the nature of injury and need for proper evaluation
Prerequisites	• Adequate exposure, light, and analgesia • Lithotomy position for adequate exposure • Hand wash—using soap and water for 2–5 minutes or using alcohol-based scrub for 20–30 seconds[2]
Skin preparation	Can be performed by scrubbing the external genitalia and inner thighs with soap and water or povidone-iodine spray; or with 4% chlorhexidine and rinsing with 1:100 savlon solutions[3]
Antibiotic prophylaxis	• Antibiotics are not recommended for repair of first- and second-degree lacerations. • Routine antibiotic prophylaxis is recommended for women with a third- or fourth-degree perineal[4] • Antibiotic prophylaxis with aerobic and anaerobic coverage, such as a second-generation cephalosporin or cefazolin and metronidazole can be given as single dose preoperatively[5]
Instruments and materials	*Instruments:* • Sponge holder • Sims speculums • Anterior vaginal wall retractor • Allis clamps • Curved artery forceps • Babcock forceps • Suture cutting scissor • Needle holder • Toothed and nontoothed forceps • Metzenbaum scissor

Contd...

Contd...

> *Materials:*
> - 10-mL syringe with 22-gauge needle
> - Irrigation solution
> - Local anesthetic solution (Xylocaine 2%)
> - Sponges
> - Sterile gloves
> - Surgical glue if available
> - Sutures as discussed

TABLE 4: Procedure of perineal examination.

Perineal examination	
Inspection	• Careful examination distal vagina, perineum, and anorectum • Evaluation of extent of tear, its apex and bleeding
Digital rectal examination	Assessment of rectal mucosa and anal sphincter
Rectovaginal examination	Place an index finger in the rectum and the thumb over the anal sphincter and by pill-rolling motion, assess the sphincter

TABLE 5: Suture material required for perineal injury.

First degree	3-0 braided polyglactin 910 (Vicryl), CT-1 needle or 3-0 monofilament polydioxanone, CT-1 needle
Second degree	3-0 braided polyglactin 910 (Vicryl), or CT-1 needle or 3-0 monofilament polydioxanone
Third degree	2-0 braided polyglactin 910 (Vicryl), CT-1 needle or 2-0 monofilament polydioxanone, CT-1 needle for external anal sphincter and 3-0 braided polyglactin 910 (Vicryl), SH needle or 3-0 monofilament polydioxanone, SH needle for internal anal sphincter
Fourth degree	4-0 braided polyglactin 910 (Vicryl), SH needle or 4-0 monofilament polydioxanone (PDS), SH needle[1]

TABLE 6: Technique of repair.

First degree	Vaginal tear is identified and anchoring stitch is taken 1 cm above the apex, followed by continuous suturing of vaginal mucosa and submucosa till the vaginal hymenal ring is reached[8] Or Surgical glue can be used
Second degree	Repaired in three stages, first layer of vaginal mucosa, and second layer of perineal muscles. Bulbocavernosus muscle is approximated with continuous stitch. Transverse perineal muscles are approximated using the same suture in continuous fashion. The repair is completed by running suture in the subcutaneous fascia ending at the hymenal ring. The knot should be directing the hymen[8] **(Figs. 8A to C).**
Third degree	EAS injury may be partial involving *incomplete loss of thickness* where the fibers are approximated using *end to end technique* rather than dividing the sphincter for an overlapping technique.[2] If *complete thickness* is lost then *either of the techniques has equal benefits*.[2] In the overlapping technique, the free muscle ends are overlapped and joined by mattress sutures; it requires dissection of the ends of the sphincter to facilitate overlap. End-to-end repair requires connecting the most posterior part of the junction of two muscles first, followed by the superior and inferior elements and ending with the anterior part of both the ends. Plain and figure-of-eight interrupted sutures can be used.[9]

Contd...

Contd...

	Internal anal sphincter when identified (thickened, pinkish white structure, and retracted laterally should be stitched using a continuous 3/0 polyglactin suture or 3/0 monofilament synthetic suture.[2] Reapproximation of this layer is important as it provides strength to the repair and helps in maintenance of anal continence.[10]
Fourth degree	The torn anal mucosa should be stitched using continuous (nonlocking) 4-0 braided polyglactin 910 (Vicryl), SH needle or 4-0 monofilament polydioxanone (PDS), SH needle.[2] Interrupted sutures result in abundance of unrequired foreign body because of multiple knots. Anal mucosa is supported by stitching layer of rectovaginal septum over it with interrupted 2/0 polyglactin suture on CT-1 needle and so contributes to anal continence and relieves tension from the sphincteric repair[11]

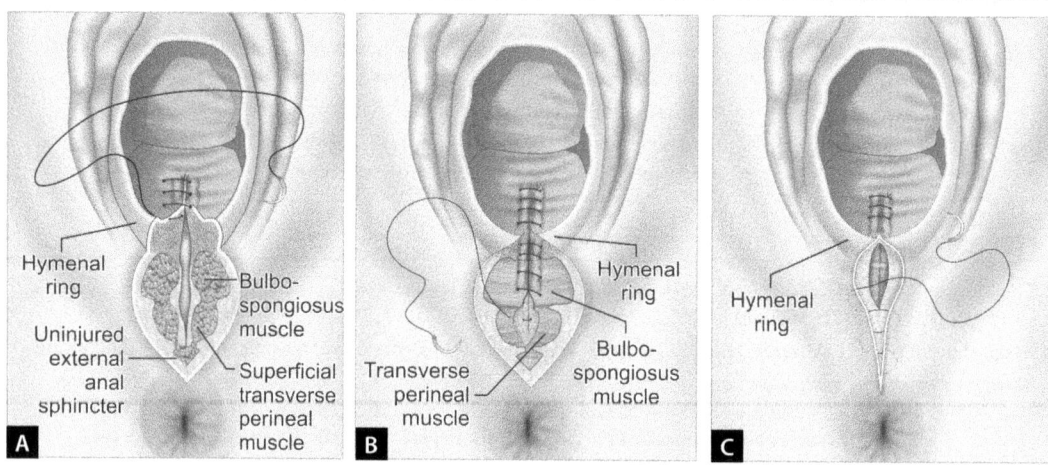

Figs. 8A to C: Stitching of second-degree perineal tear.

TABLE 7: Postoperative care.

Adequate pain control	• Local treatment as anesthetic sprays or cream, ice packs, hot-sitz baths and rectal suppositories (diclofenac and indomethacin) • Rectal suppositories should be avoided in third and fourth degree lacerations • Oral nonsteroidal anti-inflammatory can be used. Opiates should be avoided as it may lead to constipation[12]
Perineal hygiene	Perineal area is kept dry and clean by regular changing of pads[13]
Avoidance of constipation	Use of osmotic laxatives and stool softener as it leads to earlier bowel movements and less pain[14]
Prevention of urinary retention	Spontaneous voiding should be carefully checked, and women that are unable to pass urine or develop discomfort due to bladder distention require prompt evaluation
Pelvic floor exercises	Are recommended within 2–3 days of delivery in patients with obstetric anal sphincter injuries[2]
Evaluation of wound healing and counseling	Monitored frequently to avoid long-term complication as anal incontinence

◼ POSTPROCEDURE

Postoperative Care

Postoperative care is given in **Table 7**.

◼ COMPLICATIONS

Complications of perineal injury are shown in **Box 2.**

BOX 2: Early and long-term complication of perineal injury.

Early
- Excessive bleeding from laceration sites
- Hematoma formation
- Abscess formation
- Wound dehiscence

Long term
- Rectal and anal fistula
- Anal sphincter dysfunction

CONCLUSION

Perineal tears following birth are not too common provided that labor and delivery are properly managed. But if it occurs, it should be repaired by trained obstetricians to restore anal continence. As per the latest suggestions from ACOG, postpartum care should be seen as a continuous and personalized process whereby patients receive care from the physician within 3 weeks postdelivery, and are constantly monitored throughout for possible side effects.

REFERENCES

1. Committee on Practice Bulletins–Obstetrics. ACOG practice bulletin no. 198: prevention and management of obstetric lacerations at vaginal delivery. Obstet Gynecol. 2018; 132(3):e87-e102.
2. WHO Guidelines on Hand Hygiene in Health Care: First Global Patient Safety Challenge Clean Care Is Safer Care. Geneva: World Health Organization; 2009.
3. ACOG Practice Bulletin No. 195: Prevention of infection after gynecologic procedures. Obstet Gynecol. 2018;131(6):e172.
4. Royal College of Obstetricians and Gynae-cologists. (2017). Green-top guideline no. 29: The management of third- and fourth-degree perineal tears. [online] Available from http://www.acmgo.com/archivos/RCOG-2007-DESGARRO-PERINEAL.pdf [Last accessed December, 2021].
5. ACOG Practice Bulletin No. 199: Use of Prophylactic Antibiotics in Labor and Delivery. Committee on Practice Bulletins-Obstetrics Obstet Gynecol. 2018;132(3):e103.
6. Committee on Practice Bulletins—Obstetrics. Practice Bulletin No. 177: Obstetric Analgesia and Anesthesia. Obstet Gynecol. 2017;129:e73.
7. Zador G, Lindmark G, Nilsson BA. Pudendal block in normal vaginal deliveries. Clinical efficacy, lidocaine concentrations in maternal and foetal blood, foetal and maternal acid-base values and influence on uterine activity. Acta Obstet Gynecol Scand Suppl. 1974;(54):51.
8. Kettle C, Dowswell T, Ismail KM. Continuous and interrupted suturing techniques for repair of episiotomy or second-degree tears. Cochrane Database Syst Rev. 2012;(11): CD000947.
9. Meister MR, Rosenbloom JI, Lowder JL, Cahill AG. Techniques for repair of obstetric anal sphincter injuries. Obstet Gynecol Surv. 2018;73(1):33-9.
10. Mahony R, Behan M, Daly L, Kirwan C, O'Herlihy C, O'Connell PR. Internal anal sphincter defect influences continence out-come following obstetric anal sphincter injury. Am J Obstet Gynecol. 2007;196:217.e1.
11. Lindqvist PG, Jernetz M. A modified surgical approach to women with obstetric anal sphincter tears by separate suturing of external and internal anal sphincter. A modified approach to obstetric anal sphincter injury. BMC Pregnancy Childbirth. 2010;10:51.
12. Chou D, Abalos E, Gyte GML, Gülmezoglu AM. Paracetamol/acetaminophen (single administration) for perineal pain in the early postpartum period. Cochrane Database Syst Rev. 2013;(1):CD008407.
13. Goh R, Goh D, Ellepola H. Perineal tears—a review. Aust J Gen Pract. 2018;47(1-2):35-8.
14. Mahony R, Behan M, O'Herlihy C, O'Connell PR. Randomized, clinical trial of bowel confinement vs. laxative use after primary repair of a third-degree obstetric anal sphincter tear. Dis Colon Rectum. 2004;47(1): 12-7.

Vulvar Hematoma/Broad Ligament Hematoma

Monisha Singh, Narendra Malhotra

DEFINITION

A vulvar hematoma is a collection of blood in the vulva. A hematoma is defined as a collection of blood beneath an intact epidermis which may presents as a fluctuant swelling. It can be extremely tender on palpation.

REASON FOR COLLECTION

The vulva consists of smooth muscle and loose connective tissue with good arterial supply.

COURSE OF PUDENDAL ARTERY (FIG. 1)

The pudendal artery is the terminal branch of the anterior division of the internal iliac artery. Traveling inferio-lateral, this artery passes through the greater sciatic foramen and enters the ischioanal fossa (through the lesser sciatic foramen). Passing through the pudendal canal, it divides into its end branches and supplies the external genitalia and perineum. Due to restriction offered by Colles fascia and the urogenital diaphragm, hematoma thus directs toward the skin.

TYPES OF PUERPERAL GENITAL HEMATOMAS (FLOWCHART 1)

Puerperal hematomas occur in 1:300–1:1,500 deliveries and, can be potentially life-threatening complication of childbirth.

- *Infralevator hematomas*: Occur *below the levator ani muscle*, usually around vulva, perineum, and lower vagina. Usually associated with vaginal birth.

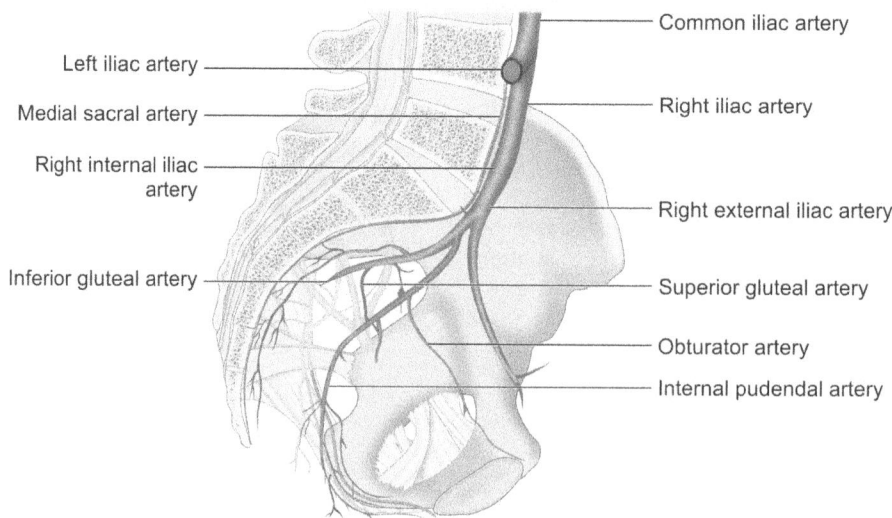

Left iliac artery

Medial sacral artery

Right internal iliac artery

Inferior gluteal artery

Common iliac artery

Right iliac artery

Right external iliac artery

Superior gluteal artery

Obturator artery

Internal pudendal artery

Fig. 1: Course of pudendal artery reaching vulva.

Flowchart 1: Puerperal genital hematoma.

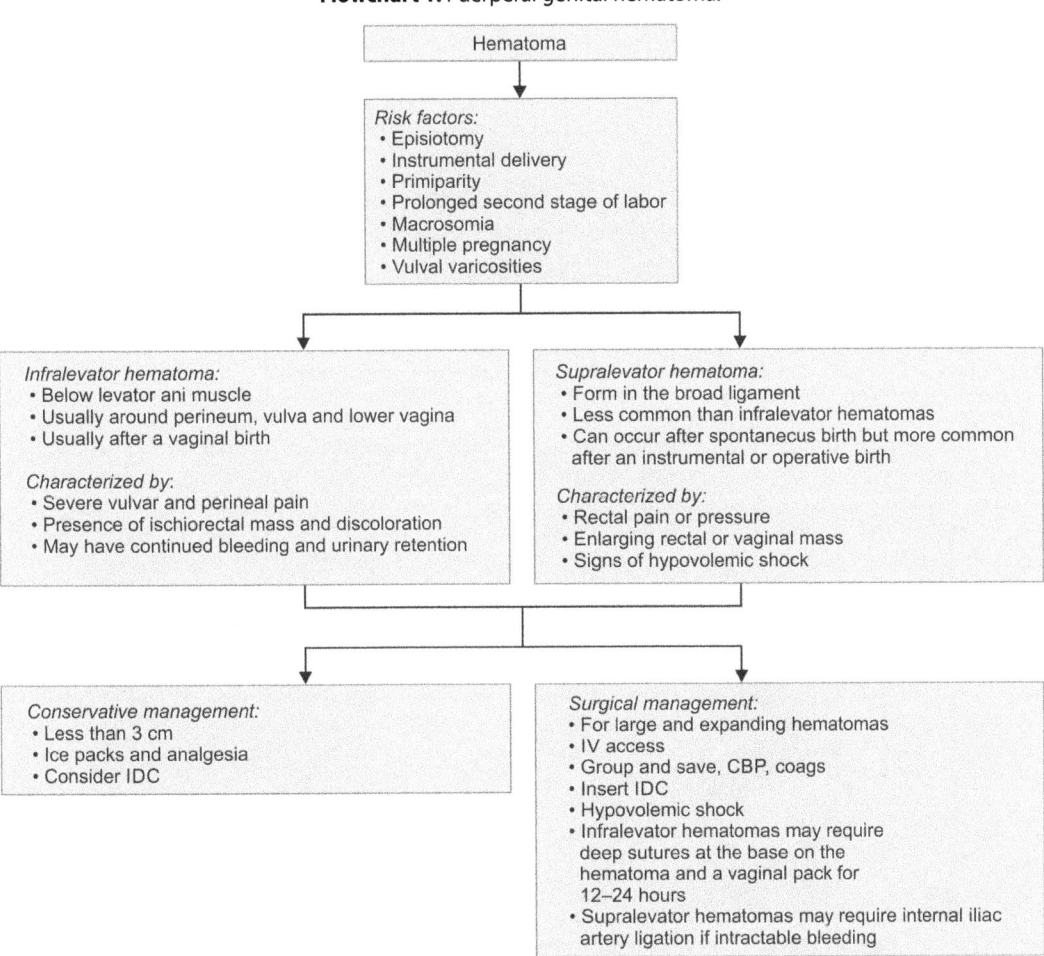

- *Supralevator hematomas*: Mentioned below as broad ligament hematoma pass stool/urine may be present.

CAUSES OR RISK FACTORS

During labor, a vulvar hematoma can result from injury directly or indirectly.

- *Direct injuries*: These include episiotomy, vaginal laceration repairs, or instrumental deliveries.
- *Indirect injury*: Extensive stretching of the birth canal during vaginal delivery.

Most vulvar hematomas are formed after a normal delivery. Risk factors for developing vulvar hematoma include instrumental delivery, episiotomy, primiparity, prolonged second stage of labor, macrosomia, use of anticoagulants, coagulopathy, hypertensive disorders of pregnancy, and vulvovaginal varicosity.

Nonobstetric vulvar hematomas can arise from any form of trauma to the perineum, from saddle injury, falling from a height, insertion of a foreign body, sexual assault, or surgery of the vulva. It is reported that *postcoital injury is the most common nonobstetric cause* of vulvar hematoma.

PREVENTION

Early recognition helps in reducing the associated morbidity and shortening the length of hospital stay **(Figs. 2A and B)**.

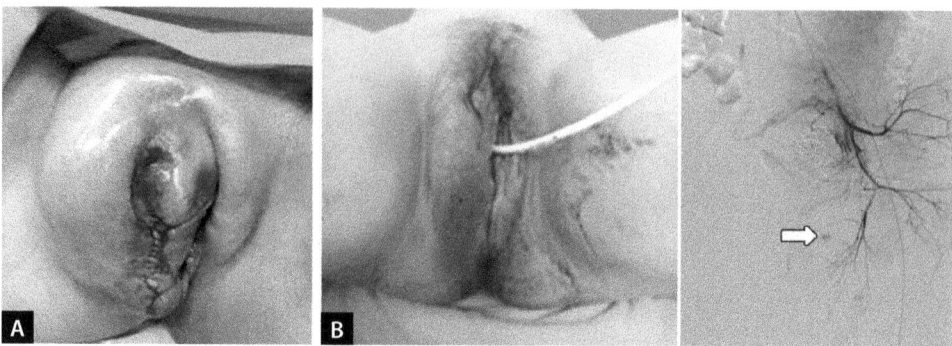

Figs. 2A and B: Infralevator hematomas; (A) infralevator hematoma; (B) Management through pelvic artery embolization.

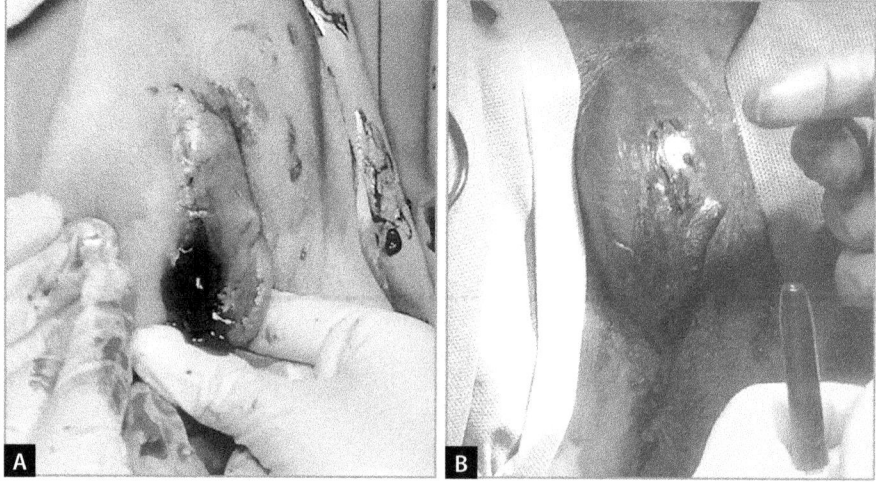

Figs. 3A and B: Infralevator hematoma; management through drainage; catching the bleeding and creating an hemostasis.

■ ASSESSMENT

History of vaginal bleeding, pain in vulval region, abdominal pain, difficulty in sitting, and unable to pass stool/urine in time are others.

Urological or neurological signs and symptoms may be present based on size and site of hematoma. Patients may present with urinary retention or micturition difficulties (mechanical urethral obstruction). In severe cases, the patient can be hemodynamically unstable and will require urgent management. Symptoms usually develop within a few hours to days of delivery.

Rule out history of connective tissue disorders or coagulopathies. Nonobstetrical causes have to assessed and managed according to extent of injuries to perineum or pelvis. Such hematomas will be visible on physical examination. This is seen as a tender fluctuant lump of variable size (**Figs. 3A and B**).

Perineal pain is the hallmark symptom that should prompt clinicians to examine the patient for a suspected puerperal genital hematoma.

General

- *General condition*: Pulse, blood pressure, respiratory rate, pallor, and urine output
- Cardiovascular and respiratory system

- *Abdominal examination*:
  - Uterus size, contracted and retracted or not.
  - Tenderness over the uterus and other areas of abdomen.
- *Pelvic examination*:
  - On inspection of vulva:
    - Presence of swelling, size of swelling, and site of swelling in relation to episiotomy
    - Bleeding from the swelling and from the vagina
  - Per speculum examination:
    - Confirmation of findings on inspection
    - Extension of swelling, margins can be defined or not, associated swelling or hematoma present
  - Per vaginal (P/V) examination:
    - Size of uterus, any fullness in the fornices
    - Confirmation of site and size of swelling. The vulval hematoma swelling is usually tense fluctuant and sensitive tumor covered by discolored skin. Bleeding present on pressing the swelling.
  - Per rectal examination:
    - Any swelling anterior to rectum and extension of swelling.

INVESTIGATIONS

- Complete blood count (CBC), blood group, coagulation screening should be performed. Cross-matching for a blood transfusion.
- Ultrasound, computed tomography (CT), or magnetic resonance imaging (MRI) of the pelvis can be done to evaluate the size, site, and growth of the hematoma.
- Magnetic resonance imaging angiography of the pelvis may help in the detection of any aneurysms.
- Transperineal sonography is also a simple, noninvasive technique that can be useful for the follow-up and monitoring of patients undergoing expectant management of a vulvar hematoma.
- Additional investigations, such as a pelvic X-ray for pelvic bone fractures in cases of pelvic trauma, should be done.

MANAGEMENT

Conservative management usually involves the *use of ice packs, local compressions, bed rest, and analgesics.*

Surgical intervention may be necessary when:
- The hematoma is expanding
- Larger than 10 cm in size
- Causing pressure necrosis
- Hemodynamic instability, or
- Suspicion for another associated pelvic injury

Surgical management includes *surgical drainage of the hematoma, evacuation of any clots present, ligation of bleeding points,* and the assessment for signs of pressure necrosis (a complication of vulva hematoma).

Alternatively, *selective arterial embolization* may be performed.

Surgeons may choose *angiographic-assisted embolization,* if bleeding continues postoperatively, or if the vulvar hematoma reforms after surgical management. Indication—where surgery is not possible, such as in patients who are hemodynamically unstable and not fit for surgical ligation procedures. Embolization occurs in internal pudendal artery and its vaginal branch as well as uterine artery.

TREATMENT

Resuscitation and exploration under anesthesia, hematoma drainage:
- Resuscitation with blood transfusion and fluid replacement
- Exploration under anesthesia—site in relation to episiotomy and size of hematoma
- *In case of hematoma at the episiotomy site*:
  - Open the episiotomy sutures
  - Evacuate clots
  - Search for active bleeder and ligate if found
  - Close the dead space and close episiotomy in layers with proper hemostasis
  - Postoperative care—Foley's catheter, cefazolin + metronidazole, analgesics
  - Angiographic embolization can be used primarily or when hemostasis is not obtained by surgical methods.

DIFFERENTIAL DIAGNOSIS

- Bartholin's gland cysts and abscesses
- Vulvar varicosities
- Folliculitis
- Vulvar cancer
- Vulvovaginal metastasis of choriocarcinoma

COMPLICATIONS

- *Pressure necrosis* can be prevented with the prompt surgical evacuation of blood clots.
- *Infection:*
  - *Recurrence of hematoma or infection*: Prophylactic antibiotics may be prescribed if clinically indicated.
- *Complications related with pelvic arterial embolization*: Postprocedural complications such as muscle pain, guidewire perforation, vaginal fistula, pelvic infection, and temporary foot drop are also possible means some degree of exposure to ionizing radiation.

POSTOPERATIVE AND REHABILITATION CARE

- *Early mobilization* reduces the risk of venous thromboembolism.
- *Attentive wound care, postoperative analgesics, and antibiotics*

- *Continued monitoring* of the patient's vital signs is important.
- *Prognosis*: Vulvar hematomas may cause serious morbidity.
- *In conclusion*, obstetric vulvar hematoma is a concern for the obstetrician, but nonobstetric vulvar hematoma may present to the emergency clinician and primary clinicians. The main presentation of vulvar hematoma is perineal pain and unilateral swelling of the vulva. If the hematoma is not large or acutely expanding, conservative management can be considered. A serious case of vulvar hematoma can lead to hemodynamic instability and should be recognized and treated early.

BROAD LIGAMENT HEMATOMA

Anatomy

The broad ligaments consist of anterior and posterior leaflets of peritoneum which cover the lateral uterine corpus and upper cervix and extend from the lateral walls of the uterus to the pelvic sidewalls. The broad ligament is bounded superiorly by the round ligament, inferiorly by the cardinal and uterosacral ligaments, and laterally by the infundibulopelvic ligament where it blends with the pelvic sidewall. The mesosalpinx of the Fallopian tube is contiguous with the broad ligament **(Fig. 4)**.

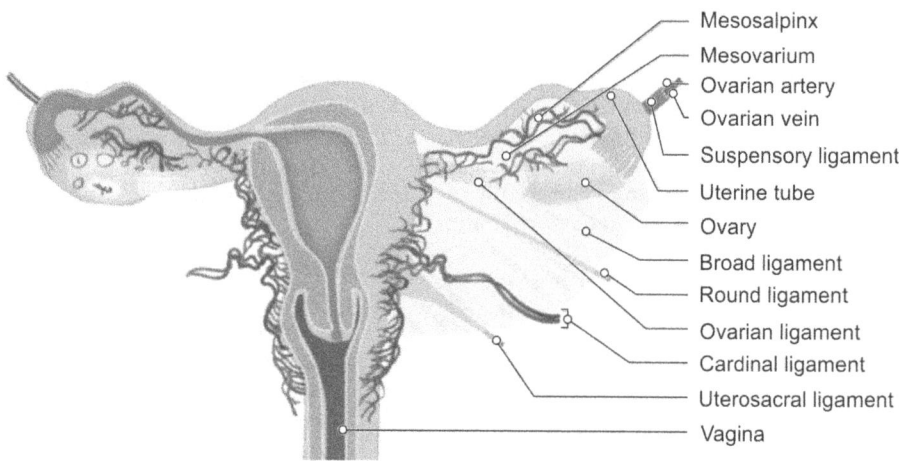

Mesosalpinx
Mesovarium
Ovarian artery
Ovarian vein
Suspensory ligament
Uterine tube
Ovary
Broad ligament
Round ligament
Ovarian ligament
Cardinal ligament
Uterosacral ligament
Vagina

Fig. 4: Anatomy of broad ligament.

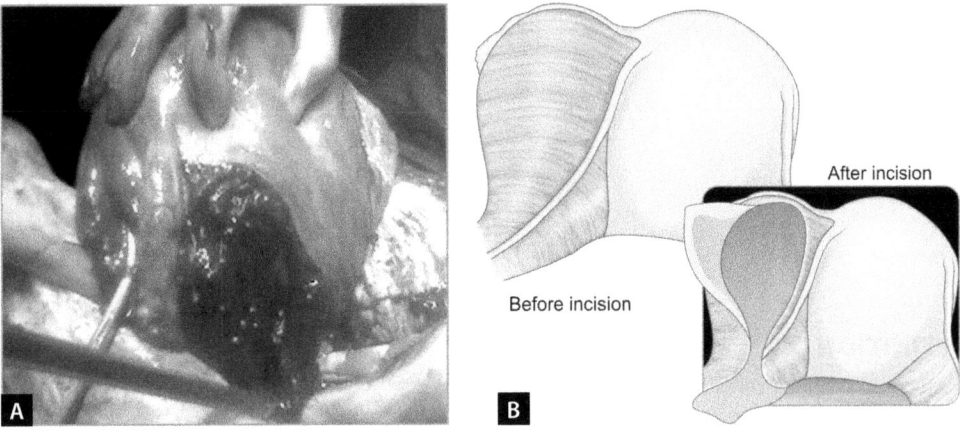

After incision

Before incision

Figs. 5A and B: Broad ligament hematoma (intraoperative and pictorial representation).

The primary blood supply to the uterus is the uterine and ovarian arteries. These vessels anastomose near the upper lateral aspect of the uterus. Blood from the upper uterus, the ovary, and upper part of the broad ligament is collected by several veins forming *a large pampiniform plexus* within the broad ligament.

Broad ligament hematomas may occur at the time of cesarean [obstetric trauma (lacerations/tear) to the cervix, upper vagina, or uterus], either trauma or extension of the hysterotomy, or accompanying tubal ligation. The diagnosis is usually late presenting *as unexplained shock with features of internal hemorrhage following delivery* raises the suspicion. Broad ligament hematomas can result in large volumes of blood loss by *dissecting into the retroperitoneal spaces* **(Figs. 5A and B).**

The source of a broad ligament hematoma can be venous, arterial, or both. Arterial bleeding usually results in a rapidly expanding hematoma and can be presented earlier. Venous bleeding typically results in slower expansion. Small stable hematomas do not require treatment and should be monitored before taking decision. If the hematoma is expanding, direct pressure should be applied to the site. This may help in hemostasis of smaller vessels and also limit blood loss while supplies are collected. It is advisable to look for the blessing and should be cauterized or suture ligated as necessary. Exteriorizing the uterus may facilitate ligation and separation from the ureter. When continued bleeding is suspected postoperatively, Interventional radiology reference for vessel embolization should be kept in mind.

Thus, strong clinical suspicion, prompt diagnosis, and timely intervention are the important factors for successful treatment.

Amniotic Fluid Embolism

Ashwini Kale, Ashish R Kale

▨ DEFINITION

Amniotic fluid embolism (AFE) is one of the most catastrophic complications of pregnancy in which it is postulated that amniotic fluid, fetal cells, hair, or other debris enters the maternal pulmonary circulation, causing cardiovascular collapse.

It was first reported by Meyer in 1926, and the syndrome was first described by Steiner and Lushbaugh in 1941.

▨ DIAGNOSIS

Symptoms

The symptoms are often sudden:
- Hypotension—most common presenting sign and symptom (100%)
- Tonic-clonic seizures are seen in 10–50% of patients.
- *Cough*: This is usually a manifestation of dyspnea.
- Altered mental state
- Rapid decline in pulse oximetry values or sudden absence or decrease in end-tidal carbon dioxide may be apparent.
- Cyanosis—sudden hypoxia and respiratory arrest. As hypoxia/hypoxemia progresses, circumoral and peripheral cyanosis and changes in mucous membranes may manifest.

Signs

- Acute pulmonary hypertension and vasospasm result in right ventricular failure, hypoxia, and cardiac arrest.
- *Coagulopathy or severe hemorrhage*: Coagulation disorders are a prominent feature of the amniotic fluid syndrome. Disseminated intravascular coagulation (DIC) is present in >83% of patients.

- *Uterine atony*: Uterine atony usually results in excessive bleeding after delivery.
- *Fetal bradycardia*—in response to hypoxia and hypotension

Four criteria must be present to make the diagnosis of AFE:
1. Acute hypotension or cardiac arrest
2. Acute hypoxia
3. Coagulopathy or severe hemorrhage in the absence of other explanations
4. All of these occurring during labor, cesarean delivery, dilation, and evacuation, or within 30 minutes postpartum with no other explanation of findings.

▨ CLINICAL FINDINGS

Continuous pulse oximetry and arterial blood gas (ABG) measurements to determine the degree of hypoxemia.

Arterial blood gas levels: Expect changes consistent with hypoxia/hypoxemia

Decreased pH and decreased pO$_2$:
- Serial complete blood counts and coagulation studies—look for hemoglobin, hematocrit, prothrombin time (PT), and activated partial thromboplastin time (aPTT)
- Chest X-ray
- 12-lead electrocardiogram (ECG)
- Decreased levels of C3, C4 levels
- Transesophageal echocardiography—may not be available everywhere.

▨ MANAGEMENT

Early recognition is very important. Hence, watchful vigilance leads to successful outcome.

General

- Maintain ABC—airway, breathing, and circulation
- Fluid resuscitation with rapid volume infusion of isotonic crystalloid and colloids solutions
- Correcting coagulopathy—with blood, blood products, fresh frozen plasma (FFP), and cryoprecipitate

Medical

- Epinephrine may be the first-line agent of choice.
- Phenylephrine, a pure α-1 agonist, is often an excellent choice early in the treatment.
- Vasopressin may be used as primary therapy or as an adjunct to other inotropic therapies and has the benefit of sparing the pulmonary vasculature from vasoconstriction, especially at low doses.
- *Hydrocortisone*: Because AFE is more similar to an anaphylactic reaction, steroids that mediate the immune responses are recommended.
- *Oxytocin*: Most commonly used uterotonic
- Recombinant factor VIIa (rfVIIa)
- Methylergonovine (Methergine) and carboprost
- Aprotinin has also been effective in reducing hemorrhage with AFE.
- Extracorporeal membrane oxygenation (ECMO) and cardiopulmonary bypass

- Hysterectomy, as a last resort, may be required in patients with persistent uterine hemorrhage to control blood loss, is the definitive management.

CONCLUSION

Early diagnosis and aggressive management, vigilant use of uterotonic agents is the key to patient survival. There is still lot to be done in terms of definitive diagnostic tests. Despite good intensive care unit (ICU) setting and management, the maternal prognosis is poor.

BIBLIOGRAPHY

1. Clark SL, Hankins GD, Dudley DA, Dildy GA, Porter TF. Amniotic fluid embolism: analysis of the national registry. Am J Obstet Gynecol. 1995;172(4 Pt 1):1158-67.
2. Gist RS, Stafford IP, Leibowitz AB, Beilin Y. Amniotic fluid embolism. Anesth Analg. 2009;108(5):1599-602.
3. O'Shea A, Eappen S. Amniotic fluid embolism. Int Anesthesiol Clin. 2007;45(1):17-28.
4. Saha R, Maharjan S, Thapa J. Amniotic fluid embolism understanding pathophysiology from a successfully managed case. N J Obstet Gynaecol. 2006;1:55-8.
5. Thongrong C, Kasemsiri P, Hofmann JP, Bergese SD, Papadimos TJ, Gracias VH, etc. Amniotic fluid embolism. Int J Crit Illn Inj Sci. 2013;3(1):51-7.

Maternal Collapse

Jyoti Bhaskar

▓ INTRODUCTION

Maternal collapse is an uncommon event but is associated with severe maternal morbidity and mortality. In the UK MBRRACE reports, substandard care continues to be a major contributory factory.[1] Hence, it is essential that the labor room and obstetric ward team are skilled in initial effective resuscitation techniques, and are able to systematically investigate and diagnose the cause of the collapse and institute cause directed ongoing management.

▓ DEFINITION

Maternal collapse is defined as an acute event involving the cardiorespiratory systems and/or central nervous systems, resulting in a reduced or absent conscious level (and potentially cardiac arrest and death), at any stage in pregnancy and up to 6 weeks after birth.[2]

▓ CAUSES: RESUSCITATION COUNCIL (UK)[3] (TABLE 1)

TABLE 1: Causes of maternal collapse.

Reversible causes (4H 4TE)	Conditions in pregnancy
4H	
Hypovolemia	Bleeding (APH, PPH, traumatic, uterine rupture, ectopic pregnancy, splenic, or hepatic rupture), dense spinal block, septic or neurogenic shock
Hypoxia	Cardiac events—peripartum cardiomyopathy, myocardial infarction, aortic dissection, and aneurysms
Hypo/hyperkalemia and hyponatremia	Indiscriminate oxytocin use
Hypothermia	
4T's	
Thromboembolism	Amniotic fluid embolus, pulmonary embolus, air embolus, and myocardial infarction
Toxicity	Local anesthetics, magnesium sulfate, anaphylaxis, and poisoning
Tension pneumothorax	Following trauma/suicide attempts
Tamponade	Following trauma/suicide attempts
Eclampsia and pre-eclampsia include intracranial hemorrhage for pregnant woman	
(APH: antepartum hemorrhage; PPH: postpartum hemorrhage)	

▦ ACTION

- Immediate action
- Secondary action
- Documentation
- Debriefing

Immediate Action

See **Box 1** and **Flowchart 1**.

Secondary Action: Identify and Correct the Reversible Causes

See **Table 2**.

BOX 1: Immediate action of maternal collapse.

- *Ensure safety*
- *Shout and summon help*
- *Stimulate and assess response*, if assessor is confident
- Open airway, check for breathing and pulse for *10 seconds—ABC*
- *Crash call—code blue. Dial your hospital assigned number*
- Adult cardiac arrest trolley and defibrillator/ automated external defibrillators (AED) to be bought to the patient
- Do not attempt to move the patient

Flowchart 1: Immediate action of maternal collapse.

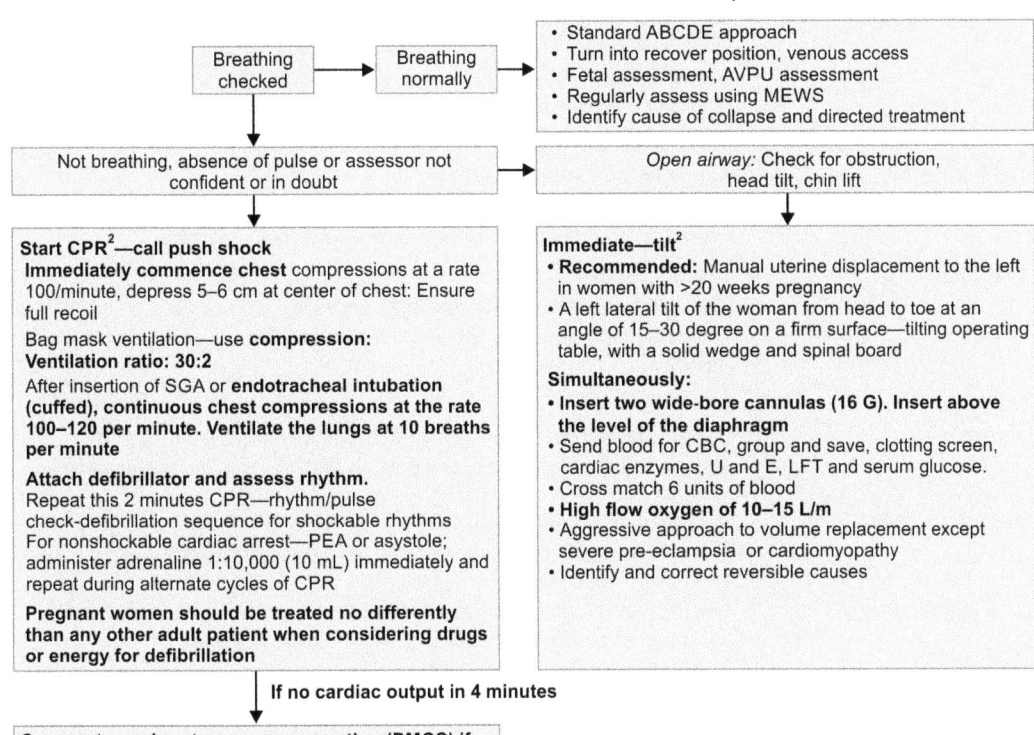

(AVPU: alert voice pain unresponsiveness, CPR: cardiopulmonary resuscitation; SGA: supraglottic airway; PEA: pulseless electrical activity)

TABLE 2: Secondary action of maternal collapse.

The reversible causes

Hemorrhage	• *APH*—deliver fetus and placenta promptly • *Massive placental abruption*: Cesarean may be indicated • *PPH*—follow guidelines of management of PPH. 1 g of intravenous tranexamic acid within 3 hours of delivery significantly reduces mortality[5]
Cardiac cause	• After initial resuscitation, the cardiac disease should be managed by cardiology team. Pain relief with morphine, 12 lead ECG should be done meanwhile • Delivery may be necessary to facilitate this management
Thromboembolism Pulmonary embolism	• Maintain airway, oxygenation, may require ventilation • Prolonged CPR may break up the thrombus. Maintain BP with normal saline, avoid fluid overload, anti-coagulate with an IV bolus of 10,000 units of heparin with senior input consider thrombolytic agents; If used CPR must continue for 90 minutes
Amniotic fluid embolism	• Supportive rather than specific • Early involvement of, anesthetists, hematologists and intensivists, is essential to optimize outcome • Monitor blood hemostatic and coagulation parameters • Treat with blood components accordingly
Accidental total spinal	• Reassurance, administer oxygen • Vasopressors (ephedrine and adrenaline) • Intubation and sedation may be required until block regresses
Anaphylaxis	• Stop offending agent • 500 µg (0.5 mL) of 1:1,000 adrenaline is given *intramuscularly* • Adjuvant therapy consists of chlorpheniramine 10 mg IV and hydrocortisone 200 mg IV
Drug toxicity Opioids	• Discontinue any opioid therapy, administer oxygen, *basic life support* • Administer intravenous naloxone (initially 0.4 mg, repeated and infusion if necessary)
Magnesium sulfate	• Stop magnesium sulfate infusion • 10 mL 10% calcium gluconate or 10 mL 10% calcium chloride given by slow intravenous injection
Local anesthetic drugs	• Give IV bolus injection of intralipid 20% 1.5 mL/kg over 1 minute followed by an intravenous infusion of intralipid 20% at 0.25 mL/kg/min
Hypoglycemia	• Blood glucose levels <72 mg/dL should be treated • Stop insulin infusion • Give 75–100 mL of 20% glucose over 15 minutes intravenously
Sepsis	As per the surviving sepsis campaign guidelines
Eclampsia	As per the eclampsia management protocol

(APH: antepartum hemorrhage; PPH: postpartum hemorrhage)

Documentation and Incident Reporting

Accurate and continuous documentation of all events, sequence, time, and steps undertaken during resuscitation has to make. After the event all those involved should write full notes and an incident form should be filled. Poor documentation has several clinical and medicolegal consequences.

Debriefing

This is a very stressful and traumatic event. It is important to debrief the staff, the woman and all her relatives.

Factors that influence the outcome:

- *Resuscitation team*:
  - Apart from the hospital CPR team, the senior most staff nurse in the maternity unit, resident obstetrician, and anesthetist should be included in this team.
  - The most senior obstetrician and senior anesthetist should be called at the time of a cardiopulmonary arrest call.
  - The neonatal team should be called early if delivery is expected soon.
  - If CPR is successful, a consultant intensivist should be involved as soon as possible
- *Ongoing training*: All the maternity staff should undergo basic life support skill training and should be regularly updated with the CPR adaptations of pregnant woman.

▊ SUMMARY

- Best outcomes for both mother and fetus are through successful maternal resuscitation.
- Planning and training of maternal collapse should be in collaboration with the obstetric, neonatal, emergency, anesthesiology, intensive care, and cardiac arrest services. All the maternity staff should be regularly updated and trained.
- Priorities for CPR in a pregnant woman include high-quality CPR and relief of aortocaval compression through left lateral uterine displacement.

- If mother is not resuscitated within 4 minutes of CPR and umbilicus is above umbilicus, perimortem cesarean section should be completed by 5 minutes at the place of resuscitation.
- Simultaneously with the CPR, investigation and diagnosis of the reversible causes should be initiated and treatment should be cause directed.
- Documentation is the most essential process and should be completed immediately after the event as poor and incomplete documentation can have severe medicolegal implication.

▊ REFERENCES

1. Confidential Enquiry into Maternal and Child Health. Saving Mothers' Lives: Reviewing Maternal Deaths to Make Motherhood Safer-2003–2005. The Seventh Report of the Confidential Enquiries into Maternal Deaths in the United Kingdom. London: CEMACH; 2007.
2. RCOG. (2019). Green top guideline No 56-Maternal collapse in Pregnancy and the Puerperium. [online] Available from http://www.missionmrcog.com/home/images/Library/Greentop_Guidelines/2019/003_Maternal_collapse.pdf [Last accessed December, 2021].
3. Resuscitation Council (UK). (2021). Adult advanced life support. [online] Available from https://www.resus.org.uk/library/2021-resuscitation-guidelines/adult-advanced-life-support-guidelines [Last accessed December, 2021].
4. Katz V, Balderston K, DeFreest M. Perimortem cesarean delivery: Were our assumptions correct? Am J Obstet Gynecol. 2005;192:1916-21.
5. WOMAN Trial Collaborators. Effect of early tranexamic acid administration on mortality, hysterectomy, and other morbidities in women with post-partum haemorrhage (WOMAN): an international, randomised, double-blind, placebo-controlled trial. Lancet. 2017;389: 2105-16.

33

Disseminated Intravascular Coagulation

Jyoti Bhaskar, Meenakshi Sharma

INTRODUCTION

Disseminated intravascular coagulation (DIC) complicates nearly 0.03–0.35%[1,2] of pregnancies, though the exact incidence is not defined. In developing countries, leading causes of DIC is due to retained stillbirth and preeclampsia[3] while in developed countries it occurs most commonly due to placental abruption especially when associated with intrauterine fetal demise.[1]

ETIOLOGY AND PATHOPHYSIOLOGY

Pregnancy is associated with a physiological procoagulant state to decrease blood loss during parturition by endothelial activation, increased liver synthesis of coagulation factors, and decreased activity of coagulation inhibitors and fibrinolysis.

Obstetric DIC can occur in settings of:
- Systemic inflammatory response and cytokine activation with subsequent activation of coagulation system, like in sepsis or trauma.

- Release of procoagulant factors in the bloodstream like in pregnancy-related complications such as eclampsia/hemolysis, elevated liver enzymes, and low platelet (HELLP) or amniotic fluid embolism.

The most common conditions which can lead to DIC are:
- Amniotic fluid embolism
- Abruptio placentae
- Acute peripartum hemorrhage
- Preeclampsia/HELLP syndrome
- Retained stillbirth
- Septic abortion and intrauterine infection
- Acute fatty liver of pregnancy
- Massive blood transfusion

CLINICAL FEATURES

The main symptoms and signs are those of the obstetric complications causing DIC.

Disseminated intravascular coagulation resulting from a wide spread activation of both clotting and fibrinolysis systems can lead to hemorrhagic or thrombotic manifestations and sequelae.

LABORATORY FINDINGS IN DIC

Laboratory tests	Normal values	Values suggestive of DIC	Comments
PT	9.5–13.5 seconds	Prolonged >1.5 mean control	Prolongation of PT may not occur until significant progression of the disease
aPTT	22.6–38.9 seconds	Prolonged >1.5 mean control	Prolongation of aPTT may not occur until the underlying condition has progressed considerably
Plasma fibrinogen	244–696 mg/dL	<150 mg/dL	Concentrations may be significantly overestimated when plasma is diluted with colloids. Some reports suggest the use of Clauss fibrinogen
D–dimer	.05–1.7 µg/mL	Elevated	Sensitive indicators of obstetric DIC but poor specificity
FDP	<40 µg/mL	Elevated	
Platelet count	150	Reduced	Some obstetrical syndromes are associated with low PLT counts that are not related to DIC
Antithrombin III	76–128%	Reduced	

(aPTT: activated partial thromboplastin time; DIC: disseminated intravascular coagulation; FDP: fibrin degradation products; PT: prothrombin time; PLT: platelets)

SPECTRUM OF DIC IN OBSTETRICS

Spectrum of DIC in obstetrics is given in **Table 1**.

DIAGNOSTIC CRITERIA

Disseminated intravascular coagulation in an obstetric patient is not clearly defined but is characterized by falling platelets and fibrinogen and rising fibrin degradation products (FDPs). Since none of the laboratory tests like platelet count, prothrombin time (PT), and activated partial thromboplastin time (aPTT) alone are specific enough to diagnose DIC, scoring criteria is used to diagnose DIC.[4]

There are several DIC scoring criteria being used but they are not specific for pregnancy (**Table 2**).

The physiological changes in hemostasis in pregnancy, with increase in fibrinogen levels and decreased platelets in the third trimester, affect the accuracy in diagnosing obstetric DIC.

Subsequently Erez et al., in 2014,[2] developed a pregnancy-specific ISTH DIC score by using only three components, platelet count, fibrinogen

TABLE 1: Spectrum of DIC in obstetrics.

Severity of symptoms	Laboratory findings	Clinical condition
Stage 1: Low grade compensated	↑FDP's ↓Platelets	Preeclampsia and related syndromes
Stage 2: Uncompensated but no hemostatic failure	↓↓Platelets ↓Fibrinogen ↓Factor V and VIII	Small abruption Severe preeclampsia
Stage 3: Rampant with hemostatic failure	As above plus ↑↑FDP Gross depletion of coagulation factors especially fibrinogen	Placental abruption Eclampsia Amniotic fluid embolism

(DIC: disseminated intravascular coagulation; FDP: fibrin degradation product)

TABLE 2: Pregnancy nonspecific DIC score.

Name of scoring criteria	ISTH DIC score[5]	JAAM DIC score[6]	SIC score 2017
Full form	International Society on Thrombosis and Haemostasis	Japanese Association for Acute Medicine	Sepsis-induced coagulopathy score
Good for scoring	Nonobstetric patients with overt DIC	Acute onset of sepsis-induced coagulopathy	Resembles JAAM
Usefulness	Severe DIC and mortality	Nonovert DIC	Simplified and better identifies patients for anticoagulant therapy
Parameters used	PT Platelets FDP Fibrinogen	SIRS criteria Platelets PT Fibrin marker	Platelets PT SOFA score
Total score to support diagnosis of DIC	5 supports DIC	4 supports DIC	4 supports DIC

(SIRS: systemic inflammatory response syndrome; SOFA: sequential organ failure assessment)

TABLE 3: Pregnancy-specific modified SSC-ISTH score.[7]			
	0	**1**	**2**
Platelet count (/mL)	>100,000	<100,000	<50,000
Increase in PT or INR	<25%	25–50%	>50%
Fibrinogen levels (mg/L)	>200	<200	

concentrations, and the PT difference based on physiological changes in pregnancy.

The diagnostic criteria as per Scientific and Standardisation Committee on DIC of the International Society on Thrombosis and Haemostasis (ISTH) 2016 are given in **Table 3**.[7]

A score of ≥3 is compatible with overt DIC. Coagulopathy must be detected before as transfusion of blood and its components, itself can account for delusional or shock-related consumptive coagulopathy.

MONITORING OF DIC

During DIC, the laboratory tests demonstrate progressively decreasing platelet count and fibrinogen, prolongation of the PT and aPTT, increasing fibrinogen-degradation/fibrin-degradation products and D-dimer concentrations.

Hemostasis may be assessed by:
- Clinical observation
- *Laboratory-based conventional coagulation tests*: They need to be repeated at a minimum interval of 6–8 hours.
- Point-of-care testing (POCT) such as thermoelectrometry (TEM), thromboelastography, and FIBTEM assay if available.

There is a good correlation between the conventional coagulation tests and POCT.

MANAGEMENT OF DIC

The successful management of DIC depends on early recognition and prompt management of underlying obstetric causes with correction of coagulopathy requiring multidisciplinary management.

The basic principles of managing obstetrical DIC are:
- Multidisciplinary approach
- Treatment of obstetrical causes

- Transfusion of blood and blood-related products
- Supportive care

Multidisciplinary Approach

The best outcome is achieved when the team managing a pregnant woman with DIC comprises an experienced obstetrician, hematologist, and intensivist experienced in transfusion medicine.

Treatment of Obstetric Cause

The clinical presentation of DIC in pregnancy is mostly hemorrhage. It is vital to identify the underlying obstetric cause and initiate immediate appropriate cause directed measures and expedite delivery.

Fluid and Blood and Blood Products

Fluid Choice

It is essential to restore fluid balance and infuse crystalloids or Hartman's solution till the blood arrives. The general principle is to transfuse two-three times the estimated blood loss till blood products are available.

Blood and Blood Products

Component therapy is the mainstay of therapy in DIC. In acutely bleeding patients where DIC is suspected, a massive transfusion protocol is to be followed as packed red blood cell (PRBC)/ fresh frozen plasma (FFP) in the ratio of 1:1 till coagulation profile is available.

Goal-directed therapy:[7] Components should be used judiciously as unmonitored components especially FFP can cause transfusion-associated circulatory overload (TACO) and transfusion-related acute lung injury (TRALI).

TABLE 4: Management of DIC.

Laboratory parameters	Component	Dose of component	Change in hemostasis/goal
Platelet <75,000/μL	Random donor platelet Single donor platelet	2/10 kg body weight 1	Platelet >50,000/μL
Prolonged PT/APTT	FFP	15 mL/kg	Goal—PT/aPTT ratio of <1.5 × normal
Fibrinogen level <200 mg/dL	Cryoprecipitate/FFP	1 cryoprecipitate 2 pools of cryoprecipitate	Increase fibrinogen level by 10 mg/dL Increase fibrinogen by 100 mg/dL
	Fibrinogen concentrate	60 mg/kg	Increase fibrinogen by 100 mg/dL (*Goal*: Fibrinogen >100 mg/dL, ongoing PPH >200 mg/dL)

Key points:
- Platelets should be transfused when the platelet count is $<75 \times 10^9$/L based on laboratory monitoring and against 1:1:1 RBC: FFP: platelet transfusion ratios.
- If no coagulation results are available and bleeding is ongoing, then, after 4 units of RBC, 4 units of FFP should be infused and 1:1 RBC: FFP transfusion maintained until hemostatic test results are known.
- In cases of massive ongoing bleeding where women have been given 8 units of RBCs and 8 units of FFP and no coagulation results or platelet count is available then two pools of cryoprecipitate and one pool of platelets may be given.

Other hemostatic agents:
- *Tranexamic acid*: Role of tranexamic acid is not clearly established. In ongoing, PPH can consider 1 g IV early on in hemorrhage and is known to reduce mortality if given within 3 hours of birth.
- *Recombinant factor VIIa*: Not licensed for use in PPH. Use in dose 60 mg/kg in cases of uncontrollable PPH unresponsive to standard treatment. Dose >90 mg/kg can cause thrombosis.

Supportive Therapy
- *Avoid tissue hypoxia*: Optimal oxygen support should be provided to maintain tissue oxygenation.
- Prevent hypothermia and acidosis
- Regular monitoring of hematocrit, urine output, and global clotting tests is essential.

KEY POINTS OF DIC MANAGEMENT: SIX CORNERSTONE PRINCIPLES

1. Remove or treat the etiological cause expeditiously
2. Restore fluid balance
3. Adequately perfuse tissues
4. Avoid tissue hypoxia
5. Multidisciplinary team approach and management
6. Communication and documentation

REFERENCES

1. Rattray DD, O'Connell CM, Baskett TF. Acute disseminated intravascular coagulation in obstetrics: a tertiary centre population review (1980 to 2009). J Obstet Gynaecol Can. 2012; 34:341-7.
2. Erez O, Novack L, Beer-Weisel R, Dukler D, Press F, Zlotnik A, et al. DIC score in pregnant women—a population based modification of the International Society on Thrombosis and Hemostasis score. PLoS One. 2014;9:e93240.
3. Naz H, Fawad A, Islam A, Shahid H, Abbasi AU. Disseminated intravascular coagulation. JAMC. 2011;23:111-3.
4. Rabinovich A, Abdul-Kadir R, Thachil J, Iba T, Othman M, Erez O. DIC in obstetrics: Diagnostic score, highlights in management, and international registry-communication from the DIC and Women's Health SSCs of the International Society of Thrombosis and Haemostasis. J Thromb Haemost. 2019; 17(9):1562-6.
5. Taylor FB, Toh CH, Hoots WK, Wada H, Levi M. Scientific Subcommittee on Disseminated

Intravascular Coagulation (DIC) of the International Society on Thrombosis and Haemostasis (ISTH). Towards definition, clinical and laboratory criteria, and a scoring system for disseminated intravascular coagulation. Thromb Haemost. 2001;86:1327-30.

6. Gando S, Iba T, Eguchi Y, Ohtomo Y, Okamoto K, Koseki K, et al. A multicenter, prospective validation of disseminated intravascular coagulation diagnostic criteria for critically ill patients: comparing current criteria. Crit Care Med. 2006;34(3):625-31.

7. Collins P, Abdul-Kadir R, Thachil J. Management of coagulopathy associated with postpartum hemorrhage: guidance from the SSC of the ISTH. J Thromb Haemost. 2016;14:205-10.

34

Diabetic Patient in Labor

Dolly Mehra

INTRODUCTION

Normal pregnancy is a state of insulin resistance. To spare glucose for the developing fetus, the placenta produces several hormones that antagonize insulin and shift the main energy source from glucose to ketones and free fatty acids.[1] Diabetes mellitus (DM) in pregnancy is a metabolic disorder because of decrease in insulin secretion or increase in insulin resistance or combination of both, resulting in carbohydrate, protein, and lipid metabolism abnormalities. It is associated with increased maternal and fetal morbidity and mortality.

PREVALENCE

The epidemic of diabetes is now becoming a pandemic affecting people in both developed and developing countries. The global prevalence of DM in 2000 was 2.8% which is likely to increase to 4.4% in 2030.[2]

In India, the prevalence of gestational diabetes mellitus (GDM) ranges from 0.25 to 5.5%.[3] However in a study by Seshiah et al. (2004),[4] a prevalence rate of 18.9% was reported. Women with GDM in a previous pregnancy are likely to have 33.5% recurrence in a subsequent pregnancy.[5]

PRECONCEPTION

Euglycemia should be maintained during the preconception period for optimal maternal and perinatal outcome in diabetic pregnancy.

ANTENATAL FETAL SURVEILLANCE

Documenting fetal wellbeing is important during the antenatal period for any woman whose pregnancy is complicated by pregestational diabetes according to White class B **(Table 1)** or higher, however, no unified opinion for fetal assessment for women with well controlled,

TABLE 1: White's classification of diabetes during pregnancy.				
		Plasma glucose level		
Class	*Onset*	*Fasting*	*2-hour postprandial*	*Therapy*
A	Gestational	<105 mg/dL	<120 mg/dL	Diet
A+	Gestational	>105 mg/dL	>120 mg/dL	Insulin
Class	*Age of onset (year)*	*Duration (year)*	*Vascular disease*	*Therapy*
B	Over 20	<10	None	Insulin
C	10–19	10–19	None	Insulin
D	Before 10	>20	Benign retinopathy	Insulin
F	Any	Any	Nephropathy	Insulin
R	Any	Any	Proliferative retinopathy	Insulin
H	Any	Any	Heart	Insulin

uncomplicated preexisting, and gestational diabetes.[6] The American College of Obstetricians and Gynecologists (ACOG) recommends that antenatal testing be performed on all pregestational diabetes, gestational diabetes with poor glycemic control, gestational diabetes with other complications such as hypertension or growth restriction.[7]

In the first trimester, aim is at accurate dating, nuchal translucency (NT), maternal serum alpha-fetoprotein (MSAFP), unconjugated estriol, and inhibin A at 11–13.6 weeks. Fetal morphology at 18–20 weeks, fetal echo at 20–22 weeks.[8] Growth scan at 28–30 weeks, scan at 34–36 weeks to look for fetal macrosomia and polyhydramnios. Doppler study useful in growth restricted fetus.[9] Daily kick count and nonstress test (NST) to be initiated twice a week from 34 weeks. Biophysical profile not very reliable in pregnant women with diabetes because of poor reliability of AFI as a predictor of fetal wellbeing.

Diabetic pregnancies have also been classified by the American Diabetes Association (ADA) and World Health Organization (WHO) based on etiology. The WHO classification differs from ADA by additionally recognizing impaired glucose tolerance even before pregnancy.

American Diabetes Association classification of diabetes in pregnancy:
- *Pregestational diabetes*:
  - Type 1 diabetes (insulin-dependent)
  - Type 2 diabetes (noninsulin-dependent)
  - Secondary diabetes
- Gestational diabetes
- Impaired glucose tolerance during diabetes

TIMING OF DELIVERY

Timing of delivery is a delicate balance in a pregnancy complicated by diabetes. The primary goal is to prevent stillbirth. The risk of unexplained intrauterine fetal death (IUFD) increases after 36 weeks of gestation in pregnant women with diabetes, on the other hand needless intervention places the women at risk for complications such as prolonged labor and operative delivery. However, elective termination has to be weighed against the risk of delayed lung maturity and acute respiratory distress syndrome (ARDS). Few trials have been undertaken with regards to optimizing delivery outcomes in diabetics. But it has been consistently

shown that the cesarean delivery rate has been higher in diabetics than in nondiabetics,[10] even when antenatal care has achieved near-normal rates of fetal growth.[11]

Factors influencing the timing of delivery are:
- Control of diabetes
- Condition of cervix
- Previous obstetric history
- Fetal compromise

Indications for delivery at any time after 37–38 weeks include the inability to achieve adequate glucose control; poor compliance with visits or prescribed treatment; prior stillbirths; and presence of chronic hypertension. Women with well-controlled GDM, good compliance with care, and an appropriately grown fetus are allowed to enter spontaneous labor, until 40–41 weeks gestation. Tighter glycemic control during the third trimester might reduce late fetal compromise and cesarean delivery for fetal indications.[12]

PLACE OF DELIVERY

Institutional delivery is ideal. Women with GDM with good blood sugar control [2-hour postprandial blood sugar (PPBS) < 120 mg/dL)] may be delivered at their respective health facility, but pregnant women with GDM on insulin therapy with uncontrolled blood sugar levels (2-hour PPBS ≥ 120 mg/dL) on medical nutrition therapy (MNT) and physical exercise and metformin or insulin requirement >20 IU/day should deliver at the higher center.

PLAN OF DELIVERY

- A proper plan of mode and timing of delivery should be ready during the antenatal period.
- The majority of patients is induced or receives a planned elective cesarean delivery.
- Proper insulin management has to be done which will be mentioned later.
- Induction by prostaglandin gel or misoprostol.
- Antibiotics should be given prophylactically to minimize infection.
- In labor, continuous cardiotocography, if available, should be performed, otherwise fetal heart monitoring by a stethoscope.
- Strict asepsis should be maintained during labor, and the number per vaginal examination

should be restricted. Careful watch for the progress of labor and maintain a partogram.

- The likelihood of diabetic women having cephalopelvic disproportion (CPD) is high, CPD should be suspected if the cervical dilatation slows down in the late first stage of labor, if the cervix is not well applied to the presenting part or there is the arrest of labor in the second stage. An early decision for cesarean should be taken.
- Active management of labor is encouraged.
- Instrumental delivery may be required.
- Obstetricians should be well-versed and well prepared with the management of shoulder dystocia while delivering a diabetic woman. A senior obstetrician should be available. The placenta with membranes should be delivered completely and checked.

INSULIN MANAGEMENT

Strict glycemic control during labor is important to prevent neonatal hypoglycemia after birth.[13] During labor, insulin requirement is less than the daily routine requirement due to fasting status and use of energy during labor.

- Usual dose of intermediate-acting insulin is given at bedtime.
- Morning dose of insulin is withheld.
- Intravenous infusion of normal saline has begun.
- Once active labor begins or glucose levels decrease to <70 mg/dL, the infusion is changed from saline to 5% dextrose and delivered at a rate of 100–150 mL/h (2.5 mg/kg/min) to achieve a glucose level of approximately 100 mg/dL.
- Glucose levels are checked hourly using a bedside meter allowing for adjustment in the insulin or glucose infusion rate.
- Regular (short-acting) insulin is administered by intravenous infusion at a rate of 1.2 U/h if glucose levels exceed 100 mg/dL.[14,16]

Another method of using insulin is according to technical guidelines of MoHFW GOI.

Intravenous (IV) infusion with normal saline to be started and regular insulin added according to the blood sugar levels as per **Table 2**.

Elective cesarean should be scheduled in morning, usual dose of intermediate-acting insulin should be given the previous night, morning dose of insulin is withheld. Fasting blood sugar levels

TABLE 2: Intravenous (IV) infusion with normal saline.

Blood sugar level	Amount of insulin added in 500 mL NS	Rate of NS infusion
90–120 mg/dL	0	100 mL/h (16 drops/min)
120–140 mg/dL	4U	100 mL/h (16 drops/min)
140–180 mg/dL	6U	100 mL/h (16 drops/min)
>180 mg/dL	8U	100 mL/h (16 drops/min)

done. Regional anesthesia used as a patient being awake permits early detection of hypoglycemia. The blood sugar levels are maintained between 70 and 100 mg/dL during surgery.

INDICATIONS FOR CESAREAN DELIVERY

- Malpresentation
- Proliferative retinopathy
- Pregnancy is complicated by preeclampsia
- Macrosomia (>4 kg)
- Previous cesarean
- Fetal distress prior to or during labor
- Bad obstetric history in elderly patients
- Poorly controlled diabetes
- Elderly primigravida

COMPLICATIONS TO BE ANTICIPATED

- Ketoacidosis
- Prolonged labor
- Shoulder dystocia
- Increased incidence of instrumental delivery
- Increased incidence of operative delivery
- Maternal soft tissue injuries, perineal tears, vaginal lacerations, and cervical tears
- Postpartum hemorrhage
- Subinvolution of uterus
- Puerperal sepsis
- Failed lactation

MANAGEMENT OF PRETERM LABOR

Drugs that can be safely used during preterm labor in a diabetic woman are nifedipine and magnesium sulfate. Tocolytic agents such as beta-mimetic, terbutaline, and ritodrine lead to maternal hyperglycemia hence used with caution. Corticosteroids used for accelerating fetal lung maturity can also cause maternal hyperglycemia and increase the risk of ketoacidosis. The blood sugar levels start rising within 6–12 hours of administration of corticosteroids and may persist up to 5 days. However, corticosteroids are indicated in women with DM and preterm labor.[17]

CARE OF NEWBORN

A neonatologist or pediatrician should be present at delivery to attend to the newborn. To look for any neonatal complications newborns are to be kept in a nursery for 48 hours.

Newborns should be carefully examined for Apgar score, any asphyxia, and congenital malformation. Any asphyxia should be energetically treated. The baby's blood sugar should be done at birth, at 6 hours, 12 hours, and then 12 hourly till 72 hours as neonatal hypoglycemia is very common in them.

Early and more frequent breastfeeding is recommended. Injection vitamin K 1 mg given intramuscularly.

Any neonatal complications such as hypocalcemia, hypokalemia, hypomagnesemia, hyperbilirubinemia, polycythemia, macrosomia, birth trauma injury, respiratory distress, hyaline membrane disease, hypertrophic cardiomyopathy, and hypoglycemia should be taken care off. Perinatal mortality has reduced significantly in recent years due to better management of diabetes during pregnancy and better neonatal care.

POSTPARTUM

All delivered patients should be hydrated properly in the postpartum period. Insulin requirement is reduced during the first 24–48 hours postpartum, hence dose of insulin should be reassessed. Blood sugar levels should be monitored every 2 hours.

Patients who have type 1 DM will remain insulin-dependent even after delivery so insulin is restarted at .5–.6 U/kg postpartum weight. Postpartum glycemic target can be relaxed to fasting and postprandial levels of 100 and 150 mg/dL, respectively.[18]

A significant fall in blood glucose levels may occur during breastfeeding, blood glucose levels should be monitored to evaluate the need for medication. In a breastfeeding mother, insulin is preferred, WHO states that oral hypoglycemic agents are not contraindicated in lactating mothers.[19] In patients on metformin monitoring of the baby for hypoglycemia is required as it is secreted in the milk.[20]

Gestational diabetes is the first warning of inherent insulin resistance. Women with GDM need to have glucose tolerance reassessed in the postpartum period. Recommendations for postpartum evaluation are based on a 50% likelihood of women with gestational diabetes developing overt diabetes within 20 years.[21] The fifth International Workshop Conference on Gestational Diabetes recommended that women diagnosed with gestational diabetes undergo evaluation with a 75-g oral glucose tolerance test (GTT) at 6–12 weeks postpartum and other intervals such as 1 year postpartum, annually, triannually, and then prepregnancy.[22]

The factors that increased the risk for abnormal GTT postpartum included: diagnosis of GDM at an earlier gestational age, higher glucose values on GTT during pregnancy, increased body mass index (BMI), and increased birth weight. Early identification of glucose intolerance gives the opportunity to institute measures such as exercise, diet control, and weight reduction which would help in preventing the progression of diabetes. Also identification and treatment of overt diabetes early in course offer opportunity to delay or avoid vascular complications associated with disease. Women with a history of GDM are at risk of cardiovascular complications associated with metabolic syndrome. Kessous and coworkers found that women with GDM were 2.6 times more likely to be hospitalized for cardiovascular morbidity.[23]

CONTRACEPTION

The barrier method is safe and ideal. Low-dose hormonal contraceptives, injectable progesterone, and intrauterine contraceptive device (IUCD can be used in women who have GDM. In overt diabetes, low dose hormonal contraceptives are used with caution; IUCD is avoided for fear of infection. Progesterone only pills can be used. The permanent method (sterilization) is done when the family is complete.

IMPLICATIONS FOR THE OFFSPRING

Diabetes during pregnancy poses health implications on children during infancy and adult life. Studies have shown that obesity, impaired glucose intolerance, and type 2 DM are more prevalent in those who were exposed to hyperglycemia during their fetal development. Long-term lifestyle modification may reduce the risk of diabetes later in life.[24]

REFERENCES

1. Felig P. Maternal and fetal fuel homeostasis in human pregnancy. Am J Clin Nutr. 1973; 26:998-1005.
2. Wild S, Roglic G, Green A, Sicree R, King H. Global prevalence of diabetes: Estimates for the year 2000 and projecting for 2030. Diabetes Care. 2004;27:1047-53.
3. Bhattacharya G, Awasthi RT, Kumar S. Routine screening for gestational diabetes mellitus with glucose challenge test in antenatal patients. J Obstet Gynaecol India. 2001;51:245.
4. Seshiah V, Balaji V, Sanjeevi CB, Green A, et al. Gestational diabetes mellitus in India. J Assoc Physicians India. 2004;52:707-11.
5. American College of Obstetricians and Gynecologists Committee on Practice Bulletins—Obstetrics. ACOG Practice Bulletin. Clinical management guidelines for obstetrician-gynecologists. Gestational Diabetes. Obstet Gynecol. 2001;98(3):523-37.
6. Landon MB, Vickers S. Fetal surveillance in pregnancy complicated by diabetes mellitus, is it necessary? J Matern Fetal Neonatal Med. 2002;12:413-6.
7. ACOG. (2001). ACOG Practice Bulletin Number 30.Gestational Diabetes.[online] Available from https://www.semanticscholar. org/paper/ACOG-Practice-Bulletin%2C-Number-30%2C-September-2001/b78b 375917f3eec740e4616ca7ab428c2bd4b85f [Last accessed December, 2021].
8. Graves LR. Antepartum fetal surveillance and timing of delivery in the pregnancy complicated by diabetes mellitus. Clin Obstet and Gynaecol. 2007;50(4):1007-13.
9. Pietryga M, Brazer J, Wender-Ożegowska E, et al. Placental Doppler velocimetry in gestational diabetes mellitus. J Perinatal Med. 2006;34:108-10.
10. Jacobson JD, Cousins L. A population-based study of maternal and perinatal outcomes in patients with gestational diabetes. Am J Obstet Gynecol. 1989;161:413-6.
11. Naylor CD, Sermer M, Chen E, Sykora K. Cesarean delivery in relation to birth weight and gestational glucose intolerance: pathophysiology of practice style? JAMA. 1996; 275:1165-70.
12. Miailhe G, Le Ray C, Timsit J, Lepercq L. Factors associated with urgent cesarean delivery in women with type 1 diabetes mellitus. Obstet Gynecol. 2003;121:983.
13. Gabbe SG, Carpenter LB, Garrison EA. New strategies for glucose control in patients with Type 1 and Type 2 Diabetes Mellitus in Pregnancy. Clin Obstet Gynecol. 2007;50(4):1014-24.
14. Coustan DR. Delivery: timing, mode, and management. In: Reece EA, Coustan DR, Gabbe SG (Eds). Diabetes in Women: Adolescence, Pregnancy, and Menopause, 3rd edition. Philadelphia (PA): Lippincott Williams & Wilkins; 2004.
15. Jovanovic L, Peterson CM. Management of the pregnant, insulin-dependent diabetic woman. Diabetes Care. 1980;3:63-8
16. ACOG Committee on Practice Bulletins. Pregestational diabetes mellitus. ACOG Practice Bulletin No 60. Americian College of Obstetricians and Gynecologists. Obstet Gynecol. 2005; 105:675-85.
17. Kaushal K, Gibson JM, Railton A, Hounsome B, New JP, Young RJ. A protocol for improved glycemic control following corticosteroid therapy in diabetic pregnancies. Diabet Med. 2003;20:73-5.
18. Kjos SZ, Brehanan TA. Postpartum management, lactation and contraception. In: Reece EA, Consten DR, Garbe SG (Eds). Diabetes in Women, 3rd edition. Philadelphia: Lippincott, Williams and Wilkins; 2004; pp. 441-2.
19. WHO. (2002). Breastfeeding and maternal medication: Recommendations for the drugs in the eleventh WHO model list of essential drugs 2002. [online] Available from https://apps.who. int/iris/handle/10665/62435 [Last accessed December, 2021].
20. Hale TW, Kristensen TH, Hackett LP, Kohan R, Ilett KF. Transfer of metformin into the human milk. Diabetologia. 2002;45:1509-14.
21. O'Sullivan JB. Bodyweight and subsequent diabetes mellitus. JAMA. 1982;248:949.
22. Metzger BE, Buchanan TA, Coustan DR, de Leiva A, Dunger DB, Hadden DR, et al. Summary and recommendations of the fifth International Workshop-Conference on Gestational Diabetes. Diabetes Care. 2007;30(Suppl 2):S251.
23. Kessous R, Shoham-Vardi I, Pariente G, Sherf M, Sheiner E. An association between gestational diabetes mellitus and long-term maternal cardiovascular morbidity. Heart. 2013;99:1118-21.
24. Dabalea D, Knowler WC, Pettitt D. Effect of diabetes in pregnancy on offspring: Follow up research in the Pima Indians. J Mat Fet Med. 1993;9:83-8.

Aarti Chitkara, Neharika Malhotra

INTRODUCTION

Maternal cardiac disease is a major cause of nonobstetric maternal morbidity and mortality due to early diagnosis and women with cardiac disease entering pregnancy as a result of improved medical and surgical care adding to their reproductive years. In addition, more women opting for delayed conception, advancing maternal age contributes to medical conditions such as hypertension, diabetes, and hypercholesterolemia and increase the incidence of acquired heart disease complicating pregnancy.

A well-coordinated multidisciplinary approach including a maternal-fetal medicine specialist, cardiologist, and obstetrical anesthesiologist is of paramount importance to bring about an optimal maternal and fetal outcome.

CARDIAC PHYSIOLOGY DURING PREGNANCY

Maternal changes in cardiac output (CO), blood pressure (BP), systemic vascular resistance, heart rate (HR), and changes in blood volume begin early in pregnancy, reach their peak during the late second trimester, and then remain relatively constant until delivery. Understanding the physiological alterations is important to correctly interpret hemodynamic and cardiovascular tests during pregnancy, labor, and delivery; to predict the effects of pregnancy on the woman with underlying cardiac disease and to understand how the fetus will be affected by maternal cardiac disorders.

A thorough understanding of hemodynamic changes related to labor and delivery is essential for better preparedness to anticipate which cardiac conditions predispose to decompensation in the peripartum period and select appropriate monitoring and interventions to minimize the risk.

Figure 1 demonstrates the change in CO during different stages of labor and **Figure 2** demonstrates hemodynamic changes with contractions.

Labor: Pain, anxiety, and autotransfusion during each contraction contribute to increase in CO during labor. Stroke volume (SV) and HR rise and fall with each contraction, with peaks as high as 50% above prelabor values.

Delivery: Cardiac output peaks immediately after vaginal delivery or cesarean delivery reaching as high as 59% and SV 71%, persist for at least 1 hour, while HR decreases and BP remains unchanged.[1,2]

During and immediately after delivery, factors that affect the hemodynamic status in patients with cardiovascular disease include:
- Underlying cardiac pathology
- Gestational age
- Intravascular fluid status
- Positioning of the patient
- Route, dose, and choice of uterotonic agents
- Anesthetic agents

RISK STRATIFICATION

Disease-specific risk assessment should be done using modified WHO (mWHO) classification as depicted in **Table 1**. This classification system is currently the most accurate system of risk assessment. Predictors identified in studies including large populations such as CARPREG (CARdiac disease in PREGnancy), ZAHARA, and ROPAC (Registry Of Pregnancy And Cardiac disease) should be used to further refine risk estimation in such patients.

MONITORING DURING LABOR

Maternal BP and HR should be monitored in all patients with cardiac disease. Intra-arterial

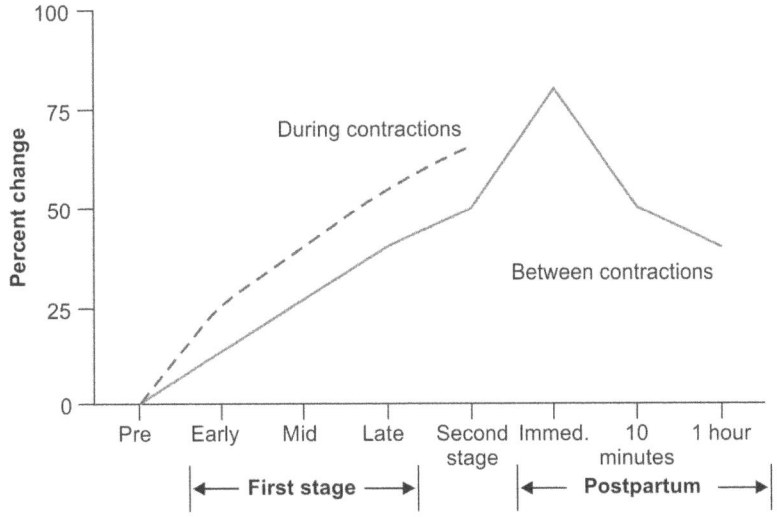

Fig. 1: Cardiac output during normal labor, delivery, and postpartum.

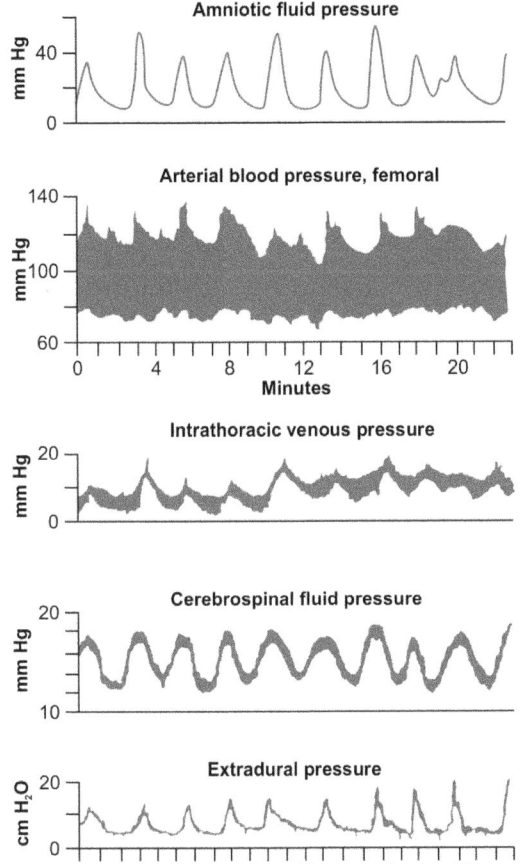

Fig. 2: Hemodynamics with contractions.

BP (IABP) monitoring may be used in women with more severe heart disease. Early signs of decompensation may be picked up with pulse oximetry and continuous ECG monitoring. A pulmonary artery catheter (PAC) is of uncertain benefit and should be avoided.[3]

OBSTETRIC CONCERNS: GENERAL PRINCIPLES

Planned Induction versus Spontaneous Onset of Labor

Risk stratification can help identify high-risk patients on case-to-case basis which can help take clinical decision with a multidisciplinary approach to schedule induction of labor. Timing of induction will depend on cardiac status, obstetric evaluation including cervical assessment, fetal well-being, and fetal lung maturity.

Monitoring: It is imperative to attach appropriate maternal monitoring devices, intravascular access, and epidural catheter for labor analgesia to help mitigate hemodynamic instability related to pain and stress of labor.

Method: Induction can be done using either mechanical or pharmacological methods. Both misoprostol (25 µg, PGE1) or dinoprostone (1–3 mg) can be used safely. Mechanical methods such as a cervical ripening balloon, artificial rupture

TABLE 1: Modified from World Health Organization (WHO) risk stratification.

WHO I	*WHO II*
• Pulmonary stenosis (small/mild) • Patent ductus arteriosus (small/mild) • Mitral valve prolapse (small/mild) • Successfully repaired simple shunt defects (ASD, VSD, PDA, APVR)	• Unrepaired ASD or VSD • Repaired tetralogy of Fallot • Turner syndrome without aortic dilatation
Follow-up during pregnancy: Once or twice in local hospital **Delivery:** Local hospital	**Follow-up during pregnancy:** Every trimester in local hospital **Delivery:** Local hospital
WHO II-III	*WHO III*
• Mild left ventricular impairment (EF>S4%) • Native or tissue valve disease not considered WHO I or IV • Marfan or other HTAD syndrome without aortic dilatation • Aorta <45 mm in bicuspid aortic valve • Repaired coarctation • AVSD	• Left ventricular impairment (30–45%) • Mechanical valve • Systemic right ventricle with good or mildly impaired function • Fontan (if otherwise well) • Unrepaired cyanotic disease • Moderate mitral stenosis • Severe asymptomatic aortic stenosis • Moderate aortic dilatation
Follow-up during pregnancy: Bimonthly in expert center **Delivery:** Expert center	**Follow-up during pregnancy:** (Bi)monthly in expert center **Delivery:** Expert center

WHO IV: Pregnancy not recommended
• Pulmonary arterial hypertension • Severe systemic ventricular dysfunction (EF<30%) • Moderate systemic right ventricular dysfunction • Severe mitral stenosis • Severe symptomatic aortic stenosis • Severe aortic dilatation • Vascular Ehlers–Dantos • Severe (re)coarctation • Fontan with any complication
Follow-up during pregnancy: Monthly in expert center **Delivery:** Expert center

(APVR: anomalous pulmonary venous return; ASD: atrial septal defect; AVSD: atrioventricular septal defect; EF: ejection fraction; HTAD: hereditary thoracic aorta disease; PDA: persistent ductus arteriosus; VSD; ventricular septal defect)

Source: Adapted and modified for congenital heart disease, from the ESC 2018 "Cardiovascular diseases during Pregnancy (management of) Guidelines" Table 3.

of membranes, and infusion of oxytocin can be safely used in women with heart disease.

A semirecumbent position with a lateral tilt is preferred during the intrapartum period with monitoring of vital signs in between contractions.

ROUTE OF DELIVERY

Vaginal delivery is the preferred mode of delivery and cesarean section is reserved for obstetric indications unless there is an underlying aortopathy such as aortic dissection, dilated aorta > 4.5 cm with Marfan syndrome or progressive aortic dilatation during gestation; severe pulmonary artery hypertension or Eisenmenger syndrome; maternal warfarin with therapeutic international normalized ratio (INR) in labor.

Vaginal-assisted Delivery

Epidural analgesia during labor in patients with cardiac disease decreases the pain and anxiety of labor. Fetal descent during second stage of labor is achieved with adequate uterine contractions and the birth can be supplemented with the help of low or outlet operative vaginal delivery (either forceps or vacuum extraction).

A preanesthetic evaluation of maternal hemodynamic tolerance of pushing using pulse oximetry waveform and saturation particularly in patients with intracardiac shunts is important.

■ ENDOCARDITIS PROPHYLAXIS

Routine antimicrobial prophylaxis to reduce the risk of infective endocarditis is not recommended following either vaginal delivery or cesarean section. However, it is reasonable to administer antibiotic prophylaxis prior to delivery (i.e., 30–60 minutes before the estimated time of delivery) in women deemed at highest risk of adverse outcomes from endocarditis such as those with prosthetic heart valves, prior infective endocarditis, or unrepaired cyanotic congenital heart disease, cardiac transplantation with valve regurgitation due to a structurally abnormal valve.

A single intravenous dose of ampicillin 2 g IV or IM or cefazolin or ceftriaxone 1 g IV or IM. In patients allergic to penicillins, cefazolin or ceftriaxone 1 g IV or IM or clindamycin 600 mg IM or IV is recommended.

■ DRUGS USED DURING PERIPARTUM PERIOD

- *Oxytocin*: Administered as a dilute solution in infusion form and not as IV bolus[4]
  Cardiovascular changes[5]
  ↓ Mean arterial pressure, total peripheral vascular resistance, ↑ peripheral vascular resistance ↓ Afterload, ↑ heart rate

Conditions at maximum risk:
  – Aortic stenosis
  – Hypertrophic obstructive cardiomyopathy
  – Ischemic heart disease
  – Aortopathy with risk of dissection
- *Misoprostol*: Few case reports suggest cardiovascular events due to coronary vasospasm due to misoprostol which were successfully resuscitated with nitroglycerine and hence should be avoided in women with a history of vasospastic angina or significant coronary artery disease.[6,7]
- *Carboprost*: It is known to cause bronchospasm, alteration in ventilation/perfusion ratio and hence should be avoided in patients with intracardiac shunt or single ventricle physiology due to significant reduction of CO.
- *Methergine*: Cardiovascular changes
  – *Vasoconstriction*: It can lead to sudden hypertension and resultant stroke
  – *Coronary vasospasm*: Potential to cause myocardial infarction (MI) in patients with ischemic heart disease (IHD)
  – ↑ *Pulmonary artery pressure*: It can cause shunt reversal and cyanosis in patients with intracardiac shunts
- *Magnesium sulfate*: MgSO$_4$ toxicity leading to respiratory arrest and hypoxia may lead to secondary cardiac dysfunction.
- *Antihypertensive agents*: Antihypertensives should be cautiously used in women with cardiac lesions sensitive to hypotension through gradual titration and more intensive monitoring.

Vasodilation, decreased SVR, decreases coronary perfusion	Reflex tachycardia
Avoid in aortic stenosis (AS) or HCM	Avoid in mitral stenosis (MS)

■ LABOR CONCERNS IN SPECIFIC CARDIAC LESIONS

- *Atrial septal defect (ASD):* Labor is generally well tolerated. Monitor the patient for arrhythmias, BP changes, and restrict the amount of fluid. Epidural analgesia is preferred as it may prevent any left-to-right shunt due to reduction in systemic vascular resistance.

- *Ventricular septal defect (VSD):* Avoid hypotension to prevent shunt reversal. Endocarditis prophylaxis is recommended by the British Society of Antimicrobial Chemotherapy.[8]
- *Pulmonary hypertension:* It is defined as mean pulmonary artery pressure > 25 mm Hg. A carefully monitored and assisted vaginal delivery can safely be allowed in centers equipped with multidisciplinary team. Intra-arterial BP monitoring with radial line in situ, oxygen on flow at 5-6 L/minute with epidural analgesia are some prerequisites. A pulmonary artery catheter is rarely necessary. Oxytocin and prostaglandin E can safely be used for induction, but avoid uterine hyperstimulation. Intravenous prostacyclin and inhaled nitric oxide should be readily available that can help improve oxygenation, decrease pulmonary vascular resistance, decrease the risk of thromboembolism by causing vascular dilatation and inhibiting platelet aggregation. Vaginal delivery with cut short second stage of labor using forceps or a vacuum to decrease maternal efforts is recommended.
- *Eisenmenger syndrome:* Right ventricular function and degree of pulmonary hypertension should be evaluated using echocardiography. Cardiac catheterization may be necessary to quantify pulmonary hypertension that can guide management in labor.
- *Pulmonary stenosis:* Monitor for signs of right heart failure (HF) during the postpartum period and cesarean section is usually reserved for obstetric indications.
- *Peripartum cardiomyopathy (PPCM):* Urgent delivery irrespective of gestation should be considered in women with advanced HF and hemodynamic instability despite optimal management. Vaginal delivery can be allowed in stable congestive HF.
- *Management of Implantable cardioverter-defibrillators (ICDs) and pacemakers:* For women with ICD in labor, the function is left on whereas the anti-tachyarrhythmia therapy is disabled during cesarean section with continuous cardiac monitoring.
- *Rheumatic heart disease in labor:* Rheumatic valvular heart disease is the most common cardiac disease encountered in pregnancy in our developing countries. The challenges posed by the severity of lesion and anticoagulants received by these women are often intriguing to the obstetrician. Multidisciplinary delivery planning with elective termination of pregnancy is important in these patients. In women with mild symptoms and good functional status, vaginal delivery with consideration of an assisted second stage of labor to reduce the need for prolonged Valsalva is appropriate. In highly symptomatic patients, planned cesarean section with the assistance of a cardiac anesthesiologist may be required.[9]

Anticoagulation should be held prior to delivery because therapeutic anticoagulation increases the risk for hemorrhagic complications with regional anesthesia, and warfarin (which crosses the placenta) increases the risk for fetal intraventricular hemorrhage.[10] Warfarin should be held after 36 weeks gestation and replaced with low molecular weight heparin (LMWH) or unfractionated heparin. Anticoagulation should be discontinued 24 hours prior to the induction of labor or cesarean section.[11] Intravenous unfractionated heparin can then be resumed 6 hours after a vaginal delivery or 12 hours after a cesarean delivery, if adequate hemostasis is achieved.[12] Warfarin may be resumed postpartum and is safe for use during breastfeeding.

■ POSTPARTUM MONITORING

The underlying cardiac disease or any peripartum event determines the intensity of postpartum monitoring in a patient with cardiac disease. International Federation of Gynecology and Obstetrics (FIGO) recommends first postpartum cardiovascular screening in women at 6-12 weeks which includes BP and proteinuria assessment, evaluation of BMI and lifestyle, smoking, and family history of cardiovascular disease (CVD). Extended cardiovascular phenotyping including investigation of macrovascular function (e.g., reactive hyperemia index, pulse wave velocity, augmentation index) structure (e.g., carotid intima thickness), microvessel structure, or cardiac echocardiography is restricted to women with high-risk CVD.[13]

REFERENCES

1. Kjeldsen J. Hemodynamic investigations during labour and delivery. Acta Obstetricia et Gynecologica Scandinavica. 1979; 58(sup89):18-249.
2. Ueland K, Hansen JM. Maternal cardiovascular dynamics: II. Posture and uterine contractions. Am J Obstet Gynecol. 1969;103(1):1-7.
3. Devitt JH, Noble WH, Byrick RJ. A Swan-Ganz catheter related complication in a patient with Eisenmenger's syndrome. Anesthesiology. 1982;57(4):335-7.
4. Jayasooriya G, Silversides C, Raghavan G, Balki M. Anesthetic management of women with heart failure during pregnancy–a retrospective cohort study. Int J Obstet Anesthesia. 2020; 44:40-50.
5. Secher NJ, Arnsbo P, Wallin L. Haemodynamic effects of oxytocin (Syntocinon®) and methyl ergometrine (Methergin®) on the systemic and pulmonary circulations of pregnant anaesthetized women. Acta obstetricia et gynecologica Scandinavica. 1978;57(2):97-103.
6. Matthesen T, Olsen RH, Bosselmann HS, Lidegaard Ø. [Cardiac arrest induced by vasospastic angina pectoris after vaginally administered misoprostol]. Ugeskrift Laeger. 2017;179(26):V02170167.
7. Owusu KA, Brennan JJ, Perelman A, Meoli E, Altshuler J. Nitroglycerin administration during cardiac arrest caused by coronary vasospasm secondary to misoprostol. Journal of Cardiology cases. 2015;12(5):166-8.
8. Crossley GH, Poole JE, Rozner MA, Asirvatham SJ, Cheng A, Chung MK, et al. The Heart Rhythm Society (HRS)/American Society of Anesthesiologists (ASA) expert consensus statement on the perioperative management of patients with implantable defibrillators, pacemakers and arrhythmia monitors: facilities and patient management: this document was developed as a joint project with the American Society of Anesthesiologists (ASA), and in collaboration with the American Heart Association (AHA), and the Society of Thoracic Surgeons (STS). Heart Rhythm. 2011; 8(7):1114-54.
9. Kela M, Buddhi M. Combined mitral and aortic stenosis in parturient: Anesthesia management for labor and delivery. J Anaesth Clin Pharmacol. 2017;33(1):114-6.
10. Hall JG, Pauli RM, Wilson KM. Maternal and fetal sequelae of anticoagulation during pregnancy. Am J Med. 1980;68(1):122-40.
11. Bates SM, Greer IA, Middeldorp S, Veenstra DL, Prabulos AM, Vandvik PO. VTE, thrombophilia, antithrombotic therapy, and pregnancy: Antithrombotic Therapy and Prevention of Thrombosis, 9th ed: American College of Chest Physicians Evidence-Based Clinical Practice Guidelines. Chest. 2012 Feb 1;141(2):e691S-736S.
12. European Society of Gynecology (ESG); Association for European Paediatric Cardiology (AEPC); German Society for Gender Medicine (DGesGM); Regitz-Zagrosek V, Blomstrom Lundqvist C, Borghi C, et al. ESC Guidelines on the management of cardiovascular diseases during pregnancy: the Task Force on the Management of Cardiovascular Diseases during Pregnancy of the European Society of Cardiology (ESC). Eur Heart J. 2011;32(24):3147-97.
13. Sheiner E, Kapur A, Retnakaran R, Hadar E, Poon LC, McIntyre HD, et al. FIGO (International Federation of Gynecology and Obstetrics) Postpregnancy Initiative: Long-term Maternal Implications of Pregnancy Complications—Follow-up Considerations. Int J Gynecol Obstet. 2019;147:1-31.

36

Obese Woman in Labor

Bhavana Mittal, Chandana S Bhat

DEFINITION

According to the World Health Organization, "overweight" is defined as a body mass index (BMI) between 25 and 30 kg/m^2 and "obesity" is defined as a BMI of 30 kg/m^2 or greater whereas according to Asian standards obesity is defined as BMI >25 kg/m^2.

CLASSIFICATION

The degree of obesity is classified into three categories:
1. Class I (BMI 30.0–34.9 kg/m^2)
2. Class II (BMI 35.0–39.9 kg/m^2)
3. Class III (BMI > 40 kg/m^2; "morbidly obese").

RISKS

Obese women are at increased risk of:
- Cesarean delivery
- Endometritis
- Wound rupture/dehiscence
- Venous thrombosis
- Twofold increased risk of maternal morbidity
- Fivefold risk of neonatal injury.

MANAGEMENT

Maternal obesity alone is not an indication for induction of labor although they are at increased risk of a prolonged pregnancy and have an increased rate of induction of labor. Obese women are at increased risk for intrapartum complications and failed induction, and this risk rises with greater degrees of obesity. With class I and II (35–39.9 kg/m^2) obesity, women who underwent an induction of labor required a cesarean delivery 20.2 and 24.2% of the time, respectively, whereas women with a BMI from 40 to 50 kg/m^2 had a failed induction rate of 31.6% and as high as 63.2% in women with a BMI

> 60 kg/m^2. Maternal age, race, and gestational age at delivery did not have an impact on obese woman's rate of requiring a cesarean delivery after induction. Favorable factors for a successful induction in obese woman include multiparity and Bishop's score at admission >5.

The length of labor in nulliparous women is proportional to maternal BMI. In overweight women, the prolongation was between 4 and 6 cm, and for obese women, labor was slower before 7 cm. TOLAC success rates are inversely related to BMI: for a BMI > 19.8, the rate is 83.1%; when BMI is between 19.8 and 26, the rate is 79.9%; between 26.1 and 29, the rate is 69.3%; and when BMI exceeds 29, the rate is 68.2%.

OUTCOMES OF DIFFERENT INDUCTION AGENTS IN OBESE WOMEN

There are only a few studies that have specifically compared the outcomes of different induction methods for obese women. Misoprostol appears to be a more effective induction agent than dinoprostone in obese women. There are differences in the labor progression and medication requirements when comparing nonobese to obese women who receive misoprostol. Obese women who receive misoprostol take longer to deliver than nonobese women by up to 4 hours which is more so for morbidly obese patients. Obese and morbidly obese women who receive misoprostol are more likely to require oxytocin for augmentation of labor, with odds ratio of 1.5 and 2.1, respectively, than their nonobese counterparts and they require 1.5–2 times the amount oxytocin for longer time periods, 15–19 hours versus 14 hours. This is in spite of the fact that an obese BMI makes a woman more likely to not achieve active labor and have a cesarean delivery for a failed induction.

LABOR AND INTRAPARTUM MONITORING

A venous access should be established early in labor and consideration should be given to the timing of epidural analgesia in labor due to increased difficulties with epidural placement, resulting in multiple attempts, and an increased risk of inadequate analgesia.

Monitoring contractions and assessing labor progress can be challenging—manual palpation and external tocodynamometry are most commonly used, but in obese women, the distance between the skin and the uterus leads to frequent signal dropout.

While there is no specific requirement for continuous electronic fetal monitoring in labor in an otherwise uncomplicated pregnancy, many obese parturients have other indications for continuous fetal monitoring, such as hypertension, or induction of labor (IOL). Abdominal adiposity can make external fetal monitoring with cardiotocography (CTG) more difficult. Internal monitoring by fetal scalp electrode should be considered if a satisfactory recording is not obtained by external monitoring.

Labor Dystocia

Obese women have longer labors, with longer duration and slower progression of the first stage of labor demonstrated in both nulliparous and multiparous women.

Though the exact mechanism of impaired uterine contractility is unknown, dysfunction in endocrine and metabolic function may lead to alterations in the normal parturition pathways in obese women. After adjusting for maternal height, pregnancy weight gain, labor induction, membrane rupture, oxytocin use, epidural analgesia, and fetal size, the median duration of labor from 4 to 10 cm is longer in obese women 6.2 hours for normal-weight women, 7.5 hours for overweight women, and 7.9 hours for obese women. The slow progression occurs mostly between 4 and 6 cm in the overweight, and up to 7 cm in obese women. No significant differences occur after cervical dilatation of 7 cm, with labor curves for women with a BMI of >30 kg/m^2 demonstrating a more gradual slope from 4 to 6 cm, and then relatively similar slopes to women with a BMI, 30 kg/m^2

thereafter in the active phase of labor, for both nulliparous and multiparous women.

When the maternal and fetal status are reassuring, increased time for cervical ripening and to progress in the first stage of labor (particularly when cervical dilatation is 7 cm) should be permitted.

Data regarding instrumental delivery in the second stage is conflicting with only few studies showing increased risk of instrumental delivery. Obese women are also more prone for shoulder dystocia with a 2.7-fold increased risk.

Cesarean Section in the Obese Woman

The risk of cesarean delivery is double for obese women compared to women with a normal BMI. Common indications for emergency cesarean section include labor dystocia and fetal distress. There is debate about the value of elective cesarean section over vaginal delivery. As the rates of cesarean section in morbidly obese women already approach 50%, and morbidity occurs with increased frequency in emergency cesarean sections, it has been argued that planned cesarean section allows the procedure to be carried out at a time where most personnel are available, potentially reducing the risks.

Risks Associated with Cesarean Section in an Obese Woman

- General anesthesia with an increased risk of difficult or failed intubation and gastric aspiration
- Increased risk of epidural failure
- Two- to fourfold increased risk of postoperative wound complications
- Postoperative venous thromboembolism (VTE).

Considerations during Cesarean in an Obese Woman

- The choice between transverse and vertical incision is controversial, and the type of skin incision should take the woman's body habitus into consideration.
- *Pfannenstiel incision*: Less postoperative pain and wound complications

- In the woman with a voluminous pannus, a supraumbilical approach allows direct access to the lower uterine segment as the umbilicus in such women is distorted caudally.
- Do not to dissect the subcutaneous tissues excessively, so that dead space is minimized.
- Closure of the subcutaneous layer in women with at least 2 cm of adipose tissue has been shown to decrease the risk of wound complications.
- Perioperative broad-spectrum antibiotics commenced before the skin incision, reduce the risk of infection, and should be given to all women regardless of BMI.

POSTPARTUM CONSIDERATIONS

Maternal

- Postpartum hemorrhage (PPH) is increased due to the association with macrosomia, or the large volume of distribution in obese women, which may reduce the efficacy of standard doses of uterotonic drugs.
- Venous thromboembolism
- Pulmonary embolism

Because cesarean delivery increases the risk of VTE, placement of pneumatic compression devices has been recommended for all patients before and after cesarean delivery by the American College of Obstetricians and Gynecologists (ACOG).

Neonatal Complications

- Macrosomia
- Increased risk of the metabolic syndrome and childhood obesity
- Asthma
- Autism spectrum disorders, childhood developmental delay, and attention-deficit/hyperactivity disorder.

CONCLUSION

The significant and consistent association between obesity and maternal, fetal, and neonatal complications indicates the need for appropriate antenatal planning, involving a multidisciplinary approach.

All pregnant women should be reminded of the importance of tempered gestational weight gain.

In an attempt to decrease the primary cesarean section rate in obese women, provided maternal and fetal status is reassuring, ample time to progress in the first stage of labor should be allowed.

In women with extremely morbid obesity and multiple risk factors for failing a trial of labor, there may be a role for individualized counseling and discussion of a planned cesarean delivery.

BIBLIOGRAPHY

1. ACOG Practice Bulletin No. 107: Induction of labor. Obstet Gynecol. 2009;114(Pt 1): 386-97.
2. Arrowsmith S, Wray S, Quenby S. Maternal obesity and labour complications following induction of labour in prolonged pregnancy. BJOG. 2011;118:578-88.
3. Crane JM, Murphy P, Burrage L, Hutchens D. Maternal and perinatal outcomes of extreme obesity in pregnancy. J Obstet Gynaecol Can. 2013;35:606-11.
4. Girsen AI, Osmundson SS, Naqvi M, Garabedian MJ, Lyell DJ. Body mass index and operative times at cesarean delivery. Obstet Gynecol. 2014;124:684-9.
5. Grasch JL, Thompson JL, Newton JM, Zhai AW, Osmundson SS. Trial of labor compared with cesarean delivery in superobese women. Obstet Gynecol. 2017;130:994-1000.
6. Hannaford KE, Tuuli MG, Odibo L, Macones GA, Odibo AO. Gestational weight gain: association with adverse pregnancy outcomes. Am J Perinatol. 2017;34:147-54.
7. Nuthalapaty FS, Rouse DJ, Owen J. The association of maternal weight with cesarean risk, labor duration, and cervical dilation rate during labor induction. Obstet Gynecol. 2004; 103:452-6.
8. Ruhstaller K. Induction of labor in the obese patient. Semin Perinatol. 2015;39(6):437-40.
9. Tipton AM, Cohen SA, Chelmow D. Wound infection in the obese pregnant woman. Semin Perinatol. 2011;35:345-9.
10. Wolfe KB, Rossi RA, Warshak CR. The effect of maternal obesity on the rate of failed induction of labor. Am J Obstet Gynecol. 2011;205:128. e1-7.

Anemic Patient in Labor

Ranjana Khanna, Parul Gupta Khanna

INTRODUCTION

Anemia in pregnancy is very common in developing nations. According to World Health Organization (WHO), the incidence of anemia in pregnancy in developing nations ranges between 35 and 75% with an average of 56%.[1] The *incidence in India* stands as high as 62–85%.[2-5]

The Government of India is spreading awareness regarding the prevention of anemia (*Anemia Mukt Bharat, PMSMA*) in pregnant females, but still, there are many patients with severe anemia who directly report late in the third trimester or in labor. So a lot of ground needs to be covered in prevention but till that time comes we have tried to give the basic outline of anemia in pregnancy with special emphasis on the management of anemic patients in labor.

ETIOLOGY[6] (TABLE 1)

Iron deficiency is one of the major etiological factors of anemia in pregnancy. Iron stores are limited and pregnancy causes an increase in demands by nearly 1,000 mg. This can be divided into the following.

The normal iron requirement during pregnancy ranges from 900 to 1,400 mg. This is equivalent to nearly 6.3 mg/day. There is an additional requirement of 1 mg/day during the lactation phase. De Leeuw et al. postulated that in case the iron supplements are not taken then it may lead to no detectable iron stores at term. This deficit requires 2 years to fill up.

During pregnancy, the iron absorption from the gut increases from 7 to 66% but then also it may not be enough. It is also essential to remember that the child acts as a parasite and maintains hemoglobin even at the expense of the mother.

Even though, the majority of cases are due to iron deficiency, other contributors of anemia should be considered. These include folate and vitamin B_{12} deficiency, infectious diseases, parasitic diseases, and hemoglobinopathies.

PHYSIOLOGICAL HEMATOGENOUS CHANGES IN PREGNANCY[7]

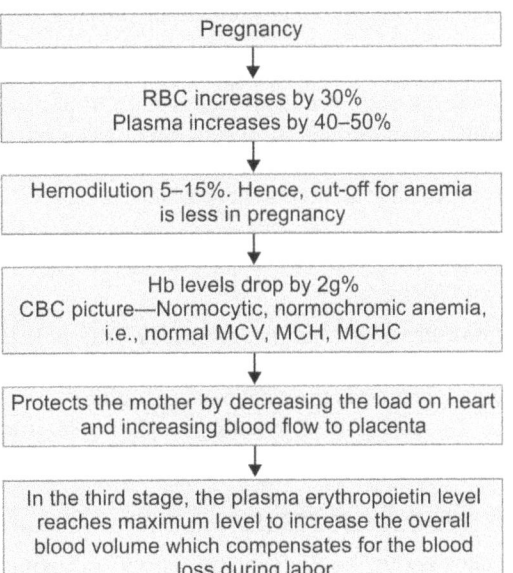

TABLE 1: Etiological factors of anemia in pregnancy.	
Increased RBC mass	450 mg
Fetal growth	225 mg
Placental development	80 mg
Blood loss during normal delivery	225 mg

DEFINITION[6,7]

Definitions	Pregnancy with hemoglobin levels
WHO	11 g/dL
WHO: Mild*	10–10.9 g/dL
WHO: Moderate	7–9.9 g/dL
WHO: Severe	<7 g/dL
CDC	11 g/dL in first trimester and 10.5 g/dL in the second trimester
ICMR: Mild	8–10.9 g/dL
ICMR: Moderate	5–7.9 g/dL
ICMR: Severe	<5 g/dL
ACOG and BCSH	11 g/dL in first trimester and 10.5 g/dL in the second and third trimester

*According to WHO, *mild anemia is a misnomer as the iron stores have already been depleted by the time the anemia is detected.* Even if there is no anemia then also there may be serious consequences of iron deficiency. Hence, the underlying depletion of iron stores should always be taken into consideration.

(ACOG: American College of Obstetricians and Gynecologists; BCHS: British Committee for Standards in Haematology; CDC: Centers for Disease Control and Prevention; ICMR: Indian Council of Medical Research; WHO: World Health Organization)

There are no recommendations by the WHO as to which trimester this cut-off should be followed. It has been seen that the fall in hemoglobin in the second trimester is around 0.5 g/dL.

EFFECT OF ANEMIA ON MOTHER[7] (TABLE 2)

Iron deficiency results in decreased erythropoiesis leading to decreased oxygen carrying capacity of blood. This leads to the following conditions.

Hence problems to anticipate during labor in an anemic patient could be (Table 3).

EFFECT ON FETUS[7]

Following are the effects on the fetus in an anemic pregnancy:
- LBW

- Increased perinatal morbidity and mortality
- Decreased adolescent growth
- Fetal hypoxia
- Anemia in fetus
- Increased NICU admissions

In anemia, due to folate deficiency there are increased chances of congenital malformations and neural tube defects in the fetus besides the other effects listed above.

BLOOD WORKUP AND CLASSIFICATION

According to NICE guidelines,[8] testing should be done at the time of first checkup and then at 28 weeks. This gives enough time for the proper assessment and management of anemia if any. Ideally, the serum ferritin levels should also be done to get an estimate of the iron stores.

In the US, there is no protocol regarding the assessment of all females for the screening of anemia. Testing is recommended in females who show signs of malnutrition or iron deficiency anemia.[9] In the UK, the measurement of serum ferritin levels is not recommended.[10]

Only performing a hemoglobin level estimation is not enough in pregnant females. It is essential to also look at the other components of complete blood picture such as mean corpuscular volume (MCV), mean corpuscular hemoglobin (MCH), and mean corpuscular hemoglobin concentration (MCHC). This is essential to differentiate between iron deficiency anemia and physiological anemia of pregnancy.[6]

Once anemia is detected then it is essential to differentiate the cause of anemia.

Complete blood count—MCV—microcytic (nutritional, hemoglobinopathies), normocytic (physiological, chronic disease, marrow suppression, or dual hematinic disease), and macrocytic (vitamin B_{12} or folate deficiency, thyroid disease, or liver dysfunction).
- Blood hematinics (iron, ferritin, vitamin B_{12}, folate)
- Reticulocytes
- Hemoglobin electrophoresis
- Lactate dehydrogenase
- Haptoglobin
- Bilirubin

In iron deficiency anemia during pregnancy, the MCV, MCH, and MCHC may be low and

TABLE 2: Effect of anemia.

Decreased exercise tolerance	Tiredness	Fatigue
Impaired cognition	Decreased mental concentration	Irritability
Depression	Palpitations	Headaches
Pallor	Glossitis	Angular cheilitis
Nail ridging	Koilonychias	Reduced immunity
Increased maternal mortality	Premature delivery and PROM	IUGR
Cardiac failure	Preeclampsia	Underperfused placenta, increased placental size, maternal hypertension

(IUGR: intrauterine growth restriction; PROM: prolonged rupture of membrane)

TABLE 3: Problems in anemic patients during labor.

PPH	Uterine inertia	Maternal exhaustion
Increased incidence of infection	Puerperal sepsis	Thromboembolism
Slow recovery and delayed wound healing	Subinvolution of uterus	Lactation failure

(PPH: postpartum hemorrhage)

on peripheral smear it shows microcytic, hypochromic with elliptocytes. However, with the increase in the erythropoietin levels of pregnancy large young blood cells may cause the MCV levels to appear normal. Hypochromic anemia may be present in hemoglobinopathies like microcytic anemias. A peripheral smear can help differentiate between iron deficiency anemia and other hemoglobinopathies. Hemoglobin electrophoresis is diagnostic for hemoglobinopathies.[6]

Serum ferritin is a measure of the iron stores in the body. It decreases early in iron deficiency anemia. However, since it is an acute phase reactant hence, C-reactive protein (CRP) should be done along with it. Serum ferritin levels if below 30 ng/mL then it indicates that the iron stores are insufficient and there is a high chance of anemia. Whereas, a level of 12 ng/mL indicates iron deficiency anemia in all stages of pregnancy.[6]

In low-resource settings, diagnosis of iron deficiency anemia can also be done with a trial therapy. If with oral iron therapy, there is an increase of Hb in 2–4 weeks then the diagnosis is confirmed.

MANAGEMENT OF ANEMIC PATIENT IN LABOR

The management of an anemic patient in labor depends on the stage of labor and the degree of anemia.

Women who are anemic twice as likely to go into labor early and three times as likely to deliver a baby with low birth weight. Anemia also increases the risk of pre-eclampsia, placental abruption, infections, postpartum hemorrhage (PPH), and cardiac failure.

Mild Anemia

For patients with mild anemia in any stage of labor, there is no active management required for managing anemia. Just have to be careful that there is no excessive blood loss during delivery. This includes the following methods such as avoidance of episiotomy, avoiding prolonged labor, suturing the episiotomy, and tears promptly. In the case of PPH, injection oxytocin intramuscularly (IM) and intravenous (IV) infusion is the first choice followed by prostaglandins either misoprostol P/R, orally, or carboprost IM can be added if bleeding continues. Injection ethylergometrine IM can be used with caution. It is also essential that in the postpartum period anemia is evaluated and treated accordingly.

Post-delivery the patient can be counseled regarding the importance of iron stores in the body and how to avoid anemia. This includes patient education regarding good eating habits and deworming. As there is iron requirement during lactation also hence, it is essential to boost up the iron stores postpartum either orally or parentally.

Appropriate contraceptive counseling should be done and a gap of minimum 2 years should be advised between subsequent pregnancies. This will help to replenish her iron stores.

Moderate Anemia[11]

Step-by-step management of moderate anemia should include the following:
- 1–2 times good IV access by 16 number cannula
- Blood grouping and cross-matching is done.
- Keep blood reserved
- Confirm the Hb levels, blood group, venereal disease research laboratory (VDRL), human immunodeficiency virus (HIV), blood sugar, hepatitis B surface antigen (HbsAg), urine analysis, thyroid stimulating hormone (TSH), and ultrasonography (USG). If not done then get the tests done stat
- Hb to be repeated if >1 month old reports.
- Obtain consent for blood transfusion
- If Hb < 8 g% then go ahead with packed red blood cells (PRBCs) transfusion
- Make the patient comfortable and prop her up if needed
- Allay her apprehensions
- Asepsis is of utmost importance.
- Oxygen inhalations if oxygen saturation is low.
- Avoid unnecessary episiotomy
- Suture episiotomy/perineal tear early
- *Lookout for PPH*: If bleeding is heavy then look for the cause—tears (cervical or vaginal) and uterine atony.
- *Uterine atony*: Look for retained placenta pieces or membrane.
- Drug of choice in PPH is oxytocin (IM or IV infusion). Oxytocin is kept at 2–8° C. Injection carbetocin an analog of oxytocin is stable at room temperature and can be given as a single dose.

- Prostaglandins (misoprostol) P/R or sublingual, or injection carboprost IM may also be used.
- If the bleeding is still uncontrolled then injection methylergometrine can be given IM with caution.
- PRBCs along with blood components fresh frozen plasma (FFP), cryoprecipitates, and platelets are transfused in the ratio 1:1:1:1.
- In the postpartum period, evaluate and treat the anemia
- Appropriate contraceptive counseling should be advised.

Severe Anemia[12]

Severe anemia (Hb < 5 g/dL) has 2 stages: (1) compensated and (2) decompensated. The latter is associated with cardiac failure which if untreated may lead to pulmonary edema and death.

Blood transfusion remains the mainstay for patients with severe anemia coming in last month or even directly in labor. However, it is essential to understand that massive blood transfusion will lead to an increase in blood volume which may push the heart toward failure. Patients with chronic anemia have severe myocardial ischemia which may be accompanied with cardiomegaly. Hence, packed cells are transfused very slowly under cover of a diuretic to maintain the blood volume. The patient should be kept in a propped up position with oxygen support. Step-by-step management of such patients includes the following:
- 1–2 times good IV access by 16 number cannula
- Send for blood grouping and cross-matching
- Keep blood reserved
- Confirm the Hb levels, blood group, VDRL, HIV, blood sugar, HbsAg, urine analysis, TSH, and USG. If not done then get the tests done stat
- Hb to be repeated if >1 month old
- Obtain consent for blood transfusion
- Give packed cell transfusion ≤ 2 units/day with administration of furosemide to prevent congestive heart failure. Target Hb level—9 g/dL
- In case of blood transfusion >2 units, it is advisable to administer injection calcium gluconate after measurement of ionized calcium in blood.

- In the second stage of labor, patient should be discouraged from straining during delivery.
- Prophylactic use of forceps and ventouse is recommended to reduce maternal exhaustion.
- Injection tranexamic acid 1 g IV slowly is recommended before the delivery of the baby in normal delivery and at the time of anesthesia before the incision. This can be repeated after 30 minutes if the bleeding is heavy.
- Replace all blood lost during delivery
- Actively manage third stage of labor
- Avoid unnecessary episiotomy
- Suture episiotomy/perineal tear early to avoid unnecessary blood loss.
- *Lookout for PPH*: If bleeding is heavy then look for the cause—tears and uterine atony
- *Uterine atony*: Look for retained placenta pieces or membrane
- Drug of choice is oxytocin (IM or IV). Injection carbetocin an analog of oxytocin is stable at room temperature and can be given as a single dose.
- Prostaglandins (misoprostol) P/R or sublingual. Injection carboprost can also be used.
- *Injection methylergometrine is however contraindicated.*
- In the postpartum period, evaluate type of anemia and treat it.
- Prophylactic antibiotics are to be given and thromboprophylaxis should be considered in appropriate cases.

It is important to understand that one packed cell transfusion contains around 240 mg of iron. This may be insufficient for boosting of the iron stores hence, a concomitant IV iron infusion helps to replete the iron stores and in the long run may help in decreasing the number of transfusions.[6]

It is essential to understand that postpartum Hb should be allowed 48 hours to settle before any further transfusions or management is planned. If the Hb concentration reached to anything above 11 g/dL nothing more needs to be done.[6]

SPECIAL CONSIDERATIONS
Thalassemia[13]

The management depends on the severity of anemia as discussed earlier. Some important points regarding the same:
- Blood reservation

- Lower segment cesarean section (lSCS) for obstetric indications only
- Active management of third stage of labor
- Breastfeeding is safe.
- Low molecular weight heparin after delivery till 7 days after discharge for normal delivery and 6 weeks for LSCS.
- The risk factors of thromboembolism in beta thalassemia include exposure of phosphatidylserine of abnormal red blood cells (RBCs), increase of platelet activation and aggregation and increased endothelial activation and decreased nitric oxide secondary to hemolysis.
- Chelation treatment with desferrioxamine which is discontinued during pregnancy in thalassemia major due to teratogenic effects on the fetus has to be restarted within the first week of puerperium.
- Contraceptive counseling should be done. However, in splenectomized women, oral contraceptives should be avoided due to high risk of thrombosis.

Sickle Cell Disease[14]

There are certain points to remember while managing a case of sickle cell disease (SCD).
- Avoid factors which precipitate sickle cell crisis (dehydration, overexertion, and extreme conditions)
- Vaginal delivery is recommended.
- LSCS if labor gets prolonged as it may lead to crisis.
- After 38 weeks induce labor or go ahead with LSCS as there is increased risk of placental abruption and stillbirth in later weeks of pregnancy.
- Keep blood reserved
- Check for atypical antibodies
- Secure good IV access
- In case if the patient has had a hip replacement due to avascular necrosis lithotomy position should be reconsidered.
- Keep patient warm and hydrated
- Continuous fetal heart rate (FHR) monitoring to check for placental abruption, mental distress, and stillbirth
- Continuous SPO_2 monitoring. Maternal SPO_2 should be maintained above 94%.

- If saturation falls below 94% arterial blood gas analysis should be done.
- Regional anesthesia is preferred for LSCS.
- Thromboprophylaxis as per thalassemia patients as there is increased risk of venous thromboembolism (VTE) in SCD patients.

CONCLUSION

Severely anemic patients coming in labor have a significantly higher incidence of perinatal and maternal morbidity and mortality. Such deliveries should be done in a tertiary care center where blood transfusion facility and intensive care facilities including neonatal intensive care unit (NICU) are available. It is essential to do active management of labor as well as of anemia to ensure the well-being of the mother and child.

REFERENCES

1. WHO. The global prevalence of anaemia in 2011. Geneva: World Health Organization; 2015.
2. Suryanarayana R, Chandrappa M, Santhuram AN, Prathima S, Sheela SR. Prospective study on prevalence of anemia of pregnant women and its outcome: A community based study. J Family Med Prim Care. 2017;6(4):739-43.
3. Agarwal KN, Agrawal DK, Sharma A, Sharma K, Prasad K, Kalita MC, et al. Prevalence of anemia in pregnant and lactating women in India. Food Nut Bulletin. 2006;27:311-5.
4. World Health Organization. The prevalence of anemia in pregnancy. WHO Technical reports, 1992-1993.
5. Prashant D, Jaideep KC, Girija A, Mallapur MD. Prevalence of anemia among pregnant women attending antenatal clinics in rural field practice area of Jawaharlal Nehru Medical College, Belagavi, Karnataka, India. Int J Community Med Public Health. 2017;4(2):537-41.
6. Muñoz M, Peña-Rosas JP, Robinson S, Milman N, Holzgreve W, Breymann C, et al. Patient blood management in obstetrics: management of anaemia and haematinic deficiencies in pregnancy and in the post-partum period: NATA consensus statement. Transfus Med. 2018;28:22-39.
7. Mishra R. Anemia. In: IAN Donald's Practical Obstetric Problems, 7th edition. Gurugram, India: Wolter Kluwer India Pvt Ltd; 2014. pp. 196-216.
8. NICE. Antenatal Care for Uncomplicated Pregnancies. Clinical guideline [CG62]. National Institute for Health and Care Excellence, London, UK; 2008.
9. Siu AL; U.S. Preventive Services Task Force. Screening for iron deficiency anemia and iron supplementation in pregnant women to improve maternal health and birth outcomes: U.S. Preventive Services task force recommendation statement. Ann Intern Med. 2015;163:529-36.
10. Pavord S, Myers B, Robinson S, Allard S, Strong J, Oppenheimer C, et al. UK guidelines on the management of iron deficiency in pregnancy. Br J Haematol. 2012;156:588-600.
11. Anemia: mild to moderate. Evidence based labour ward practical guidelines, 4th edition. India: Department of OBGY Seth G. S. Medical College & KEM Hospital, Mumbai; 2017. pp. 10-11.
12. Anemia: Severe. Evidence based labour ward practical guidelines. 4th edition. India: Department of OBGY Seth G. S. Medical College & KEM Hospital, Mumbai; 2017. pp. 8-9.
13. Beta Thalassemia in Pregnancy. Evidence based labour ward practical guidelines. 4th edition. India: Department of OBGY Seth G. S. Medical College & KEM Hospital, Mumbai; 2017. pp. 121-2.
14. Sickle Cell Disease. Evidence based labour ward practical guidelines. 4th edition. India: Department of OBGY Seth G. S. Medical College & KEM Hospital, Mumbai; 2017. pp. 123-5.

Hypertensive Patient in Labor

Prerna Keshan

INTRODUCTION

"Delivery seems to be the only cure for a whole spectrum of hypertensive disorders of pregnancy but to tackle a hypertensive patient in labor is a challenge for every obstetrician!!"

DEFINITION

Patient having a blood pressure (BP) of SBP > 140 mm Hg, DBP > 90 mm Hg in labor is called a hypertensive patient in labor.

CLASSIFICATION

- Chronic hypertension in pregnancy—SBP > 140 mm Hg, DBP > 90 mm Hg, prior to pregnancy or prior to 20 weeks of gestation, persists during labor and after 12 weeks postpartum.
- Late-onset pre-eclampsia (beyond 34 weeks) with continued manifestation during labor
- Chronic hypertension with superimposed pre-eclampsia with or without severe features during delivery such as thrombocytopenia, elevated liver enzymes, new onset renal insufficiency, pulmonary edema, cerebral, or visual disturbances.
- Labor onset hypertension[1]—solely due to the onset of labor documented for the first time over antenatal, intranatal, and postnatal period due to effect of uterine contractions, causing an increase in the stroke volume and heart rate as well as the activation of renin angiotensin system.

DIAGNOSIS

Factors leading to diagnosis as to which category of the above does the patient fit into depends a lot on whether the patient is a booked case of a particular institution or has been handled in the emergency room only during labor. An inpatient pregnant mother with hypertension in pregnancy progressing to labor is always a boon for every obstetrician as much is known about her profile and risk factors.

Antenatal records and investigations are of utmost importance to come to a conclusive diagnosis in case the patient is attending an institution only for emergency delivery. History from attendants and patient (if able to narrate) can aid in making the diagnosis of the onset and duration of hypertension. History taking must include the following points:

- Personal history of alcohol or smoke abuse
- Family history of hypertension
- Sibling history of eclampsia
- Past obstetric history and hypertension in previous pregnancy
- Fetal and perinatal outcome of previous pregnancy if had hypertension earlier.
- Baby requiring neonatal intensive care unit (NICU) care in previous pregnancy
- Medical history of any drug intake
- Fetal weight as per latest scan record
- Any history of impending signs of eclampsia such as epigastric pain, headache, or blurring of vision
- Drug history during the ongoing pregnancy
- History of monitoring BP at home
- Weight gain chart of ongoing pregnancy
- Sociodemographic profile
- Order of gestation and interpregnancy interval (birth spacing)
- Singleton or twin gestation
- History of recurrent pregnancy loss (RPL) to rule out systemic lupus erythematosus/antiphospholipid antibodies (SLE/APLAs).

INVESTIGATIONS

These investigations are targeted to differentiate between impending eclampsia, ongoing hemolysis, elevated liver enzymes, and low platelet (HELLP) syndrome or pre-eclampsia with or without severe features. In a way to investigate a hypertensive patient in labor guides us as to what should be the plan of action based on the severity of the investigation results. However note should be made that reports of the required investigations should be promptly released to decide on the mode of delivery and necessary intervention.

- *Urinary protein estimation*: Dipstick method—ranging from nil or trace to 4+ proteinuria
- *Serum uric acid estimation*: More than 6 g% strong predictor of eclampsia
- Complete blood count including platelet count (if <100,000/µL suggestive of HELLP syndrome)
- *Liver function test*: [if aspartate transaminase (AST) and alanine transaminase (ALT) elevated twice the upper limit of normal suggestive of HELLP syndrome]
- Renal function test
- Lactate dehydrogenase >600 IU/L indicative of HELLP syndrome.

MANAGEMENT

The management depends upon whether hypertension is controlled or associated with severe features and whether there are chances of seizures and developing HELLP syndrome.

The following are the prerequisite for management of a hypertensive patient in labor:
- Presence or guidance of a senior obstetrician in the team
- Informed high-risk consent from the parturient if possible for her as well as the attendants about the risk of eclampsia and severe manifestations of hypertension like HELLP syndrome.
- Strict intrapartum fetal monitoring to avoid in utero catastrophe
- Latest obstetric scan report with reassuring fetal Doppler parameters
- Proper counseling of attendants about the need for referral to tertiary level care center with facilities of high dependency unit (HDU)

even if the patient is received in active labor and shows signs of severe features during the course of treatment which cannot be tackled with available resources in the institution due to requirement of multidisciplinary approach.

With this initial workup, the actual aim in case of a hypertensive patient in labor is to deliver an active baby not in distress, uneventfully with avoidance of eclampsia in cases of severe hypertension (BP 160/110 mm Hg).

The following has to be followed:[2]
- Hourly checking of BP if >130/80 mm Hg and >160/110 mm Hg
- Every 15–30 minutes checking of BP during labor unless BP is <160/110 mm Hg in severe cases
- Continue with antenatal antihypertensives—(nifedipine and labetalol)
- Do not preload with intravenous fluids before establishing low dose epidural analgesia or combined spinal epidural analgesia.
- Management of second stage of labor—do not routinely limit the duration of the second stage of labor.
- Operative vaginal delivery can be considered in the second stage of labor in women who are not responsive to antihypertensive medications (BP > 160/110 mm Hg).

Management of Hypertensive Crisis in Labor

- Call for help
- Attain intravenous access
- Intravenous labetalol is the drug of choice if BP is >160/110 mm Hg during labor with a starting dose of 20 mg over 2 minutes and escalating dose to 80 mg until control is achieved with 10 minutes interval BP monitoring. Maternal bradycardia (pulse <60 beats) labetalol has to be withhold.

Need for cesarean section may arise due to the following reasons:
- If target BP is not achieved
- If ominous signs of impending, eclampsia is evident.
- Fetal distress on close surveillance
- Other obstetric causes such as prolonged or obstructed labor

Seizure Prophylaxis

- Magnesium sulfate bolus dose 4 g IV over 15 minutes
- Maintenance dose 1–2 g/h
- Monitor respiratory rate, urine output, and knee jerk
- Once BP threshold is achieved, BP is measured every 10 minutes for 1 hour, then every 15 minutes for next 1 hour, then every 30 minutes for next 1 hour and then once in an hour for 4 hours.

Complications that Needs Close Vigilance[3]

The eyes can see what the brain knows:
- Maternal cerebral hemorrhage
- Cardiovascular accident
- Pulmonary edema and acute respiratory distress syndrome (ARDS)
- Placental abruption
- Retinal injury
- Disseminated intravascular coagulation (DIC)
- Renal failure

Postpartum Care

- Measure BP four times a day while admitted
- Once a day between day 3 and day 5 of birth
- Every alternate days for up to 2 weeks
- Can continue with labetalol and/or nifedipine[4] if BP > 140/90 mm Hg
- Repeat laboratory investigations such as platelet count and liver function test (LFT) 48–72 hours after birth.

Criterion and Advice on Discharge

- Clinical and biochemical signs of improvement
- Follow-up care with medical review if required
- Revisit after 2 weeks

CONCLUSION

Hypertension in pregnancy being one of the leading causes of deaths in the country, emphasis should be laid on both proper antenatal care for early appraisal and timely referral in cases of severe hypertension to reduce maternal and perinatal morbidity as well as prompt and expert management during labor with multidisciplinary approach involving neonatologist, senior obstetrician, and medicine specialist. Close maternofetal surveillance during labor is the key to better obstetric outcomes.

REFERENCES

1. Di Giosia P, Giorgini P, Ferri C. Is labor-onset hypertension a novel category among hypertensive disorders of pregnancy associated with adverse events in high-risk subjects? Lights and shadows. Hypertens Res. 2016;39:401-3.
2. O' Brien L, Duong J, Winterton T, Haring A, Kuhlmann Z. Management of hypertension on the labor and delivery unit: delivering care in the era of protocols and algorithms. Perm J. 2018;22:17-170.
3. Ohno Y, Terauchi M, Tamakoshi K, Shiozaki A, Saito S. The risk factors for labor onset hypertension. Hypertens Res. 2016;39(4):260-5.
4. Briggs GG, Wan SR. Drug therapy during labor and delivery, part 2. Am J Health Syst Pharm. 2006;63(12):1131-9.

39

Eclampsia

Prerna Keshan

DEFINITION

New onset grand mal seizures/generalized tonic-clonic convulsion and/or coma during pregnancy and postpartum is not due to epilepsy or any existing abnormality in the brain.

CLASSIFICATION

- Antepartum (50%) fits occur before the onset of labor
- Intrapartum (30%) fits occur for the first time during labor
- Postpartum (20%) fits occur for the first time during puerperium within 48 hours of delivery or after 48 hours with 4 weeks (late postpartum).

DIAGNOSIS

In a patient with signs of preeclampsia, the following series of events heralds the occurrence of eclamptic fits:

- *Premonitory stage*: Unconsciousness followed by muscle twitching of face, tongue, and limbs, rolling of eyeballs—entire stage lasts for around 30 seconds
- *Tonic stage*: Entire body attains a state of tonic spasm and is called the trunk opisthotonus, limbs however remain flexed and the hands are clenched, there is cessation of breathing movements and tongue protrudes between the teeth, action if not taken during this stage the patient becomes cyanosed. This stage also lasts for 30 seconds.
- *Clonic stage*: During this stage all the voluntary muscles of the body undergo alternate contraction and relaxation, commencing from the face and then involving one side of the extremities and ultimately the whole body

is involved in the convulsive event. Tongue bite occurs during this stage, respiration becomes laborious and serosanguineous frothy fluid is accumulated in the oral cavity. Cyanosis if occurred during the third stage, now disappears and this stage lasts for around 1–4 minutes.

- *Stage of coma*: This is the last stage wherein the patient passes onto either a brief or a persistent period of coma until another convulsion occurs. Even if the coma does not persist the patient is confused and disoriented with amnesia.

These series of events may occur multiple times at different interfit duration. If it keeps occurring continuously, it is called status eclampticus. Vital parameters such as pulse, blood pressure (BP), and respiratory rate and temperature show aberrant readings in the postictal stage.

MANAGEMENT

The moment you approach an eclamptic patient—"shout out for help" aims[1] the following during management:

- Arrest ongoing convulsion
- Maintain airway, breathing, and circulation
- Prevent dreaded maternal and fetal complications

Supportive and definitive management should be done simultaneously for prompt response:

- Prevent aspiration by turning left lateral
- Get intravenous (IV) access and collect samples for necessary laboratory investigations such as liver function test (LFT), renal function test (RFT), and platelet count

- Administer magnesium sulfate (dosage discussed below)
- Shift to railed cot with tongue depressor to avoid tongue injury
- Suction oropharyngeal secretions and maintain oxygenation with 6–8 L/min via mask
- Bladder catheterization for urine output assessment
- Intravenous fluid RL/NS at 60 mL/h

Once initial management has been started the following should follow:

- Detailed history from the attendants as to duration of gestation, number of fits outside hospital, medications if any administered
- General, physical, abdominal, and vaginal examination should be done to establish obstetric diagnosis whether in labor or so.

Magnesium sulfate regime:[2]
Loading dose: 50% of 4 g diluted in 20% slow IV over 20 minutes (8 mL of drug with 12 mL of NS), 5 g (50%) intramuscular into each buttocks.

Maintenance dose: 5 g intramuscular in alternate buttocks once in 4 hours till 24 hours after delivery or last seizure whichever is later.

Recurrent seizure: If seizure recurs after 30 minutes, repeat half the loading dose 2 g in 20% solution (4 mL of drug with 6 mL NS slowly over 5 minutes)

MONITORING[3]

- Continuous pulse oximetry
- Hourly input output chart
- Hourly BP, pulse rate (PR), and respiratory rate (RR)
- Deep tendon reflexes and level of consciousness
- Continuous electronic fetal monitoring

Watch for signs of toxicity:
- SpO_2 <95% for 1 hour
- Urine output <100 mL in 4 hours
- RR < 12 breaths/min
- Loss of patellar or biceps deep tendon reflex
- Fetal heart rate (FHR) abnormalities
- Muscle weakness, slurred speech, drowsiness, and cardiac arrhythmias

Antidote: Injection 10% calcium gluconate 10 mL over 5 minutes.

Antihypertensive: Labetalol is the drug of choice—20 mg IV over 2 minutes followed by BP monitoring after 20 minutes for achievement of threshold BP.

Role of diuretics: In case of pulmonary edema furosemide is administered in doses 20–40 mg IV.

OBSTETRIC MANAGEMENT

- Antepartum eclampsia fits controlled—baby matured delivery needs to be done vaginally after induction and augmentation, if obstetric indications then cesarean section.
- Antepartum eclampsia fits controlled—baby premature delivery is recommended in neonatal intensive care unit (NICU) settings—steroid therapy and delivery
- Antepartum eclampsia fits controlled—baby dead—spontaneous expulsion or medical method of induction.
- Antepartum eclampsia fits not controlled—immediate delivery.
- Intrapartum eclampsia—in absence of any contraindications to vaginal delivery, low rupture of membrane is done to accelerate delivery once labor is established.

PROGNOSIS

Maternal

Morbidity and mortality is very high in India due to:
- Cardiac failure
- Pulmonary edema
- Aspiration and septic pneumonia
- Cerebral hemorrhage
- Acute respiratory failure (ARF)
- Cardiopulmonary arrest
- Acute respiratory distress syndrome (ARDS)
- Pulmonary embolism
- Postpartum shock
- Puerperal sepsis

Fetal Prognosis

- *Prematurity*: Iatrogenic or spontaneous
- Uteroplacental insufficiency
- Drug effects
- Birth trauma

CONCLUSION

Eclampsia being a major cause of maternal mortality in India, strategies need to be initiated to predict and prevent eclampsia which encompasses early diagnosis and treatment of preeclampsia.

However, if eclampsia is inevitable, prompt and definitive management at tertiary level care center with intensivist, physician, neonatologist, and emergency obstetric team can make a worthwhile effort toward better perinatal outcome.

REFERENCES

1. Queensland Clinical Guidelines. Hypertension and pregnancy. Guideline No. MN21.13-V9-R26. Queensland Health. February 2021. Available from [online] http://www.health.qld.gov.au/qcg [Last accessed February, 2022].

2. ACOG Committee Opinion No. 767: Emergent Therapy for Acute-Onset, Severe Hypertension During Pregnancy and the Postpartum Period. Obstet Gynecol. 2019;133(2):e174-e180. doi: 10.1097/AOG.0000000000003075. PMID: 30575639.

3. Ministry of Health and Family Welfare, Government of India. Guidelines for Antenatal Care and Skilled Attendance at Birth. New Delhi: MOHFW, GOI; 2010.

Aarti Chitkara, Neharika Malhotra

INTRODUCTION

During pregnancy, anatomic and physiologic changes in pregnancy can influence the diagnosis and management of haptic and renal disorders in pregnancy. In this chapter, we will discuss the management of these during labor.

- Common liver conditions that are specific to pregnancy:
  - Intrahepatic cholestasis of pregnancy (ICP)
  - HELLP (hemolysis, elevated liver enzymes, and low platelet count) syndrome
  - Acute fatty liver of pregnancy (AFLP)
  - Liver hematoma and nontraumatic liver rupture
- Common pre-existing hepatic disorders which can affect peripartum management of the patient are:
  - Biliary stones
  - Autoimmune hepatitis
  - Cirrhosis, including primary biliary cirrhosis
  - Esophageal varices
  - Liver transplant
  - Viral hepatitis

INTRAHEPATIC CHOLESTASIS OF PREGNANCY

0.2–2% pregnancies in USA are found to be affected by obstetric cholestasis (OC) with a heterogenous etiology. It typically begins around 25–32 weeks but can also present in the first trimester.

Clinical presentation: Pruritus and jaundice

- *Laboratory tests*: Elevated bile acids (most specific and sensitive marker), elevated transaminases, and no imaging abnormality
- *Recurrence rate*: 45–70%

- *Labor and delivery*:
  - ICP almost always resolves completely after delivery, making this the only definitive treatment.
  - This condition is dreaded with <3% risk of sudden fetal demise calling for timely and early termination of pregnancy. The algorithm has been proposed as shown in **Flowchart 1.**

ACUTE FATTY LIVER OF PREGNANCY

- This rare but serious disorder presents mainly in third trimester, but can also present in postpartum period and occurs in approximately 1 in 10,000 pregnancies.
- *Risk factors*: Multiple gestation, low maternal weight, and fetal mitochondrial gene mutation causing long-chain 3-hydroxyacyl-CoA dehydrogenase (LCHAD) deficiency.
- *Clinical presentation*: Nausea, vomiting, epigastric pain, anorexia, jaundice, or malaise
- *Laboratory findings*: Diagnosis is established using Swansea criteria mentioned in **Table 1.**
- *Labor and delivery*:
  - Maternal stabilization, intensive supportive care, and prompt delivery
  - Coagulopathy has been reported in 57% patients (A) which should be managed by transfusion of fresh frozen plasma (FFP) and cryoprecipitate, and platelets during labor.
  - The mode of delivery should be based on the likelihood of a rapid controlled vaginal delivery (<24 hours) and degree of coagulopathy, as a vaginal delivery will reduce the incidence of intra-abdominal bleeding compared to cesarean section.
  - Prophylactic antibiotics are recommended.

Flowchart 1: Timing of delivery in intrahepatic cholestasis of pregnancy (ICP).

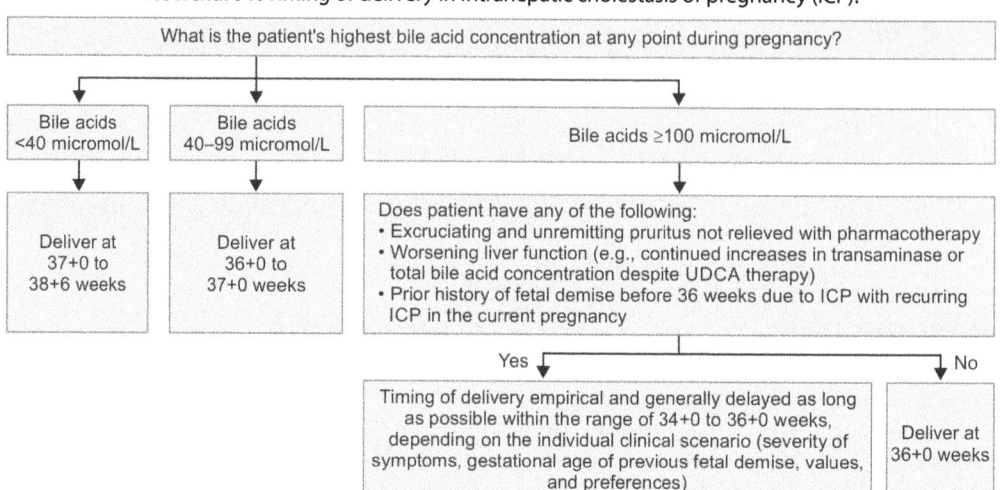

TABLE 1: Swansea criteria for diagnosis of AFLP.			
Signs and symptoms	*Laboratory findings*	*Imaging*	*Histology*
Vomiting	Elevated bilirubin (>0.8 mg/dL or >14 µmol/L)	Ascites	Microvesicular steatosis on liver biopsy
Abdominal pain	Hypoglycemia (glucose <72 mg/dL or <4 mmol/L)	Bright liver on ultrasound scan	
Polydipsia/polyuria	Leukocytosis (>11,000 cells/µL)		
Encephalopathy	• Elevated transaminases (AST or ALT) (>42 IU/L) • Elevated ammonia (>47 µmol/L) • Elevated urate (5.7 mg/dL or >340 µmol/L) • Acute kidney injury, or creatinine >1.7 mg/dL (150 µmol/L) • Coagulopathy or prothrombin time >14 seconds		

(AFLP: acute fatty liver of pregnancy; ALT: alanine aminotransferase; AST: aspartate aminotransferase)

- If labor is induced, the fetus should be monitored closely.
- Liver functions usually normalize within 1 week postpartum and recurrence in subsequent pregnancy is possible.
- *Postnatal*: Improvement/recovery should be seen by 2–3 days after delivery, though this may take up to 4 weeks.
- All infants should be tested for LCHAD deficiency, as affected infants may develop neonatal cardiomyopathy, skeletal myopathy, hepatic failure, and even sudden death.[1,2]

☐ HELLP SYNDROME

- HELLP syndrome is a severe form of pre-eclampsia in which vascular endothelial injury, fibrin deposition, and platelet activation are seen, leading to microangiopathic hemolytic anemia (MAHA).
- Maternal complications include coagulopathy, placental abruption, pulmonary failure, renal failure, ascites, subcapsular hematoma or liver rupture, and fulminant hepatic failure.

- *Labor and delivery*:
  - The decision to deliver will depend on the severity of symptoms, gestational age, and maternal and fetal condition.
  - American College of Obstetricians and Gynecologist (ACOG) (2013) states that for women with HELLP syndrome before fetal viability and at ≥34 weeks' gestation, it is advisable to induce labor after the mother is stabilized.[3]
  - If the gestational age is between fetal viability and 34 weeks, it has been suggested to delay delivery for 24–48 hours for steroid cover if maternal and fetal condition allows it.
  - The algorithm shown in **Flowchart 2** can be used for decision regarding termination of pregnancy.

CIRRHOSIS

- Hepatic cirrhosis is associated with a spontaneous abortion rate of 26%, a preterm delivery rate between 40% and 60%, and a neonatal mortality rate of approximately 15%. Maternal mortality is estimated at 10% but may be up to 50% in patients with portal hypertension who develop gastrointestinal bleeding during pregnancy.
- Outcomes are generally poor but hepatic dysfunction before pregnancy and presence of portal hypertension correlate with worse maternal/fetal prognosis.
- *Esophageal variceal bleeding*: Most common complication of cirrhosis occurring in 18–25% of pregnant women with cirrhosis.
  - Endoscopic variceal ligation is the mainstay of therapy for acute episodes of hemorrhage. Portal decompression shunt placement is required when hemorrhage cannot be controlled by endoscopy. Beta-blockers (propranolol) are recommended for therapy.
  - Vaginal delivery is preferred over cesarean delivery due to high rates of intraoperative and postoperative complications.
  - In patients with portal hypertension, however, repetitive Valsalva maneuver in the second stage of labor can increase

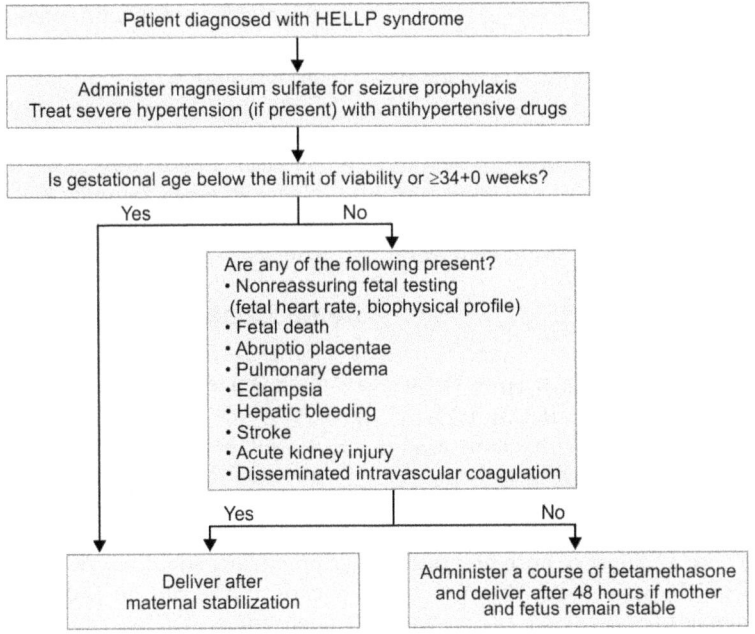

Flowchart 2: Management of patients with HELLP (hemolysis, elevated liver enzymes, and low platelet count) syndrome.

the risk of significant variceal bleeding. A passive second stage with forceps-assisted delivery may be beneficial.
- Postpartum hemorrhage is a significant source of morbidity and mortality in this patient population.

BUDD-CHIARI SYNDROME

- Budd-Chiari syndrome (BCS) is a veno-occlusive disease of the hepatic vein that increases sinusoidal pressure and can result in portal hypertension or hepatic necrosis.
- *Clinical presentation*: Abdominal pain, abrupt onset of ascites, and hepatomegaly
- *Diagnosis*: Hepatic Doppler ultrasound to identify the venous occlusion and evaluate the direction and amplitude of blood flow.
- Acute therapy includes selective thrombolytic and a surgical shunt or transjugular intrahepatic portosystemic shunt for portal hypertension.
- Chronic BCS is treated with anticoagulation therapy and careful switchover with adequate optimization prior to a planned termination of pregnancy is the key to reduce uncontrolled hemorrhage.

ACUTE VIRAL HEPATITIS

Hepatitis A Virus

Gestational complications are rarely encountered with hepatitis A virus (HAV), however a review of 80,000 pregnancies women, thirteen women with HAV were evaluated out of which 69% developed gestational complications including premature onset of labor, placental abruption, and premature rupture of the membranes. The presence of fever and hypoalbuminemia were associated with preterm delivery.

Hepatitis B Virus

The rate of perinatal hepatitis B virus (HBV) transmission has been estimated at 1.1% of newborns. Transmission was significantly associated with having a mother who was hepatitis B e-antigen (HBeAg) positive, had a HBV viral load >2,000 IU/mL. Hepatitis B immunoglobulin (HBIG) vaccine with 12 hours of birth and three complete doses of HBV vaccine has shown to be protective for neonates.

Mode of delivery: The benefit of cesarean delivery in protecting against HBV transmission has not been clearly established in well-conducted controlled trials, and available data are conflicting. Thus, cesarean delivery is not routinely recommended for carrier mothers for the sole purpose of reducing HBV transmission.[2,4,5]

RENAL DISEASE IN LABOR

Women with renal disease are increasingly becoming pregnant or contemplating on becoming pregnant as a result of:
- Increased recognition of early chronic kidney disease (CKD) because of estimated glomerular filtration rate (eGFR) reporting
- Increasing maternal age in many parts of the world
- Improved maternal outcomes from renal diseases and treatments that might have led to impaired fertility in the past.

In this chapter we will discuss few routinely encountered renal disorders with respect to labor and delivery.

Infections of the Urinary Tract

- Asymptomatic bacteriuria complicates 2–10% of pregnancies.[6] Pyelonephritis is estimated to occur in 2–4% of pregnant women.[7] Before the regular use of antibiotics, a 50% preterm birth rate was reported following an episode of pyelonephritis.
- *Labor and delivery*: Urinary tract infections (UTIs) should not interfere with the normal management of labor. However, if UTIs coincide with labor, antimicrobial therapy should be continued until the completion of the course.

Renal Stones

- Renal stones complicate around 1 in 1,500 pregnancies.[8]
- *Labor and delivery*: Renal stones presenting in labor should be managed expectantly until after delivery when there are greater options for diagnosis and management.
- Women with a history of renal stones in pregnancy should have normal intrapartum care and is not an indication for surgical delivery.

TABLE 2: Approximate risks of adverse maternal and fetal outcomes.[9]

CKD stage	Pre-eclampsia	SGA	Preterm delivery
G1	5%	13%	7%
G2	20%	18%	21%
G3	40%	19%	38%
G4-5	60%	50%	45–90%

(CKD: chronic kidney disease; SGA: small for gestational age)

Chronic Kidney Disease

Risk of adverse maternal and fetal outcomes depends on the stage of CKD (**Table 2**). Pregnancy can exacerbate the progression of CKD as a result of:

- Glomerular hyperfiltration
- Increased proteinuria
- Essential discontinuation of renoprotective medications [e.g., angiotensin-converting-enzyme inhibitors (ACEIs)]
- Increased activity of the underlying etiology [e.g. systemic lupus erythematosus (SLE)]
- Additional pregnancy-associated renal insults (e.g., pre-eclampsia, UTIs)
- Toxicity from altered pharmacokinetics of medications (e.g., calcineurin inhibitors)
- *Labor and delivery*:
  - Timing of delivery requires assessment of the progress of the pregnancy and likelihood of imminent risk. CKD itself is not an indication for early delivery, and, whenever possible, spontaneous labor at term should be the preferred option.
  - CKD is not an indication for cesarean section. The underlying CKD does not interfere with spontaneous labor. Usual analgesic options are acceptable with the exception of nonsteroidal anti-inflammatory drugs (NSAIDs), which should be avoided in all women with CKD. Opioid labor analgesia should be carefully titrated.
  - Induction of labor with prostaglandin and oxytocin is acceptable in women with CKD. Prolonged induction with oxytocin risks excessive fluid retention and electrolyte disturbance, and these risks will be higher in women with advanced CKD.
  - Accurate fluid management is essential for women with CKD in the context of operative vaginal delivery or hemorrhage to maintain renal perfusion and avoid fluid overload. Avoid methergine owing

to the risk of precipitating hypertensive complications.
  - Invasive monitoring of central venous pressure in women with CKD super-imposed with pre-eclampsia or hemorrhage should be considered for careful titration of fluid management.

Lupus Nephritis

- Lupus nephritis affects approximately 50% of patients with SLE and manifests as hypertension, proteinuria, hematuria, and/or impaired renal dysfunction. Approximately 1% of patients with lupus nephritis progress to end-stage renal failure each year after diagnosis.[10]
- *Labor and delivery*: Lupus nephritis does not affect the mode of termination of pregnancy. Some patients may warrant a preterm delivery for maternal condition after ensuring fetal lung maturity.
- *Lupus flare*: Consider increasing dose of corticosteroids and immunosuppressants [azathioprine, hydroxychloroquine (HCQ), cyclophosphamide]. Mycophenolate derivatives should be avoided throughout pregnancy due to teratogenicity. Rituximab is associated with neonatal B-cell suppression when used in later pregnancy.

▓ DIALYSIS IN PREGNANCY

- *Labor and delivery*:
  - Timing of delivery is determined by maternal or fetal complications.
  - Dialysis is not an indication for cesarean section.
  - Schedule hemodialysis (HD) within 12 hours of elective deliveries to optimize biochemistry and fluid status.

- Peritoneal dialysis can continue until labor or elective delivery commences, then drain the peritoneal cavity.
- Close attention to fluid balance during labor/operative delivery is mandatory.
- Avoid methergine or ergometrine derivatives.
- *Postnatal*:
  - Hemodialysis or peritoneal dialysis can be withheld for 24–48 hours after delivery if serum potassium and fluid status are satisfactory.
  - If the cesarean section was undertaken, peritoneal dialysis should be withheld for up to 7 days, interim HD may be required.
  - Monitor weight and blood pressure once or twice weekly during the puerperium.
  - Advice on medications with breastfeeding and contraception must be carefully discussed with the neonatologist, family panning expert taking into account patient's requirement.

SUMMARY

Hepatic and renal disorders in pregnancy are every obstetrician's nightmare. These can be dealt best involving a multidisciplinary approach involving senior obstetrician, hepatologist, nephrologist, intensivist, and neonatologist to optimize patient management and ensure a good maternal and perinatal outcome.

REFERENCES

1. Tein I. Metabolic disease in the fetus predisposes to maternal hepatic complications of pregnancy. Pediatr Res. 2000;47(1): 6-8.
2. Wang J, Zhu Q, Zhang X. Effect of delivery mode on maternal-infant transmission of hepatitis B virus by immunoprophylaxis. Chinese Med J. 2002;115(10):1510-2.
3. American College of Obstetricians and Gynecologists. Hypertension in pregnancy. Report of the American College of Obstetricians and Gynecologists' task force on hypertension in pregnancy. Obstet Gynecol. 2013;122(5): 1122-31.
4. Yang J, Zeng XM, Men YL. Elective caesarean section versus vaginal delivery for preventing mother to child transmission of hepatitis B virus–a systematic review. Virol J. 2008; 5(1):1-7.
5. Chang MS, Gavini S, Andrade PC, McNabb-Baltar J. Caesarean section to prevent transmission of hepatitis B: a meta-analysis. Can J Gastroenterol Hepatol. 2014;28(8):439-44.
6. Smaill FM, Vazquez JC. Antibiotics for asymptomatic bacteriuria in pregnancy. Cochrane Database Syst Rev. 2019;2019(11): CD000490.
7. Vazquez JC, Abalos E. Treatments for symptomatic urinary tract infections during pregnancy. Cochrane Database Syst Rev. 2011;2011(1): CD002256.
8. Meher S, Gibbons N, DasGupta R. Renal stones in pregnancy. Obstetr Med. 2014;7(3): 103-10.
9. Piccoli GB, Cabiddu G, Attini R, Vigotti FN, Maxia S, Lepori N, et al. Risk of adverse pregnancy outcomes in women with CKD. J Am Soc Nephrol. 2015;26(8):2011-22.
10. Moon SJ, Park HS, Kwok SK, Ju JH, Kim HY, Park SH. Predictors of end-stage renal disease and recurrence of lupus activity after initiation of dialysis in patients with lupus nephritis. Clin Exp Rheumatol. 2013; 31(1):31-9.

CHAPTER 41

Birth Companion

Kavita Mandrelle Bhatti

INTRODUCTION

Birth companion also known as companion of choice during labor and childbirth is one who provides continuous one-to-one support to the woman during labor and intrapartum period.

Continuous presence of the companion during labor and delivery (CSLD) is very traditional and comfortable option in alleviating the anxiety of woman in labor.

Different terms have been used including for birth companion:
- Companion of choice at birth
- Labor companion
- Emotional support during birth
- Social support during labor and delivery
- Supportive companionship
- Continuous support for women during childbirth

IMPORTANCE OF BIRTH COMPANIONSHIP

- Woman gives birth in a health facility is alone or without the support of someone she trusts.
- World Health Organization (WHO) recommends that no woman should go through pregnancy, birth, and early motherhood on her own.
- For improved quality of care during facility-based childbirth, rather than home, since institutional births are increasing throughout many low- and middle-income countries.
- WHO promotes labor companionship necessary for improving maternal and infant health.
- It is a low-cost intervention that has proved to be beneficial to the woman in labor.
- Provides emotional, psychological, and practical support to the woman in labor

- To maintain the woman's autonomy and respect her needs during the process of labor
- It is an integral component to reduce maternal mortality and morbidity
- For improved neonatal health outcome

INITIATION OF BIRTH COMPANIONSHIP

Support during childbirth differs across settings and can start at any time between conception and postpartum period. Generally, it involves the continuous presence of a companion during labor and delivery.

PREREQUISITES FOR EFFECTIVE BIRTH COMPANIONSHIP

- A female relative and preferably one who has undergone the process of labor herself
- Facilities may allow husband of the pregnant woman to be the birth companion
- Should not be suffering from communicable diseases
- She should wear clean clothes
- She should be willing to stay with the pregnant woman throughout the process of labor
- She should not interfere in the work of hospital staff and the treatment procedures
- She should not attend to other woman in the labor room
- Should be compassionate and trustworthy.

Who can be a birth companion?
- Companion of choice
- A male partner
- A family member
- A friend chosen from a woman's social network
- A non-healthcare professional (doula) trained to provide emotional and physical

support to women before, during, and after childbirth
- A healthcare professional

ROLE OF A BIRTH COMPANION

Birth companions play a number of roles in supporting woman:
- Provide information about progress of labor and advice regarding coping techniques to the laboring mother
- They provide informational support about the process of childbirth
- Bridge communication gaps between a woman in labor and the healthcare workers around her
- Provide practical support including encouraging the mother to remain mobile during labor
- Provide emotional support and continuous reassurance
- Provide nonpharmacological pain relief such as massage, hand-holding, and meditation
- Provide measures for comfort (comforting touch, massages, promoting adequate fluid intake and output) during labor and delivery
- As advocates for the women speaking up in support of her and her preferences
- Can witness and safeguard against mistreatment or neglect during labor and childbirth
- Help women, feel in control, and build their confidence through praise, reassurance, and continuous physical presence.

ADVANTAGES OF A BIRTH COMPANION DURING LABOR

- Provides respectful maternity care
- Contributes to reduced stress during labor and shortened labor
- Increased control of mother's feelings, decreased interventions, and cesareans
- Less likelihood of using pain medication while giving birth
- Improves outcome for the newborn
- Facilitates parent/infant bonding
- Decreases postpartum depression
- Enhances a positive birth experience
- Shorter length of time in labor
- More chances of a spontaneous vaginal delivery
- Decreased rate of cesarean section
- More positive health indicators for babies in the first 5 minutes after birth

Adverse and facilitating factors for implementation of birth companionship have been given in **Table 1**.

POLICY SUPPORT IN INDIA

The Ministry of Health and Family Welfare enforces birth companions during delivery in public health facilities with an aim to reduce maternal mortality ratio and infant mortality rate. Though, it is not mandatory.

What does evidence prove?

Studies suggest that women who have birth companions are less likely to experience mistreatment during childbirth. It is associated with increased satisfaction with healthcare services.

Cochrane review of CSLD found that women who received continuous labor support were more likely to have:
- Shorter labor
- Spontaneous vaginal deliveries
  - Less likely to use pain medication while giving birth
  - Babies were less likely to have low 5-minute Apgar scores.
  - The effect of CSLD differed, depending on the type of companion and the setting
  - CSLD was most effective at reducing cesarean birth when the companion was present in a doula role and in settings where epidural analgesia was not routinely available.
  - It was concluded that continuous support from a person who solely provides support, is not a member of the woman's own network, is experienced in providing labor support, and has a modest amount of training (such as a doula), appears to have the greatest impact on outcomes.
  - Compared to having no companion, support from a chosen family member or friend appeared to increase women's satisfaction with their childbirth experience.

COVID-19 AND BIRTH COMPANIONSHIP

There is increased demand for care of people who are affected by COVID-19.
- This is compounded by fear, misinformation, and limitations on movement which may hinder access to care.

TABLE 1: Adverse and facilitating factors for implementation of birth companionship.

Adverse factors	Facilitating factors
Human resource shortage	Hiring and training unemployed or retired nurses and midwives Training of lay companions
Organization of shifts and space in the facility	Provision of a private space/cubicle/lounge for short breaks
Crowding of labor rooms in resource constrained facility	Allocation of resources within the facility
Negative perceptions about the role of the companion Community culture and challenges	Clear communication with the companion about his/her duties Provision of evidence-based information Sharing of women's positive experiences with this practice to motivate their participation
Cost of hiring a doula	Involvement of family members as companions during childbirth is an inexpensive practice
Cost of transportation for volunteer companions	Cost-effective for healthcare insurers and for hospitals as it reduces the financial costs of obstetric interventions such as epidural use and cesarean sections and the time spent on complications
Nurses were considered to be "desensitized" to women's needs and less empathetic than lay companions	Influencing the attitudes of healthcare providers their sensitization and do activities including the provision of evidence-based information
Privacy for women and their companions in the labor ward	Appropriate physical space that respects women and their companion, in other words Privacy
Institutional policies	Commitment of the management of healthcare facilities
Male partners also felt they were not well integrated into the care team or decision making	Husband understands the nature of wife, and feels their participation
Introducing labor companionship may be complex and require a reorganization and restructuring of services and engagement with numerous stakeholders	Change in institutional policies
Implementation is not universal	Can start and study the pros and cons in government as well as private facilities

- Integrating human rights protection is important and essential to address public health concerns.
- WHO recommends that the emotional, practical, and health benefits of having a chosen labor companion should be respected and followed with COVID precautionary measures.
- The pandemic must not disrupt a woman's right to high-quality, respectful maternity care.

BIBLIOGRAPHY

1. Afulani P, Kusi C, Kirumbi L, Walker D. Companionship during facility-based childbirth: results from a mixed-methods study with recently delivered women and providers in Kenya. BMC Pregnancy Childbirth. 2018;18(1):150.
2. Bohren MA, Berger BO, Munthe-Kaas H, Tunçalp Ö. Perceptions and experiences of labour companionship: a qualitative evidence synthesis. Cochrane Database Syst Rev. 2019; 3(3):CD012449.
3. Bohren MA, Hofmeyr GJ, Sakala C, Fukuzawa RK, Cuthbert A. Continuous support for women during childbirth. Cochrane Database Syst Rev. 2017;7(7):CD003766.
4. Kabakian-Khasholian T, Portela A. Companion of choice at birth: factors affecting

implementation. BMC Pregnancy and Childbirth. BMC Pregnancy Childbirth. 2017;17(1):265.

5. Shakibazadeh E, Namadian M, Bohren MA, Vogel JP, Rashidian A, Nogueira Pileggi V, et al. Respectful care during childbirth in health facilities globally: a qualitative evidence synthesis. BJOG. 2018;125:932-42.

6. World Health Organization. (2016). Sexual and reproductive health. [online] Available from https://www.who.int/reproductivehealth/topics/maternal_perinatal/companion-during-labour-childbirth/en/ [Last accessed December, 2021].

Kawita Bapat, Shashibala Bhonsale Sao

INTRODUCTION

Yoga is a system devised by ancient yogis of India out of their intuitive knowledge. It understands the mysterious psychophysiology complex. According to yoga, man is not just flesh, blood and bones but a configuration of a gross body, a subtle energy body, the thinking mind, the psychological mind, the emotional mind, and the spirit or soul.

Perfect health is nothing but perfect harmony among all these aspects. Any disharmony anywhere gradually affects all the other parts and the manifestations are seen on the physical body.

All yoga techniques are extremely effective and the effects are felt almost instantaneously. Yoga is the right remedy for the sick and maladjusted modern society. Man today is a globetrotting man the long hours in the aircraft are not without perils. In the aircraft, negative blood circulation is there, especially venous return is diminished so stasis in blood vessels can lead to clot formation and they travel to the heart and cause sudden heart attack. A simple group of asanas called Pawanmuktasana maintains the optimal health. Back backpain in the neck continues bending the head forward while working resulting in cervical spondylitis causes stiffness and muscle fatigue if sitting for long. So, it is essential to release the accumulated tension in the back from time to time. Develop correct postural habits. One asana is the Tadasana and another is Bhujangasana. Lunch is very important. Have meals leisurely in cozy comforts of home with the aroma of home-cooked favorite dishes which triggers off the secretion of lot of saliva is considered luxury nowadays. Lunch has now become a hurried affair, with a mind agitated or preoccupied with various problems. Taking food under such conditions can lead to ill health. Practice relaxation before meals. Comfortably close eyes, breathe normally, visualize great picnic spot, and open your eyes and eat. According to yoga, the right nostril is connected with the left hemisphere of the brain which controls the physical actions and left nostril controls the mental actions so maintain this rhythm.

SUCCESS IN MEETINGS

Meetings are a part of a working man's daily routine. Deals are clinched differences are sorted out policies formulated and problems are solved. A tense mind is a handicap so we cannot afford to be stressed before or during an important meeting. Tense mind is a handicap. Information comes better from the highly relaxed mind. Relaxed person can influence others positively and get their cooperation which an agitated person can never achieve. Agitation spreads around and repels people. Nervousness is counterproductive. It projects weak and unattractive image, it leads to palpitations, dry mouth, and a churning stomach. This is where Pranayam helps practice abdominal breathing, chanting of powerful word "OM" with deep breathing also help.

HEALTH BOOSTER

Physical exercise is necessary to remain healthy but never overexercise. In physical exercise, O_2 consumption goes up and in asanas oxygen is conserved. Due to which there is more strength and energy through oxidation of glucose in the body. Asanas make body supple, elasticity spells better health than rigidity. Strength and vigor come not from bulky muscles but from the amount of energy in the body. Higher the energy level healthier we will feel. This energy is called prana. Prana is the vital force that keeps a man alive. Prana is bioplasmic energy said to be finer than atomic energy known to mankind since antiquity. It is called Ruach in

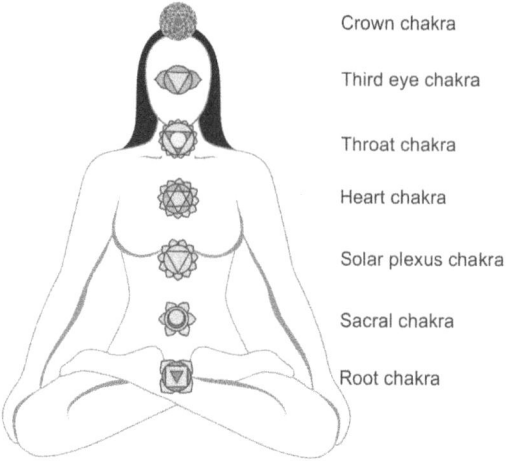

Crown chakra

Third eye chakra

Throat chakra

Heart chakra

Solar plexus chakra

Sacral chakra

Root chakra

Fig. 1: Myriad chakras.

Hebrew, Ki in Japan, Chi in China, and manna in Hawaii. According to yoga, prana is absorbed into the body from the atmosphere and then stored in the chakras or energy centers which distributes it throughout the body. There are myriad chakras for energy centers (**Fig. 1**) which also distribute it throughout the body. Surya Namaskar is complete technique suiting most people. It is dynamic slimming and highly invigorating.

ENERGETIC IN THE EVENINGS

After a busy day, invariably man heads for the bar. No harm. In the Vedas, Somras—an intoxicating drink occupied a very high place. Oxygenation of the system after a day's mental work is more effective to banish tiredness, mental work leads to stressful situation, and shallow breathing. Now try Agnisar kriya which expels the stale air and gets oxygenated air and you feel fresh and rejuvenated.

We live in momentous times, this is the best of times and perhaps also the worst. We communicate right across the world in a second. Tapping in finite information via the net, this is the bright side of the coin, the reverse side is terribly grim mindless violence stalks the world. Crime rules the roost peace of mind has become a cruel joke caught in the cesspool, it is the rising generation that is most affected, youth has immense courage and is full of optimism and is sensitive to noble ideas and ideals. But they abhor sermons. Their energy has to be channelized and there potential is to be tapped.

THE MIND

The mind is a videograph, beware the thought is the architect.

Our mind has stored innumerable pictures of the thoughts that have accumulated there over the years since our childhood. They lie dormant and in the mind and come to the surface as soon as we recall. That means that pictures in your mind or associated with every bit of your experience, our mind records our joys and sorrows experienced on different occasions, our response to these experiences, and our emotional upheavals.

Our future thoughts and experiences depend upon the thoughts and experiences that we have gathered.

Your future life is going to be shaped by the pictures you create in your mind the architect is the thought.

Thoughts and emotions are the two most important influences upon man's life whenever the thought is associated with fear and doubt leads to an action, it produces a negative result what but whenever a thought associated with self-confidence and optimism leads to an action, it has a constructive result.

Gautama Buddha about 2,000 and 500 years ago said that what we are today is the fruit of our thoughts. Speak well, good thoughts in mind, happiness is yours but if you think of evil thoughts grief pursues you.

This profound statement contains the eternal truth.

We may have swallowed so far in these debilitating and humiliating thoughts. If we are smeared with dirt, no screaming can cleanse us we have to wash ourselves with clean water. Once a thought arises upon the mind it will occur in mind again. If one repeats, I thought 5–10–20 times, it gets ingrained and lies dormant within you. Sri Aurobindo says thoughts and ideas are wandering about in the thought waves seeking a mind to that may embody them.

I simply sat down and my mind became silent as windless air and saw one thought then another coming in concrete way from outside. I flung them before they could enter and take hold of the brain and in 3 days I was free.

Finding faults with others with enthusiasm and relish will fill you with negative thoughts, your mind is becoming garbage bin where all the rubbish of others is thrown in, it is said that by meditating on God one realizes Him. By meditating on faults and shortcomings of others, you imbibe those qualities of Sri Sarada Devi divine consort of Sri Ramakrishna emphasized if you want peace of mind do not find fault with others but find fault rather with yourself. Nobody is stronger, my dear try to make the whole world your own.

BIBLIOGRAPHY

1. I am Joe's Body—J.D. Ratcliff Berkley Books, New York.
2. Introduction to Psychology—Ernest R. Hilgrad, Rita L. Atkinson and Richard C. Atkinson, Harcourt Brace Jovanorich Inc.
3. Meditation and Mantras—Vishnu Devananda.
4. Mind—It's Mysteries and Control—Swami Sivananda, Divine Life Society.
5. Sure Ways for Success in Life & God Realization—Swami Sivananda, Divine Life Society.
6. Teachings of Swami Satyananda Saraswati-Vol. 1, 4 &5 Bihar School of Yoga.
7. YOGA For Busy People.

CHAPTER

43 COVID Positive Patient in Labor

Sheeba Marwah, Chhavi Gupta, Akanksha Dwivedi

INTRODUCTION

Coronavirus disease 2019 (COVID-19) or novel coronavirus or severe acute respiratory syndrome coronavirus 2 (SARS CoV-2) has become a common discussion these days because of the havoc this virus has caused all over the world. Healthcare services including maternity care has been overwhelmed worldwide because of increased burden of cases. With new variants of virus coming in, the roots of our already dilapidated healthcare system are further getting weakened. Pregnant women constitute one of the most important categories of patients which need to be catered by healthcare system. Although pregnant women are not at an increased risk of catching the infection but they need utmost care.[1] Further, many COVID positive pregnant women may be asymptomatic at admission and may be detected during routine screening of admitted patients done within 5 days of admission. Thus, it becomes imperative for all obstetric care providers at all levels to become well versed with management and timely referral of patient to higher center as and when need arises.

TRIAGING OF PATIENTS

All patients presenting to emergency in labor should be triaged at admission, and COVID positive patients should be kept separate from negative cases to reduce the risk of transmission during hospital stay **(Flowchart 1)**.[2]

CLASSIFICATION OF PATIENTS BASED ON COVID SEVERITY

Pregnant women in labor who test positive for COVID-19 on admission, need to be further classified based on their severity and referred to appropriate facility in timely manner **(Flowchart 2)**.[3]

MANAGEMENT OF CORONA POSITIVE LABORING WOMEN IN RED ZONE

Timing of Delivery

- Timing of delivery should not be altered on basis of COVID-19 infection **(Table 1)**.
- Only patients who are not benefitting from all forms of treatment available should be offered delivery as an option to decrease extra load of pulmonary system.
- Risks and benefits should be weighed keeping in mind the gestational age, clinical condition of patient, level of healthcare available to mother, and newborn postdelivery, an informed consent from patient party along with due consideration to the fact that a surgical intervention might possibly worsen systemic status of mother in light of concurrent comorbidities.[2]

Route of Delivery

COVID-19 infection is not an indication for alteration in route of delivery especially as a measure to minimize the risk of vertical transmission from mother to baby **(Table 2)**.[4-7]

Support Person or Birth Companion

All the taboo and fear associated with the disease along with stress of labor pains takes a toll on laboring patient and presence of a birth companion may actually improve the patient's birthing experience.[1] However, birth support for COVID positive patients need to follow additional precautions.

Management of Labor (Table 3)

There still is paucity of data regarding the intricacies of disease and its pathophysiology to make a

Flowchart 1: Triaging of laboring women on admission.

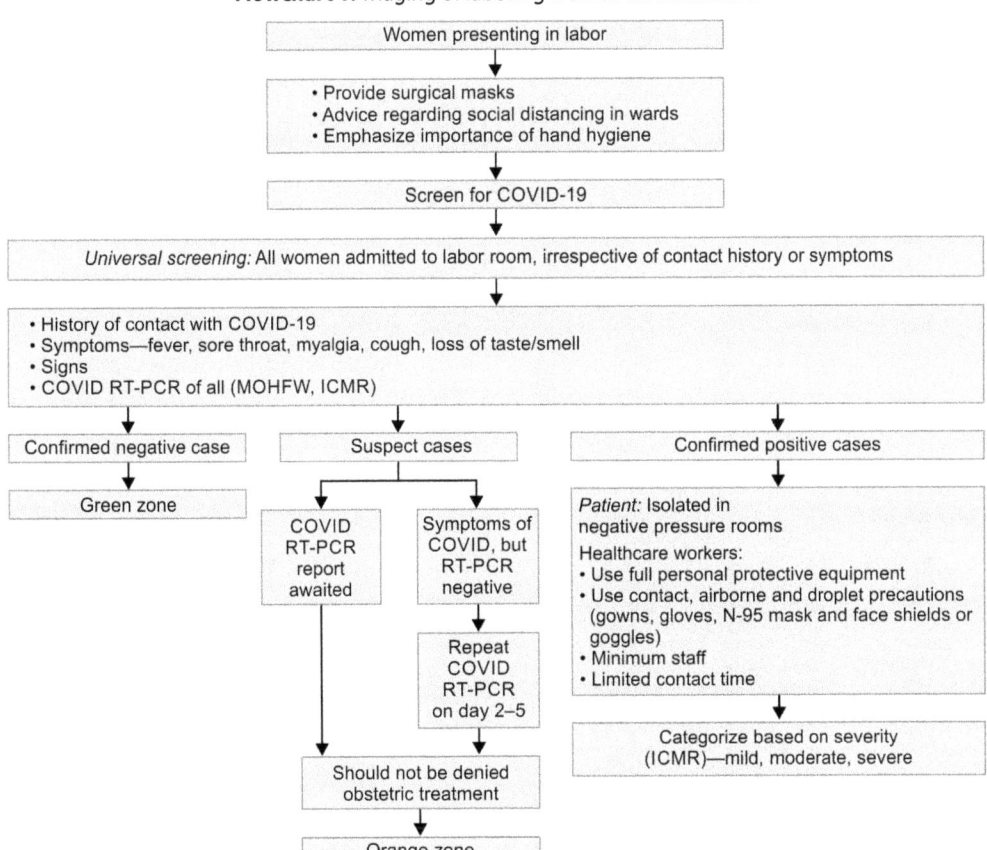

universal change in management of COVID positive cases in labor and is expected to evolve over time. Maternal and fetal monitoring during labor essentially remains similar to routine cases, with few precautions. However, COVID positive patients in labor need multidisciplinary care senior obstetrician, medical specialist, and if need arises pulmonologist and intensive care specialist as well.[1-3,8]

Management of First Stage of Labor

- Women in latent phase can wait at home, if there are no complications and transport is not an issue. Women in active phase of first stage of labor have to be admitted in dedicated labor rooms with negative pressure ventilation, individual rooms with attached bathrooms.
- All women should be examined at admission to establish baseline maternal-fetal status, as in non-COVID patients.

- COVID positive mothers may need additional testing than routine blood group, hemoglobin, screening for human immunodeficiency virus (HIV), hepatitis, venereal disease research laboratory (VDRL), such as chest X-ray, or even high-resolution computed tomography (HRCT) if indicated.
- Maternal vitals need to be monitored every hour, with special emphasis on temperature, respiratory rate, and oxygen saturation. Oxygen therapy should be given as and when needed, to maintain saturation above 94%.
- Continuous fetal heart monitoring is preferred, with review every 15 minutes, as there is increased incidence of abnormal tracings, especially in critically ill mother. However, oxygen therapy should be administered only if there is maternal hypoxia.
- Monitor the progress of labor with uterine contractions checked every 30 minutes,

Flowchart 2: Classification of COVID positive patients.

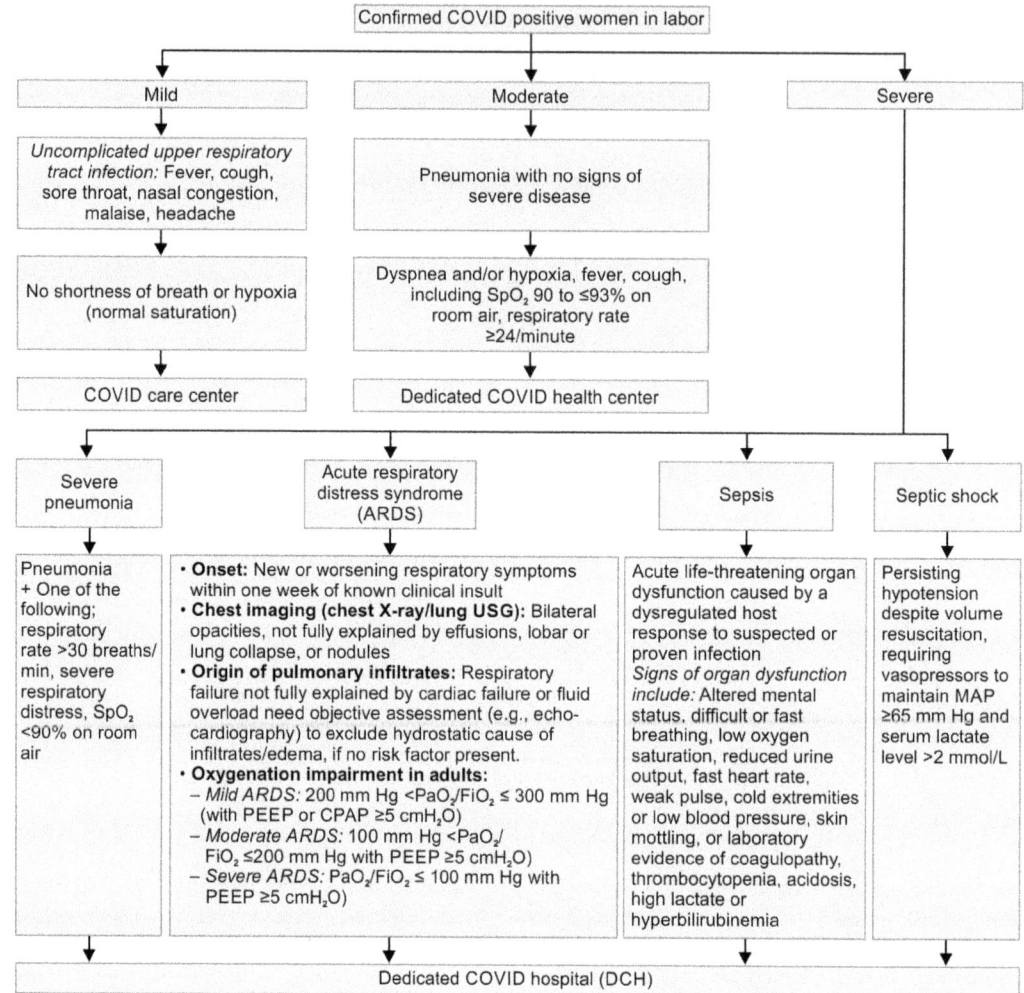

(CPAP: continuous positive airway pressure; MAP: mean arterial pressure; PEEP: positive end-expiratory pressure)

and digital vaginal examination for cervical dilation, effacement done every 4 hours.

- Oxytocin can be used for labor augmentation if contractions are inadequate, but should not be used for prolonged time as it can cause fluid overload.
- Pain relief should be offered as a distressed woman is likely to breathe heavily and increase risk of transmission. Epidural analgesia can be given as in non-COVID woman. It further offers convenience as it can serve as a substitute for general anesthesia, if need for emergency cesarean arises. However,

platelet count and coagulation profile need to be checked before as they may have received low molecular weight heparin (LMWH) for thromboprophylaxis.

- Women with mild symptoms can be allowed oral intake and mobility. Daily medications have to be continued. Routine catheterization, enema, antispasmodic agents, antacids, pubic shaving, vaginal irrigation with chlorhexidine are not recommended, as in non-COVID patients. Water birth is not a contraindication for COVID women in labor.

TABLE 1: Timing of delivery in COVID positive patients.

Asymptomatic/mild cases:	*<39 weeks:* • Based on obstetric/medical indication • Not preponed/postponed in view of COVID-19 positive status • Deliver after period of isolation is over, if time permits	*>39 weeks:* Can consider delivery to decrease risk of worsening maternal status with disease progression?
Severe or critically ill patients: Uterine distension in later months, increased oxygen consumption and decreased functional residual capacity in pregnancy may precipitate respiratory failure in pneumonia	*<32 weeks:* • In utero fetal monitoring is considered, till maternal condition is stable or improving • *Refractory hypoxemic failure or worsening clinical condition:* Delivery can be considered. Antenatal corticosteroids can be given if time permits for fetal lung maturation but tocolysis is not recommended in severely ill patients	*32–34 weeks:* Nonintubated • Termination of pregnancy may be considered in view of worsening maternal status. • Delivery is planned before worsening of maternal condition as ongoing hypoxemia may jeopardize the fetus also Intubated • *Double-edged sword:* Worsening maternal condition can compromise the fetus OR Stress of delivery may deteriorate maternal condition

TABLE 2: Route of delivery in COVID positive patients.

Asymptomatic/mild cases	• Route of delivery as per obstetric protocols • Induction can be safely done • Cesarean births are associated with increased risk of maternal deterioration and done for obstetric indications only
Severe/critically ill patients	• Decision has to be individualized • Induction can be done safely but is impractical[6,7] • Concerns of acute decompensation can be an indication for choosing cesarean as mode of delivery

TABLE 3: Birth companion for COVID positive patients.

COVID-19 negative companion (No symptoms of COVID-19 and not tested COVID positive in past 10 days)	COVID-19 positive companion
• Be present with patient throughout labor • Wear a facemask • No frequent movements in and out of the delivery room	• Cannot be physically present • But can be made available virtually via video calls

Management of Second Stage of Labor

Women can adopt birth position of their choice and comfort, if not intubated. There should be continuous electronic FHR monitoring, with review every 5 minutes. Internal FHR monitoring, digital vaginal examination, amniotomy, instrumentation can be performed, if indicated as corona virus has rarely been detected in vaginal secretions or amniotic fluid.[9] Immediate or directed pushing with Valsalva maneuver is not recommended as in non-COVID patients. Woman should be encouraged to follow her own urge to push. However, pushing often causes loss of feces, which contain the virus.[10,11] Further, during pushing woman repeated exhaling forcefully, which may generate droplets.[12-14]

Hence precautions need to be taken. Prolonged labor may cause maternal exhaustion and deteriorate general condition of the COVID positive mother, so progress of labor should be carefully monitored with active intervention when mandated. Antibiotics are not recommended routinely in view of labor or COVID infection, and are given only when bacterial infection is suspected. To reduce perineal trauma, perineal massage, warm perineal compresses, and hands on guarding of perineum are recommended and manual fundal pressure, routine episiotomy, and Ritgen's maneuver are avoided, as in non-COVID patients.

Management of Third Stage of Labor

Active management of third stage of labor to prevent postpartum hemorrhage (PPH) remains the norm in COVID positive patients as well **(Flowchart 3)**. Prophylactic oxytocin 10 U IM/IV is given before delivery of placenta. Controlled cord traction further minimizes blood loss. Sustained uterine massage is not needed, if oxytocin is given.

Delayed cord clamping can be safely performed as it is unlikely to transmit infection from mother to fetus.[15]

In case of PPH, oxytocin, misoprost can be safely used. Carboprost needs to be used with caution as it can compromise cardiovascular system, especially in women with respiratory distress. Tranexamic acid can also be used, however, some clinicians avoid it in COVID-19 patients because its antifibrinolytic properties may increase the risk for thrombosis.[16]

Management of Preterm Labor

- *Corticosteroids*: Use of corticosteroids is *not contraindicated* in these patients and should be given if preterm delivery is anticipated at 28–34 weeks of gestation.

- *Tocolytic agents*: In women presenting with preterm labor, tocolysis is *contraindicated* to avoid complications associated with a systemic illness as per general obstetric dictum. However, decision can be individualized on case-to-case basis depending on severity of disease. If there is a decision for giving tocolysis, beta-mimetic agents should be avoided if there is pulmonary involvement.

- *Magnesium sulfate*: Magnesium sulfate is used for neuroprotection in preterm labor and for seizure prophylaxis in severe pre-eclampsia and eclampsia. It can be used in pregnancy but with caution.
  - In asymptomatic or mild cases, strict *monitoring of magnesium levels* should because magnesium toxicity may cause respiratory depression thus further compromising an already overworked respiratory system.
  - In moderate or critically ill patients, especially in patients with acute kidney injury related to COVID-19 infection, *dose adjustment* is recommended instead of withholding the drug.
  - Intubated patients should be strictly *monitored for magnesium levels* because respiratory toxicity would not be evident in these cases and cardiac arrhythmias or cardiac arrest would be the first manifestation.

A multidisciplinary approach in consultation with a pulmonologist or critical care specialist is recommended in management of such cases.

POSTNATAL CARE

Additional Postnatal Care

COVID positive mothers need additional care in postnatal period, besides regular postnatal care.
- Evaluation for respiratory status is to be continued along with routine postnatal care.
- Importance of good hygiene practices including hand hygiene, perineal hygiene, and frequent disinfection of regularly used belongings should be reiterated.
- Need for frequent expression of breast milk till isolation period is over, is to be explained to patient along with risks associated with breast engorgement.

Flowchart 3: Management of labor in COVID positive patients.

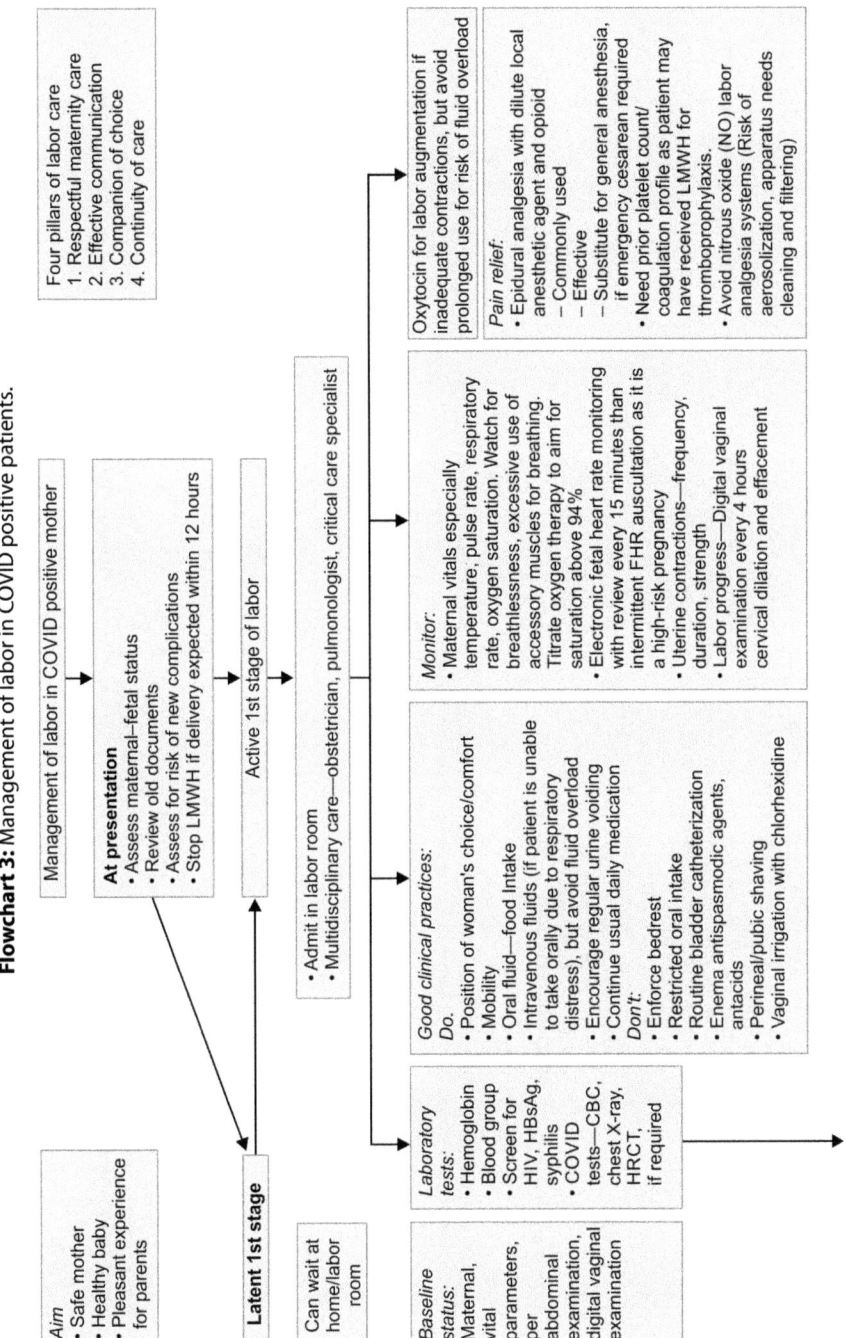

Aim
• Safe mother
• Healthy baby
• Pleasant experience for parents

Management of labor in COVID positive mother

Four pillars of labor care
1. Respectful maternity care
2. Effective communication
3. Companion of choice
4. Continuity of care

At presentation
• Assess maternal–fetal status
• Review old documents
• Assess for risk of new complications
• Stop LMWH if delivery expected within 12 hours

Latent 1st stage

Active 1st stage of labor

Can wait at home/labor room

• Admit in labor room
• Multidisciplinary care—obstetrician, pulmonologist, critical care specialist

Baseline status:
Maternal, vital parameters, per abdominal examination, digital vaginal examination

Laboratory tests:
• Hemoglobin
• Blood group
• Screen for HIV, HBsAg, syphilis
• COVID tests—CBC, chest X-ray, HRCT, if required

Good clinical practices:
Do:
• Position of woman's choice/comfort
• Mobility
• Oral fluid—food intake
• Intravenous fluids (if patient is unable to take orally due to respiratory distress), but avoid fluid overload
• Encourage regular urine voiding
• Continue usual daily medication
Don't:
• Enforce bedrest
• Restricted oral intake
• Routine bladder catheterization
• Enema antispasmodic agents, antacids
• Perineal/pubic shaving
• Vaginal irrigation with chlorhexidine

Monitor:
• Maternal vitals especially temperature, pulse rate, respiratory rate, oxygen saturation. Watch for breathlessness, excessive use of accessory muscles for breathing. Titrate oxygen therapy to aim for saturation above 94%
• Electronic fetal heart rate monitoring with review every 15 minutes than intermittent FHR auscultation as it is a high-risk pregnancy
• Uterine contractions—frequency, duration, strength
• Labor progress—Digital vaginal examination every 4 hours cervical dilation and effacement

Oxytocin for labor augmentation if inadequate contractions, but avoid prolonged use for risk of fluid overload

Pain relief:
• Epidural analgesia with dilute local anesthetic agent and opioid
  – Commonly used
  – Effective
  – Substitute for general anesthesia, if emergency cesarean required
• Need prior platelet count/ coagulation profile as patient may have received LMWH for thromboprophylaxis.
• Avoid nitrous oxide (NO) labor analgesia systems (Risk of aerosolization, apparatus needs cleaning and filtering)

Contd...

Contd...

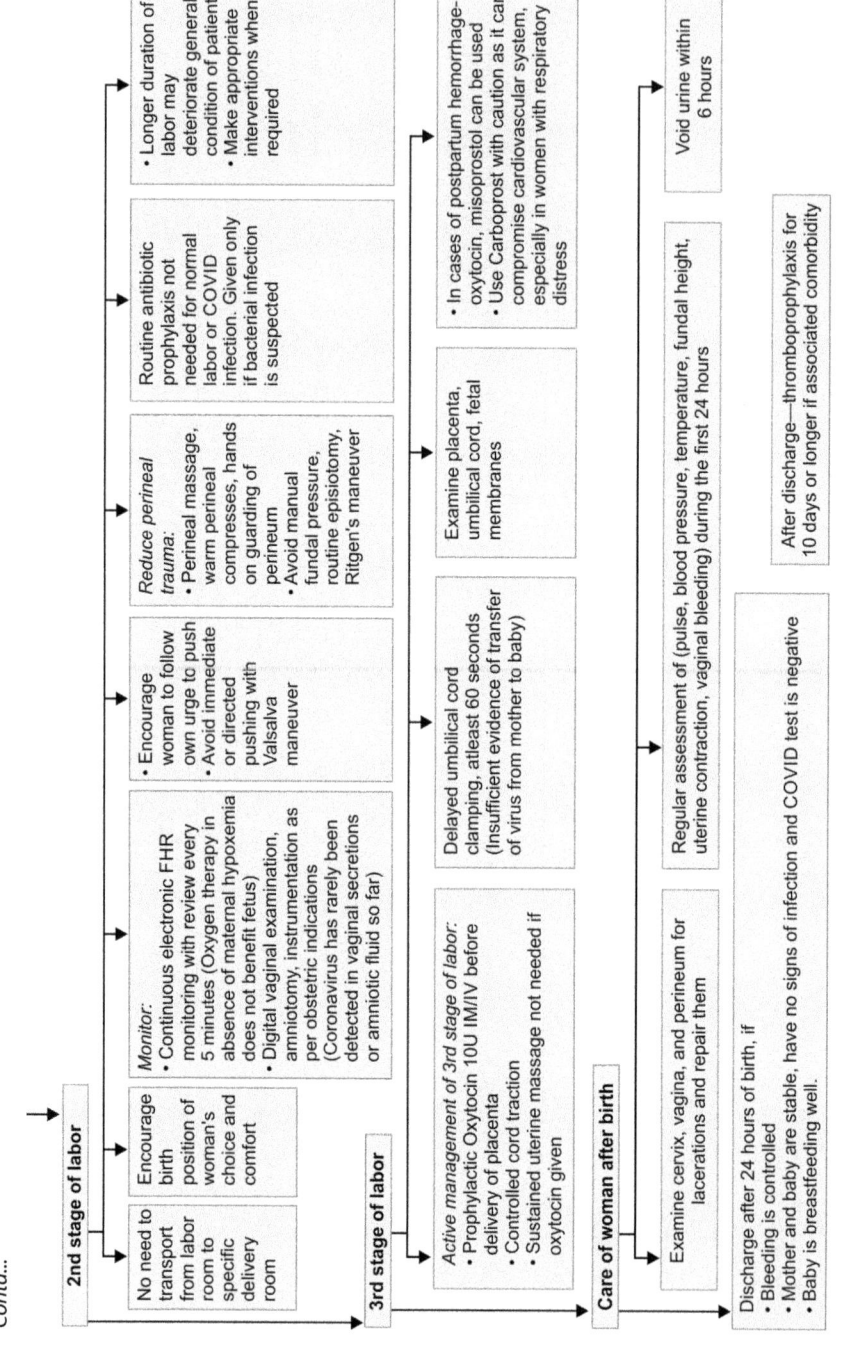

2nd stage of labor

| No need to transport from labor room to specific delivery room | Encourage birth position of woman's choice and comfort |

Monitor:
- Continuous electronic FHR monitoring with review every 5 minutes (Oxygen therapy in absence of maternal hypoxemia does not benefit fetus)
- Digital vaginal examination, amniotomy, instrumentation as per obstetric indications (Coronavirus has rarely been detected in vaginal secretions or amniotic fluid so far)

- Encourage woman to follow own urge to push
- Avoid immediate or directed pushing with Valsalva maneuver

Reduce perineal trauma:
- Perineal massage, warm perineal compresses, hands on guarding of perineum
- Avoid manual fundal pressure, routine episiotomy, Ritgen's maneuver

Routine antibiotic prophylaxis not needed for normal labor or COVID infection. Given only if bacterial infection is suspected

- Longer duration of labor may deteriorate general condition of patient
- Make appropriate interventions when required

3rd stage of labor

Active management of 3rd stage of labor:
- Prophylactic Oxytocin 10U IM/IV before delivery of placenta
- Controlled cord traction
- Sustained uterine massage not needed if oxytocin given

Delayed umbilical cord clamping, atleast 60 seconds (Insufficient evidence of transfer of virus from mother to baby)

Examine placenta, umbilical cord, fetal membranes

- In cases of postpartum hemorrhage-oxytocin, misoprostol can be used
- Use Carboprost with caution as it can compromise cardiovascular system, especially in women with respiratory distress

Care of woman after birth

Examine cervix, vagina, and perineum for lacerations and repair them

Regular assessment of (pulse, blood pressure, temperature, fundal height, uterine contraction, vaginal bleeding) during the first 24 hours

Void urine within 6 hours

Discharge after 24 hours of birth, if
- Bleeding is controlled
- Mother and baby are stable, have no signs of infection and COVID test is negative
- Baby is breastfeeding well.

After discharge—thromboprophylaxis for 10 days or longer if associated comorbidity

- Special care should be taken about maternal mental status as well. Mothers recovering from acute illness or isolation should from baby for they are at risk of developing anxiety, postpartum depression. Role of psychological support and counseling is of utmost importance and brings about desirable outcomes.

Contraception advice should be given to couple as per routine gather approach and should be given according to informed choice of couple.

Breastfeeding

Viral illnesses like CMV, HIV, etc. have been known to be transmitted from mother to baby via breast milk. However, the evidence available is less as of now in COVID cases. So, in light of current evidence WHO, AAP, ICMR, and MOHFW all recommend that nutritional benefits of breastfeeding any day exceed the risk of transmission, whatsoever, so early and exclusive breastfeeding is recommended in mothers with COVID-19 infection as well. Mother needs to be explained about the due

precautions she is supposed to take while breastfeeding.
- Importance of hand hygiene before and after touching the baby (regular hand washing and use of alcohol-based hand rubs), use of a mask (preferably a N-95 or FFP-3 or FFP-2 mask) is recommended.[17]
- The patient should avoid coughing or sneezing while breastfeeding.
- All surfaces should be thoroughly disinfected regularly.
- If mother is too unwell to breastfeed or the infant needs ICU care, expressed milk or formula milk can be given to the infant.

THROMBOPROPHYLAXIS

- All pregnant patients admitted with confirmed or suspected COVID-19 infection should be offered prophylactic LMWH for thromboprophylaxis unless delivery is expected within 12 hours or there is significant risk of hemorrhage.

TABLE 4: Infection control practices for facilities managing COVID positive patients in labor.

At triage	• Keep at least 6 feet distance between patients • Instruct all patients to cover nose and mouth during coughing or sneezing with tissue or flexed elbow for others • Perform hand hygiene after contact with respiratory secretions • Give suspect patient a triple layer surgical mask
Apply standard precautions	• Hand hygiene • Personal protective equipment (PPE) when risk of droplets, aerosols, splashes or in contact with patients' body fluids and secretions (including respiratory secretions) • Appropriate patient placement • Prevention of needle-stick or sharps injury • Safe waste management; cleaning and disinfection of equipment; cleaning of environment—linen
Apply droplet and airborne precautions	• Negative pressure rooms with minimum of 12 air changes per hour for aerosol generating procedures. If not feasible, use well-ventilated single rooms using natural or fresh air • Healthcare workers should use PPE
Apply contact precautions	• Use disposable or dedicated equipment (e.g., stethoscopes, blood pressure cuffs, and thermometers) • If equipment needs to be shared among patients, clean and disinfect between each patient use • Refrain from touching eyes, nose, and mouth with potentially contaminated gloved or ungloved hands • Avoid contaminating environmental surfaces that are not directly related to patient care (e.g., door handles and light switches) • Ensure adequate room ventilation. Avoid movement of patients or transport • Perform hand hygiene

TABLE 5: Personal protective equipment in relation to COVID-19 infection management.[2]

Protection level	Protective equipment	Scope of application
Level I protection	• Disposable surgical cap • Disposable surgical mask • Work uniform • Disposable latex gloves and/or disposable isolation clothing	• Pre-examination triage • General outpatient department
Level II protection	• Disposable surgical cap • Medical protective mask (N-95) • Work uniform • Disposable medical protective uniform • Disposable latex gloves • Goggles	• Nonrespiratory specimen • Examination and imaging • Cleaning surgical instruments of suspected/confirmed patients
Level III protection	• Disposable surgical cap, medical protective mask (N-95) • Work uniform, disposable medical protective • Uniform, disposable latex gloves • Full face respiratory protective devices or powered air-purifying respirator	Surgery, procedures, delivery, intubation, and resuscitation of suspected/confirmed patients

- Thromboprophylaxis should be given for a minimum of 10 days following hospital discharge and a longer duration should be considered if patient has an associated comorbidity.
- Confirmed or suspected cases within 6 weeks postpartum should be offered thromboprophylaxis for duration of their hospital stay and at least 10 days postdischarge.

In cases with severe illness, appropriate dosing regimen should be decided according to patient's weight following a multidisciplinary approach involving a senior obstetrician, pulmonologist and a critical care specialist.

INFECTION PREVENTION AND CONTROL PRACTICES

Infection prevention control (IPC) form a critical and integral part of clinical management of COVID positive patients **(Table 4)**.[1,3] Healthcare workers should use appropriate personal protective equipment (PPE) as per the degree and duration of exposure to COVID patients **(Table 5)**.

CONCLUSION

- Universal screening by RT-PCR is recommended for all women in labor presenting to hospital. Patients should be triaged into confirmed negative, suspected, and confirmed positive cases accordingly and managed in separate areas.
- COVID patients should be classified based on their severity of illness.
- Multidisciplinary care involving obstetrician, medical care specialist, pulmonologist, and intensive care specialist should be given in COVID positive mothers in labor, especially in severe illness.
- Infection control practices need to be followed strictly in hospital spaces, to prevent transmission among patients and healthcare workers.
- Monitor maternal vitals every hour, especially respiratory rate, oxygen saturation, and temperature. Titrate oxygen therapy to maintain saturation above 94%.
- Continuous fetal heart monitoring is preferred, with review every 15 minutes in active first stage, and every 5 minutes in second stage of labor, as there is increased incidence of abnormal tracings, especially in critically ill mother.
- Avoid prolonged oxytocin infusion as it may cause fluid overload.
- Avoid prolonged labor for risk of maternal exhaustion.
- Virus has rarely been seen in vaginal secretions or blood, but is present in feces, droplets

generated on forced exhalation during pushing.

- Magnesium sulfate, corticosteroids, oxytocin, and misoprost can be used for their usual indications.
- Delayed cord clamping and breastfeeding can be safely practiced.
- Thromboprophylaxis is given to all COVID positive pregnant women, stopped if labor is expected in next 12 hours, resumed postpartum for 10 days postpartum.

▓ REFERENCES

1. ICMR. Guidance for Management of Pregnant Women in COVID-19 Pandemic. [online]. Available from https://www.icmr.gov.in/pdf/covid/techdoc/Guidance_for_Management_of_Pregnant_Women_in_COVID19_Pandemic_12042020.pdf [Last accessed December, 2021].
2. The Federation of Obstetric and Gynecological Societies of India. (2020). FOGSI's GCPR on Pregnancy with COVID-19 Infection—for your valuable suggestions. [online]. Available from https://www.fogsi.org/fogsi-gcpr-on-pregnancy-with-covid-19-infection-version-2/ [Last accessed December, 2021].
3. Ministry of Health and Family Welfare, Government of India (2021). Clinical Management Protocol for COVID-19 (In Adults). [online]. Available from https://www.mohfw.gov.in/pdf/UpdatedDetailed Clinical Management Protocol for COVID-19 adults dated 24052021. pdf [Last accessed December, 2021].
4. Walker KF, O'Donoghue K, Grace N, Dorling J, Comeau JL, Li W, et al. Maternal transmission of SARS-COV-2 to the neonate, and possible routes for such transmission: a systematic review and critical analysis. BJOG Int J Obstet Gynaecol. 2020;127(11):1324-36.
5. Cai J, Tang M, Gao Y, Zhang H, Yang Y, Zhang D, et al. Cesarean section or vaginal delivery to prevent possible vertical transmission from a pregnant mother confirmed with COVID-19 to a neonate: a systematic review. Front Med (Lausanne). 2021;8:634949.
6. Slayton-Milam S, Sheffels S, Chan D, Alkinj B. Induction of labor in an intubated patient with coronavirus disease 2019 (COVID-19). Obstet Gynecol. 2020;136(5):962-4.
7. Liu C, Sun W, Wang C, Liu F, Zhou M. Delivery during extracorporeal membrane oxygenation (ECMO) support of pregnant woman with severe respiratory distress syndrome caused by influenza: a case report and review of the literature. J Matern Fetal Neonatal Med. 2019;32(15):2570-4.
8. Royal College of Obstetricians and Gynaecologists. (2021). Coronavirus (COVID-19) Infection in Pregnancy. [online]. Available from https://www.rcm.org.uk/media/4724/2021-02-19-coronavirus-covid-19-infection-in-pregnancy-v13.pdf [Last accessed December, 2021].
9. Schwartz DA. An analysis of 38 pregnant women with COVID-19, their newborn infants, and maternal-fetal transmission of SARS-CoV-2: maternal coronavirus infections and pregnancy outcomes. Arch Pathol Lab Med. 2020;144(7):799-805.
10. Wang W, Xu Y, Gao R, Lu R, Han K, Wu G, et al. Detection of SARS-CoV-2 in different types of clinical specimens. JAMA. 2020;323(18):1843-4.
11. Zhang W, Du RH, Li B, Zheng XS, Yang XL, Hu B, et al. Molecular and serological investigation of 2019-nCoV infected patients: implication of multiple shedding routes. Emerg Microbes Infect. 2020;9(1):386-9.
12. Berghella V. NOW!: protection for obstetrical providers and patients. Am J Obstet Gynecol MFM. 2020;2(2):100109.
13. Jamieson DJ, Steinberg JP, Martinello RA, Perl TM, Rasmussen SA. Obstetricians on the Coronavirus Disease 2019 (COVID-19) Front Lines and the Confusing World of Personal Protective Equipment. Obstet Gynecol. 2020;135(6):1257-63.
14. Boelig RC, Manuck T, Oliver EA, Di Mascio D, Saccone G, Bellussi F, et al. Labor and delivery guidance for COVID-19. Am J Obstet Gynecol MFM. 2020;2(2):100110.
15. American Academy of Pediatrics (2021). FAQs: Management of infants born to mothers with suspected or confirmed COVID-19. [online]. Available from http://services.aap.org/en/pages/2019-novel-coronavirus-covid-19-infections/clinical-guidance/faqs-management-of-infants-born-to-covid-19-mothers/[Last accessed December, 2021].
16. Ogawa H, Asakura H. Consideration of tranexamic acid administration to COVID-19 patients. Physiol Rev. 2020;100(4):1595-6.
17. Shlomai NO, Kasirer Y, Strauss T, Smolkin T, Marom R, Shinwell ES, et al. Neonatal SARS-CoV-2 infections in breastfeeding mothers. Pediatrics. 2021;147(5):e2020010918.

Human Immunodeficiency Virus-positive in Labor

Sangeeta Rai

INTRODUCTION

Human immunodeficiency virus (HIV) is ribonucleic acid (RNA) retrovirus. Its infection leads to infected person susceptible to opportunistic infection resulting in acquired immunodeficiency syndrome (AIDS). Parent to child transmission known as vertical transmission of HIV during pregnancy, delivery or breastfeeding is the primary cause of HIV infection in children.[1]

India has the third highest HIV burden in the world. NACO (National AIDS Control Organization) technical estimate report (2015) estimated that out of 29 million annual pregnancies in India, 35,255 occur in HIV-positive pregnant women.[2] In the absence of any intervention, an estimated cohort of 10,361 infected babies will be born annually. Henceforth India is committed to "ending the AIDS" epidemic as a public health threat by 2030 in line with sustainable development goals (SDGs). India is committed to the "elimination of mother-to-child transmission of HIV and syphilis" by 2020.[3]

VERTICAL TRANSMISSION OF HUMAN IMMUNODEFICIENCY VIRUS

Human immunodeficiency virus-positive mother can transmit the infection to the newborn but, as mother mostly gets infection from her partner so our national guidelines use the terminology parent-to-child transmission instead of mother-to-child transmission (**Table 1**). This vertical transmission can occur mostly during peripartum period.

Risk of HIV transmission is directly proportional to the plasma HIV RNA load. HIV is the least teratogenic virus because transplacental spread of infection to fetus in utero is very rare. But, the risk of virus transmission from infected birth canal is very high during vaginal delivery. This results in increased risk of transmission of infection to baby during peripartum period that is last few

TABLE 1: Intervention and risk of HIV transmission from mother-to-child.

Intervention	Risk of HIV transmission from mother-to-child
During pregnancy	5–10%
During labor and delivery	10–15%
During breastfeeding	5–10%
MTCT without breastfeeding	15–25%
Breastfeeding up to 6 months	20–35%
Breastfeeding up to 18–24 months	30–45%
ART with breastfeeding	2%
ART without breastfeeding	1%

(ART: antiretroviral treatment; HIV: human immunodeficiency virus; MTCT: mother-to-child transmission)

weeks of pregnancy and during delivery. The risk of parent-to-child transmission is 15–30% in nonbreastfeeding mother without any intervention while with breastfeeding this risk will be increased further by 5–10%. It is seen that timely identification of HIV and use of combination of intervention, the risk of perinatal transmission can be reduced from 30% to <1%.[2]

The risk of transmission will be reduced to 2% with use of antiretroviral treatment (ART) along with continuation of breastfeeding and which further reduced to 1% if ART given without breastfeeding.

PREVENTION OF PARENT-TO-CHILD TRANSMISSION

The Prevention of Parent to Child Transmission (PPTCT) of HIV/AIDS program was launched in the country in the year 2002. The PPTCT program aims to prevent the perinatal transmission of HIV from an HIV-infected pregnant mother to her newborn baby with four integral elements. This provides access to all pregnant women for HIV education, prevention, diagnosis, treatment, and along with care of newborn of HIV-positive mother (**Table 2**).

Essential package of PPTCT services includes:
- HIV testing is recommended in all pregnant women with opt-out approach.
- ART is recommended to all HIV-positive women irrespective of CD4 count and WHO clinical staging and once started should continue lifelong.
- Vaginal delivery is recommended. Cesarean section done only for obstetric indication (ACOG guideline recommended elective cesarean section for woman with HIV RNA load >1,000 copies/mL).
- Continue exclusive breastfeeding (avoid mixed feeding)

- Newborn HIV-exposed babies are initiated on 6 weeks of syrup nevirapine immediately after birth so as to prevent transmission of HIV from mother-to-child and is extended to 12 weeks of syrup nevirapine, if the duration of the ART of mother is <24 weeks.
- The HIV-exposed baby is initiated on cotrimoxazole prophylaxis at 6 weeks.

LABOR AND DELIVERY IN HUMAN IMMUNODEFICIENCY VIRUS-POSITIVE WOMEN

According to NACO, vaginal delivery is recommended to all HIV-positive women and cesarean section recommended for obstetric indication only.[2]

Intrapartum management has been depicted in **Flowchart 1**.

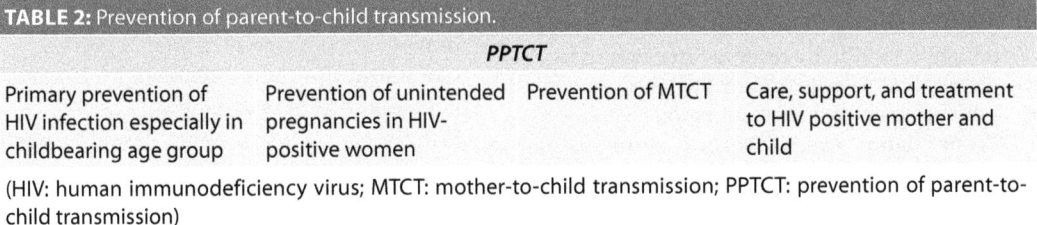

TABLE 2: Prevention of parent-to-child transmission.

PPTCT			
Primary prevention of HIV infection especially in childbearing age group	Prevention of unintended pregnancies in HIV-positive women	Prevention of MTCT	Care, support, and treatment to HIV positive mother and child

(HIV: human immunodeficiency virus; MTCT: mother-to-child transmission; PPTCT: prevention of parent-to-child transmission)

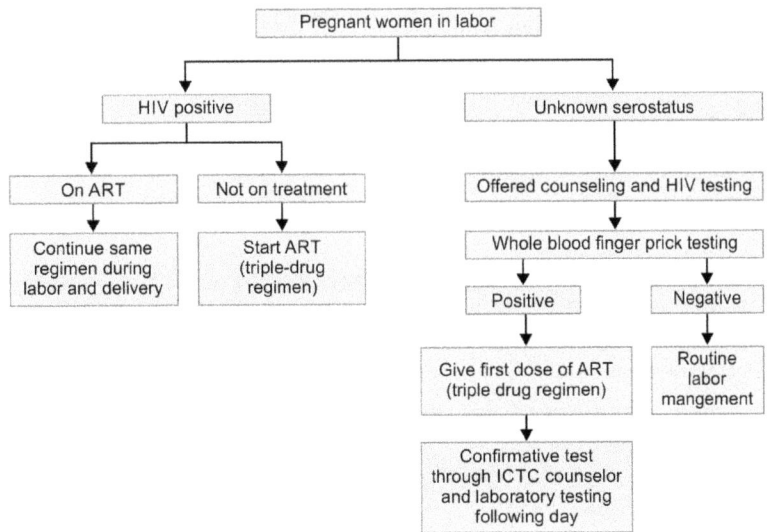

Flowchart 1: Intrapartum management.

(ART: antiretroviral treatment; HIV: human immunodeficiency virus; ICTC: integrated counseling and testing centers)

VAGINAL DELIVERY IN HUMAN IMMUNODEFICIENCY VIRUS-POSITIVE WOMEN

Highest risk of vertical transmission of HIV is during delivery.

Factors increasing risk of transmission:
- Maternal viral load
- Prolonged rupture of membranes
- Repeated per vaginal examinations
- Assisted instrumental delivery
- Invasive intrapartum fetal monitoring
- Episiotomy
- Prematurity

MANAGEMENT OF LABOR IN HUMAN IMMUNODEFICIENCY VIRUS-POSITIVE WOMEN

- Follow standard or universal work precaution
- *ARM*: Avoid artificial rupture of membrane (ARM) and keep membrane intact as long as possible, ARM to be reserved in cases of fetal distress and delay in progress of labor.
- Minimize per vaginal examination
- Proper labor event charting done using partogram or labor care guide
- Avoid invasive fetal monitoring
- Instrumental delivery is not preferred. It is reserved for fetal distress or significant maternal exhaustion. If indicated, low cavity outlet forceps preferred over ventouse.
- Unnecessary episiotomy avoided
- Safer surgical technique to be used to stitch episiotomy or lacerations.
- Standard waste disposal protocol to be followed for disposal of placenta and other medical and infectious waste.

- Counsel regarding postpartum intrauterine contraceptive device (IUCD) insertion

Cesarean Delivery in Human Immunodeficiency Virus-positive Women

Antiretroviral treatment in HIV-positive women for elective cesarean section **(Table 3)**.

Safer Surgical Techniques

Safer surgical technique for cesarean delivery:
- Standard or universal work precaution should be followed.
- Follow surgical fascial plane during surgery which would avoids unnecessary bleeding that is dry hemostatic technique.
- Use cautery judiciously
- Try to deliver head of baby by keeping membrane intact
- Immediate cord clamping after delivery
- Use round tip blunt needle and use needle holders and forceps to handle it
- Handle sharp instruments carefully while transferring to assistants

IMMEDIATE CARE OF THE NEWBORN

- Avoid nasogastric suctioning
- Wipe the blood away from the newborn
- Place infant on mother's abdomen
- Administer nevirapine to the infant within 1 hour
- Encourage exclusive breastfeeding
- Early infant testing

TABLE 3: Emergency situations and their antiretroviral treatment (ART).

Situation	ART*
Elective cesarean section	ART given prior to operation
Emergency cesarean section in women on lifelong ART	Continue standard ART regimen
Emergency cesarean section in women not on ART	Start ART prior to procedure and continue thereafter

*Standard prophylactic antibiotics to be given in all.

Immediate Postpartum Care

- Involve family and husband in postpartum care of mother and newborn
- Counsel patient and relative regarding follow-up, continuation of ART, and continuation of nevirapine prophylaxis for newborn
- Counsel regarding family planning, insertion of Cu-T at 6 weeks [if postpartum IUCD (PPIUCD) not inserted], and use of condoms (dual protection) to avoid unnecessary pregnancies
- Encourage male sterilization [nonscalpel vasectomy (NSV)] at 18 months to 2 years postdelivery.
- Breastfeeding

Exclusive breastfeeding: Breastfeeding increases risk of vertical transmission by 5–10%. This risk will be reduced to 2% if woman on ART with exclusive breastfeeding and further to 1% if woman on ART without breastfeeding. But, in our country infant mortality is higher due to poor nutrition and other infections and diseases as compare to HIV infection. So, NACO guideline recommends exclusive breastfeeding along with ART and infant nevirapine prophylaxis. If exclusive complimentary feeding is affordable to family, then it should be given.

Mixed feeding: Mixed feeding that is breastfeeding along with complimentary feeding in-between should be avoided as it has more risk of HIV transmission as compare to exclusive breast-feeding.

Exclusive breastfeeding to be given till 6 months and then complimentary feeding will be added to it. Breastfeeding can be continued up to 1 year and in early infant diagnosis (EID)-negative babies and up to 2 years in EID-positive babies.

Late Postnatal Care

- Ensure continuation of ART and nevirapine prophylaxis in infant
- Follow-up of patient for evaluation of infection and management
- Nutritious diet, adequate rest, and supplements
- Continued counseling and education regarding contraception and motivation for NSV in male
- Ensure baby linkage to EID and ART program.

TABLE 4: Different guidelines and recommendations regarding mode of delivery.

Guidelines	Recommendations
RCOG	Planned cesarean section at 38 completed weeks for HIV-positive mother on HAART therapy and vaginal delivery if viral load >50 copies/mL and CD4 count <350[4]
ACOG	Elective cesarean section if viral load is >1,000 copies/mL or unknown status[5]
NACO	Vaginal delivery[2]

(ACOG: American College of Obstetricians and Gynecologists; HAART: highly active antiretroviral therapy; NACO: National AIDS Control Organization; RCOG: Royal College of Obstetricians and Gynaecologists)

Care of Human Immunodeficiency Virus-exposed Infants

- Immediate care at birth
- Infant feeding
- Continue ART/ARV prophylaxis
- Support daily nevirapine administration to the infant
- Counsel family members to provide constant support and care
- Immunization and vitamin A supplementation
- Cotrimoxazole prophylaxis
- Monitor growth and development
- *Early infant diagnosis:* All HIV-exposed infants and children regardless of HIV status will be followed-up until 18 months of age for care, monitoring, and the final confirmatory HIV test at 18 months using three HIV rapid tests (even if HIV-1 rapid test is negative). No dried blood spot (DBS) and whole blood sample (WBS) [deoxyribonucleic acid/polymerase chain reaction (DNA/PCR)] testing to be done at or after 18 months.

Different guidelines and recommendations regarding mode of delivery have been given in **Table 4**.

ANTIRETROVIRAL TREATMENT

Lifelong triple drug regimen ART is initiated in all pregnant women with confirmed HIV infection regardless of WHO clinics staging and CD4 count at any gestational age and in labor and continued lifelong.[2]

Triple drug regimen: Tenofovir (TDF) 300 mg + Lamivudine (3TC) 300 mg + Efavirenz (EFV) 600 mg	
Pregnant woman with HIV	ART regimen
Not on any treatment	Preferred regimen: TDF + 3TC + EFV Alternative first-line treatment: AZT + 3TC + EFV AZT + 3TC + NVP TDF + 3TC + NVP
With prior exposure to NNRTIs	TDF + 3TC + LPV/r
Already on ART	Continue same regimen

(ART: antiretroviral treatment; HIV: human immunodeficiency virus; NNRTIs: non-nucleoside reverse transcriptase inhibitors)

Starting cotrimoxazole prophylaxis in pregnancy:

- Cotrimoxazole should be started if CD4 count is ≤250 cells/mm³
- *Dose*: Double strength tablet—1 tablet daily

ARV prophylaxis for infants born to mothers receiving lifelong ART:

Nevirapine prophylaxis	
Mother on ART	Continued NVP till 6 weeks
Mother not on ART or on ART < 24 weeks	Continued NVP for 12 weeks

CONCLUSION

- Preconceptional counseling of all HIV-positive women to be done, for starting ART so as to reduce viral load before conception and reducing overall risk of vertical transmission.
- HIV testing and counseling for all pregnant, women should be considered an integral component of essential care during pregnancy.

- HIV-positive women should have ART immediately after diagnosis irrespective of her CD4 count and WHO clinical staging and continued lifelong to reduce risk of transmission of infection to breastfeeding infant.
- Postpartum follow-up of patient will be done and ensure continuation of ART and linkage to ART center.
- Rapid HIV testing should be available in labor ward for unknown HIV status cases, so that HIV-positive cases identified timely and mother will be started immediately on ART and infant will receive nevirapine prophylaxis on time.

REFERENCES

1. World Health Organization. (2006). Guidelines on care, treatment and support for women living with HIV/AIDS and their children in resource-constrained settings. [online]. Available from https://www.who.int/hiv/pub/guidelines/sexualreproductivehealth.pdf [Last accessed December, 2021].
2. Government of India Ministry of Health & Family Welfare, Department of AIDS Control Basic Services Division. (2013). Prevention of Parent to Child Transmission (PPTCT) of HIV using Multi Drug Anti-retroviral Regimen in India. [online]. Available from http://naco.gov.in/sites/default/files/National_Guidelines_for_PPTCT.pdf [Last accessed December, 2021].
3. National AIDS Control Organisation, Ministry of Health and Family Welfare, Government of India. (2017). National Strategic Plan for HIV/AIDS and STI 2017–2024. [online]. Available from http://naco.gov.in/sites/default/files/Paving%20the%20Way%20for%20an%20AIDS%2015122017.pdf [Last accessed December, 2021].
4. Royal College of Obstetricians and Gynaecologists. (2010). HIV in Pregnancy, Management (Green-top Guideline No. 39), 2010. [online]. Available from https://www.rcog.org.uk/en/guidelines-research-services/guidelines/gtg39/ [Last accessed December, 2021].
5. ACOG Committee Opinion No. 751: Labor and Delivery Management of Women With Human Immunodeficiency Virus Infection. Obstet Gynecol. 2018;132(3):e131-e137.

CHAPTER

45

Preterm Labor

Vanita Jain

DEFINITION

Preterm labor (PTL) is defined as presence of regular uterine contractions that result in cervical dilation and effacement over time at 24+0 to 36+6 weeks.

DIAGNOSIS

The diagnosis of PTL is based on clinical criteria of painful, regular uterine contractions along with a change in cervical dilation, effacement, or both, or presence of regular uterine contractions and cervical effacement ≥80% or cervical dilation of at least 2 cm at admission. If and till the diagnosis of PTL is not established, the woman is classified as having "threatened preterm labor".

OUTCOME

Less than 10% of women having a clinical diagnosis of PTL actually deliver within 7 days of presentation and approximately 50% of patients with suspected PTL subsequently deliver at term. Thus, it is prudent to make efforts to identify which of the women who present with PTL are likely to deliver prematurely. This is important because if the woman is identified to be in true PTL, many interventions can be done that can improve neonatal outcome. These include administration of antenatal corticosteroid therapy, magnesium sulfate for neuroprotection, and if required transfer to a facility with an appropriate level of newborn care. Similarly, if the woman is not actually in PTL, unnecessary and sometimes costly interventions can be avoided.

GOALS OF MANAGEMENT

- To identify women presenting with PTL who are at high risk of spontaneous preterm birth.

- To identify the possible cause of PTL based on the history and physical examination although many cases are idiopathic. The cause may be an underlying obstetric complication (e.g., abruption) or medical or surgical disorder (e.g., appendicitis, pyelonephritis, and pneumonia) which would require specific treatment.

EVALUATION

History

- Suspect PTL in any patient presenting between 24 and 36+6 weeks with mild uterine contractions, menstrual-like cramping, low back ache, feeling of heaviness in the vagina or vaginal discharge of mucus, which may be clear or slightly bloody show.
- Assess the gestational age
- Review the patient's past and present obstetric and medical history, to identify the risk factors for preterm birth and to identify the possible cause.

Examination

- Maternal vital signs (temperature, blood pressure, heart rate, and respiratory rate)
- Assessment of contraction frequency, duration, and intensity
- The fetal heart rate pattern

Speculum Examination

- Estimate cervical dilation. Cervical dilation ≥3 cm supports the diagnosis of PTL.
- Assess if uterine bleeding is present and its amount. Bleeding from abruptio placentae or placenta previa can trigger PTL.
- Evaluate fetal membrane status (intact or ruptured)

Digital Vaginal Examination

- To be done after placenta previa and rupture of membranes have been excluded.
- Assess cervical dilation and effacement

Obstetric Ultrasound Examination

- Look for presence/absence of fetal, placental, and maternal anatomic abnormalities
- Confirm fetal presentation, assess amniotic fluid volume, and estimate fetal weight

This information is needed to counsel the patient about the potential causes and outcomes of preterm birth and deciding the best route of delivery.

Transvaginal ultrasound: Measure cervical length when the diagnosis of PTL is unclear. A short cervix before 34 weeks of gestation (<30 mm) is predictive of an increased risk for preterm birth, while a long cervix (≥30 mm) has a high negative predictive value for preterm birth.

Laboratory Evaluation

- *Urine culture*: Asymptomatic bacteriuria is associated with an increased risk of PTL and birth.
- Fetal fibronectin (fFN) should be performed if available when the diagnosis of PTL is doubtful. A fFN concentration ≥50 ng/mL in cervicovaginal fluid between 22+0 and 34+6 weeks of gestation in women with intact membranes correlates with an increased risk of preterm delivery within 7 days.

Management

After the above stated evaluation the patient would be classified into:
- No definitive diagnosis of PTL
- Definitive evidence of PTL

If no definitive diagnosis of PTL:
- Observe over 4–6 hours
- If uterine contractions are not increasing in frequency or intensity, cervix <2 cm dilated and cervical length >30 mm and fetal fibronectin is <50 ng/mL. The woman is at lowrisk of preterm birth.
- Confirm fetal well-being (e.g., reactive non-stress test)

- Exclude the presence of an acute precipitating event (e.g., abruption or overt infection)

Repeat per vaginum examination to see if the cervix is not progressively dilating or effacing. Discharge the patient with advice to follow-up in 1–2 weeks or if she develops signs or symptoms of PTL, or has any other pregnancy concerns (e.g., bleeding or leakage per vaginum or decreased fetal movements).

If definitive evidence of PTL:
If the woman is diagnosed as being in PTL and at high risk of spontaneous preterm birth the following interventions should be done.
1. Counseling
2. Corticosteroids
3. Tocolysis
4. Magnesium sulfate

Counseling

- The patient should be explained the inaccuracies of clinical assessment and diagnostic tests for diagnosing PTL.
- The benefits and risks of the proposed therapies
- Counseling by a neonatologist regarding the neonatal care needed and the prognosis of the neonate

Antenatal Corticosteroids

A course of steroids should be administered to all pregnant patients at 23+0 to 33+6 weeks of gestation who are at increased risk of preterm delivery within the next 7 days to reduce neonatal morbidity and mortality associated with preterm birth. At this gestational age, corticosteroids improve neonatal survival and reduce major short-term morbidity. For patients at 34+0 to 36+6 weeks most guidelines recommend administration of steroids. The options include betamethasone two doses of 12 mg intramuscularly 24 hours apart or dexamethasone four doses of 6 mg intramuscularly 12 hours apart. Transient hyperglycemia and an increase in total leukocyte count may be seen after the administration of steroids. The efficacy of steroids is maximum after 48 hours from administration of the first dose however, neonatal benefits begin to start within a few hours of administration. A single repeat course may be considered if the previous one has been administered >7 days ago.

Tocolysis

Tocolytic therapy may provide short-term prolongation of pregnancy. However, there is no evidence that tocolytic therapy has any direct favorable effect on neonatal outcomes. The upper limit of gestation for the use of tocolytic agents to prevent preterm birth is 34 weeks as beyond this gestation the perinatal morbidity and mortality are too low to justify the potential maternal and fetal complications and costs associated with inhibition of PTL.

Goals:
- Delay delivery by at least 48 hours so that antenatal corticosteroids administered to the mother have time to achieve their maximum effects.
- Provide time for safe in utero transport of the mother if required
- In patients where the cause of PTL is an underlying, self-limited condition that can cause labor, such as pyelonephritis or abdominal surgery.

Contraindications: Tocolysis is contraindicated when the maternal and fetal risks of prolonging pregnancy are greater than the risks associated with preterm birth. The contraindications include:
- Intrauterine fetal demise
- Lethal fetal anomaly
- Nonreassuring fetal status
- Severe pre-eclampsia or eclampsia
- Maternal bleeding with hemodynamic instability
- Chorioamnionitis
- Maternal contraindications to individual tocolytic agents

Choice of tocolytics:
- *Indomethacin:*
  - *Dose:* 50–100 mg loading dose (may be given orally or per rectum), followed by 25 mg orally every 4–6 hours.
  - *Side effects:* Mainly gastrointestinal such as nausea, esophageal reflux, gastritis, and emesis.
  - *Contraindications:* Platelet dysfunction or bleeding diathesis, hepatic dysfunction, gastrointestinal ulcerative disease, renal dysfunction, and asthma.
    - *Monitoring:* If continued for >48 hours, sonographic evaluation for oligohydramnios and narrowing of the fetal ductus arteriosus should be done and if either is detected the therapy should be discontinued.
    - *Caution:* It should not be given beyond 32 weeks of gestation as it may lead to premature narrowing or closure of the ductus arteriosus in the fetus.
- *Nifedipine:*
  - *Dose:* Loading dose of 20–30 mg orally, followed by an additional 10–20 mg orally every 3–8 hours for up to 48 hours, with a maximum dose of 180 mg/day.
  - *Side effects* are due to peripheral vasodilatation which may lead to dizziness, flushing, and palpitations.
  - *Contraindications* are known hypersensitivity to the drug, hypotension, and congestive heart failure. Nifedipine is a safe drug and is generally well tolerated
- *Beta-agonists (e.g., terbutaline):*
  - *Dose:* 0.25 mg is to be administered subcutaneously every 20–30 minutes for up to four doses or until tocolysis is achieved. Once labor is inhibited, 0.25 mg can be administered subcutaneously every 3–4 hours until the uterus is relaxed for 24 hours. It can also be administered as a continuous intravenous infusion started at 2.5–5 µg/min and increasing by 2.5–5 µg/min every 20–30 minutes to a maximum of 25 µg/min, or until the contractions have ceased. The infusion is then reduced to the lowest dose that maintains uterine quiescence.
  - *Side effects:* Tachycardia, palpitations, low blood pressure, hyperglycemia, and hypokalemia.
  - *Contraindications:* In women with tachycardia-sensitive cardiac disease and in women with poorly controlled hyperthyroidism or diabetes mellitus.
  - *Monitoring:* During treatment, fluid intake, urine output, and maternal symptoms, especially shortness of breath, chest pain, or tachycardia should be monitored. Glucose and potassium concentrations should be monitored every 4–6 hours. The drug should be

stopped if the maternal heart rate exceeds 120 beats/min.

- *Magnesium sulfate*:
  - *Dose*: 4–6 g IV loading dose given over 20 minutes, followed by a continuous infusion of 2 g/hour. The infusion rate is titrated based upon assessment of contraction frequency and maternal toxicity. The infusion is continued until 12-24 hours of uterine quiescence is achieved.
  - *Side effects*: Diaphoresis and flushing.
  - *Contraindications*: Myasthenia gravis and myocardial compromise.
  - *Monitoring*: The patient should be monitored for toxicity by patellar reflex, respiratory rate, and urine output if serum creatinine is >1.0 mg/dL.
  - *Caution*: The concomitant use of a calcium channel blocker and magnesium sulfate could result in respiratory depression.
- *Nitric oxide (NO) donors (e.g., nitroglycerin, NTG patch)*:
  - *Dose*: 10 mg nitroglycerin patch is applied to the skin of the abdomen. After 1 hour, if there is no reduction in contraction frequency or intensity, an additional patch is applied; a maximum of two patches are administered simultaneously. The patches are left in situ for 24 hours, after which they are removed and the patient reassessed.
  - *Side effects*: Dizziness, flushing, palpitations, and maternal hypotension.
  - *Contraindications*: No donors should not be used in women with hypotension or with preload-dependent cardiac lesions, such as aortic insufficiency.
- *Atosiban*:
  - *Dose*: Administered intravenously beginning with a bolus of 6.75 mg over 1 minute followed by a 300 µg/min (18 mg/hour) infusion for 3 hours, and then 100 µg/min (6 mg/hour) for up to 45 hours (to a maximum of 330 mg).
  - *Side effects*: Minimal side effects in the form of hypersensitivity and injection site reactions. No adverse maternal cardiovascular effects have been reported.
  - *Contraindications*: No absolute contraindications.

Discontinue tocolytics:
- If labor progresses despite treatment.
- 48–72 hours after administration of the first corticosteroid dose if contractions subside. There is no evidence to support their use for longer duration.

Magnesium Sulfate for Neuroprotection

Magnesium sulfate should be administered to women at <32 weeks of gestation, who are likely to deliver within 24 hours as it decreases the incidence and severity of cerebral palsy. In utero exposure to magnesium sulfate provides neuroprotection against cerebral palsy and other types of severe motor dysfunction in neonates born preterm. A loading dose of 4 g is given over 20 minutes followed by a maintenance dose of 1 g/hour till delivery or for a maximum of 24 hours. It is contraindicated in women with myasthenia gravis, should be avoided in women with known myocardial compromise and used cautiously in women with impaired renal function. It should be given for a maximum of 24 hours and stopped after that even if delivery has not occurred.

Ineffective therapies: There is no evidence-based role of antibiotics, progesterone, bed rest, hydration, or sedation.

If episode of preterm labor resolves:
- *Patients >34 weeks*: These patients can be discharged, as long as tests of fetal well-being are reassuring and there are no additional complications that warrant hospitalization.
- For patients <34 weeks of gestation, the duration of hospitalization should depend on patient-specific factors like gestational age, cervical status, past obstetric history, etc.
- Progesterone should be continued for patients who were candidates for therapy before their episode of PTL to reduce the risk of preterm birth because of a history of prior preterm birth or the finding of a sonographic short cervix. An episode of PTL is not an indication to start progesterone therapy if not otherwise indicated.
- Maintenance tocolysis is not recommended as it does not improve neonatal outcome.

If the labor progresses:
- Avoid early amniotomy unless indicated
- Mode of delivery to be decided by obstetric indications

- Selective use of episiotomy is recommended for rigid perineum or need to facilitate delivery of a compromised fetus.
- Instrumental delivery only if indicated, use of vacuum is to be limited to deliveries ≥34 weeks of gestation because of the risk of intraventricular hemorrhage.
- Neonatologist to be informed about the gestational age.
- Delayed cord clamping is recommended if the mother and baby are stable. Situations where immediate pediatric assistance is needed, such as thick meconium or neonatal depression cord milking is an alternative to delayed clamping for enhancing blood transfusion.
- Preterm deliveries are associated with a longer third stage than term deliveries.

CONCLUSION

Preterm labor leading to preterm birth is a leading cause of neonatal morbidity and mortality and occurs most commonly among women with no risk factors. The clinical findings of early labor are poorly predictive of the outcome. The evaluation aims to identify women who are likely to deliver preterm and would benefit from interventions to improve neonatal outcome. These interventions include counseling, antenatal corticosteroid administration, tocolysis, magnesium sulfate for neuroprotection, and transfer to a facility with appropriate neonatal services.

BIBLIOGRAPHY

1. American College of Obstetricians and Gynecologists' Committee on Practice Bulletins—Obstetrics. Practice Bulletin No. 171: Management of Preterm Labor. American College of Obstetricians and Gynecologists' Committee on Practice Bulletins—Obstetrics. Obstet Gynecol. 2016;128(4):e155-e164.
2. Lockwood CJ. (2021). Preterm labor: Clinical findings, diagnostic evaluation, and initial treatment. [online]. Available from https://www.uptodate.com/contents/preterm-labor-clinical-findings-diagnostic-evaluation-and-initial-treatment/print [Last accessed December, 2021].
3. NICE. (2015). Preterm labour and birth. NICE guideline [NG25]. [online]. Available from https://www.nice.org.uk/guidance/ng25 [Last accessed December, 2021].
4. Society for Maternal-Fetal Medicine (SMFM) Publications Committee. Implementation of the use of antenatal corticosteroids in the late preterm birth period in women at risk for preterm delivery. Am J Obstet Gynecol. 2016;215(2):B13-5.

Vaginal Birth after Cesarean

Neha Kapoor, Poonam Goyal, Pallavi Goel

INTRODUCTION

In 1916, Cragin made his famous pronouncement "once a cesarean, always a cesarean". When this statement was made, the classical vertical uterine incision was used almost universally. Although catastrophic uterine rupture developed in 4% prior classical incisions, only 0.5% transverse incisions ruptured.

In an effort to address the rising cesarean delivery rate, the American College of Obstetricians and Gynecologists (ACOG) recommended that females with one previous low-transverse caesarean delivery should be counseled to attempt labor in subsequent pregnancy **(Fig. 1)**.

ANTENATAL COUNSELING

- The antenatal counseling of women with a previous cesarean birth should be documented in the notes.
- A final decision for mode of birth should be agreed upon by the woman and members of the maternity team before the expected/planned date of delivery.
- When a date for elective repeat cesarean section (ERCS) is being arranged, a plan for the event of labor starting before the scheduled date should be documented in the notes.

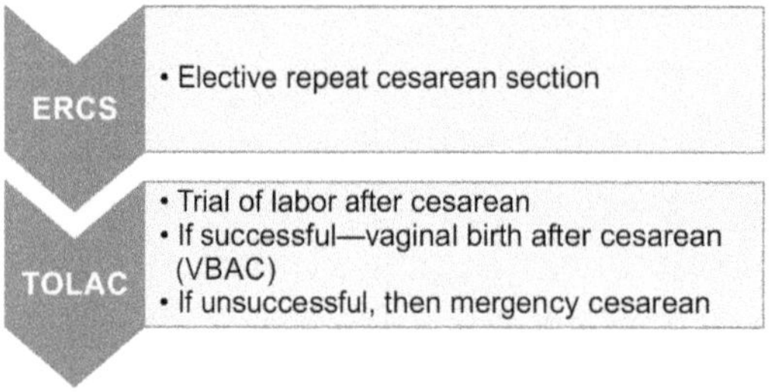

Fig. 1: Options for a patient with previous cesarean.

- The routine use of vaginal birth after cesarean (VBAC) checklists during antenatal counseling should be considered, as they would ensure informed consent and shared decision making in women undergoing VBAC.

IDEAL CANDIDATE FOR VAGINAL BIRTH AFTER CESAREAN

- Singleton pregnancy
- Cephalic presentation
- 37 +0 weeks or beyond
- Single previous lower segment cesarean delivery
- With or without history of previous vaginal birth
- Spontaneous labor

CONTRAINDICATIONS

- Previous uterine rupture (5% higher risk of rupture)
- Classical cesarean scar
- Absolute contraindication to vaginal birth—major placenta previa

CAUTION

- Complicated uterine scar (decision on case-to-case basis by senior obstetrician with access to details of previous surgery)
- Previous laparoscopic or abdominal myomectomy particularly where the uterine cavity was breached
- Hysteroscopic resection of uterine septum
- Post-dates
- Twin gestation
- Fetal macrosomia
- Antepartum stillbirth
- Maternal age >40 years or more

TABLE 1: Success and complication rates after VBAC.

	PREV 1 LSCS	PREV 2 LSCS
Success rate	72–75%	71.2%
Scar rupture	0.5%	1.36%
Hysterectomy	19/10,000	56/10,000
Transfusion	1.21%	1.99%

(LSCS: lower segment cesarean section; VBAC: vaginal birth after cesarean)

Factors associated with increased incidence of scar rupture:
- Short inter-delivery interval (<12 months), ACOG (<18 months)
- Post-date pregnancy
- Maternal age ≥40 years
- Obesity [body mass index (BMI) >30]
- Lower prelabor—Bishop score
- Macrosomia
- Decreased scar thickness [2.1–4.0 mm strong negative predictive value (NPV) for scar rupture and 0.6–2.0 mm strong positive predictive value (PPV)]

VAGINAL BIRTH AFTER CESAREAN IN PREVIOUS TWO CESAREAN

See **Table 1.**

WHERE TO CONDUCT VAGINAL BIRTH AFTER CESAREAN?

- Suitably staffed and equipped delivery suite with continuous intrapartum care and monitoring
- Resources available for immediate cesarean delivery and advanced neonatal resuscitation
- Experienced obstetrician to determine feasibility of VBAC
- Epidural analgesia is not contraindicated (increasing requirement may suggest impending uterine rupture)
- Continuous electronic fetal monitoring (EFM) commencing at onset of regular uterine contractions

Intrapartum Prerequisites
- Supportive one to one care

- Intravenous access with full blood count and blood group and save
- Continuous electronic fetal monitoring
- Regular monitoring of maternal symptoms and signs
- Regular (no <4-hourly) assessment of cervicometric progress in labor

Red Flag Signs
- Abnormal CTG present in 66–76% of scar dehiscence
- Severe abdominal pain, especially if persisting between contractions
- Acute onset scar tenderness
- Abnormal vaginal bleeding
- Hematuria
- Cessation of previously efficient uterine activity
- Maternal tachycardia, hypotension, fainting or shock
- Loss of station of the presenting part
- Change in abdominal contour and inability to pick up fetal heart rate at the old transducer site

Induction/Augmentation
- Two- to three-fold increased risk of uterine rupture
- 1.5-fold increased risk of cesarean delivery in induced/augmented labor compared with spontaneous labor
- Mechanical methods (amniotomy or Foley's catheter) are associated with a lower risk of scar rupture compared to prostaglandins.

BIBLIOGRAPHY

1. ACOG Practice Bulletin No. 205: Vaginal birth after previous cesarean delivery. Obstet Gynecol. 2019;133(2):e110-e127.
2. Royal College of Obstetricians and Gynaecologists. Birth after Previous Caesarean Birth (Green-top Guideline No. 45). London: RCOG; 2015.
3. Wu Y, Kataria Y, Wang Z, Ming WK, Ellervik C. Factors associated with successful vaginal birth after a cesarean section: a systematic review and meta-analysis. BMC Pregnancy Childbirth. 2019;19:360.

47

Episiotomy

Monisha Singh, Narendra Malhotra

DEFINITION

Episiotomy is a planned surgical incision to the perineum enlarging the vaginal orifice during the last part of the second stage of labor or delivery.

TYPES

There are only two main types of episiotomy (median and mediolateral), although seven different incisions have been described in the literature **(Tables 1 and 2).**[1]

The angle of the episiotomy does indeed affect the risk of *obstetric anal sphincter injury (OASIS)*,

together with the finding of a wide variation in the actual angle of incision **(Fig. 1)**. OASIS is a serious maternal health concern that is associated with maternal morbidities, including pelvic floor dysfunction, fecal and urinary incontinence, sexual dysfunction, and pelvic organ prolapse.[2]

ADVANTAGES OF EPISIOTOMY

- Reduced trauma to the fetal head
- Ease of repair with wound healing
- Preservation of the pelvic floor
- Prevention of anal sphincter laceration
- Prevention of shoulder dystocia

TABLE 1: Types of episiotomies with origin and direction of cut.

Types of episiotomy	Origin of the initial incision	Direction of the cut	
Median (Midline/Medial)	Within 3 mm of the midline in the posterior fourchette	Between 0 and 25 of the sagittal plane	Runs along the midline through the central tendon of the perineal body
Modified median	Within 3 mm of the midline in the posterior fourchette	Between 0 and 25 of the sagittal plane, with two transverse cuts on each side added	Claimed to increase the diameter of the vaginal outlet by 83% compared with a standard median episiotomy
"J" shaped	Within 3 mm of the midline in the posterior fourchette	At first midline, then "J" is directed toward the ischial tuberosity	Curved scissors are used starting in the midline of the vagina until the incision is 2.5 cm from the anus
Mediolateral	Within 3 mm of the midline in the posterior fourchette	Directed laterally at an angle of at least 60 from the midline toward the ischial tuberosity	
Lateral	More than 10 mm from the midline in the posterior fourchette	Laterally toward the ischial tuberosity	

Contd...

Contd...

Types of episiotomy	Origin of the initial incision	Direction of the cut	
Radical lateral (Schuchardt incision)	More than 10 mm from the midline	Laterally toward the ischial tuberosity and around the rectum	Nonobstetrical incision; may be performed at the beginning of radical vaginal hysterectomy or trachelectomy to permit easy access to the parametrium
Anterior Midline/ Anterior episiotomy or deinfibulation (the procedure of opening the scar associated with some degrees of female genital mutilation)	"Midline"	Directed toward the pubis	To free the scar, fused labia minora are incised in the midline until the external urethral meatus can be seen and the anterior flap is completely open. The clitoral remnants should not be incised

TABLE 2: Comparison of individual types of episiotomy.

Median	Mediolateral
Repair is easy	Repair is difficult
Heals easily	Chances of faulty healing is higher
Postoperative pain is minimal	Postoperative pain is higher
Blood loss is less	Blood loss is more
Dyspareunia is less	Dyspareunia is more
Extension is common	Extension is rare

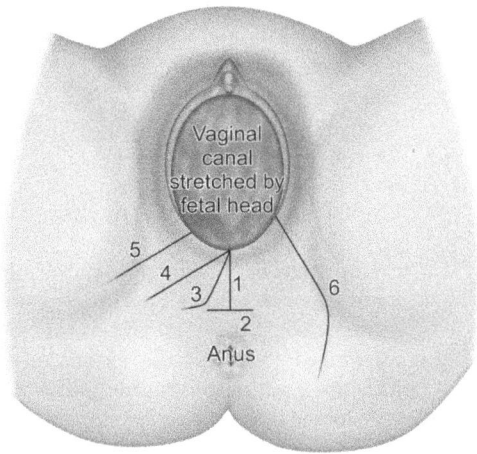

Fig. 1: Angle of episiotomy.

Following adverse outcomes:
- Extension of the incision which may lead to third- and fourth-degree tears (median episiotomy)
- Risk of unsatisfactory anatomic results
- Increased blood loss
- Higher rates of infection and dehiscence
- Increased risk of severe perineal laceration in subsequent deliveries

- *Too early episiotomy*: Extensive bleeding
- *Too late episiotomy*: Excessive stretching of a pelvic floor and lacerations
- *Location*: Approximately 5 cm long at the time of crowning. An episiotomy performed at 40° results in a postdelivery angle of 22°
- Repair of the local tissue took approximately 7 days

WHEN IS THE RIGHT TIME TO PERFORM EPISIOTOMY?

- When the presenting part is coming out of perineum and being visible during a contraction and does not recede back.

STRUCTURES INJURED DURING EPISIOTOMY

- Posterior vaginal wall
- Superficial and deep transverse-perinei muscles

- Bulbospongiosus
- Part of levator ani
- Fascia covering these muscles
- Transverse perineal branches of pudendal vessels and nerves
- Subcutaneous tissue and skin

PROCEDURE (FIG. 2)

- *Equipment*:
  - Sterile or tap water to clean area before procedure
  - 1 × 10 mL syringe
  - 1 × 22 gauge (green) infiltration needle
  - 10 mL lidocaine 1%
  - Mayo episiotomy scissors
- *Consent*:
  - Reassure woman and partner
  - Explain procedure and indications
  - Obtain and record consent
- *Technique*:
  - Ensure that the woman consents to the procedure
  - Ensure good lighting
  - Assess the perineum and decide about the type of episiotomy
  - Ensure adequate anesthesia
  - Check the equipment before starting the procedure
  - Count swabs before and after performing the episiotomy repair
  - After delivery, a rectal examination is warranted to assess the extent of the incision. A continuous running stitch with absorbable sutures is recommended.

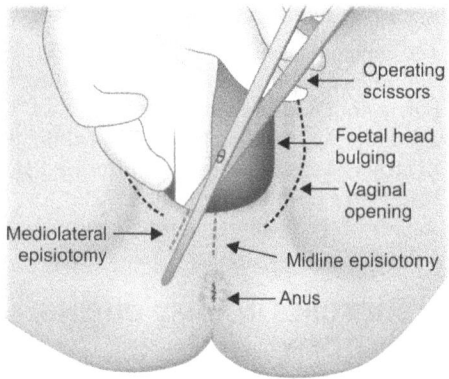

Fig. 2: Procedure of episiotomy.

  - Use a loose, continuous nonlocking method for vaginal mucosa and perineal muscles and a continuous subcuticular technique for perineal skin

POSITION AND PREPARATION OF WOMAN

- Place in comfortable legs—open position
- Cleanse perineal area
- Place index and middle fingers into vagina between presenting part and perineum
- Inject 5–10 mL lidocaine 1% slowly into center of fourchette and direct it midway between ischial tuberosity and anus (protect fetal head)
- Insert middle and index fingers into vagina and gently pull perineum away from fetal part to protect fetal head
- Perform incision when fetal head is crowning in one single straight cut to minimize damage and ensure optimal realignment
- Withdraw scissors carefully
- Control delivery of fetal head and shoulders to avoid extension
- After third stage, thoroughly inspect vagina/perineum to ascertain extent of trauma

HIGH-DEGREE PERINEAL LACERATION

Risk factors:
- Prior extensive laceration
- Fetal macrosomia
- Operative vaginal delivery
- Precipitous delivery

PERINEAL PROTECTION

Nondominant hand slowing down the delivery of the head. Dominant hand should be focused on protecting the perineum.

The best method of perineal support/protection is unclear, with the *Ritgen maneuver* (delivering the fetal head, using one hand to pull the fetal chin from between the maternal anus and the coccyx and the other on the fetal occiput to control speed of delivery), support is better.

Warm compress—a Cochrane review has found this method to reduce chances of OASIS.

Perineal massage during antenatal period and in second stage of labor. Perineal massage during the last month of pregnancy has been suggested as a possible way of enabling perineal tissue to expand more easily during birth.

▓ REPAIR (FIGS. 3 AND 4)

- Apply antiseptic solution to the area around episiotomy
- If the wound is extended, manage as third- or fourth-degree perineal tears, respectively.
- Repair in layers done after adequate anesthesia has been obtained.
- The vaginal wall is closed first with a continuous suture that starts 1 cm above the apex of the incision, including any retracted blood vessels, which may otherwise result in hematoma formation.
- Close the perineal muscles using interrupted 1-0 sutures.

- Continuous attention to anatomical approximation is important. A continuous subcuticular stitch/mattress is used for skin closure.

▓ ADVISE TO BE GIVEN TO PATIENT POSTEPISIOTOMY

- Monitor the patient for pain and urinary incontinence.
- Patients receive training on how to take sitz baths and clean the perineum.
- If there is swelling, apply ice packs which also decrease the pain.
- The sutures used to close an episiotomy do not require removal, and will reabsorb in the tissues within 6–8 weeks.
- Patients must learn how to perform Kegel exercises to help tighten up the pelvic floor muscles.
- To not resume sexual intercourse till wound has healed.

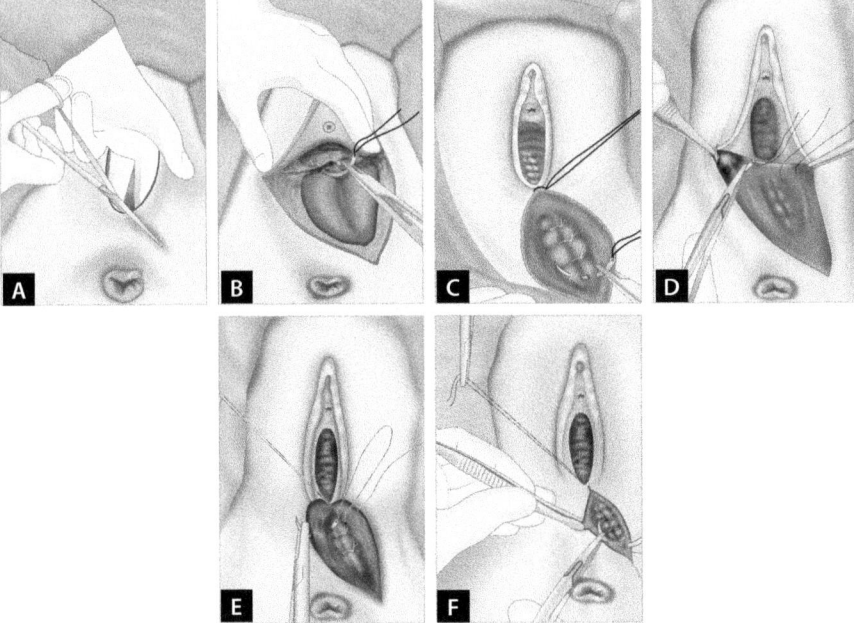

Figs. 3A to F: (A) Incision from midline toward ischial tuberosity; (B) Repair of vaginal wall; (C) Approximation of levators; (D) Approximation of bulbocavernosus muscle; (E) Reconstruction of urogenital diaphragm; (F) Skin closure.

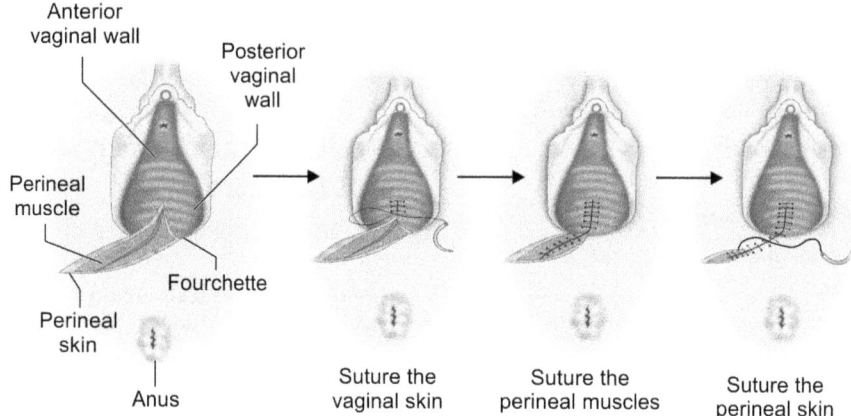

Anterior vaginal wall

Posterior vaginal wall

Perineal muscle

Fourchette

Perineal skin

Anus

Suture the vaginal skin

Suture the perineal muscles

Suture the perineal skin

Fig. 4: Perineal repair.

CONCLUSION

A basic procedure yet technical to learn and understand, episiotomy has aided in obstetrical outcomes for mothers, babies, and doctors.

REFERENCES

1. Kalis V, Laine K, de Leeuw J, Ismail K, Tincello D. Classification of episiotomy: towards a standardisation of terminology. BJOG. 2012;119:522-6.
2. Mullally A, Murphy D. Episiotomy. Glob Libr Women's Med. (ISSN: 1756-2228) 2011; DOI 10.3843/GLOWM.10128

Ruchika Garg, Pavika Lal

BACKGROUND

Antenatal fetal wellbeing is one of the *essential and integral component* for management and surveillance of high-risk pregnancies and in the past included biochemical assays (plasma and urinary estriols) and biophysical studies [antepartum fetal heart rate (FHR) tests]. The biochemical modalities had the disadvantages of questionable prognostic significance when results were abnormal, were not universally available, and did not always provide prompt, reproducible results.[1,2] FHR testing methods originated with the contraction stress test (CST) or oxytocin challenge test (OCT) and served as a tool to evaluate the fetus prior to the onset of labor which was a *natural extension of techniques of continuous intrapartum fetal heart monitoring.*[1,3]

Goals of antepartum surveillance as stated by American College of Obstetricians and Gynecologists (ACOG) and American Academy of Pediatrics (AAP) (2012).

- To prevent fetal deaths/to reduce the risk of still birth, perinatal morbidity and mortality by appropriate detection of fetal compromise accurately and effectively.
- To serve as proper guidance for necessary obstetric interventions, i.e., termination vs. justifiable continuation of pregnancy.

The available techniques of antepartum fetal testing is based on:[4-7]

- Fetal heart rate pattern
- Level of somatic activity of fetus (fetal breathing)
- Degree of muscular tone (fetal gross body movements)

} Sensitive to fetal hypoxia and acidemia

The above features of the fetus have been used as principles in nonstress test (NST)/CST, real-time ultrasonography (USG), biophysical profile (BPP), amniotic fluid volume [AFV/amniotic fluid index (AFI)] and Doppler velocimetry for evaluation of fetal well-being. These methods identify the fetuses that may be in jeopardy and thereby providing the window of opportunity for the necessary interventions before severe and progressive metabolic acidosis sets in resulting in fetal death.

Various techniques available for antepartum fetal surveillance:

- Maternal perception of fetal movements
- CST
- NST
- BPP/modified BPP
- Fetal Doppler velocimetry

The chapter reviews the indications, clinical relevance, and highlights the role of NST in the battery of techniques available for antenatal fetal surveillance.

LIMITATIONS OF ANTEPARTUM FETAL SURVEILLANCE

- *Inability to predict acute catastrophic events* [antepartum hemorrhage (APH) associated with placental abruption, placenta previa, vasa previa, cord prolapse] that bring about sudden deterioration within the fetal status. Therefore fetal deaths from such events are less amenable to prevention by use of antenatal testing.
- Although a good association exist between certain features of FHR pattern and behavior with metabolic compromise, abnormal fetal test *does not accurately reflect either the severity or duration of acidemia or hypoxemia* and even the degree of acidemia weakly correlate with adverse short- or long-term neonatal outcome.[8]

- A normal test is highly reassuring because fetal death within 1 week of a normal test is very rare, i.e., *negative predictive value is almost 99.8%* but the *positive predictive value is 10–40%* only, i.e., abnormal test result may not accurately predict the impaired fetus in utero.
- Moreover the wider application of these tests is, mainly based on circumstantial evidence as no definitive. Randomized control trial (RCT) has been conducted and therefore antenatal fetal testing forecast *fetal wellness rather than illness.*

INDICATIONS[9]

- *Fetal factors:*
  - Fetal growth restriction (FGR)
  - Multiple pregnancy
- *Maternal factors:*
  - Hypertensive disorders of pregnancy:
    - Initiate at 32 weeks
    - *Without severe features*: Twice weekly from time of diagnosis
    - *With severe features*: Daily testing
  - Gestational diabetes:
    - Initiate at 32 weeks
    - *Controlled and no comorbidities*: Once or twice weekly testing
    - *Poorly controlled*: Twice weekly testing
  - Pregestational diabetes:
    - Initiate at 32 weeks 0 day
    - Twice weekly testing
  - Systemic lupus erythematous, antiphospholipid syndrome, sickle cell disease, renal disease or thyroid disorders
  - Obesity:
    - Prepregnancy body mass index (BMI) 35.0–39.9 kg/m^2:
      - *37 weeks 0 day*: Initiate weekly testing
    - Prepregnancy BMI > 40.0 kg/m^2:
      - *34 weeks 0 day*: Initiate weekly testing
- *Obstetric factors:*
  - Previous stillbirth:
    - *Occurred at ≥32 weeks 0 day*: Initiate weekly or twice weekly testing at 32 weeks 0 day
    - *Occurred at <32 weeks 0 day*: Individualize initiation and surveillance
  - Previous FGR or preeclampsia with consequent preterm delivery:
    - *32 weeks 0 day*: Initiate weekly testing

- Cholestasis:
  - Initiate once or twice weekly testing at time of diagnosis
- Late term:
  - *41 weeks 0 day*: Initiate once or twice weekly testing
- Abnormal serum markers—pregnancy-associated plasma protein A (PAPP-A) ≤ 5th percentile (0.4 MoM) or second trimester inhibin ≥ 2.0 multiples of the median (MoM):
  - *36 weeks 0 day*: Initiate weekly testing
- *Placental factors:*
  - *Chronic placental abruption*: Initiate once or twice weekly testing at time of diagnosis
  - Umbilical cord abnormalities (velamentous cord insertion, single umbilical artery)
- *Fluid abnormalities:*
  - Isolated oligohydramnios [single deepest vertical pocket (DVP) < 2 cm]:
    - Initiate once or twice weekly testing at time of diagnosis
  - Polyhydramnios (DVP ≥ 12 cm or AFI ≥ 30 cm):
    - *32 weeks 0 day to 34 weeks 0 day*: Initiate once or twice weekly testing

NONSTRESS TEST

- *It is primarily a test of fetal condition whereas CST is a test of uteroplacental function.*
- Presently, NST is *the most widely use method* for assessment of fetal well-being and has been incorporated into the BPP testing system.
- No direct risk of maternal or fetal injury

Physiological Basis of Nonstress Test

- Physiological evolution of the fetal heart occurs across gestation and affects FHR patterns. Changes in FHR result from moment-to-moment autonomic modulation in response to factors, including input from *chemoreceptors, baroreceptors, central nervous system activities (e.g., arousal, sleep), catecholamines, and blood volume.*[10]
- Parasympathetic innervation of the heart is mediated primarily by the vagus nerve, which influences the sinoatrial (SA) and atrioventricular (AV) nodes. *Parasympathetic*

stimulation slows the FHR whereas sympathetic stimulation increases the FHR.

- *Effect of gestational age on FHR*:
    - The parasympathetic and sympathetic nervous systems exert a progressively greater influence on the FHR as gestational age advances. During early fetal development, baseline heart rate is relatively elevated, reflecting a presumptive dominant sympathetic tone. As the fetus matures, baseline FHR decreases, indicating an increasing parasympathetic influence.
    - In the first and second trimesters, cardiac contraction patterns are related to inherent myocardial rhythmicity. By the third trimester, considerable autonomic control is present, as exhibited by the periodic fluctuations (long- and short-term variability).[11]
    - Maturation of the sympathetic system causes an increase in the frequency and amplitude of FHR accelerations.[12,13]
- *Cardiovascular response to hypoxemia*: Oxygen is transferred from the maternal environment to fetal tissues along a pathway that includes the maternal lungs, heart, vasculature, uterus, placenta and umbilical cord and therefore fetal hypoxemia can result from interruption of the transfer of oxygen at any point along this pathway.

The FHR response to interrupted oxygenation depends on the cause **(Fig. 1 and Table 1)**:

- Transient fetal hypoxemia associated with uterine contractions can cause late decelerations. Stimulation of chemoreceptors

(located in carotid artery and aorta) due to decrease in arterial oxygen tension leads to a reflex increase in sympathetic outflow, causing vasoconstriction in nonvital organs and increase in blood flow to vital organs

TABLE 1: Factors influencing fetal cardiac rate and variability.

Factors influencing fetal cardiac rate

Increase:
• Atropine	Adrenergic drugs
• Increase sympathetic tone	Fetal movement
• Maternal thyrotoxicosis	Maternal fever
• Hypoxia (chronic)	

Decrease:
• Hypoxia	Hypokalemia
• Maternal hypotension	Local anesthetics
• Increase parasympathetic tone	(reflex action)
• Adrenergic blocking agents	Congenital heart block

Factors influencing fetal cardiac variability:

Increase:
• Hypoxia (acute)	Second-stage labor
• Fetal activity	

Decrease:
• Acidosis	Barbiturates
• Narcotics	Tranquilizers
• Fetal sleep (NREM)	Hypoxia (chronic)
• Tachycardia	Atropine
• Prematurity	Chronic placental insufficiency

(NREM: nonrapid eye movement)

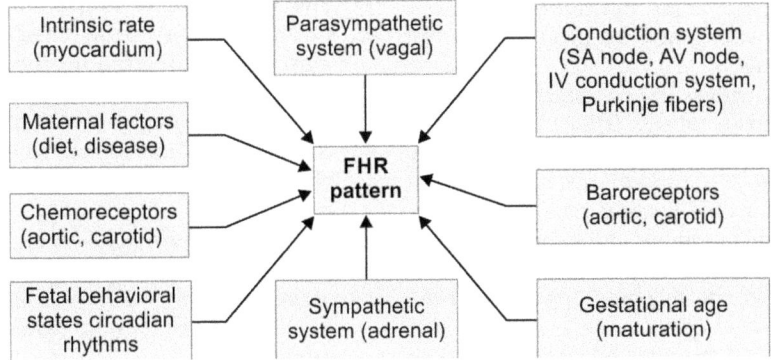

Fig. 1: Diagrammatic representation of the factors affecting fetal heart rate (FHR).
(AV: atrioventricular; SA: sinoatrial)

(e.g., adrenal glands, heart, brain). Peripheral vasoconstriction causes elevated fetal blood pressure and, in turn, stimulation of baroreceptors (located in the aortic arch and carotid sinus), resulting in reflex, vagally mediated, parasympathetic slowing of FHR shortly after the beginning of the contraction.

- Transient interruption of fetal oxygenation caused by compression of the umbilical cord can result in variable decelerations. If cord compression reduces blood flow in the umbilical vein first, transient hypovolemia may cause a reflex rise in FHR (sometimes referred to as a "*shoulder*"). Subsequent arterial compression increases blood pressure, leading to vagally mediated slowing of FHR until the cord compression resolves.

- Acute ongoing interruption of fetal oxygenation at the level of the maternal lungs (e.g., maternal hypoxemia), maternal heart (e.g., acute reduction in cardiac output), maternal vasculature (e.g., maternal hypotension), uterus (e.g., tetanic contraction, uterine rupture), placenta (e.g., abruption), or umbilical cord (e.g., prolapse) can cause prolonged decelerations.

- Early decelerations are due to fetal head compression and not fetal hypoxia, therefore not associated with adverse neonatal outcome.

- Chronic hypoxia leads to decreased variability.

Timing and Frequency

- NSTs and CSTs are initiated at the gestational age when the fetus is believed to be at increased risk of death as long as the period of gestation is advanced enough that delivery for neonatal survival would be considered.

- For the NST, fetal neurologic maturity should be sufficient enough to enable FHR accelerations.

- Pregnancy with *severe complications* (severe pre-eclampsia, severe IUGR, uncontrolled maternal blood sugars) might require testing *to begin at 26–28 weeks* gestation whereas most authorities usually recommend that testing should begin *by 32–34 weeks gestation.*

- Evidence from studies are insufficient to define the optimal frequency of testing but has been arbitrarily set at 7 days.

- *More frequent testing* is advocated (twice or thrice weekly) depending upon the severity of maternal or fetal condition.

- Testing is performed periodically as long as the indication persists, but *maternal or fetal deterioration requires reevaluation* despite recent or initial normal test results.[14]

- *A pattern of accelerations, moderate variability, and no significant decelerations during the NST and CST reliably identifies the absence of ongoing hypoxic injury* during the test, it does not preclude such injury in the future, especially if there are significant changes in clinical scenario over the time.

Performance or Significance of the Test

In 2015, a Cochrane review attempted to determine whether using the NST can improve maternal or perinatal outcome by identifying high-risk pregnancies requiring prompt induction of labor or immediate delivery by cesarean. Six randomized trials involving 2,105 participants were included. Tested patients were compared with controls who did not undergo NSTs or their test results were concealed. *No significant differences between groups were noted in:*[15]

- Maternal outcomes (frequency of induction of labor or cesarean delivery)

- Infant outcomes (perinatal mortality, low 5-minute Apgar, neonatal intensive care unit admission, and neonatal seizures)

Lastly, fetal assessment and neonatal care have changed since the 1980s; the combined use of ultrasound and FHR testing may be more predictive of fetal status and need for intervention than either test alone.

Equipment

- The electronic fetal monitor (called the cardiotocogram) is the portable equipment most commonly used for the prenatal NST (**Fig. 2**).

- The modern equipment records FHR pattern, contractions, fetal cardiac activity, maternal blood pressure, and maternal heart rate on a graph.

- It has a Doppler transducer for FHR monitoring and a pressure transducer for monitoring of uterine contractions and fetal movement which are placed on the maternal abdomen using belts.

- The complex wave generated is analyzed, and the peak is used for calculations. An internal computer then calculates the FHR by averaging several consecutive peak-to-peak frequencies to minimize artifact. This process of averaging is called "autocorrelation." It produces a FHR waveform closely resembling that derived from a fetal electrocardiogram (ECG).

• Computerized storage and interpretation of FHR records are obtainable with conventional monitors. Computerized cardiotocography provides a more detailed analysis of the FHR pattern but has not proved superior to the conventional methods.

Clinical Significance

• One should always take into account *patient's clinical condition and associated comorbid conditions, gestational age as well as general status of the fetus* at the time of observation and

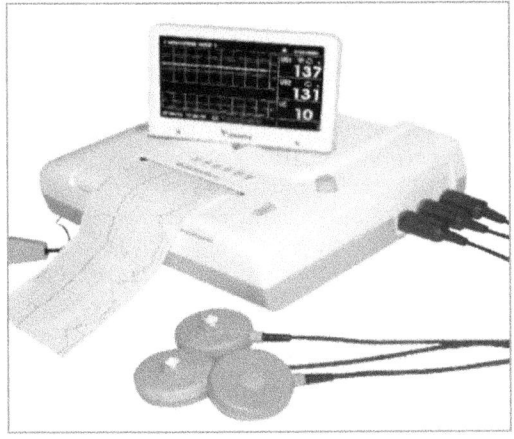

Fig. 2: Nonstress test (NST) machine with three transducers.

on the acuity and degree of a specific insult or stimulating event during proper evaluation of NST trace.

• *The presence of FHR acceleration with fetal movement is the principle behind the NST and recognizes the coupling of fetal neurological status to cardiovascular reflex responses.* It is one of the factors that tends to disappear earliest during progressive fetal compromise.

• *Interpretation of the NST includes*:
  – Baseline FHR
  – Baseline FHR variability
  – Presence of accelerations (number, amplitude, and duration of accelerations that usually correlate with fetal movement)
  – Absence of decelerations
  – Uterine contractions

• *Normal or reactive test results,* as defined by ACOG, is one in *which two or more accelerations peak at 15 bpm or more above baseline, each lasting 15 seconds or more, and all occurring within 20 minutes of beginning the test.* It was recommended that accelerations with or without perception of fetal movements or even a single acceleration is acceptable **(Fig. 3)**. A *reactive test provides reliable evidence of normal fetal oxygenation, regardless of the length of observation time needed to demonstrate reactivity.*

• *Before 32 weeks* of gestation, a reactive NST may be defined *as two accelerations that rise at least 10 beats/min above baseline and have a duration of at least 10 seconds (10 x 10).*[16] However, once a fetus has demonstrated the maturity to generate accelerations of

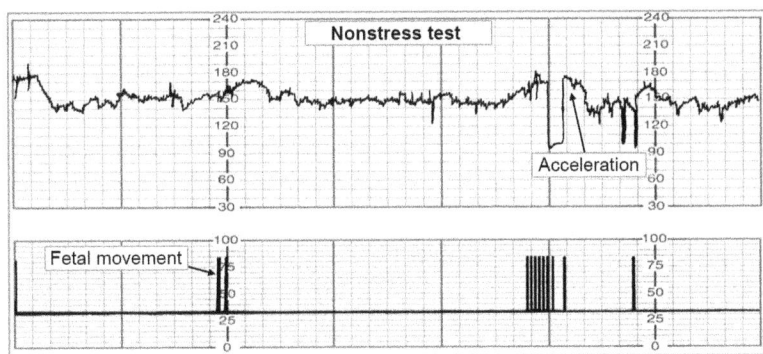

Fig. 3: Normal or reactive test results.

15 beats/min for 15 seconds, an acceleration of 10 beats/min for 10 seconds may not have the same ability to confirm normal fetal oxygenation, even before 32 weeks of gestation.

- *Extended NST*: If initially no accelerations are present in first 20 minutes of the test, *it is extended to another 20 minutes in an attempt to identify the fetus in a period of prolonged quiet sleep from those who are actually hypoxemic or asphyxiated.*

- *Vibroacoustic stimulation* (artificial larynx placed on maternal abdomen) can be used to stimulate fetal movement and shortens the average test time of NST by 7 minutes and reduce the number of nonreactive NST by 40% without decreasing its predictive value. It has been performed as soon as 5 minutes after initiation of the NST.[17] ACOG suggests positioning the device on the maternal abdomen and applying a stimulus for 1–2 seconds. If no fetal response occurs, the stimulus may be repeated up to three times for progressively longer durations of up to 3 seconds.

- *Nonreactive NST is one that lacks sufficient FHR accelerations over 40 minutes as recommended by ACOG* and some authors even extend the testing time to 60 minutes.
  - A nonreactive NST should not be assumed to indicate fetal compromise if variability remains present with absence of decelerations.
  - Moderate variability has an amplitude that ranges from 6 to 25 beats/min and is an indication of a healthy nervous system.
  - Causes for a nonreactive NST:[18]
    - Presence of a longer than average sleep cycle in a normal fetus (most common cause)
    - Fetal immaturity
    - Maternal smoking
    - Fetal neurologic or cardiac anomalies
    - Use of CNS depressant drugs (narcotics, phenobarbitone), magnesium sulfate, beta blockers
  - The fetus must undergo detailed evaluation after a nonreactive NST.
    - Repeat the test in 30 minutes.

- Perform vibroacoustic stimulation to elicit accelerations.
- Perform a back-up test, (either CST or complete BPP)
- If possible, modify factors potentially causing nonreactive results.
- Although commonly practiced, *neither maternal glucose administration nor transabdominal manual fetal manipulation significantly decreases the incidence of nonreactive test results.*[19,20]
- *Continuous nonreactive NST can indicate central nervous system depression.*
- Nonreactivity may be a sign of interrupted fetal oxygenation to the point of metabolic acidemia. The mean umbilical vein pH associated with a nonreactive NST is 7.28 ± 0.11, which is higher than the pH associated with a low BPP score, 7.16 ± 0.08.[8]

Reactive NST with Decelerations

- Multiple observational studies have described an increased frequency of intrapartum FHR decelerations and operative delivery when reactive NSTs with deceleration occurs.[21]
- Variable decelerations that are nonrepetitive, and last <30 seconds, do not require intervention and outcomes are usually good.
- *Repetitive variable decelerations at least three in 20 minutes even if mild is associated with increased risk of fetal distress and cesarean delivery during labor.*
- *Decelerations >1 minute even carries a worse prognosis.*
- Variable or prolonged decelerations observed during antepartum testing require further evaluation, which might include extended FHR and uterine activity monitoring, ultrasound assessment of fetal growth and anatomy, BPP, AFV, and/or Doppler velocimetry in the setting of FGR **(Table 2)**.
- Intermittent fetal cardiac arrhythmias can cause decelerations and therefore should be diagnosed by echocardiography and management depends on the arrhythmia and patient-specific factors.

A terminal cardiotocogram includes:[22]
- Baseline oscillation of <5 beats/min
- Absent accelerations
- Late deaccelerations with spontaneous uterine contractions

TABLE 2: Antepartum classification: nonstress test (NST).

Parameter	Normal NST (Previously "Reactive")	Atypical NST (Previously "Non-Reactive")	Abnormal NST (Previously "Non-Reactive")
Baseline	110–160 bpm	• 100–110 bpm • >160 bmp < 30 minutes • Rising baseline	• Bradycardia < 100 bpm • Tachycardia > 160 for > 30 minutes • Erratic baseline
Variability	• 6–25 bpm (moderate) • ≤ 5 (absent or minimal) for <40 minutes	≤5 absent or minimal) for 40–80 minutes	• ≤ 5 for ≥ 80 minutes • ≥ 25 bpm > 10 minutes. • Sinusoidal
Decelerations	None or occasional variable <30 seconds	Variable decelerations 30–60 seconds, duration	• Variable decelerations, > 60 seconds duration • Late deceleration(s)
Accelerations term fetus	≥ 2 accelerations with acme of ≥ 15 bpm, lasting 15 seconds < 40 minutes of testing	≤ 2 accelerations with acme of ≥15 bpm, lasting 15 seconds in 40–80 minutes	≤ 2 accelerations with acme of ≥15 bpm, lasting 15 seconds in > 80 minutes
Preterm fetus (< 32 weeks)	≥ 2 accelerations with acme of ≥ 15 bpm, lasting 10 seconds <40 minutes of testing	≤ 2 accelerations of ≥10 bpm, lasting 10 sec, in 40–80 minutes	≤ 2 accelerations of ≥10 bpm, lasting 10 seconds, in > 80 minutes
Action	Further assessment optional, based on total clinical picture	Further assessment required	Urgent action required An overall assessment of the situation and further investigation with U/S or BPP is required. Some situations with require delivery

(bpm: beats/min; BPP: biophysical profile; U/S: ultrasound)

CONTRACTION STRESS TEST

Contraction stress test initially known as oxytocin challenge test is uncommonly used now a days.
• Inconvenient to perform
• Time consuming (average time required by CST to get completed is 90 minutes)
• Sometimes interventions used to stimulate uterine contractions result in unpredictable uterine hyperstimulation and eventually fetal distress
• Limited by contraindications

Contraindications to Contraction Stress Test

• Placenta previa
• Vasa previa
• Previous classical cesarean delivery or extensive uterine surgery
• Preterm labor, patients at high risk for preterm delivery, and preterm prelabor rupture of membranes

Principle of Contraction Stress Test

Based on response of FHR with respect to uterine contractions: It is assumed that in a well-oxygenated fetus, there will be transient worsening of FHR which will recover as soon as contractions subside, but in an already compromised fetus the intermittent worsening in oxygenation during uterine contractions will lead to late decelerations of FHR pattern.

Procedure

• *Position*: Patient in lateral recumbent
• FHR and uterine contractions are simultaneously recorded with an external fetal monitor.
• An adequate uterine contraction pattern is present when at least three contractions persist for at least 40 seconds each in a 10-minute period.
• Uterine stimulation is not necessary if the patient is having spontaneous uterine contractions of adequate frequency.

- If fewer than three contractions of 40 seconds duration occur in 10 minutes, contractions are induced with either nipple stimulation or intravenous (IV) oxytocin. *Nipple stimulation usually is successful in inducing an adequate contraction pattern and allows completion of testing in approximately one half of the time required as well as cost-effective than when IV oxytocin is used.*[23.]
- For oxytocin use, a dilute IV infusion is initiated at a rate of 0.5 mIU/min and doubled every 20 minutes until a desired contraction pattern is established.
- *Nipple stimulation*: The woman is asked to rub her clothing for 2 minutes or until a contraction begins. Usually, it induces the contractions but if unsuccessful she is instructed to rub her nipples once again after 5 minutes interval, if repeat nipple stimulation fails then dilute oxytocin is used.

Interpretation of Contraction Stress Test[14]

Contraction stress test is interpreted according to the presence or absence of late FHR decelerations (**Table 3**).[24]

The presence or absence of accelerations is also noted.

- A reactive positive CST meets criteria for both a reactive NST and a positive CST.

TABLE 3: Interpretation of contraction stress test (CST).	
Negative	No late or significant variable decelerations
Positive	Late decelerations after 50% or more of contractions (even if the contraction frequency is fewer than three in 10 minutes)
Equivocal–suspicious	Intermittent late decelerations or significant variable decelerations
Equivocal	Fetal heart rate (FHR) decelerations that occur in the presence of contractions more frequent than every 2 minutes or lasting longer than 90 seconds
Unsatisfactory	Fewer than three contractions in 10 minutes or an uninterpretable tracing

- A positive (abnormal) CST indicates transient fetal hypoxemia during uterine contractions and may be an indication for delivery, depending on the clinical scenario. In one study, 50% of reactive positive CSTs were false positives, whereas 100% of nonreactive positive CSTs were true positives.[25] Thus, the presence of accelerations during the CST may reduce the need for intervention, but require additional evaluation which include a BPP and, in the setting of FGR.[26]
- A CST with variable decelerations suggests umbilical cord compression that may be due to oligohydramnios.

CONCLUSION

There is a paucity of evidence for the efficacy of antenatal fetal surveillance and for evidence-based recommendations on the timing and frequency of antenatal fetal surveillance; consequently, for most conditions, recommendations are largely based on expert consensus.

Nonstress test is a simpler, noninvasive, less time consuming and less expensive than CST without any contraindications and has a wider application than CST. It can also be conducted in an outpatient setting. Inter- and intraobserver variations with respect to the interpretation of traces can be minimized by adequate training of the staff and following uniform criteria.

REFERENCES

1. Keegan KA, Paul RH, Broussard PM, McCart D, Smith MA. Antepartum fetal heart rate testing: V. The nonstress test-an outpatient approach. Am J Obstet Gynecol. 1980;136(1):81-3.
2. Mendenhall HW, O'Leary JA, Phillips KO. The nonstress test: The value of a single acceleration in evaluating the fetus at risk. Am J Obstet Gynecol. 1980;136:87.
3. Druzin ML. Antepartum fetal heart rate monitoring: State of the art. Clin Perinatol. 1989;16:627.
4. Boddy K, Dawes GS, Fisher R, Pinter S, Robinson JS. Foetal respiratory movements, electrocortical and cardiovascular responses to hypoxaemia and hypercapnia in sheep. J Physiol. 1974;243:599-618.
5. Manning FA, Platt LD. Maternal hypoxemia and fetal breathing movements. Obstet Gynecol. 1979;53:758-60.

6. Murata Y, Martin CB Jr, Ikenoue T, Hashimoto T, Taira S, Sagawa T, et al. Fetal heart rate accelerations and late decelerations during the course of intrauterine death in chronically catheterized rhesus monkeys. Am J Obstet Gynecol. 1982;144:218-23.

7. Natale R, Clewlow F, Dawes GS. Measurement of fetal forelimb movements in the lamb in utero. Am J Obstet Gynecol. 1981;140:545-51.

8. Manning FA, Snijders R, Harman CR, Nicolaides K, Menticoglou S, Morrison I. Fetal biophysical profile score. VI. Correlation with antepartum umbilical venous fetal pH. Am J Obstet Gynecol. 1993;169:755-63.

9. Antenatal Fetal Surveillance: Indications and Timing. [online] Available from https://www.obgproject.com/2021/06/08/antenatal-fetal-surveillance-indications-and-timing/[Last accessed December, 2021].

10. Parer JT. Fetal heart rate. In: Resni CK (Eds). Maternal Fetal Medicine: Principles and Practice. Philadelphia: WB Saunders Company; 1999.

11. Lagrew DC Jr. Fetal evaluation in early gestational ages. Clin Obstet Gynecol. 1987;30: 992-8.

12. Sadovsky G, Nicolaides KH. Reference ranges for fetal heart rate patterns in normoxaemic nonanaemic fetuses. Fetal Ther. 1989;4:61.

13. Park MI, Hwang JH, Cha KJ, Park YS, Koh SK. Computerized analysis of fetal heart rate parameters by gestational age. Int J Gynaecol Obstet. 2001;74(2):157-64.

14. American College of Obstetricians and Gynecologists' Committee on Practice Bulletins—Obstetrics. Antepartum Fetal Surveillance: ACOG Practice Bulletin, Number 229. Obstet Gynecol. 2021;137:e116.

15. Grivell RM, Alfirevic Z, Gyte GM, Devane D. Antenatal cardiotocography for fetal assessment. Cochrane Database Syst Rev. 2015; 2015(9):CD007863.

16. Macones GA, Hankins GD, Spong CY, Hauth J, Moore T. The 2008 National Institute of Child Health and Human Development workshop report on electronic fetal monitoring: update on definitions, interpretation, and research guidelines. Obstet Gynecol. 2008;112(3): 661-6.

17. Tan KH, Smyth RM, Wei X. Fetal vibroacoustic stimulation for facilitation of tests of fetal wellbeing. Cochrane Database Syst Rev. 2013; (12):CD002963.

18. Oncken C, Kranzler H, O'Malley P, Gendreau P, Campbell WA. The effect of cigarette smoking on fetal heart rate characteristics. Obstet Gynecol. 2002;99(5 Pt 1):751-5.

19. Tan KH, Sabapathy A. Maternal glucose administration for facilitating tests of fetal wellbeing. Cochrane Database Syst Rev. 2012; 2012(9)CD003397.

20. Tan KH, Sabapathy A, Wei X. Fetal manipulation for facilitating tests of fetal wellbeing. Cochrane Database Syst Rev. 2013;(12):CD003396.

21. Meis PJ, Ureda JR, Swain M, Kelly RT, Penry M, Sharp P. Variable decelerations during nonstress tests are not a sign of fetal compromise. Am J Obstet Gynecol. 1986;154(3):586-90.

22. Visser GHA, Redman CWG, Huisjes HJ, Turnbull AC. Non stressed antepartum FHR monitoring implications of deceleration after spontaneous contractions. Am J Obstet Gynecol. 1980;138(4):429-35.

23. Huddleston JF, Sutliff G, Robinson D. Contraction stress test by intermittent nipple stimulation. Obstet Gynecol. 1984;63:669-73.

24. Freeman RK, Anderson G, Dorchester W. A prospective multi-institutional study of antepartum fetal heart rate monitoring. I. Risk of perinatal mortality and morbidity according to antepartum fetal heart rate test results. Am J Obstet Gynecol. 1982;143:771-7.

25. Braly P, Freeman RK. The significance of fetal heart rate reactivity with a positive oxytocin challenge test. Obstet Gynecol. 1977;50:689.

26. Farahani G, Fenton AN. Fetal heart rate acceleration in relation to the oxytocin challenge test. Obstet Gynecol. 1977;49:163.

49

Multiple Pregnancy

Alok Sharma, Aruna Singh

INTRODUCTION

- The rate and the number of twins and higher-order multifetal births have increased dramatically.
- The twinning rate rose 76% from 18.9 per 1,000 live births in 1990 to 33.2 in 2009.
- Childbearing at older age and widespread availability of assisted reproductive technologies are the two major factors accounting for these increases.
- These rates of multifetal pregnancies have a direct effect on the rates of preterm birth and its comorbidities.

PATHOPHYSIOLOGY

- Multiple gestations resulting from division of a single fertilized ovum or early embryo form monozygotic placentation. Chorionicity of monozygotic gestations is determined by the time at which division of the fertilized ovum/early embryo occurs (**Table 1**).
- The frequency of monozygotic twins is constant worldwide at 4 per 1,000 births.

- Multiple gestations resulting from the fertilization of multiple ova forms dizygotic pregnancies and by definition these pregnancies are dichorionic-diamniotic.
- The frequency of dizygotic twins varies by maternal age, parity, family history, maternal weight, nutritional state, race, and use of infertility drugs.
- In the United States, 20% of twin pregnancies are monochorionic and approximately 80% are dichorionic.

DIAGNOSIS

Early diagnosis of twin gestation is essential as delayed diagnosis can result in an increased risk of complications.

- *Clinical examination*: Multifetal gestations should be suspected if the uterine size is greater than expected or if multiple fetal heart tones are detected.
- *Ultrasonography*: It can be used to diagnose multiple gestations, to evaluate chorionicity. Chorionicity can be determined sonographically with 98% accuracy in the first trimester.
- *Early in the first trimester*:
  - Two distinct gestational sacs—dichorionic twin gestation
  - A single gestational sac with two fetal poles and two yolk sacs—monochorionic-diamniotic twin gestation
  - A single gestational sac with two fetal poles but one yolk sac—monochorionic-monoamniotic twin pregnancy
- *10–14 weeks*:
  - First trimester ultrasound scan when crown-rump length measures from 45 to 84 mm (at approximately 11 weeks to 13 weeks + 6 days) to determine gestational age, chorionicity, and amnionicity.

Timing of cleavage of fertilized ovum	Resulting placentation	Percentage of monozygotic twins
<72 hours	Diamniotic dichorionic	25–30
Days 4–7	Diamniotic monochorionic	70–75
Days 8–12	Monoamniotic monochorionic	1–2
≥Day 13	Conjoined	Very rare

TABLE 1: Determination of monozygotic twin chorionicity.

Flowchart 1: Algorithm for determination of chorionicity and amnionicity.

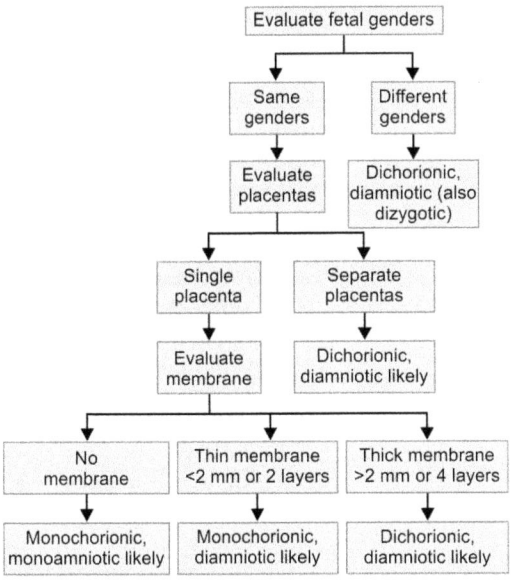

- Estimate gestational age from the largest baby in a twin pregnancy to avoid the risk of estimating it from a baby with early growth pathology.
- The chorionicity is determined by using:
  - The number of placental masses
  - The presence of amniotic membrane(s) and membrane thickness
  - The lambda or T-sign **(Flowchart 1)**
- If a woman is booked late in pregnancy, manage the pregnancy as a monochorionic pregnancy until proved otherwise.
- Assign nomenclature to babies (e.g., upper and lower, or left and right) in a twin gestation and document this clearly in the woman's notes to ensure consistency throughout pregnancy.

MATERNAL AND FETAL RISKS OF MULTIPLE GESTATION

- The various physiological adaptations that occur with multifetal gestations are typically greater than with a singleton pregnancy and this increases the likelihood of serious maternal complications.
- Virtually every obstetric complication is more common with multiple pregnancy with the exception of macrosomia and post-term gestation.
- Atypical presentations of pre-eclampsia are also more common in multifetal gestations.
- Perinatal morbidity and mortality is also increased due to preterm delivery and its comorbidities. Higher rates of neonatal and infant death and cerebral palsy.
- Approximately twofold increased risk for congenital anomalies as compared to singleton gestation.

ISSUES AND COMPLICATIONS UNIQUE TO MULTIPLE GESTATIONS

- *Monoamnionic twins:*
  - Only about 1% of all monozygotic twin gestations.
  - Perinatal mortality rates for monoamniotic twins have been reported to approach 50%.
  - Increased risk of congenital anomaly (seen in up to 25% of monoamniotic twin pregnancies), high risk of cardiac anomalies.
  - Fetal echocardiography is indicated in these pregnancies.
  - Umbilical cords frequently entangle and fetal death from cord entanglement is unpredictable. Unfortunately, no monitoring for this is effective.
  - Elective hospital admission to all patients with monoamniotic pregnancy after period of viability.
  - Elective cesarean delivery following the administration of antenatal corticosteroid therapy between 32 and 34 weeks' gestation.
- *Conjoined twins:*
  - The mortality rate is high.
    - Ultrasound can establish this diagnosis in utero as early as the first trimester based on visualization of monoamnionicity and a bifid fetal pole.
- *Monochorionic twins and vascular anastomoses:*
  - All monochorionic placentas likely share some anastomotic connection.
  - Artery-to-artery anastomoses are most frequent and are seen in 75% of the cases.
  - Vein-to-vein and artery-to-vein communications are seach found in approximately half.

- *Twin-twin transfusion syndrome (TTTS)*:
  - TTTS is exclusively a complication of monochorionic multifetal pregnancies. It is most common life-threatening complication that occurs in 10–15% of cases.
  - TTTS can present at any gestational age, but earlier onset is associated with a poorer prognosis.
  - Blood is transfused from a donor twin to its recipient sibling. The donor eventually becomes anemic and growth restricted, while the recipient sibling develops circulatory overload manifests as hydrops.
  - Fetal brain damage like cerebral palsy, microcephaly, porencephaly, and multicystic encephalomalacia are serious complications associated with placental vascular anastomoses in these cases.
  - *Diagnosis*:
    - The antenatal diagnosis of TTTS is made by ultrasound.
    - The two classic criteria are:
      - Monochorionic diamniotic twin gestation
      - Oligohydramnios, deepest vertical pocket (DVP < 2 cm) in one amniotic sac and polyhydramnios (DVP > 8 cm) in the other sac. The Quintero staging is widely used, shown in **Table 2**.
  - *Management and prognosis*:
    - Management depends on the Quintero staging and gestational age at the time of presentation.

TABLE 2: Quintero staging.

Stage	Ultrasound parameters
I	Discordant amnionic fluid volumes, but urine is still visible sonographically within the bladder of the donor twin
II	Criteria of stage I, but urine is not visible within the donor bladder
III	Criteria of stage II and abnormal Doppler studies of the umbilical artery, ductus venosus, or umbilical vein
IV	Ascites or frank hydrops in either twin
V	Demise of either twin

- *Stage I*: More than three-fourth remain stable or regress without intervention
- *Stage III or more*:
  - Worst perinatal outcome. Loss is around 70–100% without intervention
  - Various management options available are:
    - *Expectant management*:
      - In stage I cases
    - *Amnioreduction*:
      - In serial reduction amniocentesis, a needle is placed into the polyhydramniotic sac under ultrasound guidance and the fluid is withdrawn until the fluid volume normalizes (i.e., DVP < 8 cm).
      - Amnioreduction appears to offer a two- to threefold increase in overall survival compared with no intervention.
    - *Laser ablation*:
      - Laser ablation of placental anastomoses is the only therapeutic option that corrects the underlying pathophysiologic aberration.
      - It is the favored treatment option for early-onset TTTS, and is the optimal therapy before 26 weeks' gestation.
    - *Septostomy*: It involves intentional perforation of the dividing membrane, usually performed with a 20- or 22-gauge needle under ultrasound guidance.
    - *Selective feticide*: Especially if severe amniotic fluid and growth restriction occurs before 20 weeks of gestation.
- *Twin anemia-polycythemia sequence (TAPS)*:
  - Characterized by chronic and severe hemoglobin discordance in a monochorionic diamniotic twin pair in the absence of other criteria for TTTS.

- Diagnosed antenatally by middle cerebral artery (MCA) peak systolic velocity (PSV) > 1.5 multiples of the median (MoM) in the donor and <1.0 MoM in the recipient twin.
- The spontaneous form of TAPS complicates 3–5% of monochorionic pregnancies and occurs after 26 weeks of gestation.
- The iatrogenic form occurs in up to 13% of pregnancies, after laser photocoagulation of the placenta (within 5 weeks of a procedure).
- Ideal management of TAPS is not yet clear, but intrauterine transfusions—both intraperitoneal and intravenous—and laser treatment have been reported with good success.

- *Twin reversed-arterial-perfusion sequence (TRAP):*
  - Also known as an acardiac twin, a rare but serious complication of monochorionic twins with an estimated incidence is 1 case in 35,000 births.
  - In the classic TRAP sequence, there is a normally formed donor twin that shows features of high-output heart failure and cardiomegaly.
  - The recipient twin that lacks a heart (acardius) and other structures, but sustains the life due to presence of placental vascular anastomoses.
  - Color Doppler is essential to confirm diagnosis.
  - Three options are available: (1) expectant management, (2) delivery, or (3) interruption of the vascular communication between the twins.

- *Hydatidiform mole with coexisting normal fetus:*
  - This unique gestation contains one normal fetus and its cotwin is a complete molar pregnancy.
  - Reported prevalence rates range from 1 in 22,000 to 1 in 100,000 pregnancies.
  - Diagnosis is usually made in the first half of pregnancy, sonographically, a normal-appearing twin is accompanied by its cotwin, which is a large placenta containing multiple small anechoic cysts.
  - Often these pregnancies are terminated, but pregnancy continuation is increasingly adopted because of:

- The pregnancy prognosis is not as poor as previously thought, and live birth rates range between 20 and 40%.
- The risk of persistent trophoblastic disease is similar whether the pregnancy is terminated or not.

- Due to limited number of cases, robust data for firm recommendations are lacking.
- The complications of expectant management include vaginal bleeding, hyperemesis gravidarum, thyrotoxicosis, and early-onset pre-eclampsia; close surveillance is needed for those adopting continuation of pregnancy.

- *Discordant growth of twin fetuses:*
  - Fetal size inequality develops in approximately 15% of twin gestations and may reflect pathological growth restriction in one fetus.
  - *Etiopathogenesis:*
    - The cause is often unclear.
    - The etiology in monochorionic twins likely differs from that in dichorionic twins.
    - The single placenta is not always equally shared in monochorionic twins, have greater rates of discordant growth.
    - Discordancy in dichorionic twins may result from various factor, dizygotic fetuses may have different genetic growth potential.
  - *Diagnosis:*
    - Size discordancy between twins can be determined sonographically.
    - Differences in crown-rump length are not reliable predictors for birth weight discordance.
    - The weight of the smaller twin is compared with that of the larger twin, and the percent discordancy is calculated as the weight of the larger twin minus the weight of the smaller twin, then divided by the weight of the larger twin. The estimated weight difference is expressed in percentage.
      - The weight difference of 20% or more is considered as size discordancy.

- Alternatively, the abdominal circumference (AC) reflects fetal nutrition. The difference of 20 mm or more in AC measurements.
  - *Management*:
    - Serial sonographic monitoring of twin
    - Monochorionic twins are generally monitored more frequently.
    - Fetal surveillance, depending on the degree of discordancy and the gestational age
    - Fetal surveillance may be indicated, especially if one or both fetuses exhibit restricted growth.
    - Nonstress testing, biophysical profile, and umbilical artery Doppler assessment have all been recommended in the management of twins.
    - If discordancy is identified in a monochorionic twin pregnancy, umbilical artery Doppler studies in the smaller fetus may help guide management.
- *Fetal demise of one twin*:
  - Death of one fetus can occur at any time during twin gestation and the factors that affect the prognosis for the surviving twin include:
    - Chorionicity
    - Gestational age at the time of the demise
    - The duration between the demise and delivery of the surviving twin
  - Due to presence of vascular anastomoses in monochorionic twin gestations, risk of death or damage to the survivor twin is more.
  - Early in pregnancy (first trimester):
    - It may manifest as a vanishing twin and the risk of death is not increased for the survivor twin.
  - In a slightly more advanced gestation:
    - Fetus compressus, fetus papyraceus may be identified at the time of delivery.
  - In the second trimester or later:
    - Fetal demise of one twin in second trimester or later complicates about 2.4–6.8% of twin pregnancies.
    - The effect of gestational age at the time of death and the mortality risk

to the surviving twin are less clear. More severe sequelae including brain injury can also occur in the surviving fetus.
  - *Management*:
    - Decisions should be based on:
      - Chorionicity
      - Gestational age and risk to the surviving fetus
      - The cause of death
  - *First-trimester losses*—no additional surveillance
  - *After the first trimester*:
    - After the first trimester but before viability, pregnancy termination can be considered.
    - Late second and early third trimesters present the greatest risk to the surviving twin.
      - The timing of elective delivery after conservative management is debatable.
      - Although the risks of subsequent death or neurological damage to the survivor are comparatively higher for monochorionic twins at this gestational age, the risk of preterm birth is equally increased.
      - A course of antenatal corticosteroids for survivor lung maturity should be considered. Delivery generally occurs within 3 weeks of diagnosis of fetal demise.
  - In cases of single fetal death at term, especially when the etiology is unclear, most opt for delivery instead of expectant.
  - Occasionally, death of one but not all fetuses results from a maternal complication such as diabetic ketoacidosis or severe pre-eclampsia with abruption, pregnancy management is based on the diagnosis and the status of both the mother and surviving fetus.
  - Dichorionic twins can probably be safely delivered at term with no increased risk.
- *Impending death of one fetus*:
  - During antepartum surveillance, abnormal results in one twin but normal test for the other pose a particular dilemma.

- Delivery may be the best option for the compromised fetus yet may result in death from immaturity of the cotwin.
  - If fetal lung maturity is confirmed, should try to salvage both the healthy fetus and compromised fetus.
  - If twins are immature, the ideal management is controversial and should take into account the chances of intact survival for both fetuses.
    - Often the compromised fetus is severely growth restricted or anomalous, thus performing amniocentesis for fetal chromosomal analysis in women of advanced maternal age carrying twin pregnancies is advantageous.
    - Chromosomal abnormality identification in one fetus allows rational decisions regarding interventions.

PRENATAL CARE AND ANTEPARTUM MANAGEMENT

The primary objective is to provide close observation to the mother, to screen for all complications and prevent preterm birth and its morbidities.

- *Diet, lifestyle, and nutritional supplements*:
  - The increased physiologic stress of a multifetal pregnancy demands a 10% higher maternal resting energy expenditure.
  - Body mass index (BMI)-specific weight gain should be the goal.
  - The daily recommended augmented caloric intake for women with twins is 40–45 kcal/kg/day, composed of 20% protein, 40% carbohydrate, and 40% fat divided into three meals and three snacks daily.
- Uncomplicated dichorionic twin pregnancy should have at least 8 and monochorionic should have at least 11 antenatal appointments.
- Frequency of antenatal appointments may be increased depending upon complications.
- *Prenatal diagnosis and aneuploidy screening*:
  - Both first- and second-trimester serum markers have lower sensitivity compared to singleton gestations.
  - The test results typically are provided for the entire pregnancy and not for each individual fetus making interpretation of abnormal results difficult.
  - There are currently insufficient data to recommend use of the cell-free fetal DNA testing in multiple gestations.
  - Nuchal translucency measurement, which assesses each fetus independently, is a reasonable alternative to serum testing for aneuploidy screening in multiple gestations.
  - Maternal serum alpha-fetoprotein levels are approximately double in twins compared to singletons.
    - A level >4.0 MoM in twins is associated with an increased risk of neural tube and ventral wall defects and should be addressed with a detailed sonographic survey of these structures.
  - Amniocentesis can be offered if an open neural tube defect is suspected or ultrasound examination is inadequate.
  - Amniocentesis may be performed on one sac only if monozygosity is certain, otherwise, genetic amniocentesis should be performed on all sacs.
- *Preterm birth prevention*:
  - Preterm birth occurs in >40% of twin. Ultrasound surveillance of cervical length can identify those multiple gestations at increased risk of preterm delivery.
  - A transvaginal measurement of cervical length of <2.5 cm at 24 weeks is associated with an increased risk of preterm birth before 32 weeks.
  - Patient education regarding the early signs of preterm labor in multiple gestations is important.
  - Tocolysis should be reserved for women with documented preterm labor and may be administered to allow administration of antenatal corticosteroids.
  - Antenatal steroids should be administered if preterm birth is expected within 7 days and the gestational age is between 24 and 34 weeks.
  - Magnesium sulfate is also recommended for neuroprotection before anticipated delivery.

- Routine hospitalized bed rest is not associated with a decrease in preterm birth in multifetal pregnancies.
- Asymptomatic twin pregnancies in women with a reassuring cervical length and no prior history of preterm birth, cessation of work or rest at home is not recommended.
- Studies have not shown any benefit associated with the use of intramuscular 17α-hydroxyprogesterone caproate (17-OH-PC) or vaginal progesterone therapy in multiple gestation.
- Prophylactic cervical cerclage does not improve perinatal outcome in women with multifetal gestation.
  - Rescue cerclage in women with a second-trimester twin gestation and a dilated cervix may be beneficial.
  - Cerclage placement in multiple gestations should be restricted to women with either a strongly suggestive history of cervical insufficiency or objectively documented cervical insufficiency based on physical examination.
- A vaginal pessary that encircles and theoretically compresses the cervix, the silicone Arabin pessary use is not recommended at present.
- The frequency of preterm premature rupture of membranes (PPROM) rises in twin gestation and expectant management is similar to singleton pregnancies.
- *Delayed delivery of second twin*:
  - Infrequently, after preterm birth of the presenting fetus, it may be advantageous for undelivered fetus to remain in utero.
  - Maternal evaluation and thorough counseling, particularly regarding the potential for serious, life-threatening infection and abruption must be done.
  - Congenital anomalies in second twin must be ruled out.
  - The range of gestational age in which the benefits outweigh the risks for delayed delivery is likely narrow but delivery from 23 to 26 weeks should be avoided.

- *Surveillance of fetal growth and well-being*:
  - *Fetal growth assessment*:
    - Serial ultrasonography is the most accurate method to assess fetal growth in multiple gestations.
    - Serial ultrasonographic examinations should be performed every 3–4 weeks beginning at approximately 20 weeks of gestation in uncomplicated twin gestation, as shown in **Flowchart 2**.
    - More frequent examinations are required in case of any maternal or fetal complications.
    - Additionally, ultrasounds should be performed every 2 weeks in monochorionic twins beginning at 16 weeks to screen for TTTS.
  - *Antepartum testing for fetal wellbeing*:
    - Routine antepartum testing of uncomplicated dichorionic multiple gestations has not been shown to offer benefit.
    - The American College of Obstetricians and Gynecologists (ACOG) recommends that antepartum testing be performed in multifetal gestations for indications similar to those for singleton gestation.

Flowchart 2: Antenatal surveillance and delivery timing for uncomplicated diamniotic twins.

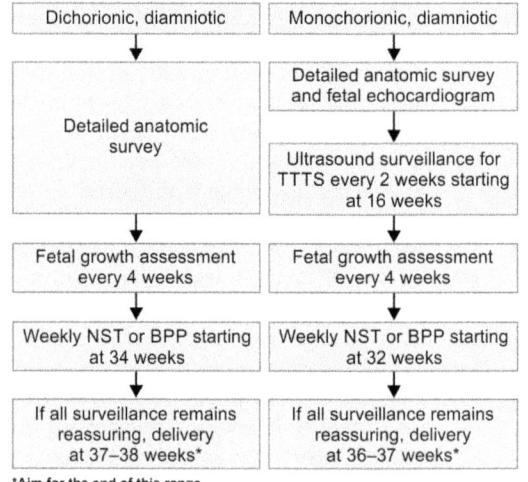

*Aim for the end of this range

(BPP: biophysical profile; NST: nonstress test; TTTS: twin-twin transfusion syndrome)

- Antenatal surveillance in the form of nonstress tests or biophysical profiles is often performed starting at 28 weeks where indicated.

LABOR AND DELIVERY

Timing of Delivery

- *The optimum time to deliver twin pregnancies depends on*:
  - Chorionicity
  - Amnionicity
  - Pregnancy complications
- Spontaneous or medically indicated preterm birth complicates over 50% of twin pregnancies.
- *Uncomplicated twin pregnancies*:
  - Elective delivery at 38 weeks in well-dated dichorionic twin pregnancies
  - Elective delivery at 34 and $37^{6/7}$ weeks for uncomplicated monochorionic diamniotic twins
  - ACOG and the Society for Maternal-Fetal Medicine (SMFM) suggest delivery of uncomplicated dichorionic twins at 38^{+0} to 38^{+6} weeks and monochorionic/diamniotic twins at 34^{+0} to 37^{+6} weeks of gestation[1]
- *Complicated twin pregnancies*:
  - Monochorionic/monoamniotic twin pregnancies are delivered between 32^{+0} and 34^{+0} weeks of gestation.
  - Other complicated twin pregnancies, timing of delivery is based on the type and severity of the disorder (e.g., TTTS, growth restriction, pre-eclampsia).

Management of Labor

- A variety of complications may be encountered during labor and delivery of twin gestation including abnormal fetal presentation, umbilical cord prolapse, placental abruption, uterine contractile dysfunction, emergent operative delivery, and postpartum hemorrhage from uterine atony.
  - Continuous electronic fetal monitoring is preferable.
  - Oral intake should be restricted to clear liquids during active labor.

- Ensure adequate intravenous access and blood product availability.
- Send blood sample for type and screen at the time of admission to labor room.
- A senior obstetrician skilled in intrauterine manipulation of a fetus should be present.
- Ideally, a portable ultrasound machine should be readily available to evaluate the presentation and position of the fetuses during labor.
- An anesthesia team should be immediately if emergent cesarean delivery or intrauterine manipulation is required.
- Pediatric staff should be available for assisting the transition of each infant, including resuscitation if needed, and the facility should be able to provide the risk-appropriate level of care for the newborn infant.
- Active management of the third stage of labor
- *Evaluation upon admission*:
  - Fetal presentation, best confirmed sonographically.
  - If active labor confirms, decision to attempt vaginal delivery vs. cesarean section.
  - Labor induction or augmentation
  - *Analgesia and anesthesia*:
    - Epidural analgesia
    - General anesthesia, if required, use halogenated inhalational agents to achieve uterine relaxation
- *Choosing the route of delivery*:
  - Amnionicity and fetal presentation at the onset of labor
  - Approximately 80% of first twins are cephalic.
  - Vaginal delivery is preferred for diamniotic twins in which the presenting twin is cephalic at the onset of labor if appropriate expertise in internal and external version and/or vaginal breech delivery is available[1]
  - Cesarean delivery is preferred for all monoamniotic twins, diamniotic twins with a noncephalic-presenting twin, and for pregnancies with standard obstetric indications for cesarean delivery (e.g., placenta previa).
  - Delivery route depends upon gestational age and fetal presentation.

- - Both twin cephalic presentation:
    - Vaginal delivery
  - *First cephalic-second noncephalic presentation*, three options are there:
    1. Vaginal delivery and intrapartum external cephalic version for second twin
    2. Vaginal delivery and internal podalic version and breech extraction—preferable to version.
       - Avoid breech extraction of second twin under following circumstances:
         - If second twin is 20% larger than presenting twin
         - If the gestational age is <28 weeks or the estimated fetal weight of the second twin is <1,500 g
    3. Vaginal delivery for first twin and cesarean section for second twin, may be required due to intrapartum complications.
  - *Breech presentation of first twin*:
    - Cesarean delivery is often preferred with a viable-size fetus.
  - *Locked twins*:
    - Cesarean delivery
- *Vaginal delivery of second twin*:
  - Following delivery of first twin, the presentation, position, and size of second twin should be identified quickly and carefully by abdominal and vaginal examination.
  - If fetal head or breech is fixed to the birth canal, moderate fundal pressure is applied to the abdomen and rupture of membranes is done.
  - Can use dilute oxytocin, if contractions do not resume within approximately 10 minutes.

- - Many reports have suggested that the interval between deliveries should ideally be 15 minutes or less and certainly not >30 minutes.
  - Obstetrician skilled in intrauterine manipulations and skilled anesthesia personnel must be present.
  - Vigilant monitoring for nonreassuring fetal heart rate or bleeding is required. Prompt cesarean delivery if indicated.
- *Special populations*:
  - *Vaginal birth after cesarean (VBAC)*:
    - VBAC in any women with previous one or more cesarean should be considered carefully.
    - According to the ACOG no evidence currently suggests an increased risk of uterine rupture, and women with twins and one previous cesarean delivery with a low transverse incision may be considered candidates for trial of labor.
    - In clinical practice, a trial of labor to women with diamniotic twin pregnancies with a cephalic-presenting twin and one prior cesarean delivery, provided they go into spontaneous labor.
    - Continuous monitoring of both fetuses should be done to look for initial sign of uterine rupture.

REFERENCE

1. American College of Obstetricians and Gynecologists' Committee on Practice Bulletins—Obstetrics, Society for Maternal-Fetal Medicine. Multifetal Gestations: Twin, Triplet, and Higher-Order Multifetal Pregnancies: ACOG Practice Bulletin, Number 231. Obstet Gynecol. 2021;137:e145.

Mohita Agarwal

DEFINITION

Fetal death means death prior to complete expulsion or extraction from the mother of a product of human conception irrespective of the duration of pregnancy and which is not an induced termination of pregnancy. The death is indicated by the fact that after such expulsion or extraction, the fetus does not breathe or show any other evidence of life such as beating of the heart, pulsation of the umbilical cord, or definite movement of voluntary muscles. Heartbeats are to be distinguished from transient cardiac contractions; respirations are to be distinguished from fleeting respiratory efforts or gasps.[1]

ETIOLOGY

Estimated risk of stillbirth is 6.4 per 1,000 pregnancies. About 25–60% of the stillbirths are attributable to unexplained causes. Of the remaining, the causes may be either or a combination of maternal, fetal, and placental.

- *Obstetric complications*: Abruption, multi-fetal gestation, ruptured membranes at 20–24 weeks
- *Placental abnormalities*: Uteroplacental insufficiency, maternal vascular disease
- *Fetal malformations*: Major structural and/or genetic abnormalities
- *Infections*: Involving the fetus or placenta
- *Umbilical cord abnormalities*: Prolapse, stricture, thrombosis
- *Hypertensive disorders*: Preeclampsia, chronic hypertension
- *Medical complications*: Diabetes, antiphospholipid antibody (APLA)

RISK FACTORS

Many factors are associated with an increased risk of stillbirth. Among others, these include advanced maternal age; obesity; African-American race; smoking; obesity; illicit drug use; maternal medical diseases—such as overt diabetes or chronic hypertension, renal disease, thyroid disorders, thrombophilias; assisted reproductive technology; nulliparity; obesity; and prior adverse pregnancy outcomes—such as prior preterm birth or growth-restricted newborn.

INVESTIGATIONS

Clinical assessment and laboratory tests should be recommended with the following aims:

- To assess maternal wellbeing (including coagulopathy)
- To determine the cause of death
- The chance of recurrence
- Possible means of avoiding further pregnancy complications (**Flowchart 1**)

The investigations are: (A) General and (B) Specific.

- *General investigations*:
  - Full blood count
  - Urine routine and microscopy
  - Urine culture and sensitivity
  - Random blood sugar
  - High vaginal and endocervical swab for C/S
  - Coagulation screen
  - Ultrasound scan for:
    - Confirmation of intrauterine death (IUD)
    - Fetal lie and presentation
    - Placental localization
    - Placental abruption or hematoma
    - Uterine pathology
    - Pelvic or adnexal pathology
- *Specific investigations*:
  - Maternal bacteriology:
    - Blood culture

Flowchart 1: Evaluation of stillbirth.

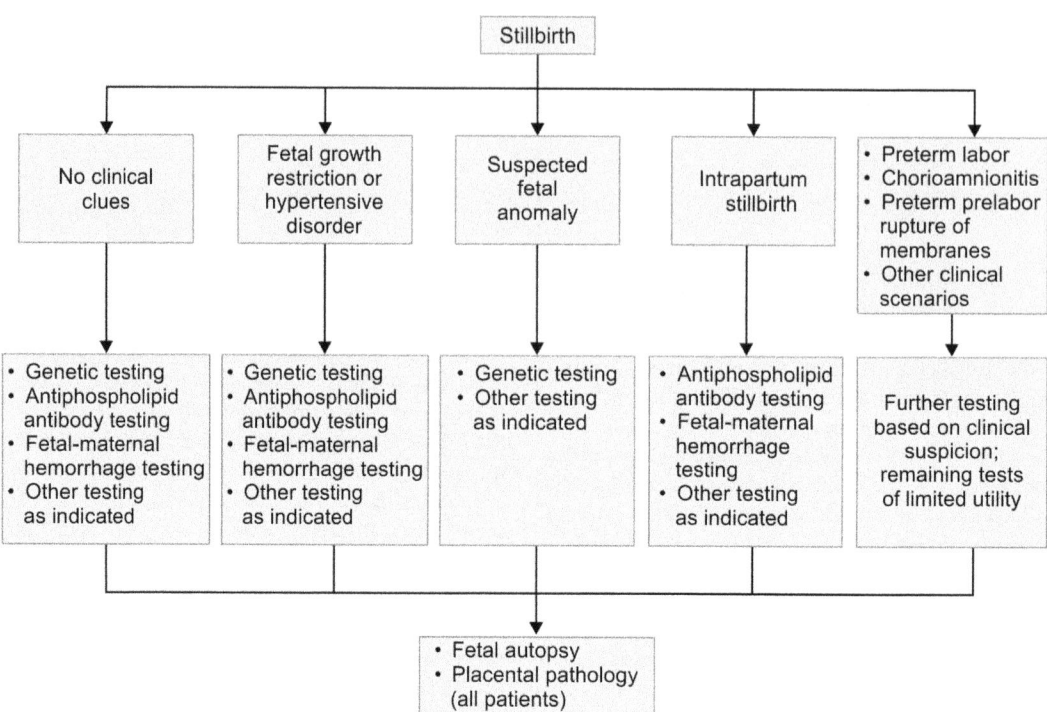

- Midstream urine
- Vaginal swab
- Endocervical swab
- Maternal serology:
  - Viral
  - Syphilis
  - Tropical infections
- Thrombophilia screen
- Kleihauer
- Thyroid screen
- Maternal HbA1c
- Anti-red cell antibody
- Anti-Ra and Anti-Lo antibodies
- Maternal alloimmune antiplatelet antibodies
- Parental karyotyping
- Fetal and placental microbiology:
  - Fetal blood
  - Fetal swabs
  - Placental swabs
- Fetal and placental tissues for karyotype:
  - Deep fetal skin
  - Fetal cartilage
  - Placenta

- Postmortem examination:
  - External
  - Autopsy
  - Microscopy
  - X-ray
  - Placenta and cord

Approach to a Patient[2]

History

- Family history:
  - Recurrent spontaneous abortions
  - Venous thromboembolism
  - Congenital anomaly or chromosomal abnormalities
  - Hereditary conditions
  - Developmental delay
  - Consanguinity
- *Maternal history*:
  - Previous venous thromboembolism
  - Diabetes mellitus
  - Raunak high potential
  - Thrombophilia
  - Systemic lupus erythematosus

- Autoimmune disease
- Epilepsy
- Severe anemia
- Heart disease
- Tobacco, alcohol, drug, or medication use

- *Obstetric history*:
  - Recurrent pregnancy loss
  - Previous child with anomaly, hereditary condition, or growth restriction
  - Previous gestational hypertension or preeclampsia
  - Previous gestational diabetes mellitus
  - Previous placental abruption
  - Previous fetal demise and pregnancy maternal age
  - Gestational age at stillbirth
  - Medical conditions complicating pregnancy
  - Pregnancy weight gain and body mass index
  - Complications of multifetal gestation
  - Placental abruption
  - Abdominal trauma

- Preterm labor or after of membranes
- Gestational age at onset of prenatal care
- Abnormality seen on ultrasound
- Infections or chorioamnionitis

Fetal Autopsy

If there is no consent for autopsy, external evaluation by a trained perinatal pathologist. Other options include photographs, X-ray imaging, ultrasonography, magnetic resonance imaging, and sampling of tissues such as blood and skin.

Placental Examination

It includes evaluation for signs of bacterial or viral infection. Discuss available test with pathologist **(Flowchart 2)**.

▓ LABOR AND DELIVERY

Recommendations about labor and birth should take into account the mother's preferences as well as her medical condition and previous intrapartum history.

Flowchart 2: Fetal and placental evaluation.

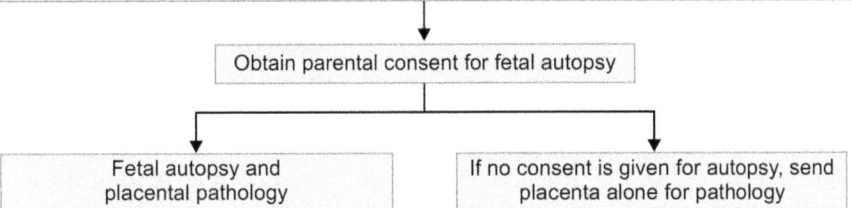

Inspect fetus and placenta:
- Weight, head circumference, and length of the fetus
- Weight of the placenta
- Photographs of the fetus and placenta
- Frontal and profile photographs of whole body, face, extremities, palms, and any abnormalities
- Document findings and abnormalities

↓

- Obtain consent from parents for cytological specimens
- Obtain cytological specimens with sterile techniques and instruments
- Acceptable cytology specimens (at least one):
  – Amniotic fluid obtained by amniocentesis at time of prenatal diagnosis of fetal demise: particularly valuable if delivery is not expected imminently
  – Placental block (1*1) cm taken from below the cord insertion site and on the unfixed placenta
  – Umbilical cord segment 1.5 cm
  – Internal fetal tissue specimen such as costochondral junction or patella; skin is not recommended
- Place specimens in a sterile tissue culture medium of lactated Ringer's solution and keep at room temperature when transported to the cytology laboratory

↓

Obtain parental consent for fetal autopsy

| Fetal autopsy and placental pathology | If no consent is given for autopsy, send placenta alone for pathology |

Source: ACOG Practice Bulletin No. 102: management of stillbirth. Obstet Gynecol. 2009;113(3):748-61.[3]

Vaginal birth is the recommended mode of delivery for most women, but cesarean birth will need to be considered with some.

More than 85% of women with an intrauterine fetal demise (IUFD) labor spontaneously within 3 weeks of diagnosis. If the woman is physically well, her membranes are intact and there is no evidence of preeclampsia, infection or bleeding, the risk of expectant management for 48 hours is low. There is a 10% chance of maternal disseminated intravascular coagulation (DIC) within 4 weeks from the date of fetal death and an increasing chance thereafter. Vaginal birth can be achieved within 24 hours of induction of labor for IUFD in about 90% of women. Vaginal birth carries the potential advantages of immediate recovery and quicker return to home. Cesarean birth might occasionally be clinically indicated by virtue of maternal condition.

Stillbirth before 24 weeks is best managed by a dilation and evacuation (D&E) by a competent provider. This involves dilation of the cervix and manual removal of the product of conception. The cervix is often predilated using laminaria placed in the cervix the night before the procedure. This risk of the procedure is greater when the fetus measures >24 weeks in size. An ultrasound estimated fetal size <24 weeks is, therefore, more important than the estimated gestational age in determining the appropriateness of a D&E. A fetus on ultrasound may measure smaller than the established gestational age due to either growth restriction caused by the underlying pathology or the stillbirth predating the diagnosis. This procedure is considered less morbid than the induction of labor because it is associated with a lower risk of infection.[4] If D&E is not desired, then a medical induction of labor is offered using misoprostol. Up to 26 weeks, give vaginal misoprostol 100 mcg every 6 hours for a maximum of four doses. If the first dose does not result in adequate contractions, the dose may be doubled up to 400 mcg. The maximum daily dosing should not exceed 1,600 mcg.[5]

Stillbirth after 24 weeks with a favorable cervix (Bishop score >6) is conducted with standard doses of synthetic oxytocin.

Stillbirth after 24 weeks with an unfavorable cervix (Bishop score <6) in the absence of a previous hysterotomy scar is achieved with misoprostol 50 mcg vaginally repeated every 4 hours for a maximum of six doses.[6] If the first dose does not result in a cervical change or over two contractions in 10 minutes, the second dose can be doubled to 100 mcg vaginally and again to 200 mcg vaginally four hours after the 100 mcg dose. The mean time to delivery is 10–11 hours. If the delivery does not occur in 24 hours, the regimen can be repeated once. Oxytocin can be substituted once the cervix reaches 4 cm if needed. Electronic monitoring is not used for induction for fetal death. Misoprostol is not repeated if there are greater than two contractions in 10 minutes due to the risk of tachysystole.[7]

Vaginal delivery is not contraindicated in pregnancies <24 weeks complicated by placenta previa.[8] Cesarean section is safer in pregnancies complicated by placenta previa and stillbirth over 24 weeks.

Women with a prior single, low transverse, cesarean delivery, and second-trimester stillbirth may receive mechanical ripening agents or misoprostol ≤200 mcg vaginally every 4 hours. The risk of rupture is 0.28% vs. 0.04% in these women with no prior cesarean section.[9]

Women with third-trimester fetal demise and an unfavorable cervix, and a prior history of a cesarean section should use a mechanical method of cervical ripening followed by oxytocin for induction. Misoprostol may be considered as an option only after rigorous informed consent. The lowest dose of 25–50 mcg vaginally should be used, and the dose should not be doubled to reduce the risk of uterine rupture.[10]

Fetal-pelvic disproportion seldom is a concern for the delivery of a stillborn, whether breech or cephalic, in the absence of macrosomia. Overlapping skull bones and fetal deterioration often allow the delivery of even large fetuses. A persistent shoulder or transverse lie may require an attempted internal or external version.[11] If unsuccessful, these fetal presentations may require a cesarean delivery.

The Royal College of Obstetricians and Gynaecologists (RCOG) Guidelines[12]

A combination of mifepristone and a prostaglandin preparation should usually be recommended as the first-line intervention for induction of labor. Misoprostol can be used in preference to prostaglandin E2 because of equivalent safety and efficacy. The use of misoprostol for induction of labor in women with IUFD has been endorsed by National Institute for Health and Care Excellence (NICE). NICE recommended that the choice and dose of vaginal prostaglandins should "take into account the clinical circumstances, availability of preparations and local protocols." A review of misoprostol use for late IUFD recommended that the dose should be adjusted according to gestational age (100 mcg 6-hourly before 26^{+6} weeks, 25–50 mcg 4-hourly at 27^{+0} weeks or more, up to 24 hours).

Mechanical methods for induction of labor in women with an IUFD increase the chance of ascending infections. In women with a single lower segment scar, induction of labor with prostaglandin is safe but not without risk. Misoprostol can be safely used for induction of labor in women with a single previous lower segment cesarean section (LSCS) and an IUFD but with lower doses (Grade C recommendation). Women with two previous LSCS should be advised that in general the absolute risk of induction of labor with prostaglandin is only a little higher than for women with a single previous LSCS (Grade C recommendation). Mifepristone can be used alone (at a dose of 600 mg) to increase the chance of labor significantly within 72 hours (avoiding the use of prostaglandin). Unless there is a pressing need to induce labor, caution should be exercised in using oxytocic agents in the presence of a uterine scar.

Medical Induction of Labor after IUFD

On the day of diagnosis of IUFD:
- Mifepristone 200 mg PO 36–48 hours after diagnosis
- 24–34 weeks misoprostol 200 mcg PV followed by 200 mcg PO 3 hourly × 4 doses
- >34 weeks misoprostol 100 mcg PV followed by 100 mcg PO 3 hourly × 4 doses

A second course may be started after 24 hours and with medical review.

Analgesia in labor is particularly important for women with an IUFD. All usual modalities should be available including regional anesthesia and patient-controlled anesthesia (RCOG, 2010). Diamorphine should be used in preference to pethidine. Regional anesthesia should be available for women with an IUFD; however, assessment for DIC and sepsis should be undertaken before

administering regional anesthesia. Women undergoing VBAC should be closely monitored for features of scar rupture. Fetal heart rate abnormality, usually the most common early sign of scar dehiscence, does not apply in this circumstance. Other clinical features include maternal tachycardia, atypical pain, vaginal bleeding, hematuria on catheter specimen, and maternal collapse (RCOG, 2007).

■ SUPPRESSION OF LACTATION

Women should be advised that dopamine agonists successfully suppress lactation in a very high proportion of women and are well tolerated by a very large majority; cabergoline is superior to bromocriptine. Dopamine agonists should not be given to women with hypertension or pre-eclampsia. Estrogens should not be used to suppress lactation.

■ PREGNANCY AFTER STILLBIRTH

Preconceptional or Initial Prenatal Visit
- Detailed medical and obstetrical history
- Review evaluation of prior stillbirth
- Determination of recurrence risk
- Discuss recurrence of comorbid obstetric complications
- Smoking cessation
- Preconceptional weight loss in obese women
- Genetic counseling if family genetic condition exists
- Diabetes screen
- *Thrombophilia screen*: Antiphospholipid antibodies (only if history indicates)
- Support and reassurance

First Trimester
- Dating sonography
- *First-trimester screen*: Pregnancy-associated plasma protein A, human chorionic
- Gonadotropin, and nuchal translucency
- Support and reassurance

Second Trimester
- Fetal sonographic anatomical survey at 18–20 weeks' gestation
- Maternal serum screening (quadruple) *or* single-marker alpha fetoprotein

- First-trimester screening elected
- Possible uterine artery Doppler studies at 22–24 weeks' gestation
- Support and reassurance

Third Trimester

- Sonographic screening for fetal-growth restriction, starting at 28 weeks
- Kick counts starting at 28 weeks
- Antepartum fetal surveillance starting at 32 weeks *or* 1–2 weeks earlier than
- Prior stillbirth
- Support and reassurance

Delivery

- Elective induction at 39 weeks
- Delivery before 39 weeks only with documented fetal lung maturity by amniocentesis
- Provides risk modification but does

REFERENCES

1. MacDorman MF, Reddy UM, Silver RM. Trends in stillbirth by gestational age in the United States, 2006–2012. Obstet Gynecol. 2015;126(6):1146.
2. Stillbirth. In: Williams JW, Bloom S, Leveno K, Leveno KJ, Hauth J, et al. (Eds). Williams Obstetrics, 25th edition. McGraw-Hill Education; 2018.
3. ACOG Practice Bulletin No. 102: management of stillbirth. Obstet Gynecol. 2009;113(3):748-61.
4. Edlow AG, Hou MY, Maurer R, Benson C, Delli-Bovi L, Goldberg AB. Uterine evacuation for second-trimester fetal death and maternal morbidity. Obstet Gynecol. 2011;117(2 Pt 1):07-16.
5. Ngai SW, Tang OS, Ho PC. Prostaglandins for induction of second-trimester termination and intrauterine death. Best Pract Res Clin Obstet Gynaecol. 2003;17(5):765-75.
6. Gómez Ponce de León R, Wing DA. Misoprostol for termination of pregnancy with intrauterine fetal demise in the second and third trimester of pregnancy - a systematic review. Contraception. 2009;79(4):259-71.
7. Bugalho A, Bique C, Machungo F, Faáundes A. Induction of labor with intravaginal misoprostol in intrauterine fetal death. Am J Obstet Gynecol. 1994;171(2):538-41.
8. Perritt JB, Burke A, Edelman AB. Interruption of nonviable pregnancies of 24-28 weeks' gestation using medical methods: release date June 2013 SFP guideline #20133. Contraception. 2013;88(3):341-9.
9. Goyal V. Uterine rupture in second-trimester misoprostol-induced abortion after cesarean delivery: a systematic review. Obstet Gynecol. 2009;113(5):1117-23.
10. Gómez Ponce de León R, Wing D, Fiala C. Misoprostol for intrauterine fetal death. Int J Gynaecol Obstet. 2007;99(Suppl 2):S190-3.
11. Chauhan AR, Singhal TT, Raut VS. Is internal podalic version a lost art? Optimum mode of delivery in transverse lie. J Postgrad Med. 2001;47(1):15-8.
12. National Institute of Clinical Excellence. (2010). Late Intrauterine Fetal Death and Stillbirth (Green-top Guideline No. 55). Greentop Guidelines 55. [online] Available from https://www.rcog.org.uk/en/guidelines-research-services/guidelines/gtg55/#:~:text=Update%2026%20July%202011%3A%20The,gestational%20age)%20when%20inducing%20labour. [Last accessed December, 2021].

51

Preterm Prelabor Rupture of Membranes

Vanita Jain, Aashima Arora

DEFINITION

Rupture of membranes (ROM) prior to onset of labor is termed as prelabor rupture of membranes.[1] It comprises of:

- *Term prelabor rupture of membranes*: ROM at/beyond 37 weeks period of gestation (POG). Affects 8% of pregnancies.
- *Preterm prelabor rupture of membranes*: ROM from period of viability to 36^{+6} weeks POG. Affects 2–3% of pregnancies.
- *Previable rupture of membranes*: ROM before period of viability (may vary between regions). Affects <1% of pregnancies.

This chapter will focus on preterm prelabor rupture of membranes (PPROM).

- PPROM should not be confused with ROM during actual preterm labor.
- The term "preterm premature rupture of membranes" used previously has been abandoned as preterm and premature can both suggest prematurity of fetus.[2]

CAUSES

Major risk factors of PPROM are a history of PPROM, short cervical length, second- or third-trimester vaginal bleeding, uterine overdistension, connective tissue disorders, low body mass index, poor socioeconomic status, cigarette smoking, and illicit drug use.

- No obvious cause is found in most cases of PPROM.
- These factors may act individually or together.
- Intra-amniotic infection is commonly associated with PPROM.

CLINICAL IMPORTANCE

Preterm prelabor rupture of membranes is clinically relevant because of the associated maternal and fetal complications.[1,2]

Maternal Complications

- *Clinically evident intra-amniotic infection*: 15–35%
- *Postpartum infection*: 15–25%
- *Abruptio placentae*: 2–5%
- Increased risk of cesarean delivery

Fetal Complications

The most significant risks to the fetus after PPROM are complications of prematurity. Overall 25% of preterm births are associated with PPROM. Globally, perinatal morbidity and mortality rate associated with PPROM exceed 20% of affected pregnancies. PPROM may lead to intrauterine death in 1–2% of cases secondary to umbilical cord accidents.

Respiratory complications of newborn are the most common complications of preterm birth; other significant ones being increased risk of sepsis, intraventricular hemorrhage, and necrotizing enterocolitis. Long-term complications include increased risk of neurodevelopmental impairment.[3]

CLINICAL EVALUATION IN A WOMAN WITH SUSPECTED PPROM

Aim: Confirmation of diagnosis and prevention of infection.

Steps in diagnosis of PPROM:

1. *History*: Besides routine medical and obstetric history, ask for time of onset of fluid leakage, amount and color of leaking fluid, presence/absence of uterine contractions, and vaginal bleeding.

   History alone does not confirm or rule out the diagnosis and examination is essential in a patient with suspected PPROM.

2. *Examination*: Important examination features are:
   - *General physical examination*: Look for pulse and temperature (signs of intra-amniotic infection).
   - *Abdominal examination*: Estimate fetal size, presentation, uterine contractions, uterine tenderness (may indicate chorioamnionitis or placental abruption)
   - *Sterile speculum examination*: Direct leakage from cervix causing "pooling" of fluid at the posterior fornix is diagnostic of ROM. Valsalva maneuver may be attempted if fluid leakage is not evident. Otherwise, the woman may be given a sterile pad and asked to walk around for some time.
   - Speculum examination can be performed at presentation or patient may be given a 30-minute period in a semi-Fowlers position to allow "pooling" of amniotic fluid in the vagina. Speculum examination may also detect umbilical cord prolapse, cervical dilation, or vaginal bleeding. Vaginal swab should be obtained for culture if infection is suspected (not recommended routinely).
   - Digital examination should be avoided unless delivery appears imminent or patient appears to be in active labor.[2]
3. *Ancillary tests*: These include ferning of dried vaginal fluid under microscopic examination, checking vaginal fluid pH (nitrazine test) and use of commercial amniotic fluid detection kits.[4]
   - These tests are not recommended routinely but may be helpful in 10–20% cases where diagnosis is doubtful based on history and examination.
   - Microscopic examination involves collecting leaking fluid from the speculum, smearing it over a clean glass slide, letting it air dry without cover and then examining it under the microscope for characteristic "ferning" pattern. Prolonged leakage causing minimal fluid collection and contamination with blood or vaginal discharge are common causes of false-negative microscopic test.
   - Nitrazine test is based on the fact that the normal pH of vaginal secretions is 3.8–4.5 whereas amniotic fluid is alkaline (pH 7.1–7.3). Therefore, conversion of pH strip to blue when it is touched onto the speculum after per speculum (P/S) examination (indicating basic pH) is suggestive of amniotic fluid leakage. False-positive test results may occur in the presence of blood or semen, alkaline antiseptics, certain lubricants, trichomonas, or bacterial vaginosis. On the other hand, prolonged ROM leading to minimal residual fluid may result in false-negative result.
   - Amniotic fluid detection kits have high negative predictive value but are expensive. These tests are based upon identification of amniotic fluid-specific proteins (like growth factor-binding protein-1 and placental alpha-micro-globulin-1) in vaginal fluid. False positive rates of 20–30% are reported and the results must be interpreted in accordance with the clinical presentation.
4. *Role of ultrasound (USG)*: USG is an essential part of examination though it is not diagnostic of PPROM.[1] In all cases of PPROM, USG must be done to confirm fetal presentation and wellbeing.
   - Assessment of amniotic fluid using amniotic fluid index (AFI) or maximum vertical pocket (MVP) is a useful adjuvant test if the diagnosis is not definite but absence of oligohydramnios does not rule out ROM.
   - There is no definitive role of cervical length assessment by transvaginal USG in cases of PPROM.

■ MANAGEMENT (FLOWCHART 1)

After clinical assessment, if diagnosis of PPROM is confirmed, check the following:
- Period of gestation
- Fetal presentation (confirmed with USG)
- Fetal wellbeing (by electronic fetal monitoring if gestation >28 weeks)
- Any evidence of intrauterine infection/abruption
- Group B *Streptococcus* (GBS) status of patient: If unknown, take appropriate swabs
- Availability of neonatal facilities

Flowchart 1: Approach to a patient with PPROM

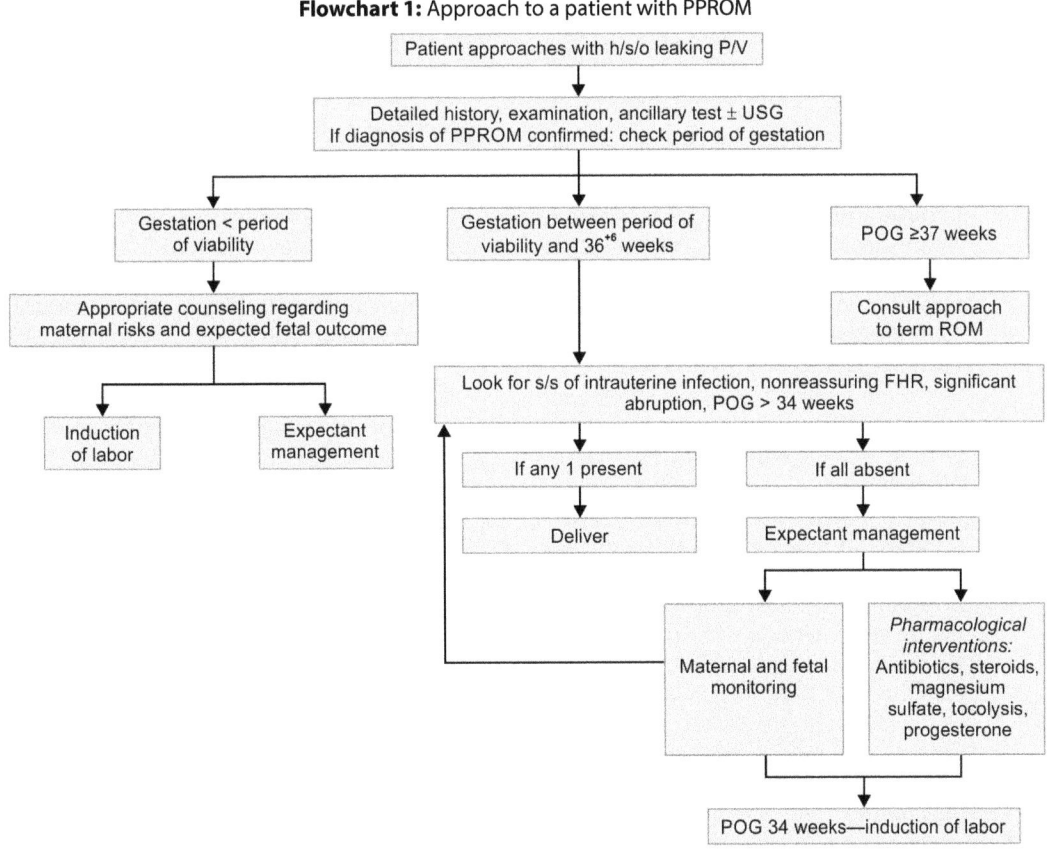

(POG: period of gestation; PPROM: preterm prelabor rupture of membranes; P/V: per vaginum; USG: ultrasound)

Indications for Delivery

Indications are abnormal fetal testing, evidence of intra-amniotic infection, and significant abruption.

Recommended Management

In absence of above indications of delivery, women with PPROM before 34 weeks POG should be offered conservative management till 34 weeks gestation.[5]

- Detailed counseling of woman must be done by obstetrician and neonatologist about management plan and expected prognosis.
- It should be informed that in spite of conservative management, 50% women will deliver within 1 week and the duration of latency is inversely proportional to the gestation at onset.

Conservative management of PPROM comprises of appropriate monitoring and pharmacological interventions.

MATERNAL AND FETAL MONITORING DURING EXPECTANT MANAGEMENT

- *Goal of monitoring*: Periodic assessment to look for chorioamnionitis/intra-amniotic infection, placental abruption, umbilical cord compression, fetal wellbeing, and labor.
- *Place of monitoring*: Hospitalization during expectant management of PPROM is standard of care and safety of home-based care is not proven.[1]
- *Method of monitoring*: During hospitalization, pregnant woman is watched closely for chorioamnionitis as PPROM is the major

risk factor for clinical chorioamnionitis. A rise in maternal temperature, tachycardia, uterine tenderness, and foul smelling or purulent vaginal discharge should raise suspicion for intrauterine infection.

- Diagnosis of chorioamnionitis is usually clinical based on a combination of maternal fever with two other signs of infection (maternal/fetal tachycardia, uterine tenderness, purulent liquor).
- Maternal fever of >100.4°F is present in 95–100% cases of chorioamnionitis while tachycardia is seen in >50% cases.
- Serial monitoring of leukocytes and inflammatory markers have not proved to be useful if there is no clinical evidence of infection.
- Culture of amniotic fluid is the gold-standard for diagnosis of intra-amniotic infection, but clinically less useful in view of prolonged report time and invasive nature of collection of amniotic fluid. However, it may be needed to confirm/exclude the diagnosis when typical clinical findings (like maternal fever) are absent or there is an overlap with other infective condition like pyelonephritis.

- *Fetal monitoring*: There is insufficient evidence to recommend a particular frequency of fetal monitoring. The fetus must be monitored with clinical examination and cardiotocography/biophysical profile daily to twice weekly depending on available resources. Fetal tachycardia is also an important sign suggesting clinical chorioamnionitis present in 40–70% cases. Periodic USG evaluation should be performed to monitor fetal growth.
- Home care in PPROM should be offered only to women who refuse prolonged hospitalization after thorough counseling, understand warning signs, agree to monitor signs of infection/abruption, and live close to a tertiary care hospital with dependable transportation.

PHARMACOLOGICAL INTERVENTIONS DURING EXPECTANT MANAGEMENT

Besides maternal and fetal monitoring, women with PPROM or their neonates may benefit from certain pharmacological interventions during conservative management. These interventions are as follows:

- *Antenatal corticosteroids*: Single course of antenatal corticosteroids after PPROM is recommended for all pregnant women with PPROM < 34 weeks of gestation. This has been proven to reduce neonatal mortality, respiratory distress syndrome, necrotizing enterocolitis, and intraventricular hemorrhage.
    - A single repeat course (rescue course) may be administered to cases of PPROM who are <34 weeks of gestation, are at risk of preterm delivery within 7 days, and whose prior course was administered >14 days back.
    - Delivery should not be delayed to achieve a rescue course.
- *Antibiotics*: Prophylactic use of broad-spectrum antibiotics has been proven to prolong pregnancy and reduce maternal and neonatal infections.[6] These are termed as "latency antibiotics."
    - Insufficient evidence to suggest optimal antibiotic regimen.
    - Intravenous ampicillin (2g every 6 hours) and erythromycin (250 mg every 6 hours) for 48 hours, followed by oral amoxicillin (500 mg every 8 hours) and erythromycin estolate or stearate (333 mg every 8 hours) for 5 days is recommended by most authorities.
    - Erythromycin may be replaced with azithromycin 1 g stat dose at admission in case of nonavailability or intolerance. It is preferred by some in view of ease of administration and better tolerance.
    - Amoxicillin-clavulanic acid must be avoided due to increased rates of neonatal necrotizing enterocolitis.
    - GBS prophylaxis must follow routine guidelines.
- Magnesium sulfate for neuroprotection: The administration of magnesium sulfate is recommended when delivery is anticipated within next 24 hours before 32 weeks of gestation in order to reduce the risk of cerebral palsy.[7]
- *Tocolytics*: Routine use of tocolytics is not recommended in all women with PPROM as

no significant maternal or neonatal benefit has been proven. Prophylactic tocolytics may lower the percentage of women delivering within 48 hours but are associated with higher chances of chorioamnionitis.[1]

- – Tocolytics can be considered in PPROM for steroid benefit to the neonate, especially at earlier gestational ages, or for maternal transport to a center with neonatal facilities.
- – Tocolytics must be avoided if there is high suspicion of infection or abruption.
- *Progestins*: These are not recommended for women with PPROM as they have not been proven to extend latency. However, they may be continued in women who are already on progestins for other indications such as history of PROM in previous pregnancy.

INDUCTION OF LABOR IN WOMEN WITH PPROM

Timing of Induction

Most guidelines recommend induction of labor at 34 weeks gestation in a woman with PPROM as the risks of conservative approach beyond this gestation outweigh the benefits.[1] The Royal College of Obstetricians and Gynaecologists (RCOG) recommends that this expectant management may be continued up to 37 weeks[8] but this must be done in consideration to patient's clinical condition, preference, and local neonatal facilities.

Method of Induction

- Intravenous oxytocin is a safe method of induction of labor in women with PPROM with a favorable cervix.
- Use of sublingual misoprostol has been found to be safe both for cervical ripening and labor induction.
- In women with poor Bishop's score, vaginal prostaglandins or mechanical methods (in form of transcervical Foley catheter) have been attempted for cervical ripening to decrease induction-delivery interval and rate of operative delivery. Though most studies have found benefit with these agents, some authors have reported increased rates of intra-amniotic infection with mechanical methods

and hence their use is discouraged in setting of PPROM.

SPECIAL CLINICAL SCENARIOS

PPROM after 34 Weeks POG (34–37 Weeks)

In women with PPROM after 34 weeks of gestation, immediate delivery has traditionally been recommended.

Recent data suggests that either expectant management or immediate delivery is a reasonable option.[9] Studies have shown no significant difference in overall neonatal morbidity or sepsis rates. Benefits of expectant management include decreased rates of respiratory distress and mechanical ventilation in neonates, causing lesser stay in intensive care unit (ICU). However, maternal adverse outcomes, such as hemorrhage and infection, are twofold higher with expectant management.

- Overall decision should be based on patient's perspective and neonatal facilities.
- Antenatal corticosteroids are recommended.
- Latency antibiotics are not recommended.[10]

Previable PPROM[11,12]

Gestation of viability varies worldwide depending on neonatal facilities available and therefore counseling must be guided by local neonatal data. Even in high-resource settings, rate of perinatal death in PROM earlier than 22 weeks is around 60%, primarily due to pulmonary hypoplasia. Neonatal outcomes are less likely to be favorable before 28 weeks of gestation in low-resource settings. Counseling must also explain that 10–15% women with previable PPROM may suffer from significant morbidity including sepsis, hemorrhage, need for transfusion, multiorgan dysfunction, etc. Life-threatening maternal infection may rarely complicate expectant management of previable PPROM.

- Expectant management or induction of labor may be chosen after counseling.
- *If expectant management is chosen*:
  - – Antibiotics may be considered as early as 20 weeks of gestation.
  - – GBS prophylaxis, corticosteroids, tocolysis, and neuroprotection are not recommended before viability.

PPROM with Cervical Encirclage in Situ

There is insufficient evidence to recommend either removal or retention of cervical encirclage after PPROM and both seem to be reasonable options.[13] Under both conditions, prolonged antibiotic use (beyond usual 7-day course) is not recommended.

PPROM after Invasive Prenatal Procedures

Preterm prelabor rupture of membranes complicates <1% of invasive prenatal procedures like amniocentesis. Pregnancy outcome in these pregnancies is usually favorable as compared to spontaneous previable PPROM, with reported perinatal survival rates around 90%. Antibiotics and monitoring for symptoms of chorioamnionitis should be advised. These patients may be managed on outpatient basis with regular USG to assess amniotic fluid volume.

PPROM with Fetal Malpresentation

There is evidence that noncephalic presentation may be associated with worse neonatal prognosis as compared to cephalic presentation at the time of diagnosis.[14]

Though the exact mechanism is not clear, cord accidents appear to be the most likely cause. Decision of termination of expectant management before 34 weeks must be in accordance to local neonatal services. External cephalic version (ECV) is contraindicated in women with PPROM.

Management in Subsequent Pregnancy (History of PPROM in Previous Pregnancy)

History of PPROM in previous pregnancy is a major risk factor for PROM and preterm birth in a subsequent pregnancy. Modifiable risk factors must be corrected and interpregnancy interval must be optimized (interval of <6 months negatively affects outcome).

Early intervention in next pregnancy is advised in the form progesterone treatment starting from 16 weeks' gestation with cervical length surveillance and placement of cervical encirclage if the length is <25 mm before 24 weeks.[1]

REFERENCES

1. Prelabor rupture of membranes. ACOG Practice Bulletin No. 217. American College of Obstetricians and Gynecologists. Obstet Gynecol. 2020;135:e80-97.
2. Shazly SA, Ahmed IA, Radwan AA, Abd-Elkariem AY, El-Dien NB, Ragab EY, et al. Middle-East OBGYN Graduate Education (MOGGE) Foundation Practice Guidelines: Prelabor rupture of membranes; Practice guideline No. 01-O-19. J Glob Health. 2020;10(1):010325.
3. Drassinower D, Friedman AM, Obican SG, Levin H, Gyamfi-Bannerman C. Prolonged latency of preterm prelabour rupture of membranes and neurodevelopmental outcomes: a secondary analysis. BJOG. 2016;123:1629-35.
4. Palacio M, Kühnert M, Berger R, Larios CL, Marcellin L. Meta-analysis of studies on biochemical marker tests for the diagnosis of premature rupture of membranes: comparison of performance indexes. BMC Pregnancy Childbirth. 2014;14:183.
5. Bond DM, Middleton P, Levett KM, van der Ham DP, Crowther CA, Buchanan SL, et al. Planned early birth versus expectant management for women with preterm prelabour rupture of membranes prior to 37 weeks' gestation for improving pregnancy outcome. Cochrane Database Syst Rev. 2017;3(3):CD004735.
6. Kenyon S, Boulvain M, Neilson JP. Antibiotics for preterm rupture of membranes. Cochrane Database Syst Rev. 2013;(12):CD001058.
7. Doyle LW, Crowther CA, Middleton P, Marret S, Rouse D. Magnesium sulphate for women at risk of preterm birth for neuroprotection of the fetus. Cochrane Database Syst Rev. 2009;(1):CD004661.
8. Thomson AJ, on behalf of the Royal College of Obstetricians and Gynaecologists. Care of Women Presenting with Suspected Preterm Prelabour Rupture of Membranes from 24+0 Weeks of Gestation. BJOG. 2019;126: e152-166.
9. Morris JM, Roberts CL, Bowen JR, Patterson JA, Bond DM, Algert CS, et al. Immediate delivery compared with expectant management after preterm pre-labour rupture of the membranes close to term (PPROMT trial): a randomised controlled trial. PPROMT Collaboration. Lancet. 2016;387:444-52.
10. Wojcieszek AM, Stock OM, Flenady V. Antibiotics for prelabour rupture of membranes

at or near term. Cochrane Database Syst Rev. 2014;CD001058.

11. Kibel M, Asztalos E, Barrett J, Dunn MS, Tward C, Pittini A, et al. Outcomes of pregnancies complicated by preterm premature rupture of membranes between 20 and 24 weeks of gestation. Obstet Gynecol. 2016;128:313-20.

12. Dotters-Katz SK, Panzer A, Grace MR, Smid MC, Keku JA, Vladutiu CJ, et al. Maternal morbidity after previable prelabor rupture of membranes. Obstet Gynecol. 2017;129:101-6.

13. Galyean A, Garite TJ, Maurel K, Abril D, Adair CD, Browne P, et al. Removal versus retention of cerclage in preterm premature rupture of membranes: a randomized controlled trial. Obstetrix Perinatal Collaborative Research Network. Am J Obstet Gynecol. 2014;211:399. e1-7.

14. Yee LM, Grobman WA. Perinatal outcomes in cephalic compared with non-cephalic singleton presentation in the setting of preterm premature rupture of membranes before 32 weeks of gestation. Obstet Gynecol. 2016;128:812-8.

Rh Incompatible Patient in Labor

Deepa Gupta, Uma Jain

DEFINITION

Rhesus (Rh) factor is an antigen present on red cell membrane (discovered by Dr Karl Landsteiner in 1937), which can stimulate an immune response in an individual who is Rh factor negative. This phenomenon is called alloimmunization or isoimmunization. If Rh –ve lady of any blood group (husband Rh +ve of any blood group) carries a Rh +ve pregnancy (of any blood group); it is Rh incompatible patient who is responsible of most cases of hemolytic disease of newborn.

POSSIBILITY OF OUTCOME

Rh negative woman if delivers a Rh positive ABO compatible infant; baby has a likelihood of isoimmunization of 16%.[1]

- 2% at time of first delivery
- 7% will have anti-RhD antibody 6 months postpartum
- 7% will be sensitized (antibody are in low concentration so not detected during or after 1st delivery; but identified early in subsequent pregnancy)

In hemolytic disease of the fetus and newborn, antibody-mediated hemolysis of fetal erythrocytes varies in severity and can have variety of manifestations.[2]

- *Mild*: Congenital anemia of the newborn (45–50%)
- *Moderate*: Icterus gravis neonatorum (25–30%)
- *Severe*: Hydrops fetalis (20–25%)

This isoimmunization can be minimized by antipartum and postpartum Rh immunoglobulin (Ig) prophylaxis[3]

- Single dose of postpartum Rh Ig reduces possibility to 1.5%
- If single postpartum RhIg is combined with single additional dose of RhIg at 28 weeks

antenatal, then possibility remains only 0.18%

The mechanism of Rh isoimmunization is shown in **Flowchart 1**.

AIMS OF INTERVENTION

- Avoid or minimize fetomaternal leak
- Prevent maternal immune system sensitization by Rh +ve cell
- Minimize fetal damage by Rh +ve antibody by timely intervention
- Timely delivery and proper neonatal care in tertiary health centers

TERMINATION OF PREGNANCY

The conditions for termination of pregnancy are described in **Flowchart 2**.

MODE OF DELIVERY

- Rh –ve pregnancy is not an indication for cesarean section
- Allow vaginal birth if
  - No obstetric or medical indication
  - Baby is term gestation
  - Cervix favorable
  - No urgency of termination as per severity of affection
- Go for cesarean section if
  - Obstetric/medical indication
  - Preterm termination [34–37 week]
  - Cervix unfavorable
  - Urgency of termination as per severity of affection (*severe form of hemolytic fetus*)
- Vaginal PGE2 gel can be safely used for cervical ripening
- Amniotomy (low rupture of membranes) quite effective for induction and augmentation of labor (avoid oxytocin if possible).

Flowchart 1: Mechanism of Rh isoimmunization.

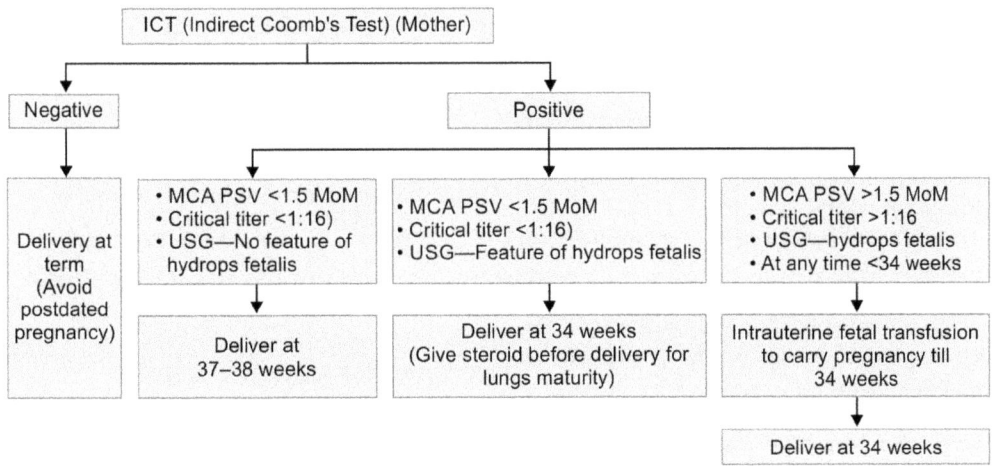

Fetomaternal hemorrhage/Leak
↓
Entry of fetal blood in maternal circulation
↓
Stimulation of maternal immune system
↓
Formation of Rh antibody (IgM, IgG)
↓
IgG cross placenta
↓
Enters fetal circulation
↓
Hemolysis of fetal RBC
↓
Hemolytic diseases of fetus and newborn
↓
Anemia in fetus
(Sinusoidal heart rate pattern)
(↑Peak systolic velocity in middle cerebral artery on Doppler study)
↓
Hepatosplenomegaly, placentomegaly, hepatic failure, portal and umbilical vein hypertension, hypoproteinemia, heart failure

| IUD | Erythroblastosis fetalis | (After birth) Antigen-antibody reaction on the RBCs surface results in hemolysis |

Anemia ... Jaundice ... Kernicterus
↓
Neonatal death

Flowchart 2: Conditions for termination of pregnancy.

ICT (Indirect Coomb's Test) (Mother)

Negative

Positive

Delivery at term (Avoid postdated pregnancy)

- MCA PSV <1.5 MoM
- Critical titer <1:16)
- USG—No feature of hydrops fetalis
↓
Deliver at 37–38 weeks

- MCA PSV <1.5 MoM
- Critical titer <1:16)
- USG—Feature of hydrops fetalis
↓
Deliver at 34 weeks
(Give steroid before delivery for lungs maturity)

- MCA PSV >1.5 MoM
- Critical titer >1:16
- USG—hydrops fetalis
- At any time <34 weeks
↓
Intrauterine fetal transfusion to carry pregnancy till 34 weeks
↓
Deliver at 34 weeks

(MCA: middle cerebral artery; PSV: peak systolic velocity)

Be Ready to Face Maternal Complications

Mother is at high risk of:
- Pre-eclampsia
- Polyhydramnios
- Big size baby and its hazards (due to hydrops fetalis)
- Coagulopathies (if dead fetus is retained for long duration)
- Postpartum hemorrhage (PPH, secondary to coagulopathy, polyhydramnios, placento-megaly, nonuse of ergometrine)

> Always keep maternal group blood (if not available then O negative) cross matched and ready in labor room

CARE DURING DELIVERY

Vaginal Delivery

The labor should be monitored carefully, and the mode of delivery and the outcome of labor should be studied in detail.
- Careful fetal monitoring (continuous electronic fetal monitoring if available) for detection of evidence of fetal distress at earliest.
- *No stripping of membrane.*
- No fundal pushing in second stage of labor.
- *Withheld prophylactic oxytocics* use in second stage of labor (do not give oxytocics at delivery of anterior shoulder).
- Placenta to be delivered spontaneously using controlled cord traction without handling or squeezing the uterus. Avoid active management of third stage of labor. Gentle handling of uterus in third stage of labor.
- Withheld manual removal of placenta, if it is required do so gently.
- Take care of PPH by prostaglandins, oxytocin instead of ergometrine
- The placenta should be examined for hyperplacentosis.
- Baby should be thoroughly examined for any obvious congenital anomaly and weight, sex and condition should be noted particularly for hydrops fetalis.
- Protect the vaginal and perineal wounds and laceration from exposure to fetal blood spill form cord.

Cesarean Section

- Avoid spillage of blood into peritoneal cavity
- *Withheld prophylactic oxytocics* use in second stage of labor
- Withheld routine manual removal of placenta (spontaneous delivery of placenta using controlled cord traction without squeezing the uterus).
- Gentle handling of uterus in 3rd stage of labor
- Proper care of PPH by prostaglandins, oxytocin.

CARE OF UMBILICAL CORD

- Quick cord clamping (to avoid even minimal amount of antibody to cross to newborn from mother. *Other conditions of quick cord clamping*:
  - Preterm baby
  - Distress baby who needs immediate resuscitation
- *Length of cord should be long* (15–20 cm) for exchange transfusion if required.
- *Cord blood collection*: For investigation
  - From placental end cut cord
  - No squeezing of cord (to avoid contamination with Wharton's Jelly)
- *Amount of blood:* 5 mL
  - Oxalated (2 ml) (nonclotted) for:
    - Hematocrit
    - Blood smear for presence of immature RBC
  - Nonoxalated (3 mL) (clotted) for:
    - ABO, Rh type
    - Bilirubin
    - Direct Coomb's test
    - Reticulocyte count

> Studies are showing that delayed cord clamping improves venous hematocrit in moderate to severe hemolytic anemia without any increase in adverse effects as exchange transfusion and hyperbilirubinemia so it may be safe, effective and cost free strategy to prevent need of exchange transfusion[4] but long-term outcomes need to be evaluated further

CARE OF NEWBORN BABY

- Conduction of delivery in tertiary care centers if
  - Baby preterm

– Positive ICT in mother with abnormal PSV in MCA on Doppler study and abnormal USG finding of hydrops fetalis
- Availability of neonatologist at the time of delivery
- Availability of advanced neonatal care unit including facilities of exchange transfusion
- Availability of Rh negative compatible blood
- Hand over baby to neonatologist just after delivery for further management

Newborn Prognosis

- *Mother unimmunized (ICT negative) baby unaffected*: Good prognosis (no hemolytic diseases)
- *Mother isoimmunized (ICT positive)*: Baby may or may not be affected with hemolytic diseases

There is a wide spectrum of clinical manifestation:
- Normal baby who develops mild jaundice who responds to conservative treatment.
- Normal baby who develops rapid jaundice and requires exchange transfusion. (Baby with hydrops fetalis, anemic with hepato-splenomegaly, generalized edema, ascites, pleural effusion).
- *In severely affected infant*: Perinatal distress factors are seen such as hypoxia, hypothermia, hypoglycemia and acidosis. They may develop disseminated intravascular coagulation. They may have leukopenia and thrombocytopenia. It should be prevented and be adequately managed if occurs. Adequate feeding, good hydration is a must.
- In extreme cases there may be a still born baby or early neonatal death due to difficulty in establishing ventilation and perfusion

Prognosis of baby depends on:
- Genotype of father
- Genotype of baby
- Maternal anti-Rh antibody titer
- History of previously affected baby with hemolytic diseases
- Availability of advanced diagnostic and therapeutic fetal medicine and neonatal care units

> With currently available advanced facilities of intrauterine and extrauterine care, neonatal survival is up to 100%

Breastfeeding

- Rh –ve pregnancy is not a contraindication for breastfeeding for both nonimmunized and isoimmunized mothers (although very small amount of antibodies pass via breast milk)
- *Breastfeeding permitted* provided no other contraindication

■ POSTPARTUM PROPHYLAXIS

Aim

To prevent subsequent pregnancies from hemolytic diseases in fetus and newborn.

Beneficiary

Rh –ve mother provided newborn is Rh +ve with negative direct Coomb's test.

Time

- *Preferred*: Within 72 hours of delivery
- *Second choice*: Within 9–10 days of postpartum
- *Last choice*: Up to 28 days of postpartum

Immunoglobulin

- IgG antibody
- Polyclonal antibody

Dose

Preferred Method[4]

- Calculate fetomaternal hemorrhage and decide dose of RhIg accordingly by:
  – Rosette test (qualitative)
  – *Kleihauer-Betke test*: Quantitative
  – Flow cytometry[5]

Standard dose of 100 µg (500 IU) will cover upto 4 mL of fetal RBC.
For every mL of fetal RBC above 4 mL give 25 µg (125 IU)
- As practically it is not possible in India, so we give standard dose of 300 µg of RhIg (1,500 IU) which will protect mother from fetal hemorrhage up to 30 mL of fetal whole blood or 15 mL of fetal RBC.[6]

Site

- Intramuscular in deltoid/anterolateral aspect of thigh
- Avoid gluteal area for delay in absorption

If newborn blood group is not available, it is better to give postpartum prophylaxis for giving benefit of doubt

AREA TO FOCUS ON

- Large number of Rh –ve women who should be protected; are not receiving anti-D[7]
- Among Indian doctors and patients, there is awareness about postdelivery prophylaxis, however prophylaxis after spontaneous abortion, MTP, ectopic pregnancy, antenatal use of Anti-D is still lacking[3]
- Antenatal prophylaxis should be recommended
- Desirable to check for fetomaternal hemorrhage; but in Indian setup standard dose will cover most of cases.
- Information and counseling of all young girls at school and college about importance of Rh group and its impact on pregnancy.
- Match blood group with Rh along with horoscope at time of marriage proposal.
- Importance of checking blood group and Rh type in each pregnancy and counseling of Rh –ve patients about importance of Rh prophylaxis and hemolytic diseases of fetus and newborn.
- Anti-D should be given into deltoid as delayed absorption if injected into gluteal muscle.

RECOMMENDATIONS

- All patients coming for MTP (medical/surgical) should have blood group available.
- Antenatal prophylaxis of single dose of 300 μg at 28 week[8]
- 50 μg of anti-D after all sensitizing events in first trimester[9,10]
- 300 μg of anti-D for late pregnancy sensitizing events and postpartum in nonsensitized Rh –ve patient
- Due to lack of quantitative estimation of fetomaternal hemorrhage; higher dose of anti-D is recommended in order to protect majority of patients in different situation. *No need of anti-D if:*
    - Partner Rh –ve
    - Patient willing for sterilization operation
- The obstetrician, maternity nurse, the labor and delivery nurse should all be familiar for diagnosis and management with Rhesus incompatibility.
- Advocacy for partnership by Government and NGOs to help for subsidizing the cost of the immunoglobulin.
- Special insurance cover for Rh-negative women to ensure ease of procurement when needed.
- Involvement of clergy as part of premarital counselors
- Creation of special forum/groups for Rh-negative people where potential Rh-negative spouses can be met.

COUNSELING

- Follow up of neonate in neonatal clinic to look for any neurological squeal or developmental delay is essential.
- Counseling of parents regarding the neonate and also about the next pregnancy should form a part of ideal management. About risks of future pregnancy, timely visit to hospital and advised for delivery at higher center where facility of fetal monitoring, intrauterine transfusion and exchange transfusion should be available and under multidisciplinary approach.
- In case of alloimmunized women with BOH following option should be given to get healthy baby.
    - IUI with Rh negative sperm donor.
    - IVF with PGD testing for selection of Rh-D negative embryo
    - Use of gestational carrier

FUTURE

- *Role of PCR*: Prenatal Rh-D genes reveal homozygosity of the partner.
- *Noninvasive prenatal testing (NIPT)*: Fetal RhD genotype and grouping can be done from fetal cell free DNA in maternal circulation in the first trimester of pregnancy which can reduce the need of invasive procedures in fetus to detect RH antigen.
- Use of noninvasive prenatal diagnostic methods coupled with delayed cord clamp at birth *(still under study)* may further improve the management of fetus of HDN and decrease the risk of neonatal morbidity and mortality

CONCLUSION

Prevention of Rh isoimmunization by using immunoprophylaxis is one such development which has brought about an astounding amount of success. But unfortunately, lack of tertiary level ultrasound (across all sections of community), unavailability of intrauterine transfusion and state-of-the-art laboratory facilities to do Kleihauer-Betke test in our country have been the major handicaps to tackle problem of Rh isoimmunization. This is further enhanced by lack of awareness of antenatal and postnatal prophylaxis program. Further the *high price* of immunoglobulin is the final blow to the problem.

Poor documentation of prior sensitizing events are the factors resulting in the isoimmunized pregnancy. A small well-knit team comprising an obstetrician, sonologists, blood bank personnel, neonatologists and nursing staff working in close coordination is necessary for successful management of Rh-isoimmunization.

REFERENCES

1. Reshma P. FOGSI and ICOG good clinical practice recommendations. Mumbai: FOSGI; 2018.
2. Virkud A. Rhesus Alloimmunization during pregnancy. In: Modern Obstetrics, 3rd edition. New Delhi: APC Publishers; 2013. pp. 371-84.
3. Deka D. Prophylaxis in India gone haywire: analysis of 200 cases presented at the 47th AICOG, 2004. Agra: AICOG; 2004.
4. McAdams RM. Delayed cord clamping in red blood cell alloimmunization: safe, effective and free. Trans Pediatr. 2016;5(2):100-3
5. Johnson PR, Tait RC, Austen EB, Shwe KH, Lee, D. Flow cytometry in diagnosis and management of large fetomaternal haemorrhage. J Clin Path. 1995;48:1005-8.
6. Costumbrado J. Rh incompatibility. Florida: StatPearls; 2020.
7. Joseph KS. Controlling RH haemolytic disease of the new born in India. Br J Obstet Gynecol. 1991;98(4):369-77.
8. NICE. Jenny Ford clinical guideline RHESUS (RHD) negative antenatal management, version 3, London: NICE; 2015.
9. Practice Bulletin No. 181: Prevention of Rh D Alloimmunization. Obstet Gynecol. 2017;130(2):e57-e70.
10. American College of Obstetricians and Gynecologist. ACOG Practice Bulletin No. 75: Management of alloimmunization during pregnancy. Obstet Gynecol. 2006;108(2):457-64.

Fetal Growth Restriction: Patient in Labor

Asmita Kaundal, K Aparna Sharma

INTRODUCTION AND TERMINOLOGIES

Fetal growth restriction (FGR) is defined as a fetus who fails to reach its genetically predetermined growth potential.[1]

Small for Gestational Age

Small for gestational age (SGA) fetus is one whose abdominal circumference (AC) or effective fetal weight (EFW) is below 10th percentile for given gestational age.[1]

The SGA babies may or may not be growth restricted.

CLASSIFICATION

Depending upon the gestation at which the condition is detected FGR is classified as early (<32 weeks) and late FGR (>32 weeks) **(Table 1)**.

TABLE 1: Classification of fetal growth restriction (FGR).

Early onset FGR	Late onset FGR
Gestational age <32 weeks, in absence of congenital anomalies with AC/EFW <3rd centile or UA-AEDF or	GA >32 weeks, in the absence of congenital anomalies with AC/EFW <3rd centile *or* at least two out of the following:
• AC/EFW <10th centile combined with	• AC/EFW <10rd centile
	• AC/EFW crossing centiles >2 quartiles on growth centiles
• UtA-PI >95th centile and/or	• CPR <5th centile or
• UA-PI >95th centile	UtA-PI >95th centile

(AC: abdominal circumference; AEDF: Absent-end diastolic flow; CPR: cerebroplacental ratio; EFW: effective fetal weight; GA: gestational age; PI: pulsatility index; UA: umbilical artery; UtA: uterine artery)

Growth restricted fetuses are at increased risk of stillbirth hence a planned induction/cesarean section is preferred over waiting for spontaneous onset of labor.[2,3] FGR babies are at increased risk of adverse perinatal outcome and these babies tolerate the stress of delivery poorly and it is important to monitor the woman with FGR babies during labor and delivery.

CRITERIA OF DELIVERY[1]

- Any maternal indication where continuing pregnancy can severely affect maternal health (severe preeclampsia, eclampsia, HELLP syndrome)
- Any fetal indication where continuing pregnancy can adversely affect the fetus **(Table 2)**

MODE OF DELIVERY[4,5]

- Absent or reversed diastolic flow in the umbilical artery (UA AREDV) delivery by cesarean section.
- Normal UA Doppler or abnormal UA Doppler with end diastolic velocities present induction of labor with continuous fetal heart rate monitoring via cardiotocograph (CTG) is recommended. If the patient goes in spontaneous labor, continuous CTG monitoring should be done if CTG is not available, fetal heart must be auscultated every 15 minutes in first stage and every 5 minutes in second stage of labor.

FGR Patient in Labor

At admission:

- Delivery of a woman with fetal growth restricted fetus should be done at a tertiary care center

TABLE 2: Recommended management of pregnancies with fetal growth restriction (FGR).

Early FGR	Late FGR
24+0 to 25+6 weeks: Management needs to be individualized	Deliver at any gestational age if there is presence of any of the following: • Repeated and persistent unprovoked fetal heart deceleration • Altered biophysical profile (BPP score score ≤ 4) • cCTG STV, 3.5 ms at 32+0 to 33+6 weeks and <4.5 ms at ≥34+0 weeks • Absent or reversed umbilical artery end diastolic flow (UA-EDF)
≥26+0 weeks, deliver if any of the following is present: • Repeated persistent unprovoked fetal heart rate deceleration • Abnormal biophysical profile (BPP score ≤4)	*Deliver at 36+0 to 37+0 weeks*: Deliver if UA-PI >95th percentile or AC/EFW <3rd percentile
26+0 to 28+6 weeks: Deliver if ductus venosus a-wave is at or below baseline or STV <2.6 ms	*38+0 weeks to 39+0 weeks*: Deliver if there is evidence of cerebral blood flow redistribution or any of the features of FGR
29+0 to 31+6 weeks: Deliver if UA-EDF is reversed or STV <3.0 ms	
32+0 to 33+6 weeks: Deliver if UA-EDF is reversed or STV <3.5 ms	
≥34+0 weeks: Deliver if UA-EDF is absent or STV<4.5 ms	
(cCTG: computed cardiotocograph; STV: short-term variation)	

- It should be a multidisciplinary approach with availability of a fetal medicine unit, trained obstetrician, pediatrician, and anesthetist. There should be a provision for emergency cesarean section, neonatal intensive care unit (NICU) and intensive care unit for high-risk mothers.
- Women who develop FGR are themselves either suffering from underlying chronic disease or are at risk of developing certain pregnancy-related complication **(Appendix I)**.[6] Every attempt should be made to elicit history from the woman or relatives to find out any risk factors associated with FGR. Review of the previous records of woman if available.
- Calculation of correct the gestational age from last menstrual period and first trimester ultrasound.
- A thorough examination general physical should be done to rule out any high-risk medical or surgical condition. A meticulous obstetrical examination to know the lie, presentation, liquor and estimated fetal weight

on abdominal examination and Bishops score. Membrane status, color of liquor (if ruptured membranes) and pelvic assessment should be done to rule out any contraindication for or normal vaginal delivery.
- Fetal heart rate should be heard for full 1 minute. Continuous monitoring of fetal heart through CTG if available.
- Record her temperature, pulse rate (PR), blood pressure (BP), respiratory rate, urine albumin and sugar.
- Keep a record of input and output of the women especially the high-risk women.
- Baseline investigation such as blood group and ABO-Rh typing, complete blood count, liver function test, kidney function test and coagulation profile.
- Consider antenatal steroids in case gestational age is between 24+0 and 35+6 weeks.

First stage:
- Woman should lie on one of her sides to avoid aortocaval compression

- Maintain hydration
- Vital charting should continue: Temperature, PR, BP every 2 hourly
- Continuous watch for progress of labor (maintain partograph)
- Continuous CTG monitoring for fetal heart rate if not available fetal heart should be monitored every 10–15 minutes in first stage immediately after the contraction is gone for full 1 minute.
- Discourage any premature bearing down
- Earliest decision for cesarean section

Second stage:
- Maintain hydration and continue vital charting as in first stage of labor
- Continuous CTG monitoring and in the absence of CTG fetal heart rate should be heart with fetal Doppler or stethoscope for full 1 minute, post contraction every 5 minutes.
- Woman should be encouraged to push down with the contractions and relax when the contraction is gone.

Early neonatal care:
- A trained pediatrician should be available at the time of delivery
- The baby should receive immediate neonatal care and should be assessed for any assisted ventilation or need for NICU care
- Early breastfeeding should be preferred as per the maternal and fetal conditions

Immediate postpartum care: Since the woman with FGR babies are already at increased risk for maternal complication such as hypertensive disorders, diabetes with vasculopathy, heart disease, restrictive lung disease monitoring should continue in the postpartum period as well.
- Check for PR, BP, RR every 30 minutes for initial 2 hours and then 4 hourly for next 24 hours
- Check for any excessive bleeding or episiotomy site hematoma formation
- Assess for pallor
- Check breast for any engorgement, motivate to breastfeed if the baby is with the mother or else express milk. Advice to wear proper breast support

Women need a continuous support through the antenatal period, labor to delivery. These women can be at increased risk of developing postpartum depression, every attempt to find any symptom suggestive for this, timely management should be done.

APPENDIX I
Causes for Fetal Growth Restriction[6]

Maternal Causes
1. Hypertensive Disorders
2. Insulin-dependent diabetes mellitus with vasculopathy
3. Congenital cyanotic heart disease
4. Restrictive pneumopathies
5. Severe renal disease.
6. Autoimmune disease.
7. Thrombophilias (hereditary and acquired)
8. Hyperhomocysteinemia
9. Severe anemia
10. Nutritional
11. Drugs use
12. Ethnicity
13. Stress, depression

Fetal Causes
1. Chromosomal abnormalities
2. Genetic syndromes
3. Intrauterine infection
4. Multiple gestations
5. Inborn error of metabolism

Placental Causes
1. Inadequate placentation
2. Bilobed placenta
3. Low insertion placenta
4. Chorioangioma
5. Velamentous insertion of umbilical cord
6. Presence of single umbilical artery

REFERENCES

1. ISUOG Practice guidelines: diagnosis and management of small for gestational age fetus and fetal growth restriction. Ultrasound Obstet Gynecol. 2020;56:298-312.
2. Gordijn SJ, Beune IM, Thilaganathan B, Papageorghiou A, Baschat AA, Baker PN, et al. Consensus definition of fetal growth restriction: a Delphi procedure. Ultrasound Obstet Gynecol. 2016;48:333-9.
3. Walker KF, Bugg GJ, Macpherson M, McCormick C, Grace N, Wildsmith C, et al. Randomized Trial of Labor Induction in Women 35 Years of Age or Older. N Engl J Med. 2016;374:813-22.

4. Cheng YW, Kaimal AJ, Snowden JM, Nicholson JM, Caughey AB. Induction of labor compared to expectant management in low-risk women and associated perinatal outcomes. Am J Obstet Gynecol. 2012;207:502.e1-8.

5. RCOG. The Investigation and management of the small for gestational age fetus. Green top Guideline No. 31, 2nd edition. London: RCOG; 2013 (Minor revisions, 2014).

6. Nardozza LMM, Caetano ACR, Zamarian ACP, Mazzola JB, Silva CP, Marcal VMG, et al. Fetal growth restriction: current knowledge. Review. Arch Gynecol Obstet. 2017;295(5): 1061-77.

CHAPTER

54

Kangaroo Mother Care

Kavita Mandrelle Bhatti, Sahir Bhatti

INTRODUCTION

"Kangaroo mother care" is the skin-to-skin contact of the neonate or infant on the chest of the mother (or another caregiver when not possible with the mother) and exclusive breastfeeding.[1]

This has been shown to prevent death in infants with low-birthweight.[2]

World Health Organization (WHO) guidelines currently recommend two types of kangaroo mother care:

1. *Intermittent Kangaroo mother care*: Short periods of kangaroo mother care when the mother visits her infant who is still being nursed in an incubator and when the infant's condition begins to stabilize.
2. *Continuous Kangaroo mother care*: When the infant's condition has stabilized and the mother provides kangaroo mother care all the time, both day and night.

Skin-to-skin contact should be the standard care for term as well as preterm babies.

For premature and low-birthweight babies it is more essential for their stability.

COMPONENTS OF KANGAROO MOTHER CARE

- Skin-to-skin contact
- Exclusive breastfeeding.

MECHANISMS BY WHICH IMMEDIATE KANGAROO MOTHER CARE MIGHT CONFER BENEFIT

Contact with the mother's skin will help the baby to get colonized by the mother's protective microbiome and more likely to receive early breastfeeding. Less handling of the baby by other persons reduces the risk of infection to the infant.

Constant monitoring of the infant by the mother and absence of stress related to mother–infant separation may contribute to reduced mortality.

TIMING OF INITIATION OF KANGAROO MOTHER CARE

- Skin-to-skin contact should start at birth.
- If separation is absolutely necessary for any reason, it should be as short as possible.

Initiation of Kangaroo Mother Care after a Cesarean Section

Skin-to-skin contact can be done in the operating room if the mother has had a spinal or epidural anesthesia. If she has received general anesthesia for cesarean, the baby can be put on father's chest.

CLOTHING OF MOTHER AND BABY DURING KANGAROO MOTHER CARE

Any front-open, light dress as per the local culture. A suitable apparel like kangaroo bag or binder that can retain the infant for an extended period of time.

The infant should be dressed in cap, socks, disposable diapers, and front-open sleeveless shirt made of a soft natural fabric.

POSITIONING OF THE BABY

- The infant should be placed between the mother's breasts in an upright position.
- The head should be turned to one side in a slightly extended position.
- The baby is held in a "frog"-like position with the hips flexed and abducted and the arms also flexed.

- The baby's abdomen should be at the level of the mother's epigastrium so that the mother's breathing stimulates the infant and reduces chances of apnea in the neonate or infant.

MONITORING OF THE INFANT

Mother should be trained to observe her infant for danger signs, like low body temperature, respiratory problem, feeding difficulty, and change in color during kangaroo mother care.

FEEDING DURING KANGAROO MOTHER CARE

Holding the infant near the breast, stimulates milk production. The mother should be able to breastfeed while the infant is in kangaroo mother care position.

Mother may express breast milk while the infant is in kangaroo mother care position.

BENEFITS OF KANGAROO MOTHER CARE

Benefits for the baby:
- Reduces risks of hypothermia
- Promotes lactation and weight gain
- Reduces infections and hospital stay
- Better bonding between mother and newborn
- Stabilizes baby's heart rate
- Improves baby's breathing pattern and makes breathing more regular
- Improves oxygen saturation levels
- Gain in sleep time
- Decreased crying

Benefits for the mother:
- Increases breast milk production
- Increases mother's confidence in the ability to care for the new born
- Increases mother's sense of control

REFERENCES

1. Chan GJ, Valsangkar B, Kajeepeta S, Boundy EO, Wall S. What is kangaroo mother care? Systematic review of the literature. J Glob Health. 2016;6(1):010701.
2. Ministry of Health and Family Welfare, Child Health Division, Government of India. (2014). Operational Guidelines – Kangaroo Mother care and optimal feeding of low birth weight infants. [online] Available from https://www.nhm.gov.in/images/pdf/programmes/child-health/guidelines/Operational_Guidelines-KMC_&_Optimal_feeding_of_Low_Birth_Weight_Infants.pdf September [Last accessed December, 2021].

Ajay Kumar Gupta, Deepa Gupta

INTRODUCTION

Neonatal resuscitation means to revive or restore life to a baby from the state of asphyxia. Ninety percent of newly born babies make the transition from intrauterine to extrauterine life without difficulty. They require little or no assistance to begin spontaneous and regular respirations. Approximately 10% of the newborn require some assistance to begin breathing at birth and only about 1% may need extensive resuscitative measures to survive. It is important to anticipate and be prepared for this eventuality in all deliveries.

Preparations should include warm and dry place to do the resuscitation, radiant warmer, clean prewarmed towels, newborn size self-inflating PPV bag, and size 0 and 1 mask. These are summarized in **Box 1.**

CONDITIONS FOR RESUSCITATION PROCEDURE (FLOWCHART 1)

As soon as baby is born, dry the baby with a clean, dry and warm towel and immediately replace the towel. Assess the baby for crying and breathing. If the baby is crying and breathing, there is no need for resuscitation.

> **BOX 1:** Essential preparations for neonatal resuscitation.
>
> - A draught free, warm room with temperature >25°C
> - A clean, dry and warm delivery surface
> - A radiant warmer/overhead lamp with 200 watt bulb if available
> - Two clean, warm towels/clothes
> - A folded piece of cloth (0.5–1 inch thick)
> - A newborn size self-inflating PPV bag and infant masks in two sizes: size "1" for normal weight baby and "0" for small baby
> - A suction device
> - Oxygen (if available)
> - A clock (with seconds' hand)

Start the resuscitation immediately if the baby is—
- Not crying
- Gasping
- Not breathing

If meconium is present and the baby is not crying, start suction immediately. First do suction from mouth by inserting the tube of suction devise not more than 5 cm beyond the lip. Stop suctioning when secretions are cleared, even if the baby is not breathing.
- *Baby is gasping or is not breathing*: Start resuscitation with ventilation immediately with PPV bag and mask.
- The mask usually is held on the face with the thumb, index, and/or while middle finger encircling the rim of the mask in shape of letter C, the ring and fifth fingers bring the chin forward to maintain a patent airway.
- Start ventilation by squeezing the bag to deliver breath. Remember, the lungs of a fetus are filled with fluid, so the first few breaths will often require higher pressures and longer inflation times than will subsequent breaths.
- Adequate pressure required to squeeze the bag should be just enough to produce gentle chest rise as it happens in normal breathing.
- During the initial stages of neonatal resuscitation, breaths should be delivered at a rate of 40–60 breaths per minute, or slightly less than once a second.
- To help maintain a rate of 40–60 breaths per minute, try saying to "Breathe – Two – Three, Breathe –Two – Three".
- If one squeezes the bag on "Breathe" and release while one says, Two, Three, one will probably be ventilating at a proper rate.
- After starting ventilation with bag and mask, one should look for chest movement after ventilating two to three times to ensure adequacy of ventilation.

Flowchart 1: Neonatal resuscitation.

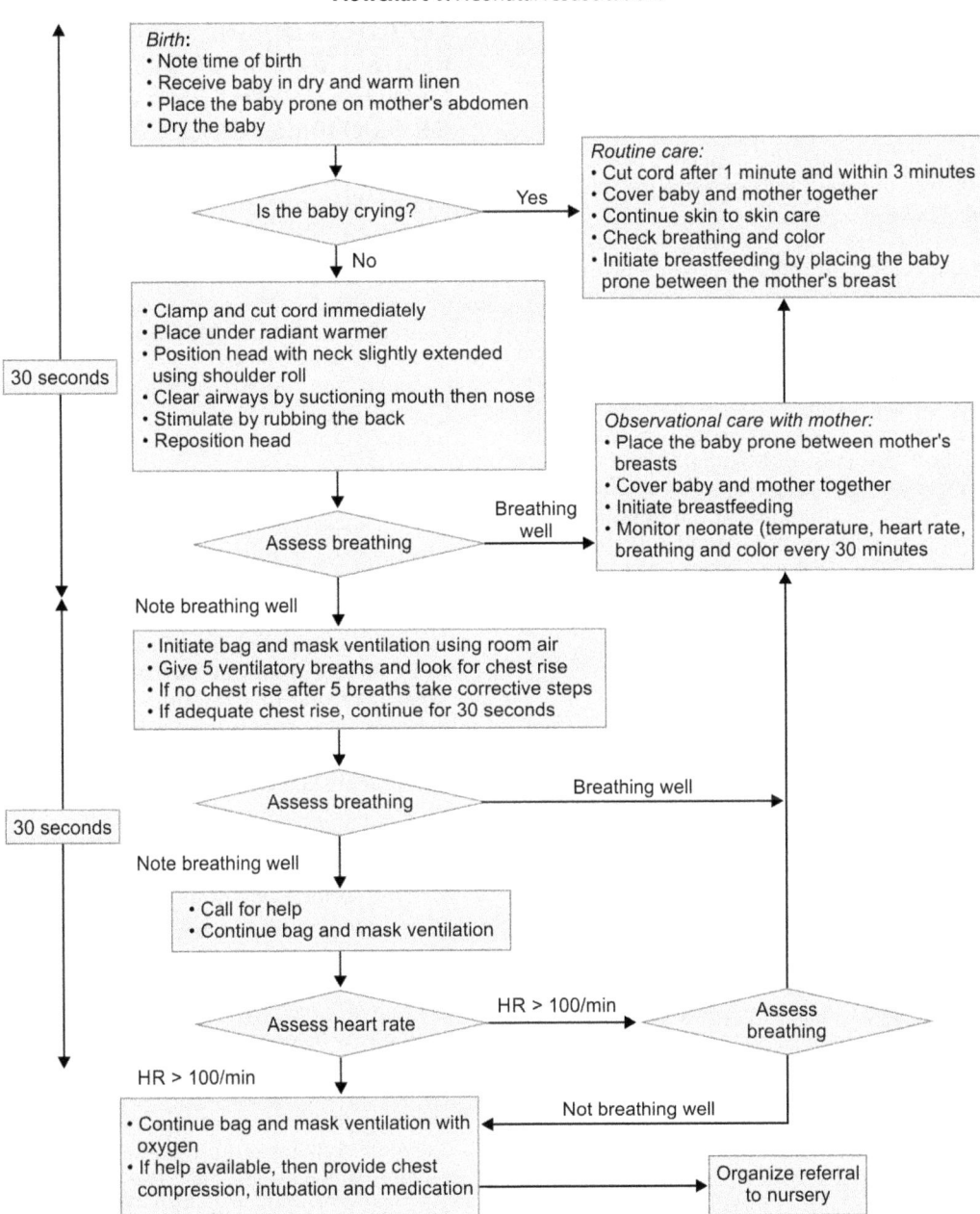

- If the chest movement is absent or inadequate then one should immediately take steps to improve ventilation.

Various reasons for inadequate or absent chest movements may be:
- The seal is inadequate

- The airway is blocked
- Not enough pressure is being given

Successful ventilation will be indicated by spontaneous breathing. Some babies improve quickly and begin breathing well after 30 seconds of adequate ventilation. Some babies may require prolonged ventilation with bag and mask. If the baby is breathing spontaneously after 30 seconds of ventilation, gradually reduce the rate and volume of breaths and watch for the baby's breathing. A baby who is breathing well will be crying or breathing quietly and regularly (chest is rising symmetrically with frequency 30–60/min. If the baby is breathing well then stop the ventilation and provide observational care.

A baby who is not breathing well (gasping or not breathing at all) after 30 seconds of adequate ventilation needs continued ventilation and further evaluation. Expert help is required.

Continue with bag and mask ventilation and provide oxygen through bag and mask. Check the heart rate of the baby.

Heart rate can be evaluated by feeling the umbilical cord pulse or listening to the heart beat with stethoscope while one stops ventilation for 6 seconds. Feel the pulse in the umbilical cord where it attaches to the baby's abdomen. If no pulse can be felt in the cord then one must listen over the left side of chest with the stethoscope and count the heartbeat. It may be necessary to stop ventilation for few seconds to listen with stethoscope.

A heart rate above 100 beats per minute is normal.

If the heart rate is normal (above 100 bpm) but the baby is still not breathing well continue to provide bag and mask ventilation and reassess after every 30 seconds until the baby is breathing well as majority of babies whose heart rate is above 100 bpm eventually start to breathe well. However if the baby still does not breathe, continue ventilation and seek expert help.

If the heart rate is slow make sure that one has taken all the steps to improve the ventilation. The chest should move gently with each breath. Continue to do bag and mask ventilation and reassess heart rate approximately after every 30 seconds, in the meantime the more skilled healthcare provider (pediatrician) should provide advanced care if possible. The baby may need more advanced support such as endotracheal (ET) intubation, chest compressions and medications. Arrange for referral if advanced care is not available. Ventilation should continue uninterrupted during the transport process.

If there are no signs of life (breathing/heart rate) even after 20 minutes of birth, ventilation may be stopped.

WHAT SHOULD BE SPECIFIC PRACTICES DURING NEONATAL RESUSCITATION FOR DELIVERY OF WOMEN WITH SUSPECTED OR CONFIRMED SARS-COV-2 INFECTION?

Infection Prevention during Resuscitation

In the absence of any clinical trials comparing various approaches to prevent infection during resuscitation, following guidelines are based on viral transmission studies, expert opinion and general infection prevention guidelines by professional organizations:

- *Personal protective equipment (PPE)*: The resuscitation team should wear an N95 mask, face shield or goggles, and full PPE for attending delivery of women with suspected or confirmed SARS-CoV-2 infection.
- *Resuscitation equipment*: A new set of disposables and disinfected reusables should be used for each delivery. Disposables such as ET tubes, suction catheter, orogastric tube, tapes for fixing ET tube, umbilical catheter, syringes placed near the resuscitation area should be discarded even if unused. Reusable equipment should be thoroughly disinfected as per hospital protocol. Wear protective clothing when dealing with contaminated equipment.
- *Airway*: Perform oral or nasal suction only if indicated to clear the airway.
- *Respiratory support*: If positive pressure ventilation is needed, self-inflating bag and mask or a T-piece resuscitator with disposable tubing may be used. If a T-piece resuscitator is used, a disposable circuit should be used. Indications for intubation are as per standard Neonatal Resuscitation Program (NRP). The use of aerosol boxes during intubation is not recommended in neonates. The use of filters attached to T-piece/bag mask devices is not recommended during neonatal resuscitation.
- The neonatal resuscitation team should doff the PPE after exiting the delivery area, discard the component in appropriate bins as per disposal policy and perform hand hygiene. Transfer of the neonate to the designated area can be performed by another healthcare

worker wearing appropriate PPE. However, if there is a shortage of personnel, the resuscitation team member can doff partially and wear a fresh outer gown and gloves to transport the neonate. If the neonate is on respiratory support, transport personnel should wear an N95 mask.

- It is recommended to continue practicing skin-to-skin contact (SSC) immediately after birth as part of the "routine care". During SSC, mother should follow the recommended infection prevention and control measures, hand hygiene, respiratory etiquette and triple-layered mask.

- Due to absence of any evidence indicating increased transmission of infection due to delayed cord clamping and well-established benefits of delayed cord clamping, the NNF-FOGSI-IAP guidelines group recommends delayed cord clamping as per-neonatal resuscitation.

Guidelines, even if mother is SARS-CoV-2 positive, and irrespective her being symptomatic, are given in **Box 2.**

> **BOX 2:** Recommendation: Neonatal resuscitation (for delivery of women with suspected or confirmed SARS-COV-2 infection).
>
> - Minimum number of personnel should attend resuscitation (one person in low-risk cases and two in high-risk cases where extensive resuscitation may be anticipated) and wear a full set of personal protective equipment including N95 mask and face-shield/goggle
> - Mother should perform hand hygiene and wear triple layer mask
> - Neonatal resuscitation should follow standard guidelines. If positive pressure ventilation is needed, self-inflating bag and mask or a T-piece resuscitator with disposable circuit may be used
> - Indications for intubation shall not change because of maternal COVID-19 status
> - Delayed cord clamping and early skin-to-skin contact should be practiced
> - Perform oral or nasal suction only if indicated to clear the airway
> - Endotracheal administration of medications should be avoided
> - Bathing is not recommended in view of risk of hypothermia and hospital-acquired infections

BIBLIOGRAPHY

1. Aziz K, Lee CHC, Escobedo MB, Hoover AV, Kamath-Rayne BD, Kapadia VS, et al. Part 5: Neonatal Resuscitation 2020 American Heart Association Guidelines for Cardiopulmonary Resuscitation and Emergency Cardiovascular Care. Pediatrics. 2021;147(Suppl 1):e20200 38505E. doi: 10.1542/peds.2020-038505E. Epub 2020 Oct 21. PMID: 33087555.

2. Berkelhamer SK, Kamath-Rayne BD, Niermeyer S. Neonatal resuscitation in low-resource settings. Clin Perinatol. 2016;43(3):573-91.

3. Chawla D, Chirla D, Dalwai S, Deorari AK, Ganatra A, Gandhi A, Kabra NS, Kumar P, Mittal P, Parekh BJ, Sankar MJ, Singhal T, Sivanandan S, Tank P; Federation of Obstetric and Gynaecological Societies of India (FOGSI), National Neonatology Forum of India (NNF) and Indian Academy of Pediatrics (IAP). Perinatal-Neonatal Management of COVID-19 Infection - Guidelines of the Federation of Obstetric and Gynaecological Societies of India (FOGSI), National Neonatology Forum of India (NNF), and Indian Academy of Pediatrics (IAP). Indian Pediatr. 2020;57(6):536-548.

4. NSSK Resource Manual. Ministry of Health and Family Welfare.

5. Sawyer T. Neonatal resuscitation: airway, breathing, and then chest compressions. Resuscitation. 2021;158:275-276.

6. Zaichkin JG. Neonatal Resuscitation: Neonatal Resuscitation Program 7th Edition Practice Integration. Crit Care Nurs Clin North Am. 2018;30(4):533-547.

Postnatal Deep Vein Thrombosis Prophylaxis

Kunal Doshi, Jaydeep Tank

INTRODUCTION

Deep vein thrombosis (DVT) is the presence or formation of blood clot in the deep vein. DVT affects lower limbs more commonly than upper limbs. Pulmonary embolism (PE) is an obstruction of pulmonary artery or its branches by a thrombus. The most likely source of thrombus in the pulmonary branches is an embolization from deep vein from the legs. This occurs in one-third of patient with DVT. Prevention of DVT thereby reduces the incidence of PE, a serious and life-threatening condition.

Venous thromboembolism (VTE) includes DVT and PE. DVT is a major preventable cause of mortality and morbidity worldwide. DVT and PE account for 60,000–100,000 deaths annually in the United States.[1]

Pulmonary embolism remains a leading direct cause of maternal mortality in the UK.

Virchow's Triad (Fig. 1): Sir Rudolf Virchow described the triad which leads to the modern day understanding of VTE. The triad consists of venous stasis (immobility), endothelial injury (surgery or trauma), and hypercoagulability of blood (thrombophilia).

Venous stasis is the most important factor, but the presence of endothelial injury and/or hypercoagulability increases the risk of DVT. Hospitalized patients are at risk of venous stasis, and with the presence of other factors, they are at increased risk of DVT compared to patients in the community.

PHYSIOLOGICAL CHANGES IN PREGNANCY

Pregnancy is a prothrombotic state; it has all components of Virchow's triad: venous stasis, endothelial damage, and hypercoagulability.

Venous stasis results from a hormonally induced decrease in venous tone and obstruction of venous flow by the enlarging uterus. A reduction of venous flow velocity of approximately 50% occurs in the legs by weeks 25–29 of gestation. This lasts until approximately 6 weeks postpartum, at which time normal venous velocities return.

The risk of DVT and PE is high during the postpartum period and is maximum at 3-6 weeks after delivery.

IDENTIFICATION OF HIGH RISK PATIENTS

Pre-existing Risk Factors

- History of DVT/VTE
- Inherited or acquired thrombophilias
- Obesity (>30 kg/m²)
- Smoking
- Paraplegia

Obstetric Risk Factors

- Multiple pregnancy
- Current pre-eclampsia

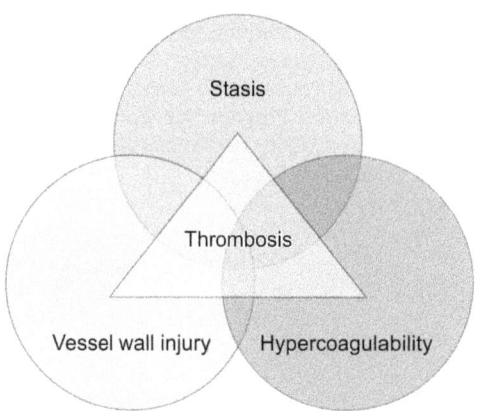

Fig. 1: Virchow's triad.

- Cesarean birth
- Prolonged labor (>24 hours)

New Onset/Transient

- Hyperemesis/dehydration
- Ovarian hyperstimulation syndrome (OHSS)
- Admission or immobility (bed rest > 3 days)
- Current systemic infection requiring IV antibiotic or admission to hospital

POSTNATAL DEEP VEIN THROMBOSIS PROPHYLAXIS

Deep vein thrombosis prophylaxis is aimed at mechanical pumping of the blood in order to prevent the stasis of blood or pharmacological agents aimed at reducing the hypercoagulability.

Although the prevention of DVT starts as soon as a patient is diagnosed with pregnancy by careful history taking and identifying high risk individuals we will be focusing on the postnatal aspects.

THROMBOPROPHYLAXIS AFTER DELIVERY

Assessment of Risk

Obesity

All women with class 3 obesity (BMI ≥ 40 kg/m^2) should be considered for prophylactic low molecular weight heparin (LMWH) in doses appropriate for their weight for 10 days after delivery.

Previous Venous Thromboembolism

All women with a previous history of confirmed VTE should be offered thromboprophylaxis with LMWH or warfarin for at least 6 weeks postpartum regardless of the mode of delivery.

Asymptomatic Thrombophilia

Women with thrombophilia without previous VTE should be stratified according to both the level of risk associated with their thrombophilia and the presence or absence of a family history or other risk factors. Women with a family history of VTE and an identified thrombophilia should be considered for 6 weeks' postnatal thromboprophylaxis.

Heritable Thrombophilia

Women with previous VTE associated with antithrombin deficiency (who will often be on long-term oral anticoagulation) should be offered thromboprophylaxis with higher dose of LMWH (either 50%, 75% or full treatment dose) antenatally and for 6 weeks postpartum or until returned to oral anticoagulant therapy after delivery. Management should be undertaken in collaboration with a hematologist with expertise in thrombosis in pregnancy and consideration given to antenatal anti-Xa monitoring and the potential for antithrombin replacement at initiation of labor or prior to cesarean section.

Acquired Thrombophilia

Women with antiphospholipid syndrome (APS) should be offered thromboprophylaxis with higher dose of LMWH (either 50%, 75%, or full treatment dose).

Table 1: Suggested thromboprophylactic doses for antenatal and postnatal LMWH.

Weight	Enoxaparin	Dalteparin	Tinzaparin (75 μ/5kg/day)
<50 kg	20 mg daily	2500 units daily	3500 units daily
50–90 kg	40 mg daily	5000 units daily	4500 units daily
91–130 kg	60 mg daily*	7500 units daily	7000 units daily*
131–170 kg	80 mg daily*	10000 units daily	9000 units daily*
>170 kg	0.6 mg/kg/day*	75 μ/kg/day	75 μ/kg/day*
High prophylactic dose for women weighing 50–90 kg	40 mg 12 hourly	5000 units 12 hourly	4500 units 12 hourly

*May be given in 2 divided doses
LMWH: low molecular weight heparin)

TABLE 2: Summary of guideline for thromboprophylaxis in women with previous VTE and/or thrombophilia.

Very high risk	Previous VTE on long-term oral anticoagulant therapy	Recommend antenatal high-dose LMWH and at least 6 weeks postnatal LMWH or until switched back to oral anticoagulant therapy
	Antithrombin deficiency Antiphospholipid syndrome with previous VTE	*These women require specialist management by experts in hemostasis and pregnancy*
High risk	Any previous VTE (except a single VTE related to major surgery)	Recommend antenatal and 6 weeks postnatal prophylactic LMWH
Intermediate risk	Asymptomatic high-risk thrombophilia homozygous factor V Leiden/compound heterozygote Protein C or S deficiency Single previous VTE associated with major surgery without thrombophilia, family history or other risk factors	Refer to local expert Consider antenatal LMWH Recommend postnatal prophylactic LMWH for 6 weeks Consider antenatal LMWH (but not routinely recommended) Recommend LMWH from 28 weeks of gestation and 6 weeks postnatal prophylactic LMWH
Low risk	Asymptomatic low-risk thrombophilia (prothrombin gene mutation or factor V Leiden)	Consider as a risk factor and score appropriately Recommend 10 days if other risk factor postpartum (or 6 weeks if significant family history) postnatal prophylactic LMWH

(LMWH: low molecular weight heparin; VTE: venous thromboembolism)
Source: RCOG Guideline 2015 Green Top Guideline 37a. London: RCOG; 2015.

Agents for Thromboprophylaxis

Low Molecular Weight Heparin

Low molecular weight heparins are the agents of choice for antenatal and postnatal thromboprophylaxis. Doses of LMWH are based on weight. It is only necessary to monitor the platelet count if the woman has had prior exposure to unfractionated heparin (UFH). Monitoring of anti-Xa levels is not required when LMWH is used for thromboprophylaxis. Doses of LMWH should be reduced in women with renal impairment. LMWH is safe in breastfeeding. The half-life of LMWH is 12 hours which is longer than UFH. LMWH should not be given for 4 hours after use of spinal anesthesia or after the epidural catheter has been removed and the catheter should not be removed within 12 hours of the most recent injection. Thromboprophylaxis can be initiated as soon as possible postdelivery as long as there is no postpartum hemorrhage (PPH) and regional anesthesia is not used.[2]

Unfractionated heparin: In women at very high risk of thrombosis (previous history of VTE who is on long-term oral anticoagulation or APS with history of VTE), UFH may be used peripartum in preference to LMWH where there is an increased risk of hemorrhage or where regional anesthetic techniques may be required. If UFH is used after cesarean section (or other surgery), the platelet count should be monitored every 2–3 days from days 4–14 or until heparin is stopped.

Danaparoid

Potential use of danaparoid should be in conjunction with a consultant hematologist with expertise in hemostasis and pregnancy.

Fondaparinux

Fondaparinux should be reserved for women intolerant of heparin compounds. Fondaparinux use in pregnancy should be in conjunction with a consultant hematologist with expertise in hemostasis and pregnancy.

Low-dose Aspirin

Aspirin is not recommended for thrombo-prophylaxis in obstetric patients. (New 2015)

Warfarin

Warfarin use in pregnancy is restricted to the few situations where heparin is considered unsuitable, e.g., some women with mechanical heart valves. Women receiving long-term anticoagulation with warfarin can be converted from LMWH to warfarin postpartum when the risk of hemorrhage is reduced, usually 5–7 days after delivery. Warfarin is safe in breastfeeding.

Dextran

Dextran should be avoided antenatally and intrapartum because of the risk of anaphylactoid reaction.

Oral Thrombin and Xa Inhibitors

Nonvitamin K antagonist oral anticoagulants (NOACs) should be avoided in pregnant women. Use of NOACs is not currently recommended in women who are breastfeeding.

Antiembolism Stockings

The use of properly applied antiembolism stockings (AES) of appropriate size and providing graduated compression with a calf pressure of 14–15 mm Hg is recommended in pregnancy and the puerperium for women who are hospitalized and have a contraindication to LMWH. These include women who are hospitalized post-cesarean section (combined with LMWH) and considered to be at particularly high risk of VTE (e.g., previous VTE) and women traveling long distance for >4 hours.

There are no trials to support the use of AES in pregnancy and the puerperium and recommendations are largely derived from extrapolation from studies using AES in the hospitalized nonpregnant population. Small studies have shown that AES significantly improve venous emptying in pregnant women and increase the blood flow while decreasing the lumen diameter of the superficial femoral and common femoral veins in late pregnancy and early postpartum patients.[3]

REFERENCES

1. Stone J, Hangge P, Albadawi H, Wallace A, Shamoun F, Knuttien MG, et al. Deep vein thrombosis: pathogenesis, diagnosis, and medical management. Cardiovasc Diagn Ther. 2017;7(Suppl 3):S276-S284.
2. RCOG Guideline 2015 Green Top Guideline 37a. London: RCOG; 2015.
3. Büchtemann AS, Steins A, Volkert B, Hahn M, Klyscz T, Jünger M. The effect of compression therapy on venous haemodynamics in pregnant women. Br J Obstet Gynaecol. 1999;106:563-9.

Postpartum Intrauterine Contraceptive Device

Bhavana Mittal, Chandana S Bhatt

DEFINITION

Postpartum intrauterine contraceptive device (IUCD) is the intrauterine device insertion within 10 minutes to 48 hours of expulsion of placenta.

WHAT IS THE DEVICE USED?

The copper bearing intrauterine contraceptive device, popularly known as IUCD, is a small, flexible plastic frame containing coiled copper impregnated with barium sulfate.
- IUCD 380 A, effective up to 10 years
- IUCD 375, effective up to 5 years

TYPES OF INSERTION

The timing of IUCD insertion are described in **Table 1**.

MEDICAL ELIGIBILITY CRITERIA FOR POSTPARTUM IUCD

The eligibility criteria for postpartum IUCD insertion are given in **Table 2**.

Clinical Technique for Insertion of the Immediate Postpartum IUCD

Steps for insertion of IUCD:
1. *Check for woman's consent:* Rule out conditions which prevent insertion of IUCD–
   a. Rupture of membranes for more than 18 hours
   b. Chorioamnionitis
   c. Unresolved postpartum hemorrhage
2. Visualize cervix by inserting a Sims speculum in the vagina and depressing the posterior wall of the vagina.
3. Clean cervix with antiseptic solution and wait for 2 minutes to allow the antiseptic to work.
4. Grasp IUCD with long placental forceps in the sterile package using a no-touch technique

and apply gentle traction on the anterior lip of the cervix using the ring forceps and insert IUCD into lower uterine cavity and avoid touching the walls of vagina.
5. Once the placental forceps is in the lower uterine cavity, lower the ring forceps that is holding the anterior lip of the cervix and move the left hand to the woman's abdomen and push the entire uterus upward.
6. Gently move placental forceps upward toward the fundus following the curve of the uterine cavity and when it reaches the uterine fundus, resistance is felt.
7. Open placental forceps and release the IUCD at the fundus. Sweep placental forceps to side wall of the uterus and stabilize the uterus.
8. Examine the cervix to ensure there is no bleeding. If IUCD is seen protruding from cervix, remove and reinsert.

TABLE 1: Timing of intrauterine contraceptive device (IUCD) insertion.

Types	Procedure
Postplacental	It is done immediately (within 10 minutes) following delivery of the placenta, following active management of third stage labor and the delivery of the placenta
Intracesarean	IUCD is introduced through the uterine incision during a cesarean section and placed at the uterine fundus
Immediate postpartum	IUCD is inserted within 48 hours following the birth of the baby
Extended postpartum/ interval IUCD	IUCD inserted 6 weeks or later postpartum.

TABLE 2: Eligibility criteria for postpartum intrauterine contraceptive device (IUCD) insertion.

Category 1 (Safely use)	Category 2 (Generally use)	Category 3 (Generally do not use)	Category 4 (Do not use)
• Immediate postplacental • Immediate postpartum <48 hours or during cesarean section • >6 weeks postpartum	No conditions	• Between 48 hours and 6 weeks postpartum • Chorioamnionitis • Prolonged rupture of membranes (ROM) >18 hours	• Puerperal sepsis • Unresolved postpartum hemorrhage

TABLE 3: Problems related to postpartum IUCD insertion and their management.

Problems at the time of insertion	
Discomfort or pain	Reassure that a moderate amount of discomfort is associated with insertion
Displacement of the IUCD	Remove the IUCD and reinsert the same IUCD if not contaminated
Cervical laceration	Repair as needed depending on size of laceration and amount of bleeding
Uterine perforation	Stop the procedure immediately and gently remove the instruments and IUCD, and monitor vitals
Problems encountered after immediate postpartum IUCD insertion	
Changes in menstrual bleeding patterns	• Determine severity of symptoms. If symptoms are mild and consistent with postpartum uterine involution, reassure • If bleeding is persistently heavy and prolonged—consider removal
Cramping or pain	Consider NSAIDs
Infection	Antibiotic treatment
IUCD string problems	• Partner can feel strings—reassure • Longer strings, shorter strings—cut short if they are long • Missing strings—localize and reassure
Pregnancy with an IUCD	
Counsel the woman and proceed accordingly: • Removing the IUCD slightly increases the risk of abortion • Leaving the IUCD in place can cause second trimester abortion, infection and preterm delivery	

(IUCD: intrauterine contraceptive device; NSAIDs: nonsteroidal anti-inflammatory drugs)

Clinical Technique for Insertion within 48 Hours of Delivery

Insert the IUCD using the placental forceps or the ring forceps. Some modification in the technique may be required to bring the uterus a little down and more pressure may be required at the cervix to allow the ring forceps with the IUCD to reach the fundus.

Clinical Technique for Intracesarean Insertion

Insertion can be done either manually or using a ring forceps. Once it is placed at the fundus, the hand should be slowly withdrawn, noting whether the IUCD remains properly placed. The strings can be pointed toward the cervix but should *not* be pushed through the cervical canal. This is to prevent uterine infection by contamination of the uterine cavity with vaginal flora, and to prevent displacement of the IUCD from the fundus by drawing the strings downward toward the cervical canal.

COMMON PROBLEMS AND THEIR MANAGEMENT

The common problems related to postpartum IUCD insertion and their management are discussed in **Table 3**.

FOLLOW-UP CARE

After postpartum IUCD insertion, follow up-after 6 weeks postpartum and is important to assess patient satisfaction and address concerns.

CONCLUSION

- Postpartum IUCD is one of the most effective, reversible contraceptive methods currently available.
- Using an IUCD immediately postpartum will not affect breastfeeding adversely and will not change the amount or quality of breast milk.
- Postpartum IUCD begins to work immediately and is effective for up to 10 years.
- Spontaneous expulsion noted in few cases most likely to occur during the first 3 months postpartum.

- Return of fertility postremoval of the IUCD is almost immediate.

REFERENCES

1. PPIUCD Reference Manual–March 2018. Family Planning Division Ministry of Health and Family Welfare Government of India.
2. World Health Organization: Medical eligibility criteria for contraceptive use. 2015.
3. National Rural Health Mission. Framework for Implementation, 2005-2012.
4. IUCD reference Manual for Medical Officers, Family Planning Division, Ministry of Health and family welfare, Govt of India (2013).
5. Mishra S. Evaluation of safety, efficacy and expulsion of post-placental and intra-cesarean insertion of intrauterine contraceptive devices. J Obstet Gynecol India. 2014;64:337-43.

58

Your Medicolegal Safety and Keeping Records

VK Goyal, Poonam Goyal, Aditee Goyal

When we talk about your safety meaning doctors medicolegal safety, patient safety is of paramount importance and broadly its duty of care toward our patient.

The medical profession is one of the noblest professions in the world. Today, the patient–doctor relationship has almost diminished. Corporatization in health care has made it like a business, and the medical profession is been considered by most as profit making rather than that of service. We all know medicine, is an inexact science; most of the time we cannot predict with certainty of an outcome of patient. It depends on the certain facts and circumstances if the patient responds to the treatment or not. While in court it depends on the personal notions of the judge concerned who is hearing the case. The best way to handle medicolegal issues is prevention.

As per Supreme Court of India version in. *Laxman Balkrishna Joshi vs. Trimbak Bapu Godbole And Anr.* 1968.

Case: A person who holds himself out ready to give medical advice and treatment impliedly holds forth that he is possessed of skill and knowledge for the purpose. Such a person when consulted by a patient, owes certain duties, namely, a duty of care in deciding whether to undertake the case, a duty of care in deciding what treatment to give, and a duty of care in the administration of that treatment. A breach of any of these duties gives a right of action of negligence against him. The medical practitioner has a discretion in choosing the treatment which he proposes to give to the patient and such discretion is wider in cases of emergency, but he must bring to his task a reasonable degree of skill and knowledge and must exercise a reasonable degree of care according to the circumstances of each case.

SAFETY MEASURES

- *Avoiding common errors*: With the growing awareness and internet being used by more and more people, the doctor no longer "knows best." Patients usually complaint of a feeling that they were not heard, that they/their patient was not properly attended, and nobody seemed to care, leading to a bad outcome. Many patients now expect to be part of the decision-making processes concerning their own care.

  To avoid these feelings and improve patient/attendants' satisfaction we have to change our routine as follows:
  - Always attend the cases properly.
  - Listen carefully, do not be in a hurry.
  - Do not interrupt.
  - Maintain eye contact.
  - Always examine the patient carefully with proper attention.
  - Always establish a good rapport.
  - Never be rough, rude or in human.
  - Be empathetic toward the patient.
  - Show your genuine concern.
  - Never look overconfident.
  - Never overreact.
  - Never over promise.
- *Inform*: About the patient's condition, also check that they have understood it.
- *Discuss*: Diagnosis and treatment options, including anticipated benefits and potential risks.
- *Better to explain* finances, at the beginning and subsequently during the continued indoor/outdoor treatment.
- *Always* give guarded prognosis especially in critical cases.
- Assure for "care and not cure."

- Never claim that you are the best; as it increases your responsibility/liability.
- *Decide* if more than one option remains, the patient will have to decide again with consultation with the treating physician and relatives/friends.
- The option of a second opinion may be given if necessary.
- *Documentation*: First go for proper consent, then document all the discussion held with the names of persons present, including details of all options and risks discussed. Always document the history, local and systemic examination findings, and vitals in your out-patient department (OPD) prescription/indoor case sheet. Do have a differential diagnosis. Always record the history of any allergy.

COMMUNICATION

It is the important part of medical safety; good communication maintains good doctor–patient relationship and is important for patient's care. Most of the time patients judge the quality of clinical competence by their interpersonal interactions. Try to maintain good communication skills leading to improved clinical effectiveness and reduce medicolegal risk. It is always important to communicate clearly and properly with all clinical, administrative, and medical colleagues. Clear communication with your subordinates.

The longer the quality time a physician spends with the patient, the less likely will that physician be sued.

Be rationale: Always avoid unnecessary investigations. If any extra or costly investigation is recommended, clearly explain to the patient/attendants about its necessity. If investigations are not advised one can put allegations of not suspecting that diagnosis. Never force for any one specific laboratory, just ask of any accredited laboratory.

TREATMENT

Better to follow any standard or accepted protocol (Bolam principle) as per availability, circumstances, and the consent of the patient and relatives.

We should always follow—do "no harm" policy and the highest standard of professional conduct to be maintained.

If the case is beyond qualification, refer to concerned specialist. As per Supreme Court (SC) [Poonam Varma vs. Ashwin Patel AIR (96) SC 2111] and other case in various courts. Practicing specialty other than the registered qualification is not allowed.

Second opinion: Never hesitate in telling the patient to go for second opinion from an equally competent practitioner.

Team approach: In all critical cases it is better to follow a multispecialty approach.

Prescriptions:
- Always write prescriptions in capital letters, preferably generic drugs (Chapter 1.5 MCI Guidelines). Printed prescription is better.
- Avoid abbreviations of drugs.
- The medicines shall be prescribed as per the requirements with proper justifications.
- Always be careful with the drugs having narrow safety margins. Always explain the likely complications/major side effects of the drugs.
- Always "look-alike" or "sound-alike" drugs to be taken into consideration to avoid errors.
- Always ask/record any history of allergy.

Group practice is advantageous as:
- Liabilities can be delegated to equally competent colleagues.
- Second opinion is easily available as different subspecialties can practice under one roof avoiding the need for referral outside.
- There is an overall decrease in stress and strain and one gets more time for family.

WHEN TO INFORM POLICE?

The police should be informed without delay where we suspect any foul play, medicolegal cases, road traffic accidents, or if there is a possibility of aggression or violence in the healthcare establishment or in nearby place. Just dial number 100 and note down the name of attending person and channel number given.

PREVENTION OF VIOLENCE IN THE HOSPITAL

The incidences of violence have increased tremendously. We have to be very alert, suspicious, and careful in preventing such mishaps.

Install CCTV cameras at recommended places specially to record time of arrival and time of attending the patient.

- Restrict the entry of relatives or unauthorized persons.
- Ask for photo identity of the visitors or relatives.
- Install alarm bells and warning systems in the hospital.
- All establishments should develop a standard operating procedure (SOP) for violence (Code Violet). We can have a "no treatment list of offenders" circulated amongst our colleagues in our local area.
- Inform the senior colleagues, med-legal organizations, and police if there are some mishaps, misunderstandings, or aggressive individuals. Have a crisis management committee.

INDEMNITY OR PROTECTION SCHEMES

Financial safety in practice can be achieved with personal professional indemnity or hospital error and omission policies. The policy should be taken with previous experiences and the reliability of the company.

RECORD KEEPING—METHODS OF RECORD KEEPING

Medical records are an essential component in modern healthcare management. It is the only reliable proof of treatment given to patient and in accessing health status.

For medicolegal safety, two important points in medical practice always to be remembered are communication and documentation. Document whatever you communicate and communicate whatever you document. The traditional method of record keeping is manual method involving papers and books; manual record needs large storage areas and difficulties in the retrieval. In the present era computerization of medical records is a better option, and can be easily stored and retrieved.

Tips for Good Record Keeping

- Write legibly
- Every entry should be timed, dated, signed/named by the person making the

entry. Deletion and alterations should be countersigned.

- Avoid abbreviations
- Do not alter an entry
- Avoid unnecessary comments

A good medical record should include:

- Proper chief complaints and detailed medical history
- Details of the examination, clinical findings, local, systemic and all vitals
- Details of any investigations requested and reports
- Details of all treatment advised/orders and provided
- Your professional opinion, meaning differential diagnosis
- All information/discussion provided to the patient
- Any decisions made by the patient and proper informed consent
- Follow up arrangements and referrals if any

Just to cite observation of court in case *Dr Anil Kumar Aggarwal v/s Hardwari Lal; Appeal No. 68 of 2008; Dated: 25 May 2017.*

Manifestly, in the instant case, there was no "diagnostic dialogue." The prescriptions/slips do not record any symptoms of the disease nor the advice for even basic clinical tests. Applying the aforestated concepts to determine the question of medical negligence, on facts at hand, we have no hesitation in coming to the conclusion that the treating doctor was clearly negligent in treating the patient.

Consent is founded on the principle of autonomy—it must be given freely by a complaint patient, on a voluntary basis, after making an informed decision.

For consent to be legally valid, the patient must be: *Capable of giving consent, sufficiently informed to make a considered decision, giving consent voluntarily.*

Advantages of Keeping Good Clinical Records

Good clinical records:

- Help sharing of relevant information, coordination, and continuity of care among team members

- Help informed decision making for patient management and for route cause analysis in the investigation of serious incidents
- Help audit capabilities
- Always help to provide informative/evidence in a court of law

Progress Notes

These are the record of a patient's illness and treatment. All medical personnel involved in patient care record their notes concerning the progress or lack of progress made by the patient in relation to the chief complaints at the time of hospitalization. Patient's condition and the investigations ordered/treatment given or planned to be documented.

Discharge Notes

This is an important document regarding the inpatient treatment of a patient. The discharge summary should reflect date and time of admission, chief complaints, diagnosis, investigations done, treatment given/operative procedure done, and patients progress. Always note the instructions to be followed by the patient after discharge including dietary advice and date of next visit. Urgent reporting instructions to be given/documented with emergency contact phone number, if an any untoward symptom arises. Always keep a carbon copy of discharge slip.

All the patients are also entitled to have a detailed discharge summary even if getting discharged against the advice of the doctor [leave against medical advice (LAMA)]. All these discharges should be signed by the doctor, patient/relative and duly witnessed.

Referral Notes

Always mention the date and time on referral note and keep the carbon copy. Also write cause of referral, treatment given, and condition at the time of referral. One medical person should always accompany the referral patient.

Certificates

A medical certificate is an important, medical document. If medical certificate is ever produced in the court and is proved to be false, the issuing doctor will be held liable. While issuing a medical certificate following things should be kept in mind:

- Medical certificate should be on institution/doctor letter pad.
- Always date, time, and place should be mentioned.
- Issue it only for legitimate purpose and only when necessary.
- It has to be true and clear without any ambiguity.
- There should be two identification marks of the patient.
- Illness period should be clearly mentioned.
- Always maintain the duplicate copy of every certificate.

How Long to Maintain the Records?

- As per Medical Council of India (MCI) guidelines patient records are maintained for 3 years. (Section 1.3.1 and Appendix 3).
- Death patients—10 years
- Cases under litigation—2 years after final disposal of the case
- PCPNDT record—2 years
  "Better to maintain all the records for longer period in digitalized form."

How to Destroy the Records?

- Public notice of destroying the records in one English newspaper and in one local language paper mentioning the specific date of destruction, with the time limit of one month.
- Records can be given if someone want, with written request by the patient.
- After 1 month destroy the records up to date specified except for following:
  - Where litigation is going on or in prelitigation stage
  - Where likely future trouble is expected.
  - Any mentally ill patient.

Always Keep Hard Copy

Digitalization of records are now widely used as electronic patient records but still hard copy is always required for following documents:
- Consent
- Referral slips
- Ongoing litigations

Request for Records

Any request for medical records by patient or his authorized attendant in writing should be acknowledged and record asked should be issued within 72 hours.

Pointers in Documentation

The primary pitfall in documentation is attempt to alter. For smaller errors, only/always draw a single line through the error with sign and date.

BIBLIOGRAPHY

1. Abdelrahman W, Abdelmageed A. Medical record keeping: clarity, accuracy, and timeliness are essential. BMJ. 2014;348:f7716.
2. Bali A, Bali D, Iyer N, Iyer M. Management of medical records: facts and figures for surgeons. J Maxillofac Oral Surg. 2011;10(3): 199-202.
3. Gutheil TG. Fundamentals of Medical Record Documentation. Psychiatry (Edgmont). 2004; 1(3):26-8.
4. Mathioudakis A, Rousalova I, Gagnat AA, Saad N, Hardavella G. How to keep good clinical records. Breathe (Sheff). 2016; 12(4):369-73.
5. Medical Protection Society. The Six C's: Common risks for new doctors (and how to avoid them) [online] Available from https://www.medicalprotection.org › view › the-six-cs-cab [Last accessed December, 2021].
6. Raveesh BN, Nayak RB, Kumbar SF. Preventing medico-legal issues in clinical practice. Ann Indian Acad Neurol. 2016; 19(Suppl 1):S15-S20.
7. Thomas J. Medical records and issues in negligence. Indian J Urol. 2009;25(3):384-8.

Breaking Bad News

Mala Srivastava, Neema Tufchi, Ankita Srivastava

▓ INTRODUCTION

Breaking bad news (BBN) to patients is one of the most difficult responsibilities in the practice of medicine. But no medical school imparts training in breaking bad news to patients and their relatives. Bad news not only refers to death but also to diagnoses that impose changes in the patient's life. Performed improperly, BBN can lead to patient's stress, anxiety, and misunderstanding of diagnosis, treatment, and prognosis, resulting in less favorable outcomes overall. Further, physicians' psychophysiological stress reaction in medical communication of bad news can lead to an increase in their anxiety, burnout, and alienation from the situation and the patient.

▓ DEFINITION OF BAD NEWS

One source defines bad news as "any news that drastically and negatively alters the patient's view of her or his future. Bad news not only means death, it may mean diagnosis of missed abortion or IUD for pregnant patients, diagnosis of multiple sclerosis for middle aged women, or type I diabetes for an adolescent. How a patient responds to bad news can be influenced by the patient's psychosocial context. It might simply be a diagnosis that comes at an inopportune time, such as unstable angina requiring angioplasty during the week of a daughter's wedding, or it may be a diagnosis that is incompatible with one's employment, such as a coarse tremor developing in a cardiovascular surgeon.

In recent years, a variety of consensus guidelines for communicating bad news to patients have been published. One of the most used protocols for delivering bad news is the SPIKES, a six-step strategy that facilitates the information flow and addresses the patient's distress.

Although the controversy over whether it is possible to develop BBN abilities, several studies have reported that training medical students and clinicians can have positive effects on their interest in acquiring the desired skills. Attitudes toward properly communicating bad news and the possibility to be trained on desirable skills by medical students and physicians are preliminary steps to develop appropriate medical courses that can effectively change their behavior.

▓ STRATEGIES FOR BREAKING BAD NEWS

Different strategies have been applied by doctors and these includes:
1. SPIKES
2. ABCDE
3. BREAKS
4. CONES

SPIKES and ABCDE appear to be the most commonly used.

ABCDE Strategy

A = Advance preparation
B = Build a therapeutic environment/relationship
C = Communicate well
D = Deal with patients and family reactions
E = Encourage and validate emotions

A—Advance Preparation

- Familiarize yourself with the relevant clinical information. At least basic information about prognosis and treatment options.
- Arrange for adequate time in a private, comfortable location.
- Mentally rehearse how you will deliver the news. You may wish to practice out loud, as

you would prepare for public speaking. Script specific words and phrases to use or avoid.

• Prepare emotionally

B—Build a Therapeutic Environment/ Relationship

• Determine the patient's preferences for what and how much they want to know.
• When possible, have family members or other supportive persons present.
• Introduce yourself to everyone present.
• Foreshadow the bad news, "I'm sorry, but I have bad news."
• Some patients or family members will prefer not to be touched. Be sensitive to cultural differences and personal preference.
• Assure the patient you will be available. Schedule follow-up meetings.

C—Communicate Well

• Ask what the patient or family already knows and understands.
• Speak frankly but compassionately.
• Allow silence and tears.
• Be aware that the patient will not retain much of what is said after the initial bad news. Write things down, use sketches or diagrams, and repeat key information.
• At the conclusion of each visit, summarize and make follow-up plans.

D—Deal with Patient and Family Reactions

• Assess and respond to emotional reactions. With subsequent visits, monitor the patient's emotional status, assessing for despondency or suicidal ideations.
• Be empathetic. Crying may be appropriate, but be reflective.
• Do not argue with or criticize colleagues; avoid defensiveness regarding your, or a colleague's, medical care.

E—Encourage and Validate Emotions

• Offer realistic hope. Even if a cure is not realistic, offer hope and encouragement about what options are available. Discuss treatment options at the outset, and arrange follow-up meetings for decision making.

SPIKES

The spikes strategy was developed by late Robert F Buckman, Walter F Baile and their colleagues in 1992.

• S—Setting up the conversation
• P—Perception
• I—Invitation by the patient (Involving the patient)
• K—Knowledge to the patient
• E—Emotions and empathy
• S—Strategy and summary + (Self-reflection)

Setting

• Privacy:
  – Some patients may or may not like to have family members or friends around with them.
  – If there are a number of people closely supporting the patient, ask your patient who will act as a spokesperson for everybody during the discussion.
  – This gives your patient support.
  – It also alleviates some of the stress you will experience when dealing with multiple people during an emotionally charged interview.
• Sit down
  – You have to be seated during an interview to break bad news
• Look attentive and calm
  – Maintain eye contact. This assures patient that you are listening.
  – If the patient becomes tearful, is a good idea to break eye contact momentarily.
• *Be in listening mode*: It involves
  – Silence
  – Repetition
  – Nodding
  – Smiling (appropriately)
  – Saying things like "hmmm"
• Availability
  – Make arrangement for the phones to be answered and do not interrupt the meeting.
  – If, however, unavoidable phone calls or interrupting do occur, courteously address them so that your patient does not feel less important than the interruption.

P—Perception

- Assess the patients understanding or the seriousness of their condition.
- Assess the patient and family member's level of understanding.
- Watch for signs of denial.

I—Invitation/Information

- Most patients want to know all the details about their medical situation, but this is not always the case.
- Accept the patient right not to want to know, but offer to answer any question he or she have later.
- Offer to answer any questions the patient/family members may have.

K—Knowledge Explaining the Facts

- Before you break bad news, give your patient a warning that bad news is coming.
- Avoid technical scientific language as much as possible, e.g., instead of "metastasized"—say spread.
- Avoid being pessimistic, over optimistic but tell the whole truth.

E—Empathy and Emotion

Have an emphatic response to patient's problem, the emphatic response is a technique or skill.
It comprises of three steps.

- *Step 1*: Listen for and identify the emotion (or mixture of emotion)
- *Step 2*: Identify the cause or source of the emotion, most likely the bad news the patient received
- *Step 3*: Show your patient that you have made the connection between the above two steps, that is, you have identified the emotion and its origin.
  - *Denials*: "It is not me, the lab must have mixed up the specimen".
  - *Anger*: "Why was this not seen earlier"?
  - Numbness

S—Strategy and Summary Strategy

- Decide what the best medical plan would be for the patient.
- Recommend a strategy on how to proceed.
- Ask the patient to repeat you their understanding of the plan
- Possibly have a clear treatment plan in writing

BREAKS

This pneumonic has been put together by Dr Naranayam, Bista and Koshi, all from India.

- B—Background
- R—Rapport
- E—Exploring
- A—Announce
- K—Kindling—Observe patient's response
- S—Summarize—Summarize just as in the SPIKES strategy

The CONES Protocol

Used in the following situations:

1. Disclosing a medical error
2. Sudden deterioration in the patient's medical condition
3. Sudden unexpected death

Note: The news should be delivered by the most senior person on the patient's treatment team.

C—Context
O—Opening slot
N—Narrative
E—Emotions
S—Strategy and summary

C—Context

- Prepare for what to say and anticipate the patient family reaction.
- Have the conversation in a quiet undisturbed area
- Seat the patient closest to you and have no barriers between you
- Have a box of tissues available.

O—Opening Slot

Alert the patient/family members of the impending bad news

N—Narrative Approach

- Explain the chorological sequence of events,
- Avoid assigning blame and or making excuses
- Emphasize that you are investigating how the error occurred

Offer a Clear Apology: Emotions

Address strong emotions with empathic responses:

Use the E—V—E protocol as soon as emotions occurs (Explore, Validate, Empathize)

"I know that it is upsetting for you and it is awful for me too", "I know this is awful", "it is very rare, but it does happen and I am sorry to say that it did".

Beware of being pushed into making promises you cannot deliver.

The angry patient:
- What to do
  - Acknowledge the person's anger
  - Try to find out the reason for his anger
  - Validate his feelings
- How to do it
  - Sit reasonable close to patient (not too close, not too far), and maintain eye contact
  - Speak calmly without raising your voice
  - Avoid dismissive or threatening body language
  - Be empathetic
  - Be aware of your safety
- What not to do
  - Glare at the person
  - Confront, interrupt or touch him or her
  - Put the blame on others or seek to exonerate yourself
  - Make unreasonable promise

BREAKING BAD NEWS OVER THE TELEPHONE

This should be avoided as much as possible until it becomes absolutely necessary.

Some patient may accept a brief phone conversation with the initial statement of bad news, a statement of sympathy, and a follow-up plan.

Acknowledge the difficulty of waiting for a follow-up appointment for extended discussion.

Gently, but firmly limit the extent of conversation.

OBSTACLES TO COMMUNICATION OF BAD NEWS

- Medical education does not teach it well enough
- Students are usually not encouraged to show emotion or feeling
- There is unrealistic expectation of the health care system by society
- Cultural differences in disclose of information
- Time limitations of medical staff
- Lack of trust in the medical system
- Lack of experience with issues related with death and dying

- Emotions such as fear of the process of dying, of blame, of not having all the answers, emotional out burst
- Sadness, guilt, failure, helplessness
- No one wants to be the bad guy
- Some families do not want the patient to hear truth as it stands"
- Some doctors feel it is a waste of their precious time so spend as little time as possible doing it
- Multiple physicians—who should perform the task
- Fear of medicolegal system, everyone has a "right" to be cured: if no cure happens, someone is to blame

CONCLUSION

Breaking bad news is frequently a tense and distressing experience for both the patient and the physician. Your patients emotional responses will be difficult to withstand unless you have a strategy with which to address them, note that more than 50% of communication of bad news is nonverbal, focus on the patients concerns. Know the facts (patient details, expectations, culture, religious inclinations). Acknowledge the limitations of a physician and medical science in general. Finally practice communicating clearly, completely and compassionately.

BIBLIOGRAPHY

1. Alies TA, Herndun JE Small EJ. Quality of the life impact of three different doses of suramin in patients with metastatic hormone–refractory prostrate carcinoma: result of intergroup 01569/cancer and leukemia group b 9480. Cancer. 2004;101(10):2202-8.
2. Back T. Mastering communication with seriously ill patients. Cambridge: Cambridge University Press; 2009.
3. Baile WF, Buckman R, Lenzi R, Glober G, Beale EA, Kudelka AP. SPIKES-A six-step protocol for delivering bad news: application to the patient with Cancer. Oncologist. 2000;5(4):302-11.
4. Bousquet G, Orri M, Winterman S, Brugière C, Verneuil L, Revah-Levy A. Breaking bad news in oncology: a meta-synthesis. J Clin Oncol. 2015;33(22):2437-43.
5. Buckman R, Korsch B, Baile WF. A practical guide to communication skill in clinical practices. Portland, Oregon: Lumen Learning; 1998.

6. Buckman R. Breaking bad news: a guide for health care professionals. Baltimore: Johns Hopkins University Press; 1992.

7. Buckman R. Breaking bad news: why is it still so difficult? BMJ. 1984 May 26; 288(6430): 1597-9.

8. Buckman R. How to break bad news: a guide for health care professionals. Baltimore, MD: Johns Hopkins University Press; 1992. p. 15.

9. Butow PN, Kazem JN. When the diagnosis is cancer; patient communication experiences and preferences cancer. 1996;77(12):2630-7.

10. Dias LM, Carvalho AEV, Furlaneto IP, de Oliveira CGS. Medical residents perceptions of communication skills, a workshop on breaking bad news. Rev Bras Educ Medica. 2018;42(4):175-83

11. Fallowfield L, Jenkins V. Communicating sad, bad, and difficult news in medicine. Lancet. 2004;363(9405):312-9.

12. Fiedrechsen MJ, Strang PM, Carlssan ME. Breaking bad news in the transition from curative to palliative cancer care – patient's view of the doctor giving the information. Support Care Can. 2000:8(6):472-8

13. Finan C, Nasr SZ, Rothwell E, Tarini BA. Primary care providers' experiences notifying parents of cystic fibrosis newborn screening results. Clin Pediatr (Phila). 2015;54(1):67-75.

14. Girgis A, Sanson-Fisher RW. Breaking bad news 1: current best advice for clinicians. Behav Med. 1998;24(2):53-9.

15. Heaven CM, Maguire P. Disclosure of concerns by hospice patients and their identification by nurses. Palliat Med. 1997;(4)284-90

16. Heaven CM, Maguire P. The relationship between patients concerns and psychological distress in a hospice setting. Psychooncology. 1998;7(6)502-7

17. Hollyday SL, Buonocore D. Breaking bad news and discussing goals of care in the intensive care unit: AACN. Adv Crit Care. 2015;26(2):131-41.

18. Jurkovich GJ, Pierce B, Pananen L, Rivara FP. Giving bad news: the family perspective. J Trauma. 2000;48(5):865-70.

19. Keefe-Cooperman K, Brady-Amoon P. Breaking bad news in counseling: applying the PEWTER model in the school setting. J Creativ Ment Health. 2013;8(3):265-77.

20. Kelley KJ, Kelley MF. Teaching empathy and other compassion-based communication skills. J Nurs Prof Dev. 2013;29(6):321-4.

21. Lamba S, Tyrie LS, Bryczkowski S, Nagurka R. Teaching surgery residents the skills to communicate difficult news to patient and family members: a literature review. J Palliat Med. 2016;19(1):101-7.

22. Ley P. Giving information to patients, New York: Wiley; 1982.

23. Lo B, Quill T, Tulsky J. Discussing palliative care with patients. Ann Intern Med. 1999;130;744-9.

24. Maguire P. Improving communication with cancer patients. Eur J Can. 1999;35(10);1415-22

25. Maynard DW. On "realization" in everyday life: the forecasting of bad news as a social relation. Am Sociol Rev. 1996: 147094466.

26. Narayanan V, Bista B, Koshy C. "BREAKS" protocol for breaking bad news. Indian J Palliat Care. 2010;16(2):61-5.

27. Nishimura K, Nonomura N, Yasunaga Y, Takaha N, Inoue H, Sugao H, et al. Low doses of oral dexamethasone for hormone-refractory prostate carcinoma. Cancer. 2000;89(12)2570-6.

28. Parie M, Jones B, Maguire P. maladaptive coping and affective disorders among cancer patients. Psychol Med. 1996;26(4)735-44

29. Parker PA, Baile WFJ, de Moor C, Lenzi R, Kudelka AP, Cohen L. Breaking bad news about cancer: patients' preferences for communication. J Clin Oncol. 2001;19(7):2049-56.

30. Ptacek JT Eberhardt TL. Breaking bad news. A review of literature. JAMA. 1996;276(6)496-502.

31. Reed S, Kassis K, Nagel R, Verbeck N, Mahan JD, Shell R. Breaking bad news is a teachable skill in pediatric residents: a feasibility study of an educational intervention. Patient Educ Couns. 2015;98(6):748-52.

32. Rider EA, Volkan K, Hafler JP. Pediatric residents' perceptions of communication competencies: implications for teaching. Med Teach. 2008;30(7):e208-17.

33. Sikstrom L, Saikaly R, Ferguson G, Mosher PJ, Bonato S, Soklaridis S. Being there: a scoping review of grief support training in medical education. PLoS One. 2019;14(11):e0224325.

34. Studer RK, Danuser B, Gomez P. Physicians' psychophysiological stress reaction in medical communication of bad news: a critical literature review. Int J Psychophysiol. 2017;120:14-22.

35. Villagran M, Goldsmith J, Wittenberg-Lyles E, Baldwin P, Creating COMFORT. A communication-based model for breaking bad news. Commun Educ. 2010;59(3):220-34.

36. Wolfe AD, Frierdich SA, Wish J, Kilgore-Carlin J, Plotkin JA, Hoover-Regan M. Sharing life-altering information: development of pediatric hospital guidelines and team training. J Palliat Med. 2014;17(9):1011-8.

Manyata Accreditation

Jaideep Malhotra, Raji Cheriyan

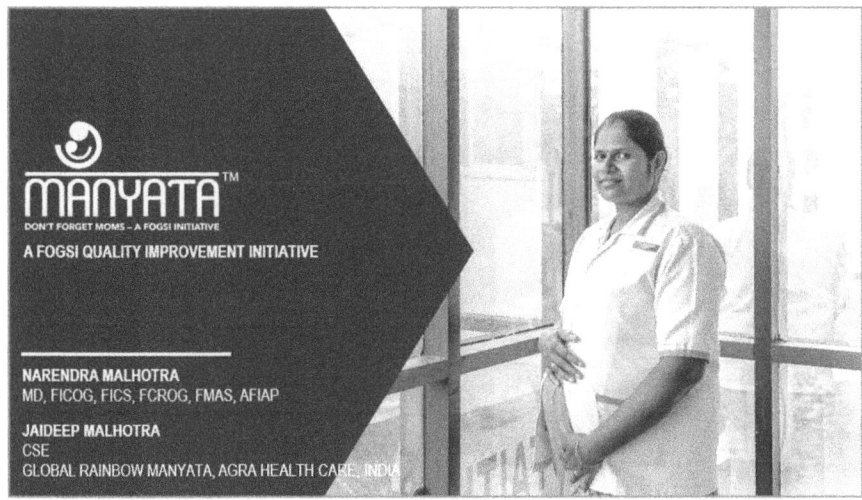

QUALITY OF PRIVATE MATERNITY CARE IN INDIA

 32,000 women die in India, every year, due to complications related to pregnancy and childbirth

 India has a mixed health system; when women deliver in facilities, a quarter of rural women and half of urban women choose private maternity providers

 The ripple effects of a mother's death are enormous—devastating families, communities, nation's economies

 Clinical maternity care in the local private sector is inconsistent

 Lack of quality care can make it difficult to manage complications arising of childbirth

 Lack of quality standards puts pregnant women and new mothers' health at risk

So, what can we do to ensure that no mother has to die giving life, no matter where she seeks care? → Evidence shows that one of the most powerful ways to prevent maternal deaths is to provide high-quality, evidence-based care to mothers during pregnancy and childbirth = THAT'S WHERE MANYATA COMES IN

ABOUT MANYATA

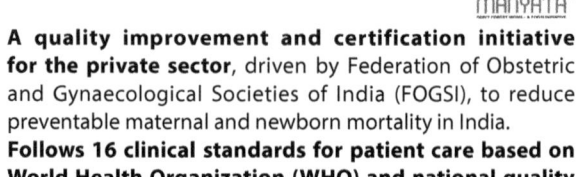

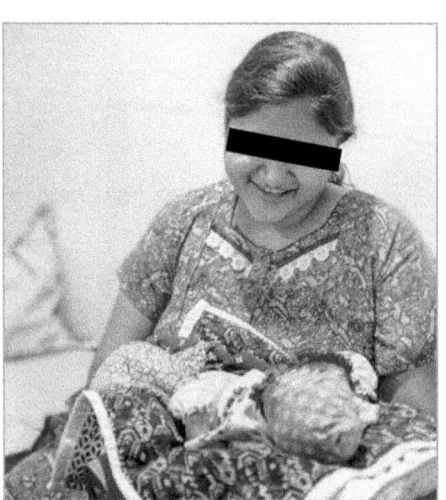

It's time to bring back focus on mothers.
#DONTFORGETMOMS

- **A quality improvement and certification initiative for the private sector**, driven by Federation of Obstetric and Gynaecological Societies of India (FOGSI), to reduce preventable maternal and newborn mortality in India.
- **Follows 16 clinical standards for patient care based on World Health Organization (WHO) and national quality care standard**, for antenatal, intrapartum and postpartum care to ensure that women receive quality maternity care to ensure consistent, safe, respectful, and quality care during and after pregnancy.
- **Applies innovative methods** that combine classroom such as virtual sessions, mentoring visits, drills and simulation to train and equip private healthcare providers.
- **Present in 15 states** covering low and middle income regions
- **Complements India's national efforts** toward achieving Universal Health Coverage (UHC) and national maternal health priorities.
- **Bringing quality care to the remotest areas of India** by working in Niti Aayog's "Aspirational Districts"

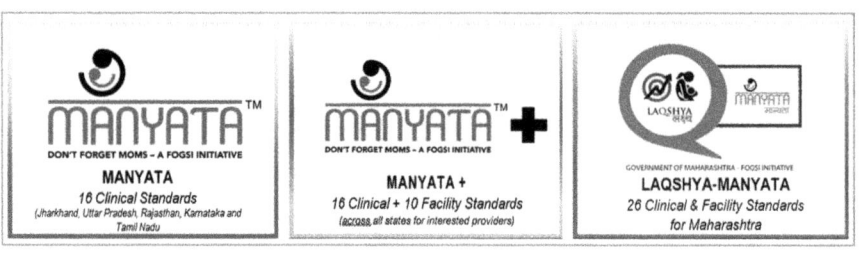

PROGRAM PROCESS AT A GLANCE

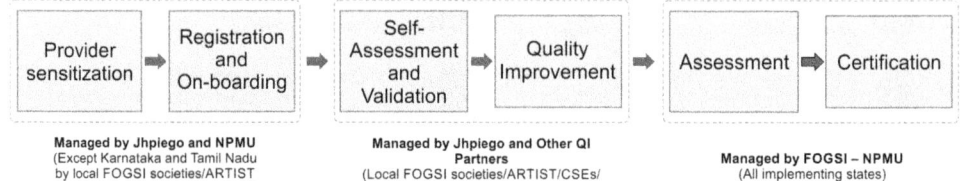

Provider sensitization → Registration and On-boarding → Self-Assessment and Validation → Quality Improvement → Assessment → Certification

Managed by Jhpiego and NPMU
(Except Karnataka and Tamil Nadu by local FOGSI societies/ARTIST and Rajasthan by PSI and HLFPPT)

Managed by Jhpiego and Other QI Partners
(Local FOGSI societies/ARTIST/CSEs/PSI and HLFPPT)

Managed by FOGSI – NPMU
(All implementing states)

ABOUT LAQSHYA-MANYATA (FOGSI-GOM)

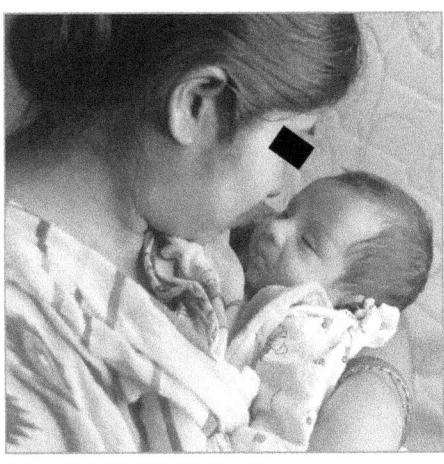

- **LaQshya-Manyata** is a joint initiative between the Public Health Department, Government of Maharashtra and The Federation of Obstetric and Gynaecological Societies of India (FOGSI)
- **Aims to improve the quality of private maternity care** in Maharashtra by building skilled and capable teams ensuring consistent, safe and respectful care for mothers during and after childbirth
- **Follows 16 clinical and 10 facility standards** for patient care aligned with national government's LaQshya program and WHO standard guidelines
- **Covers 34 districts and 27 corporations in Maharashtra** including low and middle income regions such as aspirational districts such as Nandurbar

OVERVIEW OF CLINICAL STANDARDS

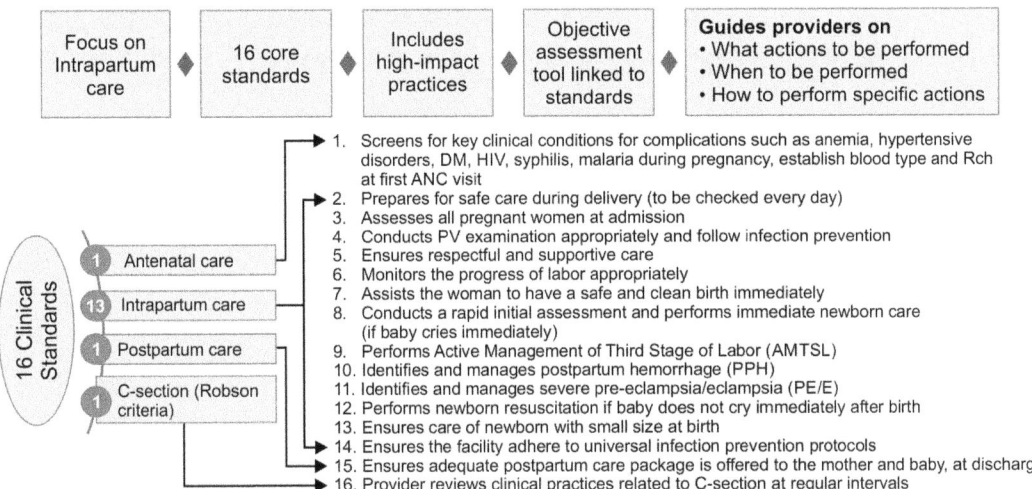

OVERVIEW OF FACILITY STANDARDS

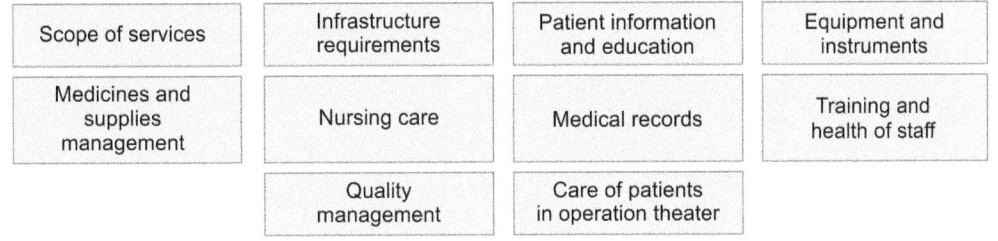

PROVIDER'S JOURNEY TO QUALITY CARE

Quality assurance →

Registration	Self-assessment and validation	Learner quality improvement	Assessment	Certification
• Provider identification and sensitization • Online registration and payment through Manyata portal	• Online self-assessment • Validation and orientation by program team • Action planning	• Trainings at FOGSI centers for skill enhancement (CSEs) • Mentoring visits • Virtual trainings through ECHO clinics • Additional training and mentoring visits (optional)	• Assessment by FOGSI lead assessors	• Recognition by FOGSI

← Quality improvement →

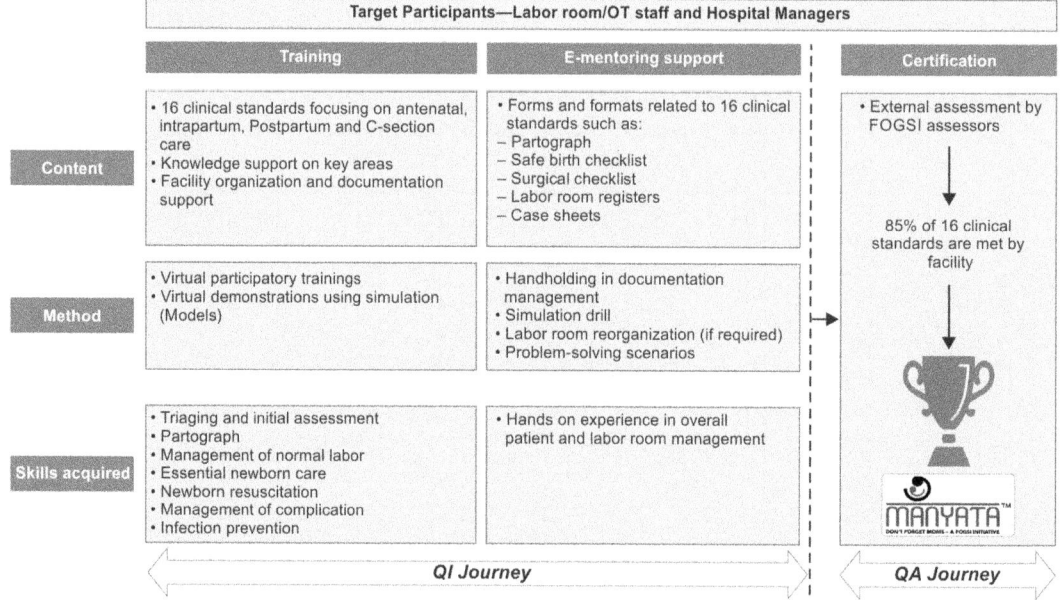

Target Participants—Labor room/OT staff and Hospital Managers			
	Training	**E-mentoring support**	**Certification**
Content	• 16 clinical standards focusing on antenatal, intrapartum, Postpartum and C-section care • Knowledge support on key areas • Facility organization and documentation support	• Forms and formats related to 16 clinical standards such as: – Partograph – Safe birth checklist – Surgical checklist – Labor room registers – Case sheets	• External assessment by FOGSI assessors 85% of 16 clinical standards are met by facility
Method	• Virtual participatory trainings • Virtual demonstrations using simulation (Models)	• Handholding in documentation management • Simulation drill • Labor room reorganization (if required) • Problem-solving scenarios	
Skills acquired	• Triaging and initial assessment • Partograph • Management of normal labor • Essential newborn care • Newborn resuscitation • Management of complication • Infection prevention	• Hands on experience in overall patient and labor room management	MANYATA™ DON'T FORGET MOMS – A FOGSI INITIATIVE
	← QI Journey →		← QA Journey →

Center for Skill Enhancement (CSEs)

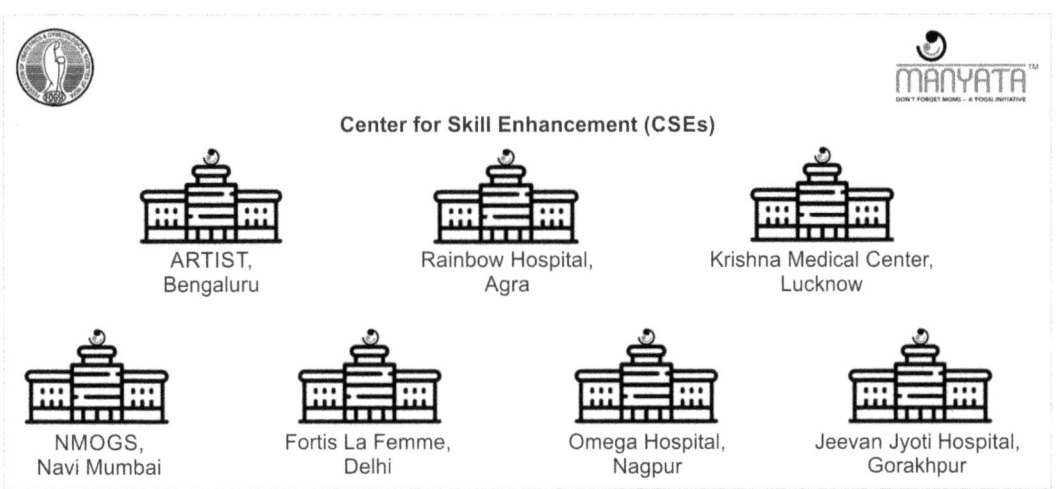

ARTIST, Bengaluru

Rainbow Hospital, Agra

Krishna Medical Center, Lucknow

NMOGS, Navi Mumbai

Fortis La Femme, Delhi

Omega Hospital, Nagpur

Jeevan Jyoti Hospital, Gorakhpur

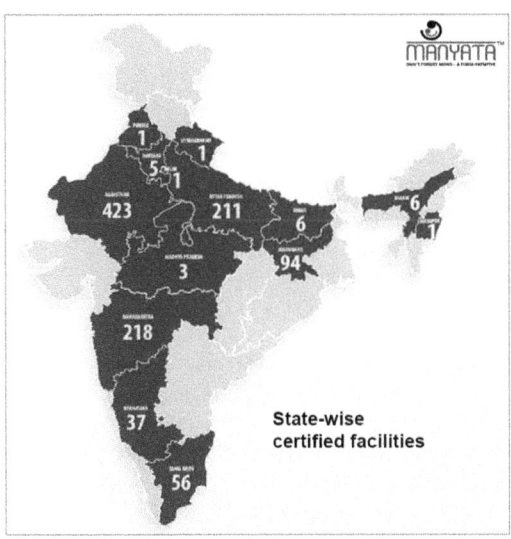

State-wise certified facilities

Coverage and impact

549,384 Safer deliveries	**12,779** Providers trained
1486 Registered facilities	**1109** Certified facilities
550+ Virtual assessments	**100+** LM virtual assessments

MANYATA CLINICAL STANDARDS

S. No.	Standard	Verification criteria		Remarks
Antenatal Care				
1	**Provider screens for key clinical conditions that may lead to complications during pregnancy. (To be verified only among booked cases)**			
1.1a	Screens at the point of reception/waiting area	1.1a.1	Ask questions on ruling out infection and exposure to infection during pandemic. Availability of infrared thermometer and pulse oximeter at the point of use Record temperature and SPO$_2$	
1.1b	Screens for anemia Screens for height/weight/BMI/nutritional checklist available	1.1b.1	Estimates Hb at least once in every trimester	
1.2	Screens for hypertensive disorders of pregnancy	1.2.1	Functional BP instrument and stethoscope at point of use are available	
		1.2.2	Records BP at each ANC visit	
		1.2.3	Performs proteinuria testing during all ANC contacts if a pregnant woman is hypertensive	
1.3	Screens for DM	1.3.1	Uses/Refers for standard single step 75 g OGTT for screening of GDM at first ANC visit and repeats OGTT test at second ANC visit (24–28 weeks) if negative in first screening	
1.4	Screens for HIV	1.4.1	Screens/refer for HIV during first ANC visit in all cases, and repeat HIV testing, considering window period if the spouse is positive or s/he has high-risk behavior	
1.5	Screens for syphilis	1.5.1	Screens/refer for syphilis in first ANC visit in all cases, and again in the third trimester or at the time of delivery if she has high-risk behavior or untested earlier.	
1.6	Screens for malaria	1.6.1	Screens for malaria (only in endemic areas)	
1.7	Establishes blood group and Rh type during first ANC visit	1.7.1	Establishes blood group and Rh type during first ANC visit	
1.8a	Screens for asymptomatic bacteriuria	1.8.1	Screens for asymptomatic bacteriuria using urine culture/urine Gram staining/dipstick test for nitrite during each scheduled ANC contact	
1.8b	Screen for COVID-19		RT-PCR or RAT report	

Contd...

Contd...

S. No.	Standard	Verification criteria		Remarks
1.9	Establish standard operating procedure for ANC clinics for pregnant woman during pandemic	Restricting physical visits of pregnant mother to reduce risk of infection		(4 minimum physical visits or need based and continuing teleconsultation for subsequent visit.
		Allow limited woman with prior booking in consideration of accommo-dating mothers with danger signs		
		Following MOHFW/State protocol for ANC clinic		
		The facility has displayed IECs related to preventive, promotive, and therapeutic care		
		Established procedure of educating mothers on health promotive behaviors and BPCR		
	Standard 1 final response (Yes/No):			**0**
At Admission:				
2	**Provider prepares for safe care during delivery (to be checked every day)**			
2.1	Ensures sterile/HLD delivery tray is available	2.1.1	Ensure availability of uterotonics agents—IM/IV oxytocin (preferred), misoprostol, PPH box, and eclampsia kits are ready	Y
2.2	Ensures functional items for newborn care and resuscitation	2.2.1	Designated newborn corner is present	Y
		2.2.2	Ensures functional items for newborn care and resuscitation	Y
		2.2.3	Switches radiant warmer "on" 30 minutes before childbirth	N
2.3	If facility provides services to infectious disease		Ensures demarcation of routine care area and designated care area for COVID-19	
			Availability of appropriate signages	
			Ensures availability of sterile equipment	
	Standard 2 final response (Yes/No):			**0**
3	**Provider assesses all pregnant women at admission**			
3.1	Takes obstetric, medical, and surgical history	3.1.1	Takes obstetric, medical, and surgical history	
			Screen all mothers on admission in a designated area	

Contd...

Contd...

S. No.	Standard		Verification criteria	Remarks
3.2	Assesses gestational age correctly	3.2.1	Assesses gestational age through either LMP or fundal height or USG (previous or present is available)	
3.3	Records fetal heart rate	3.3.1	Functional Doppler/fetoscope/stethoscope at point of use is available	
		3.3.2	Records FHR	
3.4	Records mother's BP and temperature	3.4.1	Functional BP instrument, stethoscope, pulse oximeter, and functional thermometer at point of use are available	
		3.4.2	Records temperature, pulse, RR, BP, and SPO_2.	

Standard 3 final response (Yes/No):

4	**Providers conduct PV examination appropriately**			
4.1	Conducts PV examination as per indication	4.1.1	Conducts PV examination only as indicated (4 hourly or based on clinical indication) *(Ask Doctor/Nurse as per facility protocol)*	
4.2	Conducts PV examination following infection prevention practices and records findings	4.2.1	Soap, running water, antiseptic solution, and sterile gauze/pads are available	
		4.2.2	Performs hand hygiene (washes hands and wears sterile gloves on both the hands with correct technique)	
		4.2.3	Cleans the perineum appropriately before conducting PV examination	
		4.2.4	Alert specialist/doctor if liquor is meconium stained	
		4.2.5	Records findings of PV examination	

Standard 4 final response (Yes/No):

5	**Provider monitors the progress of labor appropriately**			
5.1	Undertakes timely assessment of cervical dilatation and descent to monitor the progress of labor	5.1.1	Partograph is available in labor room	Y
		5.1.2	Initiates partograph plotting when cervical dilatation is ≥4 cm.	N
5.2	Interprets partograph (condition of mother and fetus and progress of labor) correctly and adjusts care according to findings	5.2.1	If parameters are not normal, identifies complications, records the diagnosis, and makes appropriate adjustments in the birth plan *(Ask Doctor/Nurse as per facility protocol)*	

Contd...

Contd...

S. No.	Standard	Verification criteria		Remarks
5.3	Obstructed labor	5.3.1	Staff knows diagnosis and management of **obstructed labor** (Interpreting partograph, rehydrates the patient, check vitals, gives broad spectrum antibiotics, perform bladder catheterization, and takes blood for Hb and grouping)	
			If the facility is a designated COVID hospital, plan the C-section in designated time to reduce cross infection to other noninfected cases	
5.4	Unnecessary augmentation and induction of labor are not done using uterotonics.	5.4.1	Oxytocin and misoprostol inductions are done only for clear medical indication and the expected benefits outweigh the potential harms. Outpatient induction of labor is not done.	
			COVID-positive mothers' fetal parameters should be checked frequently to detect fetal distress	
	Standard 5 final response (Yes/No):			0
6	**Provider ensures respectful and supportive care**			
6.1	Encourages and welcomes the presence of a birth companion during labor	6.1.1	Encourages and welcomes the presence of a birth companion during labor	Y
6.2	Treats pregnant woman and her companion cordially and respectfully (RMC), ensures privacy and confidentiality for pregnant woman during her stay. Behavior of labor room staff is dignified and respectful.	6.2.1	There are provisions for privacy in LR (curtains/partition between tables and non-see through windows	Y
		6.2.2	Treats pregnant woman and her companion cordially and respectfully. Confidentiality of patient's records and clinical information is maintained.	Y
6.3	Explains danger signs and important care activities to pregnant woman and her companion	6.3.1	Explains danger signs and important care activities to mother and her companion	Y
6.4	Ensures staff health surveillance during pandemic		All staff should be vaccinated	
			Ensure screening using health index checklist during pandemic to provide safe care	

Contd...

Contd...

S. No.	Standard		Verification criteria	Remarks
6.5	Ensures counseling of COVID suspect and COVID-positive mother		Ensures counseling on danger sign, skin to skin contact, early breastfeeding, and rooming in for COVID-suspect and COVID-positive mother	
6.6	Ensure services for all mothers		The facility has policy of delivering all mothers including COVID-19-positive cases	
			The facility does not refuse any patient during emergency or head on perineum	
			If time permits and facility has limited services then the facility link the patient with nearest DCH	
	Standard 6 final response (Yes/No):			1

At Delivery:

S. No.	Standard		Verification criteria	Remarks
7	**Provider assists the pregnant woman to have a safe and clean birth**			
7.1	Provider ensures six "cleans" while conducting delivery	7.1.1	Sterile gloves are available	**Y**
		7.1.2	Antiseptic solution (Betadine/Savlon) is available	**Y**
		7.1.3	Sterile cord clamp is available	**Y**
		7.1.4	Sterile cutting edge (blade/scissors) is available	**Y**
7.2	Performs an episiotomy only if indicated with the use of appropriate local anesthetic	7.2.1	Performs an episiotomy only if indicated and uses local anesthesia *(Ask doctor/nurse as per facility protocol)*	Y
7.3	Allows spontaneous delivery of head by maintaining flexion and giving perineal support; manages cord round the neck; assists in delivery of shoulders and body	7.3.1	Allows spontaneous delivery of head by maintaining flexion and giving perineal support; manages cord round the neck; assists in delivery of shoulders and body	Y
	Standard 7 final response (Yes/No):			1
8	**Provider conducts a rapid initial assessment and performs immediate newborn care (if baby cried immediately)**			
8.1	Delivers the baby on mother's abdomen	8.1.1	Two towels at normal room temperature or prewarmed to room temperature	Y
		8.1.2	Delivers the baby on mother's abdomen	Y
8.2	Ensures immediate drying and assess breathing	8.2.1	If breathing is normal, dries the baby immediately and wraps in second warm towel	Y

Contd...

Contd...

S. No.	Standard	Verification criteria		Remarks
8.3	Performs delayed cord clamping and cutting	8.3.1	Performs delayed cord clamping and cutting (1–3 minutes) unless medical indication otherwise	Y
8.4	Ensures early initiation of breastfeeding	8.4.1	Initiates breastfeeding within one hour of birth	Y
8.5	Assesses the newborn for any congenital anomalies	8.5.1	Provider immediately assesses the newborn for any congenital anomalies	Y
		8.5.2	Provider ensures specialist care if required	Y
8.6	Weighs the baby and administers vitamin K. **OPV/BCG/Hepatitis B vaccinations are given within 24 hours of birth**	8.6.1	Baby weighing scale is available	Y
		8.6.2	Vitamin K injection is available	Y
		8.6.3	Weighs the baby and administers Vitamin K. **OPV/BCG/Hepatitis B vaccinations are administered within 24 hours of birth**	Y
	Standard 8 final response (Yes/No):			1
9	**Provider performs Active Management of Third Stage of Labor (AMTSL)**			
9.1	Performs AMTSL and examines the placenta thoroughly	9.1.1	Palpates mother's abdomen to rule out second baby	N
		9.1.2	Administers uterotonics. Preferred is Injection. Oxytocin 10 IU IM/IV within one minute of delivery of baby (use Misoprostol 600 µg if oxytocin is not available)	Y
		9.1.3	*Performs controlled cord traction (CCT) during contraction*	N
		9.1.4	*Performs uterine massage*	N
		9.1.5	Checks placenta and membranes for completeness before discarding	N
	Standard 9 final response (Yes/No):			0
10	**Provider identifies and manages postpartum hemorrhage (PPH)**			
10.1	Assesses uterine tone and bleeding per vaginum regularly after delivery	10.1.1	Assesses uterine tone and bleeding per vaginum regularly	
10.2	Identifies shock	10.2.1	Identifies shock by signs and symptoms (pulse > 110 per minute, systolic BP < 90 mm Hg, cold clammy skin, respiratory rate > 30 per minute, altered sensorium and scanty urine output < 30 mL per hour)	

Contd...

Contd...

S. No.	Standard	Verification criteria		Remarks
10.3	Manages shock	10.3.1	Ensures availability of wide bore cannulas (No. 14/16), IV infusion sets and fluids and containers for collection of blood for hemoglobin, blood grouping, and cross matching	
		10.3.2	Shouts for help, follows ABC approach, monitors vitals, elevates the foot end and keeps the woman warm	
		10.3.3	Starts IV infusions, collects blood for Hb and grouping and cross matching, catheterizes the bladder and monitors I/O, gives oxygen at the rate of 6–8 liters per minute	
		10.3.4	Identifies specific cause of PPH	
10.4	Manages atonic PPH	10.4.1	Initiates 20 IU oxytocin drip in 1,000 mL of ringer lactate/normal saline at the rate of 40–60 drops per minute Initiates tranexamic acid, administered at a fixed dose of 1 g in 10 mL (100 mg/mL) IV at 1 mL per minute (i.e., administered over 10 minutes), with a second dose of 1 g IV if bleeding continues after 30 minutes (WHO protocol)	
		10.4.2	Continues uterine massage	
		10.4.3	If uterus is still relaxed, gives other uterotonics as recommended	
		10.4.4	If uterus is still relaxed, performs mechanical compression in the form of bimanual uterine compression or external aortic compression or balloon tamponade *(Ask doctor/nurse as per facility protocol)*	
		10.4.5	If uterus is still relaxed, refers to higher center while continuing mechanical compression	
10.5	Manages PPH due to retained placenta/ placental bits	10.5.1	Identifies retained placenta if placenta is not delivered within 30 minutes of delivery of baby or the delivered placenta is not complete	
		10.5.2	Initiates 20 IU oxytocin drip in 1,000 mL of ringer lactate/normal saline at the rate of 40–60 drops per minute	
		10.5.3	Refers to higher center if unable to manage	
		10.5.4	Performs manual removal of placenta (MRP) *(Ask Doctor)*	

Contd...

Contd...

S. No.	Standard		Verification criteria	Remarks
			Standard 10 final response (Yes/No):	0
11	**Provider identifies and manages severe pre-eclampsia/eclampsia (PE/E)**			
11.1	Identifies mothers with severe PE/E	11.1.1	Dipsticks for proteinuria testing in labor room are available	Y
		11.1.2	Records BP at admission	Y
		11.1.3	Identifies danger signs or presence of convulsions	N
11.2	Gives correct regimen of Inj. MgSO$_4$ for prevention and management of convulsions	11.2.1	MgSO$_4$ in labor room (at least 20 ampoules) is available	Y
		11.2.2	Inj. MgSO$_4$ is appropriately administered	Y
11.3	Facilitates prescription of antihypertensive	11.3.1	Antihypertensives are available	Y
		11.3.2	Facilitates prescription of antihypertensive	Y
11.4	Ensures specialist attention for care of mother and newborn	11.4.1	Ensures specialist attention for care of mother and newborn	Y
11.5	Performs nursing care	11.5.1	Performs nursing care	
			Standard 11 final response (Yes/No):	0
12	**Provider performs newborn resuscitation if baby does not cry immediately after birth**			
12.1	Performs steps for resuscitation within first 30 seconds	12.1.1	Suction equipment/mucus extractor is available	Y
		12.1.2	Shoulder roll is available	Y
		12.1.3	*Performs following steps on mothers abdomen:* Dries the baby; immediate clamps and cuts the cord and shifts the baby to radiant warmer if still not breathing	N
		12.1.4	*Performs following steps under radiant warmer:* **Positioning, Suctioning, Stimulation, Repositioning (PSSR)**	N
12.2	Provider initiates bag and mask ventilation for 30 seconds if baby still not breathing	12.2.1	Functional Ambu bag with mask for preterm baby is available	Y
		12.2.2	Functional Ambu bag with mask for term baby is available	Y
		12.2.3	Initiates bag and mask ventilation using room air, If not breathing well: • Applies appropriately sized mask correctly • Gives 5 ventilatory breaths and looks for chest rise	
		12.2.4	If there is no chest rise after 5 breathes, takes corrective measures (Corrects the position/sucks mouth and nose/checks the seal/gives ventilation with increased pressure). If there is adequate chest rise, continues bag and mask ventilation for 30 seconds and reassess	

Contd...

Contd...

S. No.	Standard	Verification criteria		Remarks
12.3	Provider takes appropriate action if baby does not respond to Ambu bag ventilation after golden minute	12.3.1	Functional oxygen cylinder (with wrench) with newborn mask is available	
		12.3.2	Functional stethoscope is available	
		12.3.3	Assesses breathing, if still not breathing continues bag and mask ventilation	
		12.3.4	Checks heart rate/cord pulsation	
		12.3.5	If heart rate is <100/≥100/min and baby is still not breathing, continues bag and mask ventilation and connects oxygen. *(Ask doctor/nurse as per facility protocol)*	
		12.3.6	If heart rate is ≥100 and baby is breathing well or at any point, if baby starts breathing, provides observational care with mother *(Ask doctor/nurse as per facility protocol)*	
		12.3.7	If baby is still not breathing and advance help is not available, then refers to higher center continuing bag and mask ventilation with oxygen *(Ask doctor/nurse as per facility protocol)*	
	Standard 12 final response (Yes/No):			0
13	**Provider ensures care of newborn with small size at birth**			
13.1	Preterm labor	13.1.1	Facility staff adheres to standard protocol for identification and management of preterm labor. Correctly estimates gestational age to confirm that labor is preterm.	
		13.1.2	Administration of corticosteroid is ensured between **24 and 34 weeks.**	
13.1	Facilitates specialist care in newborn weighing <1,800 g	13.1.1	Facilitates specialist care in newborn <1,800 g (refer to FBNC/seen by pediatrician)	
13.2	Facilitates assisted feeding whenever required	13.2.1	Facilitates assisted feeding whenever required	
13.3	Facilitates thermal management including kangaroo mother care (KMC)	13.3.1	Facilitates thermal management including KMC	
	Standard 13 final response (Yes/No):			1

Beyond Delivery:

14   The facility adheres to universal infection prevention protocols

Contd...

Contd...

S. No.	Standard	Verification criteria	Remarks
14.1	Instruments and reusable items are adequately and appropriately processed after each use	14.1.1 Facilities for sterilization of instruments are available	
		14.1.2 Instruments are sterilized after each use	
		14.1.3 Delivery environment such as labor table, contaminated surfaces, and floors are cleaned after each delivery	
14.2	Biomedical waste is segregated and disposed of as per the guidelines	14.2.1 Color-coded bags for disposal of biomedical waste are available	
		14.2.2 Biomedical waste is segregated and disposed of as per the guidelines	
14.3	Performs hand hygiene before and after each procedure, and sterile gloves are worn during delivery and internal examination	14.3.1 Performs hand hygiene before and after each procedure, and sterile gloves are worn during delivery and internal examination	
14.4	Personal protective equipment (PPE)	14.4.1 Availability of masks, caps and protective eye cover, sterile gloves, elbow length gloves, disposable gown/ Apron, utility gloves for housekeeping staff.	
14.5	Infection control protocols	14.5.1 Separation of routes for clean and dirty items; availability of disinfectant and cleaning agents, standard practice of mopping and scrubbing are followed.	
14.6	Microbiological surveillance	14.6.1 Provision for passive and active culture surveillance of critical and high-risk areas. Microbiological surveillance: Swab is taken from infection prone surfaces such as delivery tables, door, handles, procedure lights, etc.	
14.7	Facilitates prevention of mother to child transmission of HIV	14.7.1 Facility staff adheres to standard protocols for management of HIV in pregnant woman and newborn.	
	Providers follow appropriate PPE	Providers select appropriate PPE as per care area	
		Follows strict donning and doffing technique following checklist	
		Appropriate IECs and audit checklist's are used in both areas	
	The health care facility has a dedicated Infection Control Committee	The health care facility has a dedicated Infection Control Committee	

Contd...

Contd...

S. No.	Standard	Verification criteria		Remarks
			The Infection Control Committee meets on a monthly basis or earlier to discuss on infection prevention practices and take necessary action	
			A nurse has been designated as "Infection Control Nurse" at the health care facility to ensure monitoring of infection prevention practices and provides necessary trainings	
	Standard 14 final response (Yes/No):			

Postnatal Care Standard:

S. No.	Standard	Verification criteria		Remarks
15	**Provider ensures adequate postpartum care package is offered to the mother and baby—at discharge**			
15.1	Conducts proper physical examination of mother and newborn during postpartum visits	15.1.1	*Conducts mother's examination*: Breast, perineum for inflammation; status of episiotomy/tear suture; lochia; calf tenderness/redness/swelling; abdomen for involution of uterus, tenderness or distension	
		15.1.2	*Conducts newborn's examination*: Assesses **feeding** of baby; **checks weight, temperature, respiration, color of skin, and cord stump**	
			Assess the mothers' willingness and newborn's condition for breastfeeding	
15.2	Identifies and appropriately manages maternal and neonatal sepsis	15.2.1	Checks mother's history related to maternal infection	
		15.2.2	Checks mother's temperature	
		15.2.3	Gives correct regimen of antibiotics *(**Ask doctor/nurse as per facility protocol**)*	
		15.2.4	Checks baby's temperature and look for other signs of infections	
		15.2.5	Gives correct regime of antibiotics/ refers for specialist care *(**Ask doctor/ nurse as per facility protocol**)*	
15.3	Correctly diagnoses postpartum depression based on history and symptoms	15.3.1	Provides emotional support and refers woman to specialist care	
15.4	Counsels on importance of exclusive breastfeeding	15.4.1	Provides counseling and assistance on the importance of exclusive breastfeeding and techniques of breastfeeding	

Contd...

Contd...

S. No.	Standard	Verification criteria		Remarks
15.5	Counsels on danger signs, postpartum family planning	15.5.1	Counsels on return of fertility and healthy timing and spacing of pregnancy—Counsels on postpartum family planning to mother at discharge, home-based COVID care	
	Standard 15 final response(Yes/No):			1

C-Section Standard: (Procedural steps are not mentioned)

S. No.	Standard	Verification criteria		Remarks
16	**Provider reviews clinical practices related to C-section at regular intervals**			
16.1	Provider determines the need of C-section as per indication	16.1.1	Provider determines the need of C-section as per indication	
		16.1.2	Informs pregnant woman and her family on the need of C-section	
		16.1.3	Documents the indication/s for C-section	
		16.1.4	Ensures all C-section cases are classified as per modified Robson's criteria	
		16.1.5	Obtains written informed consent from pregnant woman/her family for C-section and anesthesia	
16.2	Operation theater is adequately equipped for conducting C-section	16.2.1	Number of OT tables in the OT are appropriate as per the C-section delivery load	
		16.2.2	Adequate supplies and equipment are available in the OT for C-section	
		16.2.3	Anesthesia tray with functional Boyle's apparatus is available	
		16.2.4	OT has adequate lighting, ventilation, and temperature control	
		16.2.5	OT complex has provision for separate washing area with 24-hour running water supply and soap	
		16.2.6	OT complex has functional toilet and staff resting/changing area	
		16.2.7	Functional newborn care area is available in the OT	
		16.2.8	Adequate supplies and equipment are available for conducting adult/newborn resuscitation	
16.3	Provider ensures adequate care for pregnant woman and newborn	16.3.1	Starts prophylactic antibiotics for mother (ampicillin 2 g IV; OR cefazolin 1 g IV) (WHO – MCPC, 2017)	
		16.3.2	Gives antenatal corticosteroids to all women for CS between 24 and 34 weeks gestation prior to the procedure	
		16.3.3	Ensures availability of anesthetic plan with anesthesiologist	

Contd...

Contd...

S. No.	Standard	Verification criteria		Remarks
		16.3.4	Ensures availability of pediatrician (practitioner skilled in the resuscitation of the newborn)	
		16.3.5	Performs ENBC in all babies crying after birth	
		16.3.6	Prepares uterotonics to be given to mother after delivery of the baby	
16.4	Provider ensures appropriate postpartum care of mother and newborn	16.4.1	Performs monitoring of mother and newborn every 15 minutes for 2 hours to detect early signs and symptoms of complications	
		16.4.2	Ensures initiating breastfeeding within an hour	
		16.4.3	Ensures appropriate thermal care for the newborn	
16.5	Reviews C-section cases through a clinical audit once every quarter	16.5.1	Reviews C-section cases through a clinical audit with team once every quarter in facility	
		16.5.2	Ensures that rate of complications of C-sections is periodically monitored in facility	

Standard 16 final response (Yes/No):

Index

EU GSPR Authorised Reprsentative
Logos Europe, 9 rue Nicolas Poussin
1700, La Rochelle, France
Phone: +33 (0) 6 67 93 73 78
E-mail: contact@logoseurope.eu

www.ingramcontent.com/pod-product-compliance
Ingram Content Group UK Ltd.
Pitfield, Milton Keynes, MK11 3LW, UK
UKHW051420270526
12721UKWH00014B/1132